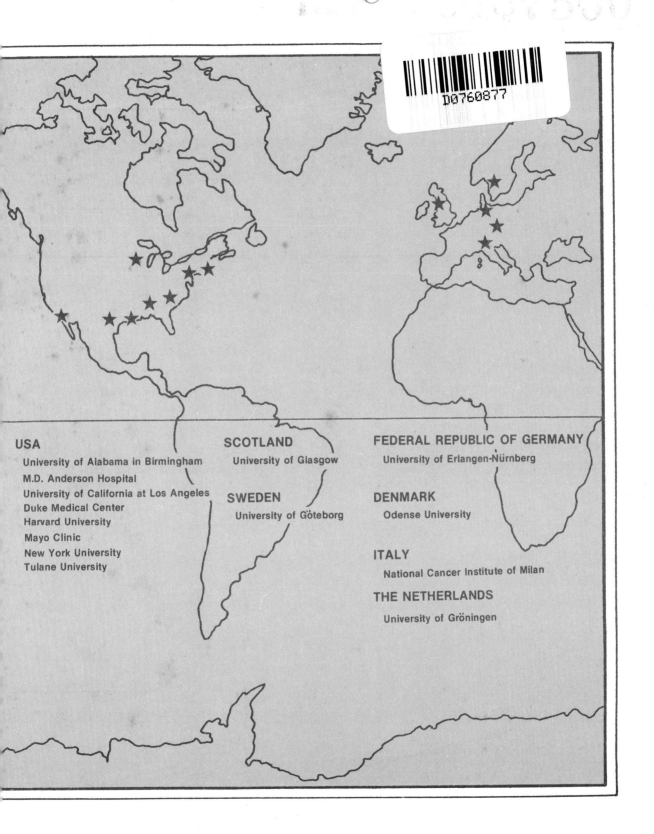

USA

University of Alabama in Birmingham
M.D. Anderson Hospital
University of California at Los Angeles
Duke Medical Center
Harvard University
Mayo Clinic
New York University
Tulane University

SCOTLAND

University of Glasgow

SWEDEN

University of Göteborg

FEDERAL REPUBLIC OF GERMANY

University of Erlangen-Nürnberg

DENMARK

Odense University

ITALY

National Cancer Institute of Milan

THE NETHERLANDS

University of Gröningen

Cutaneous Melanoma

J. B. Lippincott Company

Philadelphia

London   Mexico City
New York   St. Louis
São Paulo Sydney

Associate Editors

HELEN M. SHAW, PH.D.

Senior Investigator
Sydney Melanoma Unit
Sydney, New South Wales, Australia

and

SENG-JAW SOONG, PH.D.

Professor of Biostatistics and Biomathematics
Chief, Biostatistics Unit
Comprehensive Cancer Center
University of Alabama in Birmingham
Birmingham, Alabama

Cutaneous | Melanoma

Clinical Management and Treatment Results Worldwide

Editors

CHARLES M. BALCH, M.D., F.A.C.S.

American Cancer Society Professor of Clinical Oncology
Chief of Surgical Oncology, Department of Surgery
Associate Director for Clinical Studies
Comprehensive Cancer Center
University of Alabama in Birmingham
Birmingham, Alabama

and

GERALD W. MILTON, M.D., F.R.C.S.

Professor of Surgery
University of Sydney
Director, Sydney Melanoma Unit
Royal Prince Alfred Hospital
Sydney, New South Wales, Australia

With a foreword by Umberto Veronesi, M.D.

81 Contributors

2 Color Plates

Editorial Assistant:
  Peggy J. Hunter
  Surgical Oncology Unit
  University of Alabama in Birmingham
  Birmingham, Alabama

Illustrators:
  Samuel K. Collins, M.S., A.M.I.
  Medical Illustrator
  Medical Media Production Service
  Veterans Administration Medical Center
  Birmingham, Alabama

  Amy P. Collins, M.S., A.M.I.
  Graphics Coordinator
  Department of Photography & Instructional Graphics
  University of Alabama in Birmingham
  Birmingham, Alabama

Graphics Coordinator:
  Maxine Aycock
  Comprehensive Cancer Center
  University of Alabama in Birmingham
  Birmingham, Alabama
Sponsoring Editor: Darlene D. Pedersen
Manuscript Editor: Patrick O'Kane
Indexer: Ann Cassar
Art Director: Maria S. Karkucinski
Designer: Arlene Putterman
Production Supervisor: J. Corey Gray
Production Coordinator: Charlene Catlett Squibb
Compositor: Circle Graphics
Printer/Binder: Halliday Lithograph

6 5 4 3 2 1

Library of Congress Cataloging in Publication Data
Main entry under title:

Cutaneous melanoma

  Includes index.
  1. Melanoma. 2. Skin—Cancer. I. Balch, Charles M.
II. Milton, Gerald W. (Gerald White), 1924–
[DNLM: 1. Melanoma. 2. Skin Neoplasms. WR 500 C988]
RC280.S5C82   1985   616.99′277   84-7913
ISBN 0-397-50587-6

The authors and publisher have exerted every effort to ensure that drug selection and dosage set forth in this text are in accord with current recommendations and practice at the time of publication. However, in view of ongoing research, changes in government regulations, and the constant flow of information relating to drug therapy and drug reactions, the reader is urged to check the package insert for each drug for any change in indications and dosage and for added warnings and precautions. This is particularly important when the recommended agent is a new or infrequently employed drug.

To our wives, Carol and Janet, for their love and understanding,
and to our children, Glen, Alan, Laura, and Mark Balch,
and John, Christopher, and Claire Milton—our investment in the future

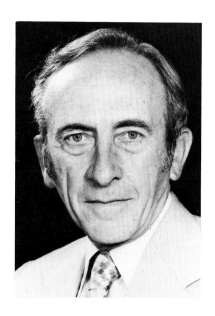

VINCENT JOHN McGOVERN died tragically in an automobile accident on December 30, 1983. The chapter that he wrote in this book with Dr. Tariq Murad (Chapter 3) was one of his last manuscripts. Dr. McGovern spent most of his life studying the pathology of melanoma and made numerous substantive contributions. In addition to multiple publications about melanoma, he has written three books addressing the pathology of melanoma.

A member of the Department of Pathology of the University of Sydney for 37 years, he was Professor of Pathology at the University of Sydney and Royal Prince Alfred Hospital until he retired in 1980 and was also President of the Royal College of Pathologists of Australia. He was undoubtedly one of Australia's most distinguished pathologists and was known nationally and internationally for his academic pursuits. Dr. McGovern was both a scholar and a dedicated pathologist. He was a personal and generous friend to many authors of this book, and we will miss him greatly.

Contributors

RIKIYA ABE, M.D., PH.D.
Associate Professor
Department of Surgery
Tohoku University
Sendai
Japan

ANNELORE ALTENDORF, M.D.
Department of Surgery
University Hospital Erlangen–Nürnberg
Federal Republic of Germany

PER KRAGH ANDERSEN, LIC. SCIENT.
Senior Statistician
Statistical Research Unit
Danish Medical and Social Science Research
    Council
Copenhagen
Denmark

CHARLES M. BALCH, M.D., F.A.C.S.
American Cancer Society Professor of Clinical
Oncology
Chief of Surgical Oncology
Professor of Surgery and Microbiology
Associate Director
Comprehensive Cancer Center
University of Alabama in Birmingham and the
    Birmingham Veterans Administration Medical
    Center
Birmingham, Alabama

ARTHUR W. BODDIE, JR., M.D.
Associate Professor of Surgery
The University of Texas M. D. Anderson
    Hospital and Tumor Institute at Houston
Houston, Texas

BERNT BOERYD, M.D.
Associate Professor
Department of Pathology
University of Linkoping
Sweden

DONN J. BRASCHO, M.D.
Professor and Vice Chairman
Radiation Oncology Department
University of Alabama in Birmingham
Birmingham, Alabama

R. DAVILENE CARTER, M.D.
Professor of Surgery
Tulane University School of Medicine
New Orleans, Louisiana

NATALE CASCINELLI, M.D.
Director, Division of Clinical Oncology E
National Cancer Institute
Milan
Italy

DAVID CHANT, M. SC., PH.D.
Department of Mathematics
University of Queensland
Queensland
Australia

DOUGLAS H. CLARK, M.D., CH.M., F.R.C.S.
Consultant Surgeon (retired)
Western Infirmary/Gartnavel General Hospital
Glasgow
Scotland

CLAUDIO CLEMENTE, M.D.
Associate Director, Department of Pathology
National Cancer Institute
Milan
Italy

ALAN S. COATES, M.D., F.R.A.C.P.
Senior Specialist in Medical Oncology
Ludwig Institute for Cancer Research
University of Sydney
Sydney, N.S.W.
Australia

ALISTAIR J. COCHRAN, M.D.
Professor of Pathology and Surgery
Division of Surgical Oncology
UCLA School of Medicine
Los Angeles, California

EDWIN B. COX, M.D.
Assistant Professor of Medicine
Duke University Medical Center
Durham, North Carolina

EDWARD T. CREAGAN, M.D.
Associate Professor of Medical Oncology
Mayo Clinic
Rochester, Minnesota

**NEVILLE C. DAVIS, A.O., M.D., HON. D.S.,
F.R.C.S., F.R.A.C.S., F.A.C.S.**
Chairman
Queensland Melanoma Project
Princess Alexandra Hospital
Brisbane, Queensland
Australia

CALVIN L. DAY, JR., M.D.
Clinical Assistant Professor of Medicine
Department of Dermatology
University of Texas Medical School at San
    Antonio
San Antonio, Texas

KRZYSZTOF T. DRZEWIECKI, M.D.
Head of Department of Plastic Surgery
Rigshospitalet/Finseninstitutet
Copenhagen
Denmark

JOHN R. DURANT, M.D., F.A.C.P.
President
Fox Chase Cancer Center
Philadelphia, Pennsylvania

JAN ELDH, M.D.
Associate Professor
Department of Plastic Surgery
University of Göteborg
Sweden

THOMAS B. FITZPATRICK, M.D.
Professor and Chairman
Department of Dermatology
Harvard Medical School
Boston, Massachusetts

ADELE GREEN, M.B.B.S.
Research Fellow
Queensland Institute of Medical Research
Brisbane, Queensland
Australia

IRENE GUGGENMOOS-HOLZMANN, M.D.
Department of Medical Statistics and
    Documentation
University Hospital Erlangen–Nürnberg
Federal Republic of Germany

PAUL HERMANEK, M.D.
Department of Clinical Oncology
Department of Surgery
University Hospital Erlangen–Nürnberg
Federal Republic of Germany

PETER HERSEY, F.R.A.C.P., D. PHIL.
Clinical Immunologist
Royal Newcastle Hospital
Newcastle, N.S.W.
Australia

HANS HOLMSTROM, M.D.
Associate Professor
Department of Plastic Surgery
University of Göteborg
Sweden

TAIZO KATO, M.D., PH.D.
Department of Dermatology
Tohoku University School of Medicine
Sendai
Japan

ALFRED S. KETCHAM, M.D.
Professor of Surgery
Chief of Surgical Oncology
University of Miami School of Medicine
Miami, Florida

HOWARD K. KOH, M.D.
Melanoma Fellow
Massachusetts General Hospital
Departments of Dermatology,
    Hematology-Oncology
Boston, Massachusetts

ALFRED W. KOPF, M.D.
Professor of Dermatology
New York University
Skin and Cancer Hospital
New York, New York

EDWARD T. KREMENTZ, M.D.
Professor of Surgery
Chief, Section of Surgical Oncology
Tulane University School of Medicine
New Orleans, Louisiana

CHRISTIAN LADEFOGED, M.D.
Chief Resident
Institute of Pathology
University Hospital
Odense
Denmark

KAM-HING LAM, M.S., F.R.C.S.ED.
Professor of Surgery
University of Hong Kong
Queen Mary Hospital
Hong Kong

JOHN A. H. LEE, M.D.
Professor of Epidemiology
Department of Epidemiology
University of Washington
Seattle, Washington

ROBERT A. LEW, PH.D.
Biostatistician
Massachusetts General Hospital
Laboratory of Computer Science
Boston, Massachusetts

**JOHN H. LITTLE, M.B.B.S., D.PH., D.C.P.,
F.R.C.PATH., F.R.C.P.A.**
Director of Pathology
Princess Alexandra Hospital
Brisbane, Queensland
Australia

JOSEPH R. LOGIC, M.D.
Associate Professor
Department of Diagnostic Radiology
University of Alabama in Birmingham
Birmingham, Alabama

RONA MacKIE, M.D.
Professor of Dermatology
University of Glasgow
Glasgow
Scotland

WILLIAM A. MADDOX, M.D., F.A.C.S.
Clinical Professor of Surgery
University of Alabama in Birmingham
Birmingham, Alabama

RAFFAELE MAROLDA, M.D.
Research Fellow
Division of Clinical Oncology E
National Cancer Institute
Milan
Italy

CHARLES M. McBRIDE, M.D.
Professor of Surgery
The University of Texas M. D. Anderson
    Hospital and Tumor Institute at Houston
Houston, Texas

WILLIAM H. McCARTHY, F.R.A.C.S., M.ED.
Associate Professor of Surgery
The Sydney Melanoma Unit
Royal Prince Alfred Hospital
Camperdown, N.S.W.
Australia

VINCENT J. McGOVERN, M.D.[†]
The Sydney Melanoma Unit
Royal Prince Alfred Hospital
Camperdown, N.S.W.
Australia

**G. RODERICK McLEOD, F.R.C.S. (ENGL. AND
EDIN.), F.R.A.C.S.**
Coordinator
Queensland Melanoma Project
Princess Alexandra Hospital
Brisbane, Queensland
Australia

CURTIS METTLIN, PH.D.
Director
Department of Cancer Control and Epidemiology
Roswell Park Memorial Hospital
Buffalo, New York

MARTIN C. MIHM, JR., M.D.
Professor of Pathology
Harvard Medical School
Massachusetts General Hospital
Boston, Massachusetts

GERALD W. MILTON, M.D., F.R.C.S.
The Sydney Melanoma Unit
Royal Prince Alfred Hospital
Camperdown, N.S.W.
Australia

[†] Deceased

DONALD L. MORTON, M.D.
Professor of Surgery
Chief, Division of Surgical Oncology
UCLA School of Medicine
Los Angeles, California

TARIQ M. MURAD, M.D.
Chief of Surgical Pathology
Northwestern University Medical Center
Chicago, Illinois

MAURIZIO NAVA, M.D.
Assistant Director
Division of Clinical Oncology E
National Cancer Institute
Milan
Italy

JAN OLDHOFF, M.D.
Department of Surgical Oncology
State University of Groningen
The Netherlands

J. WOLTER OOSTERHUIS, M.D.
Department of Pathology
State University of Groningen
The Netherlands

LARS-ERIK PETERSON
Associate Professor
Department of Statistics
University of Göteborg
Sweden

HENRIK POULSEN, M.D.
Head of Department of Plastic Surgery
University Hospital
Odense
Denmark

RICHARD J. REED, M.D.
Clinical Professor of Pathology
Tulane University School of Medicine
New Orleans, Louisiana

DENISE J. ROE, M.S.
Division of Surgical Oncology
Departments of Biomathematics and Surgery
UCLA School of Medicine
Los Angeles, California

DARIO ROVINI, M.D.
Assistant Director
Division of Clinical Oncology H
National Cancer Institute
Milan
Italy

ROBERT F. RYAN, M.D.
Professor of Surgery
Chief, Section of Plastic Surgery
Tulane University School of Medicine
New Orleans, Louisiana

MARIO SANTINAMI, M.D.
Research Fellow
Division of Clinical Oncology E
National Cancer Institute
Milan
Italy

HEIMAN SCHRAFFORDT KOOPS, M.D.
Department of Surgical Oncology
State University of Groningen
The Netherlands

HILLIARD F. SEIGLER, M.D.
Professor of Surgery and Immunology
Duke University Medical Center
Durham, North Carolina

MAKOTO SEIJI, M.D., PH.D.†
Department of Dermatology
Tohoku University School of Medicine
Sendai
Japan

HELEN M. SHAW, PH.D.
The Sydney Melanoma Unit
Royal Prince Alfred Hospital
Camperdown, N.S.W.
Australia

FRANKLIN H. SIM, M.D.
Professor of Orthopaedics
Mayo Clinic
Rochester, Minnesota

ARTHUR J. SOBER, M.D.
Associate Professor of Dermatology
Harvard Medical School
Massachusetts General Hospital
Boston, Massachusetts

SENG-JAW SOONG, PH.D.
Professor of Biostatistics and Biomathematics
Director of Biostatistical Unit
Comprehensive Cancer Center
University of Alabama in Birmingham
Birmingham, Alabama

EDWARD SOULE, M.D.
Emeritus Staff
Mayo Clinic
Rochester, Minnesota

CARL M. SUTHERLAND, M.D.
Professor of Surgery
Tulane University School of Medicine
New Orleans, Louisiana

MART SUURKULA
Associate Professor
Department of Pathology
University of Göteborg
Sweden

† Deceased

MASAAKI TAKAHASHI, M.D., PH.D.
Department of Dermatology
Tohoku Rosai Hospital
Sendai
Japan

HIDEAKI TAKEMATSU, M.D.
Department of Dermatology
Tohoku University School of Medicine
Sendai
Japan

WILLIAM F. TAYLOR, PH.D.
Professor of Biostatistics
Mayo Clinic
Rochester, Minnesota

YASUSHI TOMITA, M.D., PH.D.
Department of Dermatology
Tohoku University School of Medicine
Sendai
Japan

JÜRGEN TONAK, M.D.
Department of Surgery
University Hospital Erlangen–Nürnberg
Federal Republic of Germany

MARSHALL M. URIST, M.D.
Associate Professor of Surgery
University of Alabama in Birmingham
Birmingham, Alabama

MAURIZIO VAGLINI, M.D.
Assistant Director
Division of Clinical Oncology E
National Cancer Institute
Milan
Italy

UMBERTO VERONESI, M.D.
Director
National Cancer Institute
Milan
Italy

PETER VIBE, M.D.
Resident
Department of Plastic Surgery
University Hospital
Odense
Denmark

ROBIN T. VOLLMER, M.D.
Surgical Pathologist/Clinical Assistant Professor
    of Pathology
Veterans Administration Hospital
Duke University Medical Center
Durham, North Carolina

FRANK WEIDNER, M.D.
Department of Dermatology
Hospital Bad Cannstadt
Stuttgart
Federal Republic of Germany

JOHN WONG, PH.D., F.R.A.C.S.
Professor and Head
Department of Surgery
University of Hong Kong
Queen Mary Hospital
Hong Kong

JOHN E. WOODS, M.D.
Professor of Plastic Surgery
Mayo Clinic
Rochester, Minnesota

Foreword

One can say that the history of melanoma, its recognition, and its management symbolize the history of oncology. The obscurity of its nature, the inability to give it a clear connotation, and the sad acceptance of its incurability were the expression of the bewilderment suffered by the medical community, confronted for centuries with the mystery of cancer growth. The first sporadic successes at the end of the 19th century and the perception that extensive surgery was the only way to control melanoma were at the root of the new philosophy summarized in the dogma "small cancer, large operation" that influenced cancer surgeons for nearly a century. Finally, the entrance into clinical research of the controlled therapeutic trial was, in melanoma more than in other types of cancer, the starting point for the development of a rational approach to the disease.

The history of melanoma can, therefore, be divided into three major periods. The "pioneer" period, which goes from the first description of melanoma, by John Hunter in 1787, to the end of the following century, is the period of the first recognition of this uncommon disease seen mainly as a pathological curiosity. The scattered anecdotal reports and the absence of case series large enough to provide data on the natural history of the disease prevented the establishment of a treatment policy such as that which was possible at the end of the 19th century. If one were to identify a starting date for the second period, which may be defined as "surgical radicalism," it would be 1892, when E. Snow published an article in *The Lancet* advocating extensive surgery in melanoma, consisting of the large excision of the primary lesion associated with the dissection of the regional lymph nodes. With alternating enthusiasm and disenchantment, the "extensive surgery" policy went on for decades, being applied without any discrimination to all proliferative pigmented lesions. Three important events occurred, however, in the last twenty years that are at the root of the new course in the fight against melanoma. The first was the constitution of the WHO International Melanoma group for clinical research, whose main activity was focused on the conduct of clinical trials, not only to verify how much the established ruling should be confirmed, but also to test hypotheses for new types of treatment. The second event was the establishment in Australia of an integrated multidisciplinary study, the Queensland Melanoma Project, whose aim was the evaluation of the results of a structural joint action that would mobilize epidemiologists, pathologists, clinicians, and educators. The third occurence was the recognition by a few pathologists, like Clark, McGovern, and Breslow, of different prognostic values connected with histologic patterns. The three events all occurred in the second half of the 1960s and gave origin to the present period of development, which may be defined as "clinico-pathological experimentalism." Although pathologists and clinicians have produced data that elucidated the role and the limits of the present therapeutical resources and have clarified the weight of the various prognostic factors, it is likely that within a not overlong period all these problems will be addressed. It is now possible to predict a new period in the history of melanoma in which the leading role will be taken by the new developments in the area of laboratory research. The exciting new information coming from virology (human retroviruses), molecular biology (oncogenes), and immunology (monoclonal antibodies) will certainly deeply influence the research on melanoma in the next few years. The great expectation for radical improvements are in that direction.

What are the more immediate needs of melanoma research? On the one hand, I think there is an urgent need for clarification of etiologic factors and their mechanism of action in order to establish appropriate rules for primary prevention. The sunlight hypothesis being unconvincing, we do not, in fact, have serious recommendations for prevention. On the other hand, the drugs available at present to control the metastases of melanoma, both overt and occult, are of limited efficacy, and it is imperative that new molecules be produced and tested against melanoma cells. Apart from research, the acquired information that the improvement of survival rates is strictly correlated with early detection of the disease imposes the implementation of extensive educational plans to reach both the practitioners and the public. The present educational means for the de-tection of melanoma are still rudimentary and occasional; very rarely has an integrated program been conducted with the optimal use of the mass communication media. After all, the detection of melanoma appears to be the simplest among the different types of cancer, since it does not require any complicated equipment but only the naked eye and, of course, the necessary information. Once clear visual information is provided and people are convinced that they should look periodically at their own skin, the signs cannot be missed.

But to give appropriate information to the population, the knowledge of melanoma among physicians and among specialists must be of high quality. The discovery of a melanoma must be followed by the most appropriate and scientifically proven treatment. Therefore, the preparation and dissemination of high-quality textbooks on melanoma is of fundamental importance. This is such a book, for it represents a rational attempt to transfer to its pages the enormous clinical experience of thousands of patients seen, treated, and followed up for years in many centers throughout the world. The fact that its content is based more on analytic data from melanoma patients than on reviews from the literature reflects, in my opinion, the great originality of the efforts of Charles Balch, Gerry Milton, and their collaborators. This is a book whose logical sequence of chapters will lead the reader into the intricate pathways of the epidemiologic, pathological, and clinical aspects of this difficult and challenging disease, a disease for which the many still-undefined connotations are being unveiled by research with ever-increasing clarity.

Umberto Veronesi, M.D.
Director
National Cancer Institute
Milan, Italy

Preface

Cutaneous Melanoma is a comprehensive text about the clinical management of melanoma. It has a special accent on data presentation and collectively incorporates the clinical experience of over 20,000 patients treated at major melanoma centers throughout the world. The book spans the entire spectrum of the disease, from *in situ* melanoma to advanced stages of metastatic disease. It incorporates the basic principles of diagnosis, pathologic examination, and various treatment approaches that can be selectively employed for the many clinical presentations of metastatic melanoma. Each facet of clinical management is backed by statistical data about natural history, prognosis, and treatment results. Many aspects of melanoma management are presented in a comprehensive fashion for the first time. The chapters about diagnosis and treatment of advanced melanoma, for example, represent an exhaustive review of the literature and a presentation of a management approach that has not been previously synthesized into a single treatise.

Cutaneous Melanoma compiles the clinical experience of five surgeons and two pathologists whose careers have largely been concentrated on the management of over 4,000 melanoma patients treated over a 25-year span of time. Other melanoma authorities have generously contributed chapters in their areas of special expertise, such as isolated limb perfusion, epidemiology, and childhood melanoma. Many issues about the management of melanoma are still being debated. For this reason, we have tried to present a balanced perspective wherever possible. The most important controversy involves the pros and cons of elective lymph node dissection. Prominent authorities representing each side of the issue present their cases in a debate format. The text also places considerable emphasis on delineating those prognostic features that can most reliably predict the melanoma patient's clinical course. The clinician should be able to use these factors to group patients into risk categories according to the degree of probability that they harbor microscopic disease. We have stressed this approach because in treatment planning it is vitally important for the clinician to consider not only the disease he can see macroscopically but also the microscopic disease he cannot detect. Dr. Soong has brilliantly organized an enormous amount of data and reduced its essence into a computerized mathematical model that has been useful at UAB in day-to-day clinical management.

Cutaneous Melanoma is also unique because it includes, for the first time, a comprehensive comparative analysis involving prognostic factors and treatment results from most of the major melanoma treatment centers in the world. This collaborative study was based on the hypothesis that there are genetically determined differences in the biologic behavior of melanoma among different ethnic groups, perhaps because of immunologic responses to host defense mechanisms that have not been accounted for. Many of these centers have spent considerable time reanalyzing their data for presentation in the most comparable format possible. For example, level I melanomas were excluded from the analysis to enhance the comparability. Although many basic tenets are common to all of these centers, there is also considerable heterogeneity of disease among different populations. It is hoped that this initial attempt to analyze data on a global scale will stimulate further studies to enhance the comparability of results and to understand the biologic variability of this disease in a more sophisticated manner.

Melanoma has an incredible array of clinical presentations, which makes it a fascinating and stimulating disease to study and to treat. The management of melanoma thus embodies all the principles of cancer care, so readers who understand the strategies and rationale for treatment applied to melanoma can apply them to other forms of cancer as well.

Cutaneous Melanoma is oriented to the surgeons, oncologists, dermatologists, and other physicians who diagnose and treat melanoma patients. We have attempted to give a balanced perspective of the risks and benefits involved in each treatment modality and how these can be optimized in various clinical settings. This book is also directed to the general physician or internist who desires to know more about how to recognize cutaneous melanomas at the earliest possible stage and how to biopsy them properly both for diagnosis and for microstaging, and who desires a reference source for the subsequent clinical management of the patient. Those who are interested in the epidemiologic, immunologic, and pathologic features of melanoma will also find pertinent information in this treatise.

Acknowledgments

So many colleagues and coworkers have contributed to this project over the years that it is difficult to select only a few for specific recognition. The medical staff, nursing staff, and office staff at both the University of Alabama in Birmingham Hospital and the Birmingham Veterans Administration Hospital, as well as at the Sydney Hospital and the Royal Prince Alfred Hospital, have shared our dedication to the treatment of this disease. The support staff in the medical library, photography, medical graphics, and surgical pathology departments at all of these institutions have also been enormously helpful.

Specific recognition is given to those who directly assisted in the preparation of this book at the University of Alabama in Birmingham. The Biostatistical Unit of the Comprehensive Cancer Center has pored over these data repeatedly. A unique dimension of this book is the statistical data base, which has been assembled in a meticulous and dedicated fashion by Dr. Seng-jaw Soong, Chief of the Biostatistical Unit, and his staff, especially Mrs. Gretchen Cloud and Ms. Kathy Hecht. He has assembled data from UAB and from the Sydney Melanoma Unit, as well as raw data from a number of other melanoma centers for collaborative studies. The Surgical Oncology Office staff has shown a special dedication to the completion of this book. Mrs. Peggy Hunter, as Editorial Assistant, probably spent more time on this book than anybody else. She supervised its processing in every detail and personally checked all of the reference citations. Mrs. Hunter and Mrs. Sharon Garrison laboriously typed numerous drafts of each chapter. We are also grateful to others in the office who provided invaluable assistance, including Mrs. Judy Smith (Data Manager), Ms. Noelle Nicholls (who assisted in the editing), and our Surgical Oncology nurses who helped with the data management (Mrs. Anna Lee Ingalls and Ms. Beth Kennedy). Sam and Amy Collins, medical illustrators, and Maxine Aycock, medical graphics artist, made a special effort to provide excellent artwork, often despite short deadlines for completion. The Medical Media Production Service at the Birmingham Veterans Administration Medical Center generously provided support for this effort. Others who helped were those in the Department of Dermatology (Dr. Mitchell Sams and Dr. Emily Omura), the Department of Pathology (Dr. Sonia Kheir and Dr. James Wilkerson), and the Department of Radiology (Dr. Robert Stanley and Dr. Robert Koehler). I (C.M.B.) could never say enough about the close professional relationship of my colleagues, Drs. William Maddox and Marshall Urist and their dedication to excellent patient care. They have graciously contributed their patient material, participated in the research efforts, and helped care for my patients while I was on sabbatical leave in Sydney to prepare this book. On a personal note, there are two individuals who have played a very meaningful role in the direction of my professional career through the years. Dr. John W. Kirklin, former Chairman of the UAB Department of Surgery, has guided and supported my career in innumerable ways. He taught me the fundamental principles of surgical research and patient management as well as a standard of excellence to strive for. Anyone who examines his systematic and quantitative approach to the surgical treatment and natural history of cardiovascular disease will see that our methodological approach in melanoma research closely resembles his. Dr. John R. Durant, formerly Director of the UAB Comprehensive Cancer Center, was a major stimulus in the formative years of my surgical oncology career. He encouraged me to study melanoma and provided the unstinting support that enabled us to launch our melanoma project.

The Sydney Melanoma Unit has been helped for 25 years by the staff of the Royal Prince Alfred Hospital and by the St. Vincent's Hospital during its early years. I (G.W.M.) am especially grateful to the staff at Sydney Hospital, who supported us for 15 years with cordial and dedicated assistance. There are too many contributors to this effort to mention individually. I would like to place on record my personal indebtedness to the late Dr. James Molesworth and the late Dr. John Belisario, both eminent dermatologists, and the late Professor Jon Loewenthal, Chairman of the Department of Surgery, University of Sydney, all of whom developed my early interest in melanoma. We have learned a great deal from nurses, other paramedical staff, and students who have worked in the Unit over the years. We are particularly indebted to Sister Kerrie Ferguson, whose passion for accuracy has greatly increased the value of literally hundreds of patient records. Finally, Mr. Garth Maxwell, head technician and a veritable "jack-of-all-trades," has proved invaluable.

Research from the UAB Surgical Oncology Unit and from the Sydney Melanoma Unit would not have been possible without financial assistance from a number of sources. Much of the UAB research described in this book was supported initially from the Core Grant of the UAB Comprehensive Cancer Center (CA-13148) and by a melanoma grant from the National Cancer Institute (CA-27197). Dr. Balch received an Eleanor Roosevelt International Fellowship from the International Union Against Cancer and the American Cancer Society, that provided some of the travel funds for a sabbatical leave at the Sydney Melanoma Unit to work on this book. Support for the Sydney Melanoma Unit through the years has come from the New South Wales Cancer Council, the Bill White Memorial Research Fund, and other sources.

The editorial staff at the J. B. Lippincott Company has assisted us in the preparation of this book in an extremely professional and expeditious manner. We want particularly to acknowledge Mr. John deCarville (Vice President and Editorial Director), Ms. Darlene Pedersen (Associate Editor), Maria Karkucinski (Art Director) and Patrick O'Kane (Manuscript Editor).

Our families have provided vital emotional support and graciously forfeited some of their time with us because of the additional effort required to complete this book. As only they know, there were considerable personal sacrifices required that they willingly made. For this reason, we have chosen to dedicate this book to them.

Finally, we have been sustained through our professional careers by the courage and warmth of the large number of patients whom it has been our privilege to care for. Personal rewards from these relationships and our desire to help improve the care of other patients are the main reasons we wrote this book.

Contents

Cutaneous Melanoma

NEVILLE C. DAVIS
G. RODERICK McLEOD

The History of Melanoma from Hunter to Handley (1787–1907)

1

This brief history of the early development of melanoma focuses on the period from John Hunter to William Sampson Handley (1787–1907). A great deal of our contemporary foundation of knowledge was learned during that exciting period of medical discovery. The important aspects of the contributions of these pioneer workers will be quoted verbatim, for they are often misquoted in the modern literature.

JOHN HUNTER (1728–1793)

The first published account of a patient with a melanoma (a secondary deposit) was reported by John Hunter in 1787, although Hunter never described the disease as such. Hunter's original specimen, No. 219, preserved in the Hunterian Museum of the Royal College of Surgeons of England, was from a 35-year-old man with a recurrent mass behind the angle of the lower jaw (Fig. 1-1). The lump was excised, only to recur locally 3 years later. The metastasis enlarged slowly until it was struck with a stick during a drunken brawl, after which it doubled in size over the next few weeks. After removing the lump, John Hunter described that "part of it was white and part spongy, soft and black"; he labeled it as a "cancerous fungous excrescence." In 1968, Bodenham[1] reported that microscopic examination confirmed that the specimen was a melanoma—presumably a secondary deposit with no known primary tumor.

RENÉ LAENNEC (1781–1826)

In an unpublished memoir presented to the Faculté de Médecine de Paris in 1806, René Laennec (Fig. 1-2) was the first to describe melanoma as a disease entity, although Breschet[2] and Pemberton[23] gave the credit to Dupuytren instead. Six years before he became famous for inventing the stethoscope, Laennec first used the word *melanosis* in an 1812 issue of the Bulletins de la Faculté de Médecine de Paris.[18] Melanosis was derived from the Greek word meaning "black." Laennec stated, "The condition had apparently escaped the notice up to then of anatomists and of doctors who ordinarily do *post mortems*."[18] He noted that melanoma metastases in the mediastinal and hilar lymph nodes were different from the more common black bronchial glands, the color of which he recognized resulted from a

FIG. 1–1   A recurrent mass from the angle of the lower jaw in a man aged 35 years. This is John Hunter's original specimen of 1787, preserved in the Hunterian Museum of the Royal College of Surgeons of England.

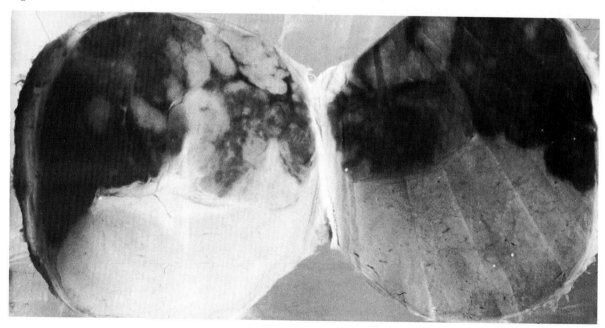

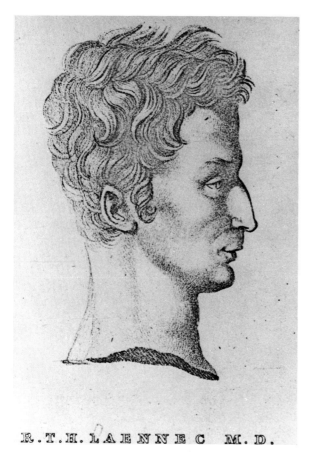

R.T.H. LAENNEC M.D.

FIG. 1–2 René Laennec, who in 1806 was the first to describe melanoma as a disease entity and, in 1812, to use the word *melanosis*.

large quantity of carbon. He also described melanomas involving the liver, lungs, eye, pituitary gland, wall of the stomach, and surface of the peritoneum. He further noted that melanotic deposits in the lungs did not cause the same hectic fever as tuberculosis, which was a common cause of death at the time.

WILLIAM NORRIS (1792–1877)

In 1820, William Norris described the first case of melanoma recorded in English literature.[19] He referred to it as a "Case of Fungoid Disease," but he actually described a patient who died from disseminated melanoma. Subsequently, he declared that this patient was "the first genuine good case of melanoma," as the following description will attest:

Mr. D., aged 59 years, of light hair and fair complexion presented to Dr. Norris on February 6, 1817 with a tumour of his abdominal wall midway between umbilicus and pubes. There had always been a mole on this position but nine months previously, it began to grow and tumour developed. It was half the size of a hen's egg, of a deep brown colour, of a firm and fleshy feel, ulcerated, and discharging a highly foetid ichthorous fluid. The apex of the tumour was broader than its base.* Some months after the tumour appeared, several distinct brown nodules sprang up around it (satellites).

The primary tumour was removed by the knife but then recurred in the scar in less than six weeks. The glands of the groin were swollen and slightly tender to the touch. In spite of the disseminated nature of the tumour the general health of the patient was not so much impaired as to interfere with his exercise or business. Multiple subcutaneous deposits developed with a distressing cough and dyspnoea before he died.[20]

Dr. Norris performed the autopsy himself and found the primary tumour to be "dark brown and reddish not unlike the internal portions of a nutmeg." A thick, black fluid discharged from the subcutaneous deposits after they were punctured. Metastases were found in the sternum and throughout the abdomen, which contained a quart of ascites fluid. The lumbar glands were "in a shockingly morbid condition"; the liver was enlarged and "studded with large oval masses of the disease." The spleen and bladder were the only abdominal organs free of the disease. The lungs were grossly involved, and the heart was literally encrusted with numerous specks varying in size from a pin's head to that of a pea. The dura mater was studded with metastases, but the brain was apparently uninvolved.

Subsequently, in 1857, Norris wrote a colorful and fascinating description of metastatic melanoma involving the abdomen at an autopsy.[20] His account speaks of

...thousands and thousands of coal black spots, of circular shapes and various sizes on the shining mucous, serous and fibrous membranes of the vital organs as the most dazzling sight ever beheld by a morbid anatomist. I shall never forget the pleasing thrill that came over me when I first beheld them. It would have puzzled the most powerful descriptive talent to have done full justice to such a novel and striking disease, displayed so beautifully in endless profusion everywhere.[20]

Mr. Causer, a surgeon in the town and a previous house surgeon of John Hunter, was told by

*Today we would describe this as pedunculated melanoma.

Dr. Norris that this patient's father had also died of melanoma. He remarked that "he was not acquainted with any case affording so strong a probability of the hereditary nature of the disease."[7]

Since William Norris was the first to study melanoma in depth, some further biographical information is of interest. Norris was born in Stourbridge, England, in 1792. After training at St. Bartholomew's Hospital under Abernathy[3] and subsequently at the University of Edinburgh, he was admitted as a Licentiate of the Society of Apothecaries of London in 1816. In 1823, he was awarded a Doctorate of Medicine degree by the University of St. Andrews in Scotland. The Vice-Chancellor of that University stated that it was common practice at that time for the M.D. degree to be awarded "on the production of testimonials from physicians of credit known to the University and on the payment of the appropriate fees."

Norris commenced general practice in Stourbridge in 1817 and served this district for an unbroken period of 60 years, dying in his hometown on March 23, 1877, from hemiplegia and apoplexy. He published his initial case report on melanoma in 1820 in the *Edinburgh Medical and Surgical Journal,* which claimed to exhibit "a concise view of the latest and most important discoveries in medicine, surgery and pharmacy."[19] It certainly did on this occasion.

What an outstanding general practitioner he must have been! He was, in the words of William Sampson Handley,[13] "a country practitioner who loved his profession well enough to ride 20 miles to see a patient who had died from melanoma and then do a complete necropsy in private practice."[8] Norris subsequently reported in 1857 "Eight Cases of Melanosis With Pathological and Therapeutical Remarks on That Disease," and this included a report on the first patient previously seen in 1820 (Fig. 1-3). In this paper, Norris referred to the condition as "melanosis," a term still used in the literature, although Robert Carswell had earlier coined the term *melanoma* in 1838.

Norris stated in his later article (1857) that melanoma often occurred "in those persons who have moles on various parts of the body." He stated that most of his cases occurred in patients "residing in very smoky iron and coal districts . . . in men, who have smoked immoderately." He referred to a case he reported "in former years, where melanosis affected almost every organ, the first tumour was not black—it was more of a scirrhous character. A second tumour sprang from the cicatrix, and, dur-

EIGHT

CASES OF MELANOSIS,

WITH

PATHOLOGICAL AND THERAPEUTICAL
REMARKS

ON THAT DISEASE.

BY WILLIAM NORRIS, M.D.,

CORRESPONDING MEMBER OF THE EPIDEMIOLOGICAL SOCIETY, &c., &c., &c.,
STOURBRIDGE.

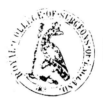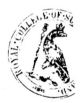

LONDON:
LONGMAN, BROWN, GREEN, LONGMANS, AND ROBERTS.
MANCHESTER:
J. AND T. CORNISH.
BIRMINGHAM:
CORNISH BROTHERS, 37, NEW STREET.
MDCCCLVII.

FIG. 1–3 The first comprehensive study of a series of melanoma patients. These observations, on his own patients, were published by William Norris in 1857.

ing life put on a similar appearance to the first, yet after death, it looked perfectly black." The patient's daughter had a cancer of the breast and his son a cancer of the lip and mouth.* He claimed that there was "a strong tendency to hereditary predisposition, and that melanosis is a disease allied to cancer."

One of his patients, a 26-year-old woman of fair and freckled appearance, provided him with "the most perfect specimen of melanotic tumour I had ever seen, which originated in a mole." Three years before, her brother, who was much annoyed at the mole's unsightly appearance, "ran a pair of scissors through it with the hope of removing it."

*This may be an example of a cancer family.

Three months later the mole began to grow and was "oval, flat, black and soft, situated between the shoulders. There was also a small tumour, the size and colour of a black grape near its upper surface." Dr. Norris removed "all the disease with abundance of the surrounding substance." The wound healed satisfactorily, and there was no return of the disease within 8 years. Another interesting patient was a 15-year-old with a probable ocular melanoma who died without an autopsy. The only case he encountered in a rural district was a 68-year-old man ("a desperate smoker") with a black ulcerated tumor of a cheek with "several black tubera around it."

If Norris suspected a malignant change in a mole, he recommended that the physician or surgeon "should immediately not only remove the disease, but cut away some of the healthy parts. I would, after excising the part, touch the wound with caustic so as not to leave an atom of the disease, if possible, and occasionally apply the same remedy to the skin in the vicinity." He used arsenic in this third case of melanosis, and the disease had not returned for 8 years. "In the present state of our knowledge, when the disease appears in several parts of the body, physic will, I fear, uniformly fail and surgery will be foiled."

Norris was jealous of his priority in describing the first case of melanoma, and he complained about subsequent authors not alluding to his case. "It is singular that Cullen, Carswell and Fawdington should have written on the disease some years after I first published and never alluded to my case." He claimed that he had seen more cases of melanosis than most provincial medical men and thought it was probably "owing to my residing near one of the great coal and iron districts in England, where persons are frequently breathing air clouded with black smoke."

A number of principles involving the clinical management and the epidemiology of melanoma were pointed out by Norris more than a century ago.[7] Some of these tenets are as follows.

First, the epidemiological features included: (1) that there is a relationship between moles and melanoma, (2) that the disease was more common in industrial than in rural areas, (3) that his patients had light-colored hair and a fair complexion, (4) that there was a family history in some cases and probably a hereditary disposition to the disease, (5) that cancers may run in families, and finally, (6) that trauma may accelerate the growth of the tumor.

Second, some pathologic features included: (1) while melanoma was often black in color, the degree of pigmentation varied, and it could be amelanotic; (2) it was often nodular and pedunculated; (3) satellite tumors might develop around the primary growth; (4) subcutaneous deposits may develop elsewhere; and (5) widespread dissemination could involve the lungs, liver, bone, heart, and dura mater.

Third, clinical features about the patient included: (1) they were more often men and heavy smokers, (2) they usually remained in good health until a very late stage of the disease, and (3) fever was not a feature, in contrast to tuberculosis.

Finally, regarding treatment, Norris (1) reported that local recurrence occurred following minimal excision; (2) was the first to advocate wide excision of the tumor and surrounding tissues, reporting an 8-year survival with this treatment; and (3) noted that neither medical nor surgical treatment was effective when the disease was widely disseminated.

OTHER EARLY 19TH-CENTURY DESCRIPTIONS

In 1823, Sir Andrew Halliday[12] reported an autopsy on a patient with "several black spots on the skin and on the surface of the dura mater. On opening the thorax and abdomen, all the viscera were found to be perfectly studded with these little black tumors."

In 1834, David Williams[25] described the primary tumor in the following manner: "On his right shoulder . . . he had a purple or dark brown stain-like connate [*i.e.,* congenital] spot or spilus [*i.e.,* mole] about the size of a section of a pea . . . his wife noticed this . . . mark . . . was increasing in size. The spilus continued to spread gradually, and after it had attained the circumference of a shilling, an excrescence, similar in color to itself, began to rise in its center." Williams's observation may be the first description of what we now refer to as horizontal and vertical growth phases of a superficial spreading melanoma.

In 1837, Isaac Parrish[22] formally reported the first case of melanoma in America. It concerned a 43-year-old woman with a "fungous tumor on the ball of the great toe . . . about half the size of a pigeon's egg. It had a red . . . smooth ulcerated surface. On the upper surface of the toe, about half an inch from the nail, there was a black tubercle, slightly elevated above the skin and about the size of a shilling. The lymphatic glands [were] tender and inflamed. At autopsy, melanose bodies [were] scattered over the surface of the peritoneum."

In 1838, Robert Carswell[4] described melanoma in his *Illustrations of the Elementary Forms of Disease*. He subdivided it into two groups—true melanosis and spurious melanosis. He described four modifications of true melanosis—punctiform melanosis, tuberiform melanosis, stratiform melanosis, and liquiform melanosis. He illustrated melanotic tumors in the liver, brain, small intestine and omentum.

In 1840, Samuel Cooper[6] gave a good description of the "black cancer." Cooper remarks that "no remedy is known for melanosis. The only chance for benefit depends upon the early removal of the disease by operation, when the situation of the part affected will admit of it. An eye affected by melanosis has been extirpated without any relapse having followed the operation at the end of two or three years; so have melanotic tumors of the skin and cellular tissue."

A case report published in 1851 in *Lancet*[24] describes a secondary melanoma of the groin in a 45-year-old woman that occurred 2 years after excision of a dark tumor on the mons veneris. Mr. Fergusson removed the secondary deposit, "the patient having been rendered insensible by chloroform. The tumour was about the size of an orange and when cut into presented all the characters of melanosis. The patient progressed favorably and was discharged well about six weeks after the operation." This is apparently the first recorded case involving surgical excision of a metastatic melanoma.

JAMES PAGET (1814–1899)

In 1853, Sir James Paget wrote in one of his best works, *Lectures on Surgical Pathology*, that "spurious melanosis" described by previous authors were "blackenings of various structures whose only common character is that they are not tumours."[21] He emphasized that "melanotic cancers [were] . . . medullary cancers modified by the formation of black pigment in their elemental structures." He referred to amelanotic tumors: "even in cancers that look colourless to the naked eye, I have found, with the microscope, single cells or nuclei having the true melanotic characters." Paget was the first to report a relatively large series of 25 patients with "melanoid cancer." Of the 17 women and 8 men, 20 were between 20 and 60 years of age. Fourteen of the cases involved the skin, nine were in the orbit, and one each involved the vagina and testicle. Eleven oc-

curred in relation to a preexisting mole or wart. The primary lesion was removed in 18 patients, 5 of whom survived for more than 2 years. All the others died in less than 2 years. Paget described what we now call superficial spreading melanoma in the following words: "The patient is usually aware of a time at which a mole, observed as an unchanging mark from birth or infancy, began to grow. In some instances the growth is superficial, and the dark spot acquires a larger area and appears slightly raised by some growth beneath it: in other cases, the mole rises and becomes very prominent or nearly pendulous."

OLIVER PEMBERTON (1825–1897)

In 1858, Pemberton referred to melanosis in his *Observations on the History, Pathology and Treatment of Cancerous Diseases*.[23] He noted that melanotic cancer is very frequently "located near a congenital mole or wart, or the congenital marks themselves undergo melanic degeneration." He remarked that "in colour, melanosis has many shades. In its primary form in the skin it is almost always brownish. Later the brown shade assumes every intensity of black. Sometimes, especially in the alteration of warts, the first change is of a slate colour." Pemberton collected 60 cases (33 men, 27 women) of cutaneous and ocular melanomas and noted the postmortem appearances in 33 cases in detail. The autopsy studies demonstrated that the liver, lungs, pleura, peritoneum, lymph glands, and bones were commonly involved. He noted that "it is a disease of adult, middle-aged and even advanced life, rather than of childhood." Pemberton also reported the first case of melanoma in a black man. The man was a 29-year-old native of Madagascar, and it is not surprising that the lesion was located on the side of the foot, a common site in dark-skinned melanoma patients. The patient died of disseminated disease, despite amputation below the knee. In this extensive review, Pemberton reports 25 cases in detail, some of which had been previously published. He concluded that none of the treatments used at that time were effective.

SIR JONATHAN HUTCHINSON (1828–1913)

Hutchinson is given credit for the first description of subungual melanoma, which he described in 1857 in an article entitled "Melanotic Disease of the Great

Toe, following a Whitlow of the Nail."[14] It is of interest that in the same year Fergusson[9] also described a melanoma on the great toe. Hutchinson referred to this entity of melanotic "whitlow" again in 1886, stating that "early amputation is demanded."[15]

In 1892 and 1894, Hutchinson[16,17] described and illustrated a series of cases from which the name "Hutchinson's Melanotic Freckle" has been applied. He described "Sir A.D. . . . (aged 56 years) with a large black stain on his left cheek, present for many years but increasing in size of late." It was not one continuous patch but a "number of separate spots, many of them confluent. An ugly nonpigmented ulcer developed above the black patch, close to the edge of the eyelid. This ulcer was epitheliomatous in some cases, and sarcomatous in others."

OTHER LATE 19TH-CENTURY DESCRIPTIONS

In 1885, Tennent[27] reported in the *Glasgow Medical Journal* that "the urine has presented a somewhat peculiar colour . . . said to have a greenish black tint" in a patient with advanced melanoma. He believed that the peculiar colour of the urine was probably caused by the absorption of melanin. He also noted that the color of multiple secondary tumors varied considerably in degree. He mentioned that a few of the tumors had "no appearance of color or pigmentation of any kind." Tennent noted that "meddlesome interference with a mole has been spoken of as highly dangerous."

Surgical excision of the primary melanoma was more widely recommended by this time. For example, Joseph Coats,[5] writing in the same issue of the *Glasgow Medical Journal,* recommended that "the operation should be so executed as to remove the tissue for some distance outside the apparent limits of the growth."

Controversies regarding lymph node dissection are not new, for its indications were debated almost a century ago. For example, Snow[26] wrote in an 1892 issue of *Lancet* about "the utter futility of operative measures which are addressed to the primary lesions only. We further see the paramount importance of securing, whenever possible, the perfect eradication of those lymph glands which will necessarily be first infected; before enlargement takes place, radical removal . . . is a safe and easier measure."

Finally, Gilchrist[11] reported, in 1899, the first case of a microscopically confirmed melanoma in an American black man. It commenced on the sole of the foot and disseminated widely before he died.

EARLY 20TH-CENTURY ARTICLES

In 1903, Frederic Eve[8] delivered a lecture about 45 melanoma patients treated at the London Hospital during the previous 20 years. Cutaneous melanomas comprised 73% of his series, and most of these growths (80%) apparently originated in pigmented moles. Eve described a melanoma on the sole of the foot and illustrated one on the palm of the hand. He remarked that "it is generally stated that the melanomata are the most malignant of tumours" but referred to "certain remarkable exceptions," including one patient who survived 20 years. The clinical management at that time also addressed surgery of the primary melanoma and the regional lymph nodes. In his words: "The treatment of melanoma of the skin can be given in a few words (*i.e.,* free excision or amputation), in accordance with the position and extent of the disease. The removal of the nearest chain of lymphatic glands, whether palpably enlarged or not, should never be omitted; for it may be taken as a matter of certainty that in the great majority of cases they are infected." During the previous 6 years at the London Hospital, he identified 3 cases of subungual melanoma and 3 cases of melanoma arising on mucosal surfaces.

In 1906, Fox[10] noted that melanoma could arise in a nevus or on blemish-free skin, "although moles are by far the commonest situations from which melanotic growths arise, yet they can originate in a skin entirely devoid of naevus tissue."

WILLIAM SAMPSON HANDLEY (1872–1962)

In 1907, William Sampson Handley (Fig. 1-4) gave two Hunterian Lectures on "The Pathology of Melanotic Growths in Relation to their Operative Treatment."[13] He demonstrated both the anatomical pathways involving the spread of melanoma and centrifugal lymphatic permeation. He based his study on a single autopsy examination of a patient with a very advanced melanoma. On this somewhat slender data base, he advocated wide local excision of the primary lesion, regional lymph node dissection, and amputation in selected cases. This is an important historic document, for Handley's recom-

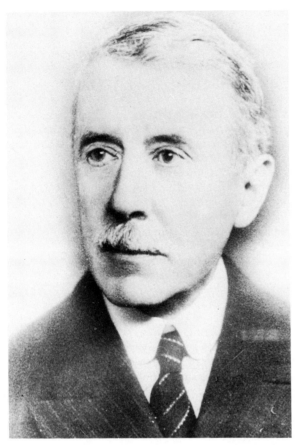

FIG. 1–4   William Sampson Handley, whose 1907 recommendations formed the basis for the treatment of melanoma for the following 50 years.

mendations formed the basis for melanoma treatment for the ensuing 50 years or more, until the extensive resections of the primary melanoma and the effectiveness of lymphadenectomy began to be questioned.

Handley recommended and illustrated operations for "melanotic sarcoma of the skin (Fig. 1-5). When malignant melanoma arises in the digits, amputation should be performed at once. The flaps should never be cut so as to include any skin within, at least, one inch of the tumour." For tumors elsewhere Handley recommended that

. . . a circular incision should be made through the skin around the tumour at what is judged by present standards to be a safe and practicable distance. The incision, situated as a rule about an inch from the tumour, should be just deep enough to expose the subcutaneous fat. The skin with a thin attached layer of subcutaneous fat is now separated from the deeper structures for about two inches in all directions around the skin incision. At the extreme base of the elevated skin flaps, a ring incision down to the muscles surrounds and isolates the area of deep fascia and overlying deeper subcutaneous fat to be removed. This fascial area is next to be dissected up centripetally from the muscles beneath up to a line which corresponds with that of the circular skin incision. Finally, the whole mass with the growth at its center is removed by scooping out with the knife a circular area of the muscle immediately subjacent to the growth. The excision of the [lymphatic] gland must . . . be carried out on exactly the same principles as the excision of the primary tumour. In late cases it may even be right to remove an area of skin over the infected glands.

FIG. 1–5   The original basis for a "wide local excision" of melanoma probably emanated from this figure in Dr. Handley's Hunterian Lecture. This diagram was used to illustrate the method of removing a malignant cutaneous melanoma. He stated that "a circular incision should be made through the skin round the tumor at what is judged by present standards to be a safe and practicable distance. The incision, situated as a rule about an inch from the edge of the tumor, should be just deep enough to expose the subcutaneous fat, is now to be separated from the deeper structures for about two inches in all directions round the skin incision...The dotted line commencing at *HH* represents in section the planes of division of the subcutaneous fat, deep fascia, and muscle. The knife should nowhere divide any of the permeated lymphatics; it will almost certainly do so unless the skin flaps are freely undermined." (Handley WS: The pathology of melanotic growths in relation to their operative treatment. Lancet 1:927, 996, 1907)

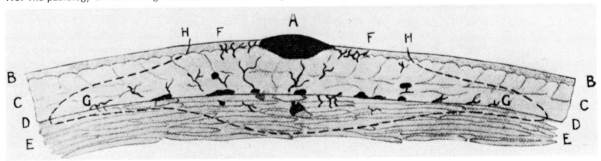

CONCLUSIONS

There have been many advances concerning the epidemiology, pathology, and treatment of melanoma since the beginning of this century. It is clear, however, that accurate and insightful observations were made during the 18th and 19th centuries that are still relevant to modern-day care of melanoma. The contemporary physician and researcher should respect (and cite) the contributions of their forebears made in the last century.

REFERENCES

1. Bodenham DC: A study of 650 observed malignant melanomas in the southwest region. Ann R Coll Surg Engl 43:218, 1968
2. Breschet D: Considerations sur line alteration organique appeleé degénérescence noire. Paris, Chez Bechet Jeune, Libraire, 1821
3. Cameron JRJ: Melanoma of skin. J R Coll Surg Edinb 13:233, 1968
4. Carswell R: Illustrations of the Elementary Forms of Disease. London, Longman, Orme, Brown, Green and Longman, 1838
5. Coats J: On a case of multiple melanotic sarcoma. Glasgow Med J 24:92, 1885
6. Cooper S: First Lines of the Theory and Practice of Surgery, 7th ed. London, Longman, Orme and Co, 1840
7. Davis NC: William Norris, M.D.: A pioneer in the study of melanoma. Med J Aust 1:52, 1980
8. Eve F: A lecture on melanoma. Practitioner 70:165, 1903
9. Under the care of Mr. Fergusson: Lancet 1:289, 1857
10. Fox W: Research into the origin and structure of moles and their relation to malignancy. Br J Dermatol 18:1, 83, 1906
11. Gilchrist TC: Are malignant growths arising from pigmented moles of a carcinomatous or sarcomatous nature? J Cutan Dis 17:117, 1899
12. Halliday A: Case of melanosis. London Medical Repository 19:442, 1823
13. Handley WS: The pathology of melanotic growths in relation to their operative treatment. Lancet 1:927, 996, 1907
14. Hutchinson J: Melanotic disease of the great toe, following a whitlow of the nail. Trans Pathol Soc London 8:404, 1857
15. Hutchinson J: Melanosis often not black: Melanotic whitlow. Br Med J 1:491, 1886
16. Hutchinson J: On tissue dotage. Arch Surg 3:315, 1892
17. Hutchinson J: Lentigo melanosis. Arch Surg 5:253, 1894
18. Laennec RTH: Sur les melanoses. Bulletins de la Faculté de Médecine de Paris 1:2, 1812
19. Norris W: Case of fungoid disease. Edinburgh Medical and Surgical J 16:562, 1820
20. Norris W: Eight Cases of Melanosis with Pathological and Therapeutical Remarks on That Disease. London, Longman, Brown, Green, Longman, and Roberts, 1857
21. Paget J: Lectures on Surgical Pathology, Vol 2. London, Longman, Brown, Green and Longman, 1853
22. Parrish I: Case of melanosis. Am J Med Sci 20:266, 1837
23. Pemberton O: Observations on the History, Pathology and Treatment of Cancerous Diseases. London, J Churchill, 1858
24. Recurrence of a melanotic tumor: Removal. Lancet 1:622, 1851
25. Silvers DN: On the subject of primary cutaneous melanoma: An historical perspective. In Fenoglio CM, Wolff M (eds): Progress in Surgical Pathology, Vol IV, p 277. New York, Masson, 1982
26. Snow H: Melanotic cancerous disease. Lancet 2:872, 1892
27. Tennent GP: On a case of multiple melanotic sarcoma. Glasgow Med J 24:81, 1885

Part I
The Primary
Melanoma

GERALD W. MILTON
CHARLES M. BALCH
HELEN M. SHAW

Clinical Characteristics

2

Melanoma can be cured with simple surgical treatment in the vast majority of patients if it is detected early in its clinical course. A skin lesion should be suspected of being a melanoma first on the basis of the clinical history. In over 90% of cases, it can also be recognized clinically as malignant by very experienced observers.[20,26] It therefore behooves the physician (both the general physician and the specialist) to know the clinical characteristics of melanoma so that suspicious moles or skin lesions will be biopsied at the earliest possible time. Histologic verification and microstaging is essential before embarking on surgical treatment as described in Chapters 6 to 8. This chapter describes the clinical characteristics and differential diagnosis of melanoma. The experience in the clinical diagnosis of melanoma, involving over 4000 melanoma patients treated at the Sydney Melanoma Unit (SMU) and the Surgical Oncology Unit at the University of Alabama in Birmingham (UAB), are summarized in this chapter.

HIGH-RISK POPULATIONS

The typical melanoma patient has a fair complexion and a tendency to sunburn rather than tan, even after a relatively brief exposure to sunlight.[10,22] The importance of these features was delineated in a case-control study conducted at the SMU, where 287 women with melanoma were compared with 574 age-matched controls.[10] Red hair color was associated with a tripling of relative risk (RR = 3), blond hair with a 60% increase (RR = 1.6), and fair skin with a doubling of risk (RR = 2.1). Women with melanoma also reported that they tended to sunburn (RR = 1.4) and to freckle (RR = 1.9) after exposure to sunlight. Of these risk factors, hair color, especially red hair, proved to be the major determinant, followed by skin color (Table 2-1). It is interesting to note that over two thirds of melanoma patients at both the SMU and UAB had red hair, blond hair, blue eyes, or some combination thereof.[7] However, eye color had no independent influence on risk.[10] At the SMU, there was a greater than threefold increase in risk (RR = 3.4) associated with those patients with an increased number of nevi on the body (i.e., > 20 nevi). The presence of multiple nevi was also found more frequently in the melanoma patients compared to the control group (8.1% versus 2.4%).

A patient with a melanoma has a higher risk for developing a second primary melanoma than does a person in the general population.[51] This risk varies from 3% to 5% in different series,[9,31,41] which is a 900-fold increased risk compared to that of the general population.[56] Each of the subsequent primary tumors normally has the appearance of the original lesion, and the patient, having once had a melanoma, will usually present with an early stage of the subsequent lesions.[41] Some patients have up to eight primary lesions at various anatomical sites. The patient who has multiple dysplastic nevi or has a familial form of melanoma has an even greater risk of

TABLE 2–1
RELATIVE RISKS ASSOCIATED WITH HAIR, SKIN, AND EYE COLOR IN CLINICAL STAGE-I MELANOMA PATIENTS

Hair	Skin Color	Eye	Cases	Controls	Relative Risk*
Red	Fair	Green or brown	22	18	4.5‡
Red	Fair	Blue	17	15	4.2‡
Red	Medium or olive	Green or brown	10	11	3.4‡
Red	Medium or olive	Blue	2	3	2.5
Blond	Fair	Green or brown	33	48	2.6‡
Blond	Fair	Blue	48	63	2.8‡
Blond	Medium or olive	Green or brown	23	72	1.2
Blond	Medium or olive	Blue	27	51	2†
Brown or black	Fair	Green or brown	28	56	1.9†
Brown or black	Fair	Blue	20	30	2.5‡
Brown or black	Medium or olive	Green or brown	41	151	1
Brown or black	Medium or olive	Blue	13	50	1

*Relative to those with brown or black hair and medium or olive skin.

†p <0.05

‡p <0.01

(Adopted from Beral V, Evans S, Shaw H, Milton G: Cutaneous factors related to the risk of malignant melanoma. Br J Dermatol 109:165, 1983)

developing multiple primary melanomas than do other patients.[9,18,58]

Familial melanomas are an uncommon occurrence, but such a clustering has been well documented and constitutes an identifiable high-risk group.[2,3,4,23,30,31,49,57,58] Among the SMU patients, 9% gave a history of melanoma occurring within their first-degree relatives. A familial occurrence among first-degree relatives was observed in 4% of the UAB patients[2] and in 10% of patients in the Queensland Melanoma Project.[57] Anderson[3] estimated that first-degree relatives of melanoma patients are 1.7 times more likely to develop melanomas than will the general population. Such persons have an onset of the disease at an early age, an increased number of multiple primary melanomas, and multiple atypical dysplastic nevi. Clark[15] described an autosomal dominant hereditary occurrence of melanoma, originally termed the B–K mole syndrome and now referred to as the dysplastic nevus syndrome, familial type.[19] Such patients typically have between 10 and 100 pigmented lesions, located predominantly over the trunk, buttocks, or lower extremity (Fig. 2-1). It is interesting to note that immune abnormalities are more frequent in familial melanoma patients and their relatives than in nonfamilial melanoma patients.[24] A positive family history of melanoma should therefore increase the suspicion of melanomas developing in other relatives, and frequent skin examinations should be made on all relatives so that an early diagnosis can be made in patients who may be so predisposed. It is also important to explain the clinical features of early melanoma to high-risk persons so that they can recognize suspicious moles. At the SMU, a pamphlet explaining the clinical features of melanoma in lay language is distributed to these persons.

Genetic factors may also play an important role in the predisposition to melanoma, perhaps by genes controlling some aspect of immune response to melanoma antigens.[1,2,12] Melanoma-prone patients appear to have an increased frequency of certain ABO, Gm, complement, and HLA phenotypes as listed below[1,2,8,11,25,45,59]:

GENETIC MARKERS ASSOCIATED WITH
MELANOMA OUTCOME

I. Increased Risk
 O blood type
 Gm[2] blood type
 DR4 histocompatibility type
 Properdin factor B (Bf–S allele)

II. Decreased Risk
 Properdin factor B (Bf–F allele)
 DR3 histocompatibility type

SIGNS AND SYMPTOMS

The cardinal feature observed in a skin lesion that proves to be a melanoma is a *change* observed over a period of months. The time scale of the observed change is important. If a lesion grows so that it doubles its size within about 10 days, it is usually an inflammatory condition such as a pyogenic granuloma. If the lesion grows so slowly that the patient or his relatives are unsure of any change, the lesion is often benign. However, medical advice should be

FIG. 2–1 Two typical B–K nevi, one of which is larger than most junctional nevi. The patient obviously has multiple pigmented nevi, larger ones being variegated in color.

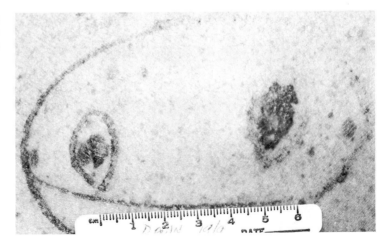

sought regarding a lesion that doubles its size in 3 to 8 months. These symptoms may include growth in the diameter or contour of a mole (either horizontally, vertically, or both), a change in color (usually darker, but sometimes lighter), bleeding, itching, ulceration, the development of a palpable lymph node, or some combination thereof (Table 2-2).[38,39,53] In the SMU patients, the median duration of first symptoms was about 5 months, with women having a slightly longer duration than men (6.2 months versus 4.5 months). Some of the typical changes of malignancy are usually observed by a relative or a friend, particularly for melanomas located on the back.

Growth (*i.e.*, increased size) and color change are the symptoms most commonly seen first (see Table 2-2). They occur in over 70% of early, curable melanomas.[40,60] Most patients may have been aware of a relatively static pigmented lesion on their skin for up to 5 years before changes developed. Of the SMU patients, the lesion arose from a pre-existing nevus in 89% of men with melanomas on the anterior trunk and in 71% of women with melanomas on the anterior leg. The growth of the melanoma observed by the patient takes two forms. The most common initial growth is horizontal or radial growth as a superficial lesion spreads out close to the surface. After this has progressed for some time (usually a few months), a nodular or vertical growth develops as a second stage. Less frequently, the nodule arises *de novo*.

In less than 20% of the patients, trauma to a mole was considered by the patient to cause a change in the lesion. It is interesting to note that symptoms that prompted the patients to visit their physicians often differed from the first observed symptom of a melanoma as described by the patient when asked about its clinical history (see Table 2-2). In fact, more than one third of patients (38%) claimed that they had noted no change in the lesion. In the majority of these patients, it was a friend or a spouse who noticed the lesion and suggested that the person seek medical attention (see Table 2-2). This occurred irrespective of whether the lesion was on the front or the back of the body. This may be attributable in part to active melanoma education programs for both the medical profession and the public that have been launched in Australia. As a result, the proportion of patients presenting for melanoma treatment with lesions in which they claimed to have noticed no change increased from 6% prior to 1960 to 38% in 1980.

The color change associated with tumor growth is most frequently a progressive darkening that increases especially as the nodular growth develops. A minority of patients describe a developing pallor associated with the growth. This may be an amelanotic nodule developing in an otherwise pigmented melanoma (Fig. 2-2). Another form of pallor develops when the melanoma is undergoing spontaneous regression. When this occurs, the pa-

FIG. 2–2 A malignant melanoma arising on the heel of a 12-year-old girl, who later died of the disease. The most actively growing part of the tumor is amelanotic and glossy and grew to this size in 3 months. The peripheral part of the tumor, which is also malignant, is deeply pigmented.

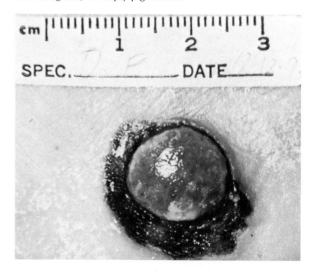

TABLE 2–2
SYMPTOMS IN CLINICAL STAGE-I MELANOMA PATIENTS TREATED AT THE SYDNEY MELANOMA UNIT BETWEEN 1977 AND 1980

Description of Symptom	First Symptom	Symptom Prompting Medical Attention
Increase in width	21%	9%
Increase in height	16%	16%
Got darker	18%	10%
Bled	9%	15%
Got lighter, itched, developed lump or blister, ulcerated	14%	12%
Noticed by patient, physician, spouse, or friend	22%	38%

tient describes how part of a flat, dark patch seems to melt into the skin (Fig. 2-3).

Itching occurs less frequently as a symptom of melanoma (see Table 2-2), but its presence may draw the patient's attention to an otherwise unnoticed lesion. The physician should consider this an important symptom of possible malignancy.[39,60] This itch caused by melanoma has definite characteristics. It is usually mild and often perilesional, and patients do not scratch the area but rub it with the pulp of their fingers.

Bleeding is not a common symptom of melanoma, since it usually occurs in a more advanced lesion. Bleeding is uncommon before a nodular growth develops and is rare in flat tumors. The bleeding from a melanoma is usually an insignificant amount that is caused by a trivial injury. This may be illustrated by two typical histories: (1) A taxi driver noticed a 2-cm spot of congealed blood on his shirt at the end of the day. This bleeding was caused by friction between the car seat and a melanoma on his back. (2) A woman noticed that when she dried herself after a shower, there were a few spots of blood on the towel. The slight friction between the towel and the melanoma on her back had been enough to damage the surface of the lesion.

In short, a melanoma will change in its physical characteristics and cause progressive signs and symptoms as it grows. A definite change in a mole, however trivial, should alert the patient and the physician to the possibility of a melanoma.

CLINICAL FEATURES OF MELANOMA

Several journal articles have described an some of the clinical characteristics of melanoma.[6,13,17,36-39,53] Melanomas can be located anywhere on the body, but they occur most commonly on the lower extremity of women and on the trunk of men (see Chap. 19).

It is helpful to examine suspicious skin lesions under a bright light (at a tangential angle with the skin) to highlight distinctive coloration and surface changes. Some of the typical features of cutaneous melanoma are shown in Plates 1 and 2 and in Figures 2-2 to 2-4. These include (1) variegation in color; (2) an irregular, raised surface; (3) an irregular perimeter with indentations; (4) ulceration of the surface epithelium; and (5) crusting. These features are generally distinct from those seen in benign nevi. The melanoma in Figure 2-4 demonstrates a multicolored lesion with a raised, irregular, and ulcerated surface. It should be emphasized, however, that not all melanomas are pigmented or evenly pigmented. The only indication of potential malignancy in the lesion depicted in Figure 2-2 is its noticeable growth. An irregular, raised surface may develop with nodularity that may be "tabletop," "dome," or "polypoid" in configuration. An irregular perimeter develops either because of uneven radial growth or because of patchy spontaneous regression. In either event, the patient or his family may have no-

FIG. 2–3 An unusual form of melanoma, sometimes referred to as a ring melanoma. The patient described the black ring as extending slowly outward over a period of about 10 months, and as this was happening, the central part faded. Note also that this lesion shows at least four different relationships between host and tumor: (1) spreading superficial melanoma, (2) black nodular melanoma (in the lower part), (3) spontaneous regression in the central area, and (4) amelanotic tumor growth.

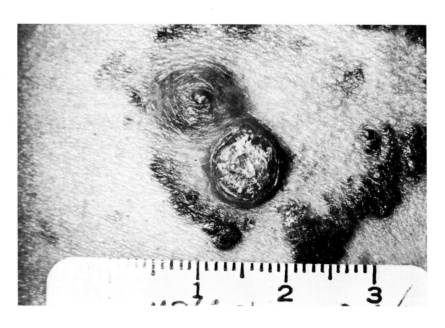

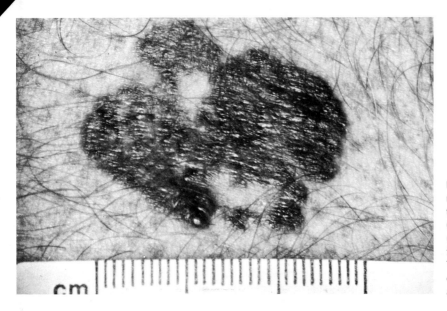

FIG. 2—4 A 3-cm-diameter melanoma showing irregular pigmentation, with small areas of regression (*above*) and a darkly pigmented nodular mass. A lighter area of superficial spreading tumor is also seen. The patient's wife had noted these changes in color for about 6 months and the nodular growth for 2 months.

ticed the changing configuration of the lesion. The ulceration of the surface may be partly concealed by a crust or blood clot (or an ooze of seropurulent discharge if the lesion has become infected secondarily).

Crusting of the surface takes one of two forms, the more severe being a scab of congealed blood. However, early in the vertical growth phase of melanoma, the malignant cells expand into the epidermis, which causes the keratin cells at the surface to shed. To the clinician, this can be seen as a fine scaling on the surface. If neither of these typical features is noted, the surface of the melanoma may appear glossy.

A majority of patients with melanomas observe a pre-existing "mole" at the site of the malignancy. The reliability of the patient's observation is influenced by the site and size of the benign precursor. A small junctional nevus on the back is less likely to be noticed by either the patient or spouse than a similar lesion on the face or chest.

Melanomas may have a variety of clinical appearances, but a common denominator is their changing nature. Therefore, any single pigmented lesion that undergoes a change in size, configuration, or color should be considered a melanoma, and an excisional biopsy should be performed (see Chap. 6 for details). It should be noted that benign nevi of various kinds tend to enlarge and become slightly darker during puberty and pregnancy and sometimes when women take contraceptive pills.

However, in most instances the change is slight and applies to all the patient's moles. Hence, it is important for diagnostic purposes that the clinical features of malignancy apply to a single lesion, except in the rare case when more than one primary melanoma may develop simultaneously. However, if genuine doubt still exists, one useful way of avoiding unnecessary excisions, particularly in teenage children, is to measure the lesion to the nearest millimeter and ask the patient or relative to repeat the measurement every 2 to 4 weeks. If the lesion remains static, biopsy can be avoided.

GROWTH PATTERNS

A convenient way of categorizing melanomas is by their growth patterns.[13,14,39] Although these are distinct pathologic entities, they also have unique clinical features that can be distinguished by the experienced clinician (Table 2-3). This is relevant, because these different categories are all distinct from benign lesions and each of them portends a different prognosis. Obviously, histologic confirmation is essential before making any definitive treatment plans.

The four major growth patterns of melanomas are superficial spreading, nodular, lentigo maligna, and acral lentiginous (see Plate 1). Their clinical features are described below, and their histologic features are summarized in Chapter 3.

Color Plates

MELANOMA GROWTH PATTERNS

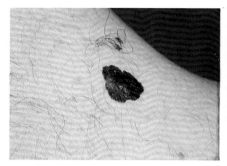

Superficial spreading

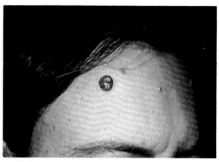

Nodular

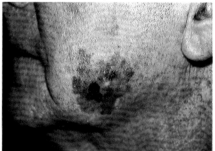

Lentigo maligna

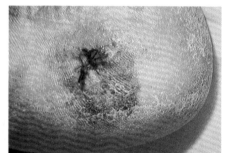

Acral lentiginous

DIFFERENTIAL DIAGNOSIS

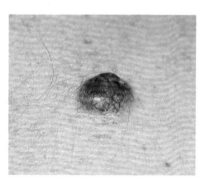

Pigmented basal cell carcinoma

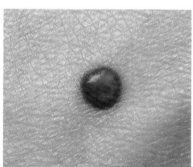

Blue nevus

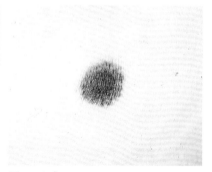

Pigmented nevus

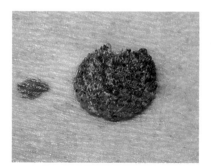

Seborrheic keratosis

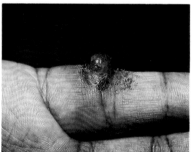

Pyogenic granuloma

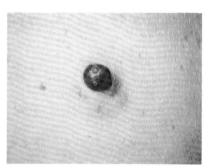

Hematoma

THE CLINICAL SPECTRUM OF CUTANEOUS MELANOMA

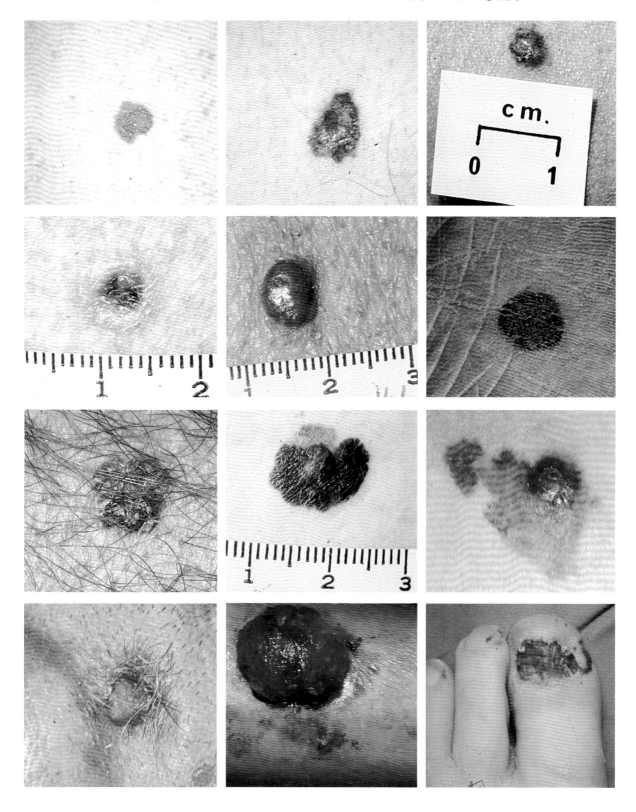

TABLE 2–3
DISTINGUISHING FEATURES OF MELANOMA GROWTH PATTERNS IN CLINICAL STAGE-I PATIENTS*

	Superficial Spreading		Nodular		Lentigo Maligna		Acral Lentiginous	
Proportion of Melanomas	70		26		3		1	
Sex (male)	44		65		55		35	
Age (years)								
8–30	24		15		2		20	
31–40	20		19		5		15	
41–50	23		17		6		8	
51–60	18		22		26		14	
61 +	15		27		61		43	
Anatomical Site	Men	Women	Men	Women	Men	Women	Men	Women
Head and Neck	13	8	15	12	95	83	0	0
Arm	7	18	15	9	5	6	0	0
Trunk	62	28	51	25	0	0	0	0
Leg	17	45	17	42	0	0	0	0
Hand and Foot	1	1	2	2	0	11	100	100
Predominant Growth Phase	Radial		Vertical		Radial		Radial	
Duration of Evolution (years)	1–5		0.5–1.5		3–15		N/A	
Maximum Diameter (mm)								
1–5	20		20		29		12	
6–10	45		39		36		51	
11–20	29		34		23		27	
20 +	6		7		12		10	
Color	Tan, brown, and black; multi-colored—can have shades of red, gray, or purple		Usually black or blue–black		Tan or brown stain		Tan or black	
Surface	Flat at first, some nodules or plaques		Dome-shaped		Flat		Flat at first, some nodules or plaques	
Perimeter	Notching or indention		"Punched-out"		Convoluted		Irregular	
Ulceration	12		55		23		42	

*All numbers are percentages unless otherwise stated.

SUPERFICIAL SPREADING MELANOMA (SSM)

Superficial spreading melanoma constitutes the majority of the melanomas (about 70% in most series).[13,14,32,36,37] The lesions generally arise in a pre-existing nevus. A history of slowly evolving change of the precursor lesion over 1 to 5 years is not uncommon, with more rapid growth developing months before diagnosis. They can occur at any age after puberty. In some patient series, there is a predilection for SSM to occur on the legs of women and on the backs of men.[14] However, in the SMU series, such a predilection was not observed, the anatomical distribution of SSM and nodular melanoma (NM) being very similar in both men and women (see Table 2-3). The average diameter of an SSM is 2 cm,[60] while more deeply invasive melanomas are even larger. Any pigmented lesion that is 5 mm to 10 mm or greater in diameter is more commonly malignant than benign. The converse is not always true, since smaller lesions may also be SSMs.

The typical appearance of an SSM when it first appears is a deeply pigmented area in a brown junctional nevus (Fig. 2-5). The initial growth of the melanoma is above the basement membrane, and for a time, the fine skin markings in many junctional nevi remain intact. As the dark areas expand, there can be variegation in color, ranging from a deep blue or jet black to a pale gray or white color. The lesion may take on a "lacy" appearance. Often there are patches of regression recognizable by areas of amelanosis (see Figs. 2-3 to 2-5).

Early in their evolution, SSMs are generally flat lesions. They may develop an irregular surface, usually asymmetrically, depending on the vertical growth phase that develops as they enlarge. They

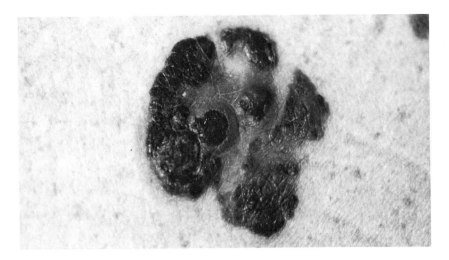

FIG. 2–5 A superficial spreading malignant melanoma with small patches of regression. It has pale superficial tumor over most of the area and patches of more darkly pigmented areas. The patient had noted the enlargement for 8 months and the darkening for 6 weeks.

sometimes have a fine crust or a scaly surface initially. As the lesion grows, the surface may be glossy. Characteristically, there is notching or indentation of the perimeter, especially as the SSM enlarges. The edge of the lesion abutting normal skin sometimes shows a fine (1-mm) pink rim or halo; presumably, this represents a form of host response with lymphocyte infiltrate. A much larger red rim surrounding the tumor develops if the lesion becomes infected or ulcerated secondarily.

NODULAR MELANOMA (NM)

Nodular melanoma is the second most common growth pattern (15%–30% of patients).[12,14,32,36,37] These melanomas are more aggressive tumors and usually have a shorter clinical onset than SSMs. They can occur at any age (but usually at middle age) and are more common on the trunk or head and neck. Men tend to have more NMs than women, whereas the opposite is true for SSM. They are usually 1 cm to 2 cm in diameter, but they can be much larger. It is more common for NMs to begin *de novo* in uninvolved skin, rather than from a pre-existing nevus (Fig. 2-6).

Nodular melanomas are generally darker than SSMs and more uniform in coloration. The typical NM is a blue–black lesion that often resembles a blood blister or a hemangioma. It may have other shadings of red, gray, or purple. About 5% of NMs lack pigment altogether (*i.e.*, amelanotic) and have a fleshy appearance (Fig. 2-7).

In contrast to SSMs, most NMs are raised or dome-shaped. Their shape is often symmetrical, but sometimes they appear as an irregularly shaped plaque. They lack the radial (horizontal) growth

phase that is so typical of the other growth patterns. They therefore have a discrete, sharply demarcated ("punched out") border, often with an irregular perimeter. Those NMs that are polypoid, with a stalk or cauliflower appearance, are particularly aggressive lesions (see Fig. 2-7).[33,35]

LENTIGO MALIGNA MELANOMA (LMM)

Lentigo maligna melanoma appears to be separate from the other growth patterns, because LMMs do not have the same propensity to metastasize as melanomas of other growth patterns.[34] They constitute a small percentage of patients (usually 4%–10%)

FIG. 2–6 A 1.5-cm nodular melanoma that developed *de novo* over 2 months. Note the glossy surface and some small keratin flakes at one edge.

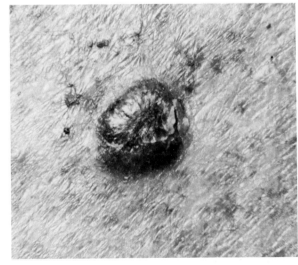

and are typically located on the face of Caucasian women.[14] Usually, LMMs have been present for long periods of time (5–15 years). They are generally large (> 3 cm), flat lesions that occur in an older age group, being uncommon before the age of 50 years. Almost all are located on the face or neck, while a few may occur on the dorsal aspect of the hands or the lower legs. They are more common in women than in men.

These lesions are likened to a stain on the skin. They are typically tan-colored with differing shades of brown. Irregular mottling or flecking may appear as the lesion enlarges, with areas of dark brown or black in some parts and areas of regression in others (Fig. 2-8).

A striking characteristic of LMM is its flatness, especially in early lesions. This is because the horizontal growth phase is very prolonged (the average history being 10 years or longer). A portion of the lesion may acquire a vertical growth phase with the appearance of a nodule or a plaque within the lesion as it grows. LMM can have extremely convoluted borders with prominent notching and indentation, which generally represent areas of regression.

ACRAL LENTIGINOUS MELANOMA (ALM)

Acral lentiginous melanoma characteristically occurs on the palms or soles, or beneath the nail beds.[5,16,27,44,52,54] This does not mean that all plantar or volar melanomas are ALMs, for a minority are SSMs or NMs.[21,44,47] They occur in only 2% to 8% of Caucasians[29] but in a substantially higher proportion (35%–60%) of dark-skinned patients, such as Negroes, Orientals, and Hispanics.[50,52]

The majority of ALMs are located on the sole.[27] They are generally large, with an average diameter of about 3 cm.[16] They usually occur in older people, with an average age in the 60s. Their evolution is relatively short, ranging from a few months to several years, with an average of 2.5 years. However, because the site of the ALM usually cannot be readily observed and the patients are often old, the symptom duration is not always accurate.

Initially, these lesions often resemble an LMM with a tan or brown flat stain on the palm or sole. The haphazard array of color is characteristic. A minority of such lesions take on a flesh-colored appearance that can be misdiagnosed as "corns" or pyogenic granulomas.

Usually, ALMs are flat at first, and there may be only minimal elevation in the presence of a deeply invasive lesion. The surface can become hyperkeratotic. Ulceration is not uncommon, and fungating masses can result from neglected lesions. As with LMM, these lesions often have a very irregular, convoluted border (Fig. 2-9). However, the ALM lesions are much more aggressive than LMM lesions and are more likely to metastasize.

SUBUNGUAL MELANOMA

Subungual melanoma is an infrequent type of cutaneous melanoma.[21,43,44,46,47] It develops in only 2% to 3% of Caucasian patients but a higher proportion of dark-skinned patients. It is evenly divided between men and women and is most often diagnosed in older patients (median 55–65 years). Over three fourths of subungual melanomas involve either the

FIG. 2–7 A polypoid, amelanotic melanoma developing in an area of superficial spreading melanoma. The raised growth had developed in 2 months.

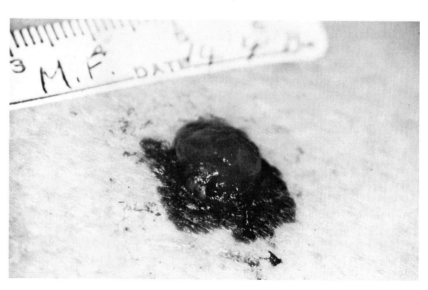

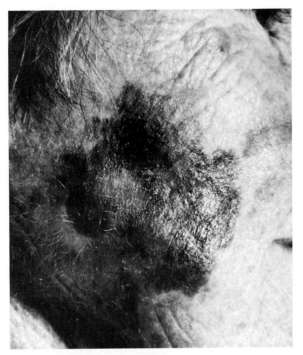

FIG. 2–8 A classic lentigo maligna melanoma on the cheek of an elderly woman. The edge and pigmentation are both irregular. Also, note the evidence of acute solar cutaneous damage on her face. This lesion was thought to have been present for more than 10 years.

great toe or the thumb. The most common sign of an early subungual melanoma is a brown to black discoloration under the nail bed. The nail plate may become detached from the nail bed and stop growing. In some cases, the melanoma may mask as a paronychial infection, ingrown toenails, or an ulceration.[28] Amelanotic tumors sometimes resemble pyogenic granulomas. The median duration of symptoms for subungual melanomas is much longer than for other cutaneous melanomas (about 18 months versus 5 months). Not uncommonly, this results from a delayed diagnosis on the part of the patient or physician.

A subungual hematoma is the most important benign lesion to differentiate from a melanoma. Subungual hematomas may appear as black lesions or multi-colored lesions (from hemoglobin breakdown products) beneath the nail bed or matrix. Usually, there is a history of sharp trauma to this area. The hemorrhage is sharply localized and does not show pigmentation in the adjacent cuticle or skin (Hutchinson's sign). If the diagnosis is in doubt, a large-bore needle or the heated tip of a paper clip can be used to drill a hole slowly in the

nail plate to reveal blood. If so, the lesion should still be watched to be sure that the damaged area continues to move distally as the nail plate grows out. Two other conditions that may cause some confusion in the differential diagnosis are fungal infections and pyogenic granulomas. Fungal infections respond generally to appropriate antibiotic treatment. Pyogenic granulomas are usually soft, pliable, and vascular, with a sharp line of demarcation between the lesion and normal skin. They develop much more quickly than a melanoma does.

It must be remembered that 10% to 15% of subungual melanomas may be nonpigmented and have a fleshy appearance. A delay in diagnosis may decrease the chances for cure. Therefore, any persistent lesion must be biopsied.

Clinically, a helpful aspect in differential diagnosis is examination of the regional lymph nodes (including epitrochlear nodes) in patients with suspicious lesions, for at least one third of patients with subungual melanomas present with nodal metastases.

Papachristou and Fortner[46] identified four factors that adversely influenced prognosis in a study of

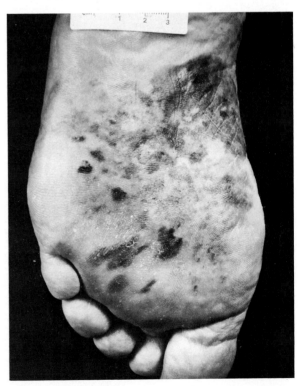

FIG. 2–9 An acral lentiginous melanoma on the sole of a 75-year-old man who did not know how long it had been present. This lesion shows all the features described in the text.

52 patients: (1) destruction of the nail, (2) subungual melanomas of the toes (as opposed to the fingers), (3) invasion of the underlying bone, and (4) lack of pigmentation.

DIFFERENTIAL DIAGNOSIS

Simply stated, malignant pigmented lesions exhibit disorder, while benign pigmented lesions show order in color, symmetry of border, and uniformity of surface characteristics.[37] This section reviews some characteristics of benign pigmented lesions with an emphasis on some of the characteristics that distinguish them from melanomas. A biopsy should be performed whenever the clinical diagnosis is suspicious for melanoma, for the features of the malignancy are usually subtle when it is in its more curable stage.

The clinical features of LMM are so typical that clinical differentiation of this condition from others usually poses no serious difficulty. However, in the early stages, simple freckles, solar lentigines, or small patches of seborrheic keratosis may cause some confusion.

On the other hand, the differential diagnosis of SSM or NM from other pigmented lesions is an important clinical problem. Some of the characteristic features are shown in Plate 1. Lesions that should be considered in the differential diagnosis are described below.

SEBORRHEIC KERATOSIS

The clinical history together with the characteristic appearance of seborrheic keratosis should lead to the correct clinical diagnosis. The lesions are commonly multiple, are waxy in appearance, and usually re-

main unchanged for long periods. When a seborrheic keratosis is thin, it resembles a smudge on the skin with a scaly surface. As it becomes thicker, it is firm to the touch and exhibits a slightly waxy surface. It is sometimes described as resembling the end of a dirty paintbrush or appearing "stuck" to the skin surface.

JUNCTIONAL, COMPOUND, AND DERMAL NEVI

These are the most common pigmented lesions in Caucasians. In one Australian survey there was an average of 15 such lesions per person.[42] The risk that any one junctional nevus will become malignant is very small. Hence, the wholesale excision of junctional nevi is unjustified.

A junctional nevus is characteristically impalpable, is pale to dark brown, and may be as large as 1 cm in diameter.[48] Usually it is smaller, while most melanomas are larger (*i.e.,* 1.5 cm or greater). Most junctional nevi remain the same size for years or else change very slowly over a period of years. They may appear after 4 years of age or at puberty. If they enlarge at all, the rate of growth is slow (about 1 mm per year) as the child grows. In contrast to melanomas, their color is orderly, and normal skin markings are usually preserved.

Compound nevi are palpable because the collected nevus cells in the papillary dermis stretch the overlying epidermis to form a palpable nodule. Compound nevi may be slightly darker brown than typical junctional nevi are. However, these two lesions commonly form part of a single nevus, one area being junctional and another darker part being compound. The flat component of a compound nevus usually has an orderly pattern of coloration and marginal integrity (Fig. 2-10).

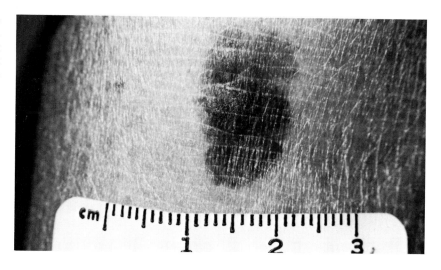

FIG. 2–10 Part of this lesion is paler than the rest, with little distortion of the fine skin creases. This part is a junctional nevus. The central part is a compound nevus, which is darker and with a slightly deformed skin surface. The patient thought the lesion had changed very little in the preceding years.

A halo nevus is a compound nevus surrounded by a depigmented halo. It is most noticeable in the summer when the surrounding skin is tanned. Halo nevi occur most frequently in the young, especially around the age of puberty, although some occur in the late 20s and early 30s. The natural course for halo nevi is to remain unchanged for a few years and then to gradually fade away, leaving little trace of either the halo or the central compound nevus.

Dermal nevi have a collection of melanocytes deeper in the dermis, rather than at the dermal–epidermal junction. They are usually dome-shaped, lack pigment, and can cause a notable distortion of the fine anatomy of the skin. The most common variety do not contain hairs, although thick, bristle-like hairs are fairly frequent in those that have been present since birth. Small congenital dermal nevi occasionally can become inflamed, swollen, and tender over a period of a few days. This is not caused by malignant degeneration but by infection or obstruction in abnormal hair follicles associated with the nevus (Fig. 2-11).

HEMANGIOMA

Hemangiomas contain large vascular spaces in the skin that usually remain static for years. If injured, they may be surrounded by a small bruise (Fig. 2-12), or they may bleed, usually more profusely than the typical melanoma. Cavernous hemangi-

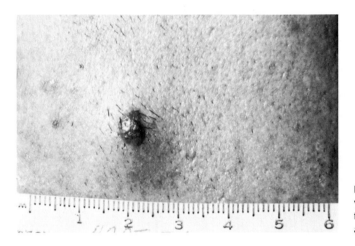

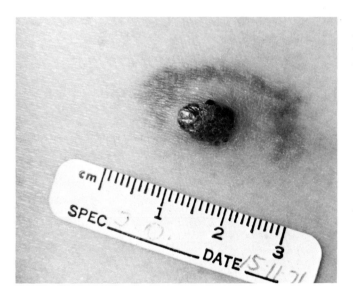

FIG. 2–11 A congenital dermal nevus on the face of a young man, which had become swollen in the preceding few days. The swelling was caused by a retention cyst in a gland, the duct of which passed through the nevus.

FIG. 2–12 A hemangioma that had been injured. Note the surrounding bruise and the small nodules of the surface. Apart from the injury, the patient was unaware of any change in the lesion in the preceding years.

omas are often blue–black in color; less often they may have a slightly red tinge. If the contained blood has clotted, a hemangioma will feel firm and the emptying sign on pressure will not be demonstrable.

A venous hemangioma, especially on the lip, may cause anxiety by being moderately large (up to a centimeter), but the patient will have noted the lesion present for years without change. The lesion can be emptied with direct pressure but may refill so rapidly that the compression sign is not easy to demonstrate without pressing it with a glass slide.

Sclerosing hemangioma or histiocytoma is a common cutaneous lesion, often multiple on the trunk and legs. It changes slowly over the years, if at all. It is rust-colored, feels both firm and slightly warm to touch, is slightly raised, the surface is intact, and it is not tender. The firmness is caused by the formation of scar tissue and the warmth of dilated blood vessels in the substance of the tumor.

BLUE NEVUS

Blue nevi consist of a collection of melanocytes in the dermis with a normal or slightly thinned epidermis stretched over the surface. The most common variety is small (usually less than 0.5 cm in diameter), blue–black in color, and palpable as a small lump. If a blue nevus is injured with sufficient violence to rip off the covering epidermis, the black collection of melanocytes has an alarming glossy surface. However, the severity of the injury, to-

gether with the observation that the lesion has been unchanged previously for years, should distinguish it from a melanoma. A less common but more unsightly form of blue nevus is the cellular blue nevus (Fig. 2-13). A blue nevus usually remains static, but rarely malignant degeneration and active growth supervene.

PIGMENTED BASAL CELL CARCINOMA AND SQUAMOUS CELL CARCINOMA

These lesions develop coloration because of excessive melanin production by melanocytes in the substance of the tumor. Pigmented squamous cell carcinomas (SCCs) are rare, while pigmented basal cell carcinomas (BCCs) are quite common. The long and slowly changing nature of a BCC over many months or several years gives a clue to its diagnosis. This lesion is usually raised from early in its development, and it may have a peripheral ring of small nodules that is not found in melanomas. It rarely bleeds, also distinguishing it from melanoma, which can sometimes bleed. The appearance of a pigmented BCC, if examined carefully, is similar to its nonpigmented counterpart. Indeed, there are often small areas of pale, pearly tumor, interspersed with areas of a dark brown color. The appearance of a pigmented BCC can mimic exactly that of a melanoma, so a tissue diagnosis will have to be established before definitive treatment. Frozen section examination may be adequate to make this distinction.

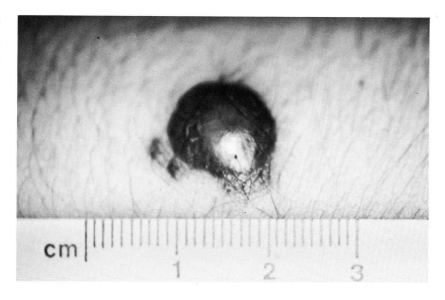

FIG. 2–13 A cellular blue nevus noticed by the patient's family physician. The patient was not worried by the lesion, because it had not changed in years. The high gloss on the surface of this blue nevus is unusual for such lesions.

PYOGENIC GRANULOMA

Pyogenic granuloma is a form of hemangioma that, although most common on the fingers, can occur at other sites. The lesion is characteristically irritated, hence its apparent growth. The cause of the irritation and inflammation is not always infectious. The history often given by the patient is that a small lesion (up to 0.5 cm) developed rapidly over several days or weeks. It can be a blood-colored lesion, often with a semiglossy surface, with an area of inflammatory reaction extending up to 1 cm or more around the lesion. The lesion may have itched; and despite the marked inflammatory halo that may surround it, the lesion is not painful. A pyogenic granuloma is raised above the level of the surrounding skin, and the surface is usually intact unless it has been injured (Fig. 2-14). The rapid history and the marked inflammatory reaction are features that distinguish it well from melanoma.

SPITZ NEVUS

Another type of nevus that may be confused with melanoma in children is called a Spitz nevus, also referred to as compound melanocytoma or a juvenile melanoma.[55] This lesion occurs most frequently in children at the age of 5 to 10 years and rarely occurs after the age of about 25 to 30 years. Typically, the lesion develops more rapidly than other nevi on growing children. A Spitz nevus is not usually darkly pigmented, although there may be spots of brown in the main pink tumor mass. The surface is usually smooth, flat, or dome-shape, and is not ulcerated.

DOUBTFUL DIAGNOSIS

In spite of care to establish the diagnosis of melanoma, there is a small proportion of patients in whom the true nature of the condition is doubtful after interpretation of an initial biopsy. The following procedures should be adopted in such situations:

1. Care is taken to ensure that the initial biopsy was an excisional biopsy and that the pathologist has examined the entire lesion with step sections. If the original biopsy was not excisional, the remainder of the skin lesion should be excised for further histologic evaluation.
2. An independent opinion is obtained from two or more pathologists.
3. The clinical history given by the patient and relatives is reviewed to ascertain whether these features support the diagnosis of malignancy. If they do, the lesion is more likely to be malignant than benign and vice versa.
4. When real doubts of the diagnosis persist, in spite of the above, the patient is told of the situation. If the previous biopsy was close (*i.e.,* less than 1 mm) to the edge of the tumor, a slightly wider excision is recommended, since the morbidity of the procedure is generally negligible. The tissue is examined for residual tumor, and the patient is asked to report for regular checkups.

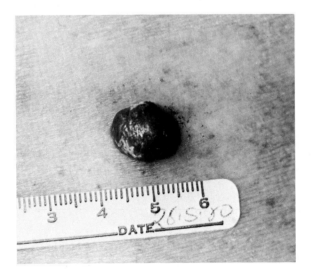

FIG. 2–14 This pyogenic granuloma had developed in 2 weeks. It is slightly unusual because it was situated on the back and because the inflammatory halo around it is more extensive than usual.

REFERENCES

1. Acton RT, Balch CM, Barger BO, Budowle B, Go RCP, Soong S–j, Roseman JM: The occurrence of melanoma and its relationship with host, lifestyle and environmental factors. In Costanzi JJ (ed): Malignant Melanoma 1, p. 151. The Hague, Nijhoff, 1983
2. Acton RT, Balch CM, Budowle B, Go RCP, Roseman JM, Soong S–j, Barger BO: Immunogenetics of melanoma. In Reisfeld RA, Ferrone S (eds): Melanoma Antigens and Antibodies, p. 1. New York, Plenum, 1982
3. Anderson DE: Clinical characteristics of the genetic variety of cutaneous melanoma in man. Cancer 28:721, 1971
4. Anderson DE, Smith JLJ, McBride CM: Hereditary aspects of malignant melanoma. JAMA 200:741, 1967
5. Arrington JH III, Reed RJ, Ichinose H, Krementz ET: Plantar lentiginous melanoma: A distinctive variant of human cutaneous malignant melanoma. Am J Surg Pathol 1:131, 1977
6. Balch CM: Oral and cutaneous melanoma: Clinical recognition, pathological features, and prognostic factors. Ala J Med Sci 17:51, 1980
7. Balch CM, Soong S–j, Milton GW, Shaw HM, McGovern VJ, Murad TM, McCarthy WH, Maddox WA: A comparison of prognostic factors and surgical results in 1,786 patients with localized (stage I) melanoma treated in Alabama, USA, and New South Wales, Australia. Ann Surg 196:677, 1982
8. Barger BO, Acton RT, Soong S–j, Roseman J, Balch C: Increase of HLA–DR4 in melanoma patients from Alabama. Cancer Res 42:4276, 1982
9. Bellet RE, Vaisman I, Mastrangelo MJ, Lustbader E: Multiple primary malignancies in patients with cutaneous melanoma. Cancer 40:1974, 1977
10. Beral V, Evans S, Shaw H, Milton G: Cutaneous factors related to the risk of malignant melanoma. Br J Dermatol 109:165, 1983
11. Budowle B, Barger BO, Balch CM, Go RCP, Roseman JM, Acton RT: Associations of properdin factor B with melanoma. Can Genet Cytogenet 5:247, 1982
12. Clark DA, Necheles T, Nathanson L, Silverman E: Apparent HL–A5 deficiency in malignant melanoma. Transplantation 15:326, 1973
13. Clark WH Jr, Ainsworth AM, Bernardino EA, Yang C–H, Mihm MC Jr, Reed RJ: The developmental biology of primary human malignant melanomas. Semin Oncol 2:83, 1975
14. Clark WH Jr, From L, Bernardino EA, Mihm MC: The histogenesis and biologic behavior of primary human malignant melanomas of the skin. Cancer Res 29:705, 1969
15. Clark WH Jr, Reimer RR, Greene M, Ainsworth AM, Mastrangelo MJ: Origin of familial malignant melanomas from heritable melanocytic lesions: "The B–K mole syndrome." Arch Dermatol 114:732, 1978
16. Coleman WP III, Loria PR, Reed RJ, Krementz ET: Acral lentiginous melanoma. Arch Dermatol 116:773, 1980
17. Davis NC, McLeod GR, Beardmore GL, Little JH, Quinn RL, Holt J: Primary cutaneous melanoma: A report from the Queensland Melanoma Project. CA—A Journal for Clinicians 26:80, 1976
18. Elder DE, Goldman LI, Goldman SC, Greene MH, Clark WH Jr: Dysplastic nevus syndrome: A phenotypic association of sporadic cutaneous melanoma. Cancer 46:1787, 1980
19. Elder DE, Greene MH, Guerry D IV, Kraemer KH, Clark WH Jr: The dysplastic nevus syndrome: Our definition. Am J Dermatopathol 4:455, 1982
20. Epstein E, Bragg K, Linden G: Biopsy and prognosis of malignant melanoma. JAMA 208:1369, 1969
21. Feibleman CE, Stoll H, Maize JC: Melanomas of the palm, sole and nailbed: A clinicopathologic study. Cancer 46:2492, 1980
22. Gellin GA, Kopf AW, Garfinkel L: Malignant melanoma. A controlled study of possibly associated factors. Arch Dermatol 99:43, 1969
23. Greene MH, Reimer RR, Clark WH Jr, Mastrangelo MJ: Precursor lesions in familial melanoma. Semin Oncol 5:85, 1978
24. Hersey P, Edwards A, Honeyman M, McCarthy WH: Low natural-killer-cell activity in familial melanoma patients and their relatives. Br J Cancer 40:113, 1979
25. Jörgensen G, Lal VB: Serogenetic investigations on malignant melanomas with reference to the incidence of ABO system Rh system, Gm, Inv, Hp and Gc systems. Humangenetik 15:227, 1972
26. Kopf AW, Mintzis M, Bart RS: Diagnostic accuracy in malignant melanoma. Arch Dermatol 111:1291, 1975
27. Krementz ET, Reed RJ, Coleman WP III, Sutherland CM, Carter RD, Campbell M: Acral lentiginous melanoma. A clinicopathologic entity. Ann Surg 195:632, 1982
28. Leppard B, Sanderson KV, Behan F: Subungual malignant melanoma: Difficulty in diagnosis. Br Med J 1:310, 1974
29. Lopansri S, Mihm MC Jr: Clinical and pathological correlation of malignant melanoma. J Cutan Pathol 6:180, 1979
30. Lynch HT, Frichot BC III, Lynch JF: Familial atypical multiple mole-melanoma syndrome. J Med Genet 15:352, 1978
31. Lynch HT, Frichot BC III, Lynch P, Lynch J, Guirgis HA: Family studies of malignant melanoma and associated cancer. Surg Gynecol Obstet 141:517, 1975
32. McGovern VJ, Mihm MC Jr, Bailly C, Booth JC, Clark WH Jr, Cochran AJ, Hardy EG, Hicks JD, Levene A, Lewis MG, Little JH, Milton GW: The classification of malignant melanoma and its histologic reporting. Cancer 32:1446, 1973

33. McGovern VJ, Shaw HM, Milton GW: Prognostic significance of a polypoid configuration in malignant melanoma. Histopathology 7:663, 1983

34. McGovern VJ, Shaw HM, Milton GW, Farago GA: Is malignant melanoma arising in a Hutchinson's melanotic freckle a separate disease entity? Histopathology 4:235, 1980

35. Manci EA, Balch CM, Murad TM, Soong S-j: Polypoid melanoma, a virulent variant of the nodular growth pattern. Am J Clin Pathol 75:810, 1981

36. Mihm MC Jr, Clark WH Jr, From L: The clinical diagnosis, classification and histogenetic concepts of the early stages of cutaneous malignant melanomas. N Engl J Med 284:1078, 1971

37. Mihm MC Jr, Clark WH Jr, Reed RJ: The clinical diagnosis of malignant melanoma. Semin Oncol 2:105, 1975

38. Mihm MC Jr, Fitzpatrick TB, Lane–Brown MM, Raker JW, Malt RA, Kaiser JS: Early detection of primary cutaneous malignant melanoma: A color atlas. N Engl J Med 289:989, 1973

39. Milton GW: Clinical diagnosis of malignant melanoma. Br J Surg 55:755, 1968

40. Milton GW, Lewis CWD: The presentation of malignant melanoma (melanoblastoma). Med J Aust 1:239, 1963

41. Moseley HS, Giuliano AE, Storm FK, Clark WH Jr, Robinson DS, Morton DL: Multiple primary melanoma. Cancer 43:939, 1979

42. Nicholls EM: Development and elimination of pigmented moles, and the anatomical distribution of primary malignant melanoma. Cancer 32:191, 1973

43. Pack GT, Oropeza R: Subungual melanoma. Surg Gynecol Obstet 124:571, 1967

44. Paladugu RR, Winberg CD, Yonemoto RH: Acral lentiginous melanoma. A clinicopathologic study of 36 patients. Cancer 52:161, 1983

45. Pandey JP, Johnson AH, Funderberg HH, Amos DB, Gutterman JV, Hersh EM: HLA antigens and immunoglobulin allotypes in patients with malignant melanoma. Hum Immunol 2:185, 1981

46. Papachristou DN, Fortner JG: Melanoma arising under the nail. J Surg Oncol 21:219, 1982

47. Patterson RH, Helwig EB: Subungual malignant melanoma: A clinical–pathologic study. Cancer 46:2074, 1980

48. Reed RJ, Ichinose H, Clark WH Jr, Mihm MC Jr: Common and uncommon melanocytic nevi and borderline melanomas. Semin Oncol 2:119, 1975

49. Reimer RR, Clark WH Jr, Greene MH, Ainsworth AM, Fraumeni JF Jr: Precursor lesions in familial melanoma. A new genetic preneoplastic syndrome. JAMA 239:744, 1978

50. Reintgen DS, McCarty KM Jr, Cox E, Seigler HF: Malignant melanoma in black American and white American populations. A comparative review. JAMA 248:1856, 1982

51. Scheibner A, Milton GW, McCarthy WH, Nordlund TT, Pearson LJ: Multiple primary melanoma—a review of 90 cases. Aust J Dermatol 23:1, 1982

52. Seiji M, Takahashi M: Acral melanoma in Japan. Hum Pathol 13:607, 1982

53. Sober AJ, Fitzpatrick TB, Mihm MC, Jr, Wise TG, Pearson BJ, Clark WH, Jr, Kopf AW: Early recognition of cutaneous melanoma. JAMA 242:2795, 1979

54. Sondergaard K, Olsen G: Malignant melanoma of the foot. A clinicopathological study of 125 primary cutaneous malignant melanomas. Acta Pathol Microbiol Scand [A] 88:275, 1980

55. Spitz S: Melanomas of childhood. Am J Pathol 24:591, 1948

56. Veronesi U, Cascinelli N, Bufalino R: Evaluation of the risk of multiple primaries in malignant cutaneous melanoma. Tumori 62:127, 1976

57. Wallace DC, Beardmore GL, Exton LA: Familial malignant melanoma. Ann Surg 177:15, 1973

58. Wallace DC, Exton LA, McLeod GRC: Genetic factor in malignant melanoma. Cancer 27:1262, 1971

59. Walter H, Brachtel R, Hilling M: On the incidence of blood group O and Gm phenotypes in patients with malignant melanoma. Hum Genet 49:71, 1979

60. Wick MM, Sober AJ, Fitzpatrick TB, Mihm MC, Jr, Kopf AW, Clark WH, Jr, Blois MS: Clinical characteristics of early cutaneous melanoma. Cancer 45:2684, 1980

VINCENT J. McGOVERN
TARIQ M. MURAD

Pathology of Melanoma: An Overview

3

Most of the advances in our understanding of melanoma in recent years have concerned the relationship of prognosis with histologic features. Consequently, it is most important that the clinician and the pathologist be thoroughly aware of this relationship so that the surgical specimen submitted for examination will be one from which the pathologist can supply the maximum amount of information required in planning and management of the patient.

PRECURSORS OF MELANOMA

It was not so long ago that every melanoma, apart from that arising in lentigo maligna, was thought to have arisen in a junctional or compound nevus of childhood type. Lesions that are now classified as melanoma precursors, either dysplastic nevus[18,19] or melanoma *in situ,* were then called by a variety of names such as active junctional (or compound) nevus, atypical melanocytic hyperplasia, premalignant melanocytic hyperplasia, and premalignant melanosis.

Invasive melanoma may progress in a stepwise fashion from a nonmalignant precursor, the dysplastic nevus, to melanoma *in situ,* to invasive melanoma; or it may begin as melanoma *in situ.*[42] Both the dysplastic nevus and melanoma *in situ* may appear in the epidermis overlying a benign intradermal nevus. More commonly, however, they occur *de novo.* Precursor lesions of either type may be present for many years before progressing to invasive melanoma.

Clark and associates[15,53] in 1978 described nonmalignant lesions that were the precursors of familial or hereditary melanoma. These lesions were, on the average, larger than the ordinary junctional and compound nevi of childhood, though it was common for patients to have both types of nevus. The lesions often appeared in crops and varied in number from a few to hundreds. Clark called them B-K nevi after the first two families he investigated. Later, Elder and co-workers[18,19] described similar lesions in patients with no family history of melanoma. Again, these lesions often appeared in crops and varied from a few to many. They called the lesion a dysplastic nevus and the condition, dysplastic nevus syndrome. Sagebiel[55] made a histologic study of borderline lesions in which he noted gradations ranging from melanocytic hyperplasia up to mela-

noma *in situ;* he applied the term *atypical melanocytic hyperplasia* for all these gradations. The early stages of Sagebiel's atypical melanocytic hyperplasia correspond to the B-K nevus of Clark and associates and to the dysplastic nevus of Elder and co-workers.

Elder and co-workers[19] noted that a proportion of superficial spreading melanomas had an adjacent component consisting of a dysplastic nevus. In a series of 723 melanomas with an adjacent component of superficial spreading type (SSM), McGov-

FIG. 3–1 (A) Melanoma with an adjacent component of superficial spreading type. There is a nodule of invasive melanoma that has macular pigmentation with irregular borders spreading out from it. (B) In this case, the superficial spreading component consists of a pagetoid invasion of the epidermis of melanoma cells (*i.e.,* melanoma *in situ*).

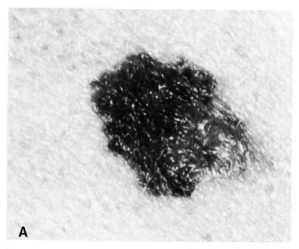

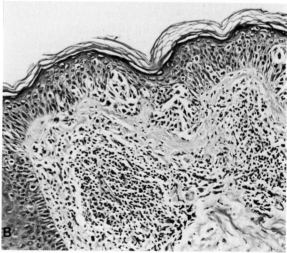

ern and associates[42] found that the superficial spreading component consisted wholly of melanoma *in situ* in 61% of cases (Fig. 3-1). The remaining 39% was composed of wholly dysplastic nevus (Fig. 3-2) or melanoma *in situ* close to the invasive tumor and dysplastic nevus peripherally.

From this, it is concluded that the common SSM arises in one of two ways: either by direct malignant transformation of epidermal melanocytes or by malignant transformation in a dysplastic nevus. It is quite likely that the proportions of these two modes will vary from country to country according to the intensity of the carcinogenic agent in the environment and the susceptibility of the population.

Dysplastic nevi are usually, but not invariably, larger than the ordinary junctional and compound nevi of childhood. A junctional nevus is seldom more than 3 mm in diameter, while it is common for the dysplastic nevus to be more than 5 mm in diameter, and often as large as 1 cm (Fig. 3-3). Junctional and compound nevi often have well-circumscribed margins and uniform color, whether dark or light brown. The dysplastic nevus is usually irregular in outline and color. In addition to shades of brown, there can also be pink areas. Whereas the

ordinary nevi of childhood look remarkably alike, dysplastic nevi have great variation in shape and color, even in each individual patient. Dysplastic nevi occur most frequently on the back and, less commonly, below the waist and on the buttocks, the scalp, and the chest. Not infrequently, a dysplastic nevus will develop over an intradermal nevus dating from childhood. The age when dysplastic proliferation of melanocytes first occurs is not known, but it has been encountered in childhood.[39] Sagebiel found that the average age of his patients with atypical melanocytic hyperplasia (including melanoma *in situ*) was 38 years, while the average age of patients with melanoma having a superficial spreading component that was unequivocally invading the papillary dermis of the skin was 44 years.[55] One might infer from this study that an average of 6 years may elapse before a premalignant lesion becomes invasive; however, such an inference is valid only if dysplastic nevi invariably undergo malignant transformation. As with other premalignant conditions, it is unlikely that more than a minority do so. Furthermore, it is conceivable that only 40% of melanomas with a superficial spreading component begin as a dysplastic nevus, the other 60% commencing as melanoma *in situ*.[42] Dysplastic

FIG. 3–2 *(A)* Flat melanoma with invasion. *(B)* The peripheral noninvasive component has the pattern of a dysplastic nevus; there is irregular proliferation of melanocytes chiefly on and in the ridges with fusion of adjacent proliferating groups. There is condensation of collagen around affected rete ridges but no inflammatory component at the periphery of the lesion in this field.

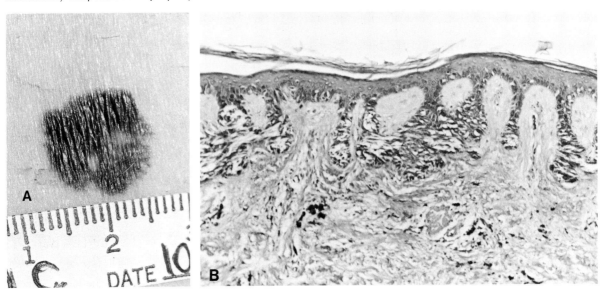

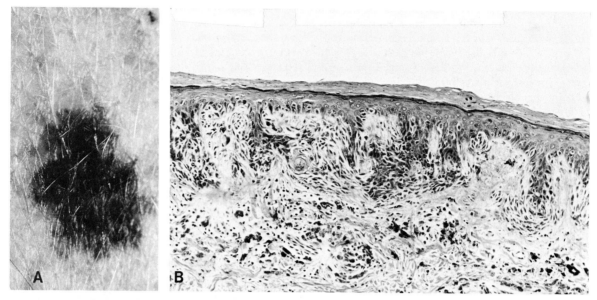

FIG. 3–3 (*A*) Dysplastic nevus from the back of a man whose brother died from melanoma. The typical features are irregular outline and nonuniform color. The lesion was roughly 0.8 cm × 0.6 cm in maximum dimensions. (*B*) There is elongation of rete ridges and irregular proliferation of melanocytes on the ridges with fusion of adjacent masses of proliferating melanocytes. There is a reactive perivascular lymphocytic infiltrate in the dermis.

nevi cannot be distinguished by the naked eye from lesions that are composed entirely of melanoma *in situ*.

Jones and colleagues[28] studied a large number of lesions from various institutions diagnosed as junctional nevi between 1959 and 1968. Of these, 169 specimens were from patients older than 40 years. The diagnosis of junctional nevus, including dysplastic nevus, was confirmed in 74 instances. Thirty-four were reclassified as melanoma *in situ*, of which 11 recurred, 5 with invasive melanoma. This study emphasizes the importance of recognizing melanoma *in situ* and of adequate excision, and is a strong argument in favor of using the term *melanoma in situ* instead of a euphemism that may mislead a surgeon into neglecting to re-excise an incompletely removed "nevus."

CLASSIFICATION OF MELANOMA

Melanoma is classified according to its noninvasive component, because it is impossible to do so on the invading portion, which looks similar in each growth pattern. The classification recommended by an international group of pathologists in 1982 is still based on that of Clark,[12] but it is a clarification and an expansion of that recommended in 1972.[40]

MELANOMA WITH NO ADJACENT COMPONENT

Melanoma with no adjacent component, also called nodular melanoma (NM), has the clinical appearance of a nodule with perhaps an inflammatory flush surrounding it but no spreading pigment. It tends to be larger and thicker than SSM, and it has, more frequently, an ulcerated surface and a polypoid configuration (Fig. 3-4). Microscopically, there is some overlap between this type of melanoma and SSM. This is because there is often a tapering off into melanoma *in situ*, and if this tapering extends for more than three rete ridges, it should then, according to the 1972 classification, be classified as SSM.[40] In an unpublished study of 333 melanomas of this type from the Sydney Melanoma Unit (SMU), there were 27 (8.1%) with remnants of dysplastic nevus within three rete ridges of the invasive tumor. Melanoma of this growth pattern is a faster growing tumor with more mitotic activity than SSM has.

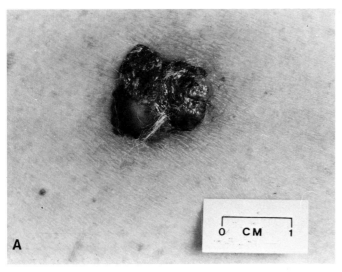

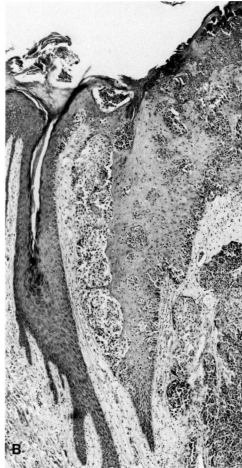

FIG. 3–4   (*A*) A melanoma consisting of a polypoid nodule with no adjacent pigmentation (NM) but surrounded by an inflammatory flush. (*B*) Microscopically, the melanocytic proliferation stops abruptly.

MELANOMA WITH ADJACENT COMPONENT OF THE SUPERFICIAL SPREADING TYPE

Melanoma in which there is an adjacent component of the superficial spreading type is the most common type and is also the variety that is increasing in incidence throughout the world. It has a characteristic clinical appearance, there being an impalpable or barely palpable component adjacent to our surrounding a focus of dermal invasion. Occasionally, there is quite deep invasion, although the surface is flat. More commonly, however, the invasive component is represented by a nodule.

Not only is it recognizable clinically, but its adjacent component is recognizable histologically. Clark and associates[13] used the term *radial growth phase* for the superficial spreading component. The reason for the use of this term rather than "non-invasive" component is that frequently there is some microinvasion, which most pathologists include with *in situ*. As mentioned above, the superficial spreading component may consist of melanoma *in situ* (see Fig. 3-1), or a nonmalignant proliferation of melanocytes at the periphery with the pattern of a dysplastic nevus (see Fig. 3-2).

MELANOMA WITH ADJACENT COMPONENT OF THE LENTIGO MALIGNA TYPE

Lentigo maligna (LMM), a term first introduced in English by Becker[9] to describe a flat pigmented lesion likely to become malignant, is now commonly used in Europe and the United States to denote the lesion first described by Hutchinson in 1892 as senile freckle and subsequently known as Hutchinson's melanotic freckle (HMF).[27] The proportion of HMF that develops into melanoma is quite small. In the absence of a population survey to determine its incidence, one can only guess how often malignancy occurs; however, most estimates are in the vicinity of 5%. The duration of the benign phase before the advent of malignancy may be as short as 5 years or longer than 40 years. The histologic distinction between the benign phase and the *in situ* melanoma phase of LMM is generally regarded as impossible or too difficult to be practicable.

LMM occurs more frequently in women than in men, and the most common sites are the malar and temple regions of the face. It occurs mainly in persons aged 50 years or more and in skin exhibiting very severe solar degeneration (Fig. 3-5). Less common sites are the neck and dorsal aspects of the wrists and hands. Very occasionally, it occurs in skin of other sites, such as the limbs, but only when there is severe solar damage. There are several reports in the literature in which melanomas are classified as LMM when they are located on normally covered parts of the body, such as the trunk and thighs. Such a diagnosis should be viewed with circumspection, since it is generally accepted that the diagnosis of LMM requires the presence of severe solar change in both the epidermis and dermis.[14,44] It is most important that LMM be accurately diag-

nosed, since it has a much better prognosis than other melanomas, especially in women. Consequently, its management is different.[14,44]

MELANOMA WITH ADJACENT COMPONENT OF THE ACRAL LENTIGINOUS TYPE

Melanoma with an adjacent component of the acral lentiginous type involves the soles of the feet, the palms of the hands, and the subungual regions (*i.e.*, in glabrous skin).[4,21,51] Other histogenetic types can also occur in these antomical areas. Ordinary junctional and compound nevi also occur in glabrous skin, but they seldom exceed 3 mm in extent and are not as common as in the skin of other parts of the body.

The lesion that gives rise to melanoma of this type is usually more than 2 cm in diameter and has a smooth surface. In color, it may have tones of brown or black with paler areas. Its smooth surface is deceptive, as there can be quite extensive melanoma invading the dermis and which is impalpable because of the thick layer of keratin (Fig. 3-6). Nevertheless, nodules with ulceration can occur.

Subungual melanomas can masquerade as inflammatory conditions. Hutchinson drew attention to this feature, and, consequently, this lesion is sometimes termed Hutchinson's melanotic whit-

FIG. 3–5 (*A*) Melanomatous nodule arising in LMM (Hutchinson's melanotic freckle). Note the irregular crescentic outline and its variable pigmentation. (*B*) The characteristic features are epidermal atrophy and severe solar elastosis with homogenization. At the periphery of the lesion, there is a lentiginous proliferation of atypical melanocytes in the basal layer, extending down the hair follicles, without much pagetoid invasion of the epidermis. There is a lymphocytic infiltrate in the dermis.

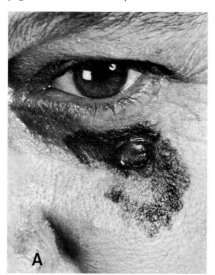
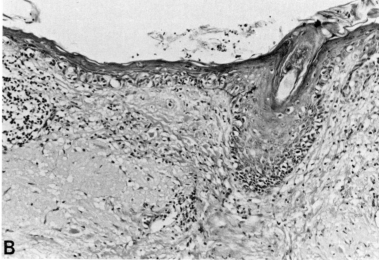

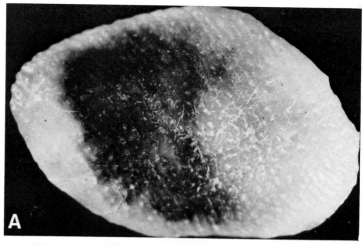

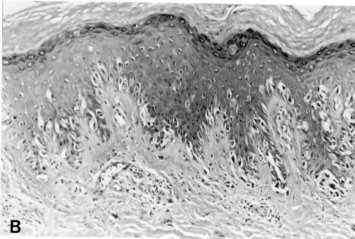

FIG. 3–6 (A) ALM from the sole of the foot. This is an invasive lesion, but because of the thickness of keratin, this was not clinically discernible. The irregular outline is characteristic. (B) The adjacent lentiginous component of an ALM (not that of A). There is irregular acanthosis, elongation of rete ridges, and proliferation of very atypical melanocytes in the basal region with little attempt to form clusters.

low.[26] The lentiginous component emerging from the subungual region may not contain much pigment, and, because of its resemblance to an inflammatory condition, there is often delay in applying appropriate treatment.[50] The adjacent lentiginous component in each of these sites has the same typical appearance. Occasionally, SSM and NM may also occur on the soles and palms.

MELANOMA WITH ADJACENT COMPONENT OF THE MUCOSAL LENTIGINOUS TYPE

Although SSM and NM can occur in the mucosa, the characteristic melanoma has an adjacent lentiginous component that is very similar to the acral lentiginous lesion. These lesions occur rarely, but, when they do occur, the most common site is the vulva[11] and, occasionally, the glans penis and the oral cavity.

MELANOMA OF UNCLASSIFIABLE TYPE

There are various reasons for melanoma being unclassifiable. The specimen may not be representative, or there may be technical faults. A common cause, however, is spontaneous regression, which destroys the epidermal component of the tumor so that it becomes impossible to detect the presence of an adjacent component.

MELANOMA WITH SPECIAL PATTERNS

DESMOPLASTIC

Melanomas with this type of stromal reaction can occur in any of the growth patterns discussed above, most commonly LMM, acral lentiginous melanoma, and locally recurrent melanoma.[16,39] The chief characteristic is a cellular and fibrous reactive stroma (Fig. 3-7). The stroma may have a pattern resembling that of a fibrous histiocytoma, or it may be nonspecific. When the pathologist faces the problem of making the diagnosis of desmoplastic melanoma, electron microscopy may be of help. Electron microscopy has revealed a fibrous histiocytic stroma in some cases, a nonspecific fibroblastic reaction in others, and in some the stroma has the appearance of a schwannoma.* The desmoplastic reaction may involve part or the whole of the tumor because the neoplastic cells occur singly or in small groups between the collagen bundles.

Desmoplastic melanoma presents problems both for the clinician and for the pathologist. These tumors are very difficult to delineate, both clinically and microscopically. Consequently, they frequently recur. Often, the pathologist cannot see any junctional component, and he is therefore reluctant to diagnose melanoma. This is especially true for amelanotic tumors. In some cases, he will be able to see that the malignant melanocytes are originating from epidermal appendages. In others, the appendages may have all been destroyed, but additional blocks of tissue and step-sectioning may reveal remnants of involved hair follicles or sweat ducts. The prognosis for desmoplastic melanoma is generally poor.[16]

MALIGNANT BLUE NEVUS

An excellent study of cellular blue nevi is that of Rodriguez and Ackerman.[54] Some cellular blue nevi metastasize to the local lymph nodes and proceed no farther. It is likely that these are not metastases but are derived from errant melanocytes that migrated from the neural crest at the same time as those giving rise to the cutaneous blue nevus, since blue nevi occur in lymph nodes independently of cutaneous lesions.[2,39] Also in favor of this theory is the fact that the majority of these are in young people in the second or third decade.

Malignant blue nevi that disseminate widely are very uncommon. Sometimes there is a portion of the primary growth resembling the common desmoplastic blue nevus, but more often the diagnosis is one of exclusion. If there is no fibrosis between the melanoma and epidermis, the possibility is that the lesion is a metastasis. If there is fibrosis, the possibility is that the junctional connection has been

lost by spontaneous regression. The pathologist may also have difficulty in determining possible malignancy in a cellular blue nevus. The ordinary criteria can be misleading, and the diagnosis of malignancy is probably made too frequently.

MULTIPLE PRIMARY MELANOMAS

The genetic studies of Anderson[3] convincingly demonstrated a hereditary basis for the development of melanoma in some families. He regards the occurrence of two or more melanomas in a family as hereditary. Wallace and associates[58] came to the same conclusions. They found that close relatives of men with melanoma had a greater risk of developing the lesion themselves than did close relatives of women with melanoma. They also noticed that in Queensland, persons of Celtic background had a much greater likelihood of showing a familial aggregation of cases. No other particular inherited features, such as the color of the skin, hair, eyes, or the susceptibility to sunburn, could be demonstrated.

Clark and associates[15,53] showed that patients with hereditary melanoma had distinct precursor lesions (B-K nevus, dysplastic nevus). These precursors could occur singly or could be multiple and had a tendency to occur in crops. The histologic features of these have already been discussed. Patients with the hereditary melanoma syndrome may have multiple tumors either synchronously or sequentially; and, furthermore, they occur earlier than nonfamilial melanomas.

Multiple melanomas may also occur sporadically in persons not belonging to a melanoma family but, nevertheless, having dysplastic nevi similar to those in members of the familial melanoma group.[18,19]

Occasionally, a patient may be thought to have multiple primary melanomas both clinically and histologically, when all the cutaneous tumors developing subsequently to the first tumor are, in fact, metastatic. These epidermotropic metastases push up and invade the epidermis to resemble primary melanomas with no adjacent component.[31]

MELANOMA ARISING IN CONGENITAL NEVI

There has always been a problem in classifying congenital nevi. Kopf and associates[30] classified them according to their largest diameter (small: 1.4 cm or

---

*E. J. Wills, unpublished data. Staff specialist electron microscopist, Royal Prince Alfred Hospital, Sydney, Australia.

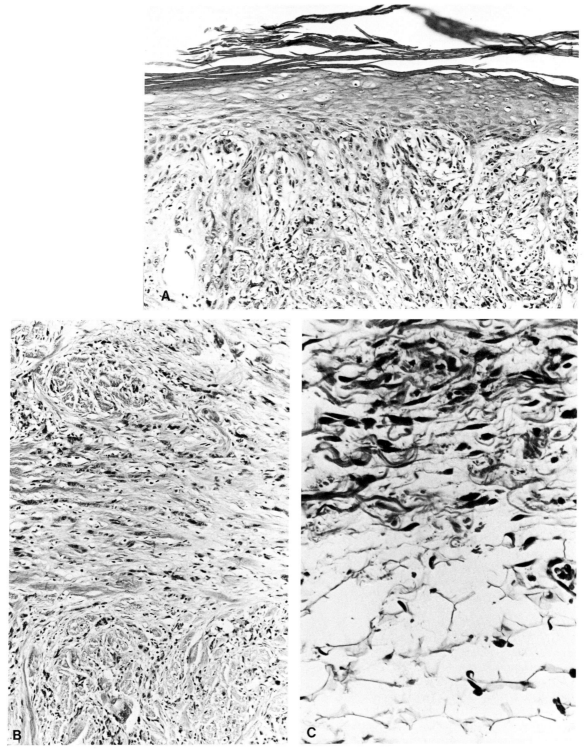

FIG. 3–7 Desmoplastic melanoma. (*A*) Proliferating melanoma cells are becoming mixed with spindle fibroblastic cells. Edema obscures the junctional origin of the melanoma. (*B*) Melanoma cells and spindle cells in a dense fibrotic stroma. It is difficult to identify the melanoma cells. (*C*) The tumor extends into the subcutaneous fat, where isolated melanoma cells are scattered deeply among the fat cells.

less; medium: 1.5 cm–19.9 cm; and large [giant]: 20 cm or more). Greeley and co-workers[23] suggested that an area larger than 900 mm² or any major part of an anatomical region (*e.g.*, face or hand) should be the criterion for giant nevi. Giant congenital nevi tend to have a dermatomal distribution; and when they involve the dorsal region, there may be a midline orientation.[52] When the nuchal region and the scalp are involved, there may also be meningeal melanocytosis. Giant nevi often have satellites, and indeed there may be numerous congenital nevi of varying sizes scattered over the body. All congenital nevi can be hairy and large, while medium-sized lesions may have a lumpy pachydermatous surface.

Histologically, congenital nevi are similar to any other intradermal nevi except that the nevus cells tend to be scattered singly throughout the dermis; often extended into the septa of the subcutaneous fat; and may be found in the arrectores pilorum muscles, in the walls of blood vessels, and in cutaneous nerves. Sometimes, there is a desmoplastic stromal reaction in the dermis that is responsible for the pachydermatous appearance. In addition to the intradermal nevus cells, there may be a proliferation of junctional nevus cells. In giant nevi, there may be foci of cellular blue nevus. The lumpiness found in some large congenital nevi is caused by horn cysts with or without a foreign body reaction and occasionally with calcification.

There is a good deal of controversy as to how often melanoma occurs in congenital nevi. From the authors' personal experience, melanoma arising in small or medium congenital nevi is extremely rare. Melanoma arising in a giant nevus is much more common, varying in different reports from 2% to 31%. Kopf and associates estimated that by the age of 80 years, 8% of patients with giant congenital nevi would have developed melanoma.[30] Melanomas in congenital nevi have been found at birth, and most cases occurred before the age of 20 years.[52] When melanoma appears, it is often difficult to locate its origin; and in some cases, it has to be assumed that the melanoma commenced in the blue nevus component.

Kaplan[29] recommended biopsy as the guide to management. When the specimen showed junctional melanocytic proliferation, blue nevus, or what he called "neuronevus," there was an enhanced likelihood that melanoma would supervene. Neuronevus is presumably the lesion described by Masson,[48] which is now usually classified with cellular blue nevi. They occur as isolated lesions, as well as in giant congenital nevi, usually on the buttocks. Kaplan urges that congenital nevi with any of these components be completely removed.

SPONTANEOUS REGRESSION OF MELANOMA

A feature of primary cutaneous melanoma is the phenomenon of spontaneous regression.[37,39,56] This is an inflammatory process in that it is characterized by a dense infiltrate of lymphocytes among the melanoma cells that undergo degeneration and disintegration (Fig. 3-8). Unlike dermatitis, in which chronic inflammation is expressed by a perivascular lymphocytic and histiocytic infiltrate, the infiltrate of the regression process does not have a perivascular orientation, though there may be vessels present. Pigment liberated by the disintegrating melanoma cells is phagocytosed. As new blood vessels appear, the process abates and fibrosis becomes apparent. The regression process may affect the entire melanoma, or it may affect only a part; and it may halt at any time, leaving a focus of melanoma cell dropout and fibrosis (Fig. 3-9). It is possible that partial regression is caused by an immunologic attack on a single clone, there being evidence that melanoma, as well as being frequently multiclonal in its cellular composition, is also multiclonal immunologically.[22]

The histologic features of regression were initially described by Smith and Stehlin[56] from the M. D. Anderson Hospital, where their incidence of complete regression (*i.e.*, metastatic melanoma with no demonstrable primary growth or occult primary melanoma) was 8.3%. In a series from Sydney in 1966, occult primary melanoma comprised 7% of 613 patients.[36]

Partial regression of primary cutaneous melanoma affects men more frequently than women and is more common in thin melanomas. More than 50% of lesions up to 0.7 mm thick recorded at the SMU exhibited foci of regression.[42] This incidence is much higher than the 10% incidence for all melanomas in the Alabama series[5] or that of Gromet and co-workers,[24] who recorded partial regression in 19% of lesions up to 0.75 mm thick. Excluding lesions that had metastasized when first seen, the overall figure for partial regression in melanomas seen at the SMU was 35%.[43] This is higher than that of any other published series and probably results from the particular interest of the pathologist (V. J. McGovern), who records quite small foci.

There are certain clinical problems arising out of regression of melanoma.

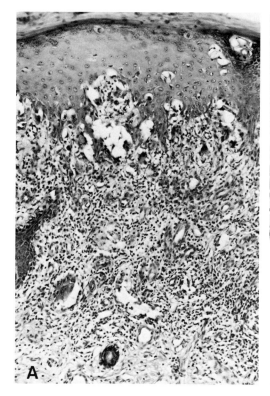

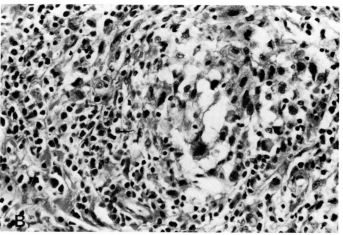

FIG. 3–8 (A) Melanoma infiltrated by lymphocytes with disintegration of the neoplastic cells. (B) Melanoma cells among the lymphocytes that are undergoing destruction.

METASTATIC MELANOMA IN ABSENCE OF A DEMONSTRABLE PRIMARY LESION

The inference from metastatic melanoma when there is no demonstrable primary lesion is that the primary lesion regressed completely after giving rise to a metastasis. If the metastasis is in a lymph node, a thorough search should be made of the drainage area for a small scar, either pigmented or unpigmented. The scar should be excised, as it may still harbor viable melanoma cells. If the metastasis is in an internal organ, the search for a scar must be much more widespread.

PIGMENTED LESION WITH A DEPIGMENTED HALO

Regression in SSM may predominantly affect the noninvasive component, resulting in a lesion that simulates a halo nevus. The cenral nodule, however, should give rise to suspicion that the lesion is, in reality, a melanoma. Furthermore, the regression process may not extend to the limits of the superficial spreading component, and a peripheral ring of pigment may persist around the depigmented halo. This is occasionally encountered in regressing nevi,

but it is rare. A regressed nevus does not usually leave a scar, but a regressed melanoma almost always leaves a scar. Many patients with regressing benign nevi have more than one such lesion.

APPEARANCE OF SATELLITES

The regression process may divide a melanoma with a large superficial spreading component into several discrete islands with one or more nodules in it that simulate satellitosis. Although histologically there may be pigment-containing phagocytes in the regressed areas, these may not be apparent clinically because the scar tissue from past regression may not permit light to penetrate or be reflected from the pigment-containing phagocytes. Therefore, skin between the unregressed islands can appear almost normal to the naked eye.

APPEARANCE OF AN INFLAMMATORY NODULE

A regressing NM may, if pigment is scanty, have the appearance of a simple inflammatory nodule. A melanoma precursor, even before the stage of melanoma *in situ*, can have a fairly dense lymphocytic

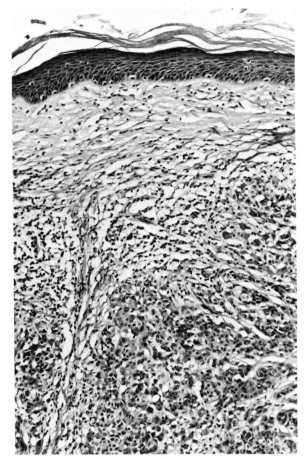

FIG. 3–9   Partially regressed melanoma. In the lower part of the photomicrograph, there are surviving melanoma cells. The junctional connection has been lost, and there is fibrosis of the upper dermis with lymphocytes mixed with the subjacent melanoma cells, which are undergoing dissolution.

infiltrate together with pigment–containing phago-cytes, prominent vessels of the superficial vascular plexus, and fibrosis, thus simulating regression. A careful examination, however, will show that the lymphocytic infiltrate is perivascular, that the fibrosis is laminated around rete ridges, and that the proliferated melanocytes in the junctional region are not degenerating.

Although spontaneous regression usually commences in the peripheral regions, it can affect any part of the tumor. Occasionally, it completely obliterates the junctional component. While the process of regression is active, there should be no difficulty in interpretation, but when it has subsided, the lesion may simulate a metastasis. The correct diagnosis depends on recognizing that the normal collagen

of the papillary dermis has been replaced by horizontally oriented fibrosis.

Cells that have survived the regression phenomenon may proliferate to form a nodule in the dermis that can be mistaken for a metastasis. Again, recognition of the pattern of fibrosis enables the pathologist to arrive at the correct diagnosis.

REGRESSION IN THIN LESIONS

The study of Gromet and associates[24] suggests that patients with thin, partially regressed melanomas have a worse prognosis than patients with thin unregressed lesions. Similarly, the earlier figures for 5-year survival rates for patients in these categories from the SMU also indicated that this may be so.[41] However, when 10-year survival rates were recently calculated, it was found that regression did not influence prognosis in patients with thin lesions (see Chap. 19). Most of the regressed lesions that recurred did so within 5 years, while the majority of unregressed thin lesions that recurred did so after 5 years. Sixteen of 353 patients with lesions up to 0.7 mm thick died from melanoma—10 (5%) with partially regressed lesions and 6 (4%) with unregressed lesions. Partial regression also did not affect the survival rates of patients with thicker lesions.[43]

PROGNOSTIC SIGNIFICANCE OF HISTOLOGIC FEATURES OF MELANOMA

TUMOR THICKNESS

The thickness of a tumor is the single most important indicator of prognosis in patients with SSM and NM but not LMM.[5,6,10,43] For melanomas of other histogenetic types, the significance of thickness has not yet been determined.

The measurement of tumor thickness is objective and reproducible, and any errors in thickness measurement usually result from malorientation of the tissue block or from miscalculation of the ocular micrometer reading. Breslow[10] recommended that measurements be made vertically from the upper level of the granular layer of the epidermis to the deepest part of the tumor (Fig. 3-10). Lateral extensions from hair follicles deep to the main mass of tumor should be ignored except when there is no measurable tumor from the surface. If the lesion is ulcerated, measurement should be made vertically from the surface of the ulcer to the deepest part of the lesion. Measurements should not be made to

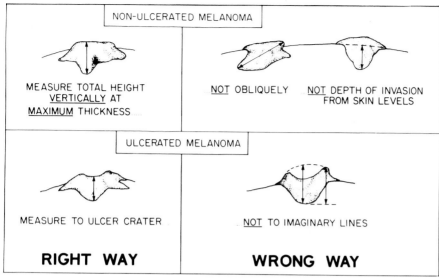

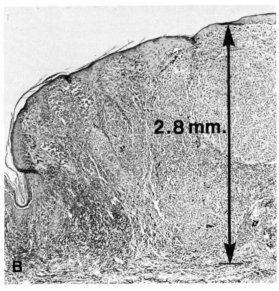

FIG. 3–10 (A) Method of measuring nonulcerated and ulcerated melanomas using the Breslow microstaging criteria. (Balch CM: Pathology, prognostic factors and surgical treatment of cutaneous melanoma. Curr Concepts Oncol 4:8, 1982. Reprinted by permission.) (B) A melanoma 2.8 mm in thickness as measured by the ocular micrometer. (Balch CM, et al: Cutaneous melanoma. In Hardy JM (ed): Textbook of Surgery: Basic Principles and Practice, p 304, Philadelphia. J B Lippincott, 1983)

deep areas of tumor within vessels, or to tentacular extensions or intradermal satellites, which probably represent vascular or lymphatic permeation. Melanomas associated with pseudoepitheliomatous hyperplasia should not be measured, as they will give a false impression of the thickness.

ULCERATION

One would be inclined to regard ulceration as a function of thickness of the lesion. Up to a point this is so, but there is, in addition, an enhancement of the adverse prognosis related to thickness.[8,20,32,47] This is more marked in women with ulcerated lesions, so that their prognosis is very similar to that of men with ulcerated lesions (Fig. 3-11). McGovern and colleagues[47] found a correlation between the rate of growth and ulceration. In every degree of thickness, melanomas with grade 3 mitotic activity were more likely to be ulcerated.

LEVEL OF INVASION

The first attempt at histologic staging of melanomas was that of Mehnert and Heard.[49] The method of Clark and associates[12] was similar, but they added

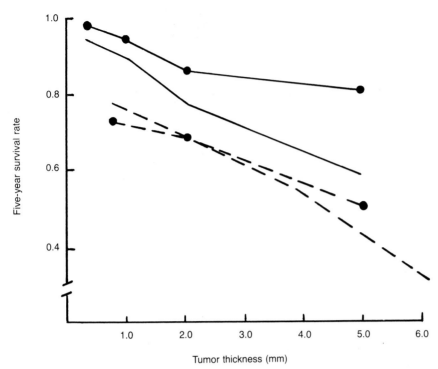

FIG. 3–11 Five-year survival rates according to thickness of primary tumors in 1654 patients with clinical stage I melanoma with or without ulceration. Men with ulceration, (–––––); men without ulceration, (———); women with ulceration, (●–––●); women without ulceration, (●—●)

level III for neoplasms that filled the papillary dermis and depressed the papillary-reticular dermal interface without actually invading the reticular dermis (Fig. 3–12). It was shown that level III melanomas had a prognosis worse than that of level II and almost as poor as that of level IV.

Skin varies in thickness from person to person and according to anatomical site; consequently, the various levels are not comparable at different sites or in different persons. Apart from this, since this is a very subjective feature, pathologists often have difficulty in determining levels. This difficulty can be minimized by using a polarized light through the microscopic slide, by which the birefringent pattern of collagen of the papillary dermis can be readily distinguished from that of the reticular dermis. Although determinations of levels are less discriminating than direct measurements of thickness by the ocular micrometer,[10] it is recommended that they be recorded in addition to measurements of thickness, as they may well be of biological significance. Clark's levels cannot be determined for polypoid lesions and mucosal lesions that do not have microanatomical levels. Furthermore, they cannot be determined in cases where there has been regression followed by fibrosis that obliterates the microanatomical landmarks.

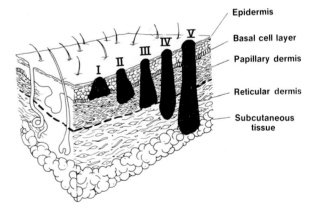

FIG. 3–12 A schematic illustration of the anatomy of the skin demonstrating the locations of different levels of invasion using the Clark microstaging criteria.

GROWTH PATTERN

There is a certain degree of overlap between SSM and NM, so that the Committee of Pathologists that met in 1972[40] recommended that when the adjacent component involved no more than three rete ridges, the lesion should be categorized as NM. Involvement of more than three rete ridges should put the tumor into the category of SSM. The overall survival rate of patients with SSM is better than for patients with NM, but SSMs are, on the average, thinner and have less mitotic activity than NMs, so that for similar degrees of thickness, the survival rates are comparable.[43]

Patients with the less common LMM have a much better survival rate than those with the other growth patterns (see Chap. 19). The incidence of LMM varies from country to country and seems to be the only variety that is solely due to the effects of the sun. While the overall survival is much better for this form of melanoma, no criteria, other than its histogenetic type, have been established for prognosis. McGovern and associates[44] found that clinical stage I women had a a 100% 5-year survival rate, while for men the corresponding figure was 92%. Nevertheless, it has been reported that a few women do die from LMM. No series of LMM patients has been sufficiently large for a significant analysis of prognostic features to be made; furthermore, many series include lesions of the covered parts of the body, which should not be included in this category.

Factors influencing survival rates for acral and other lentiginous types of melanoma have not been determined. These types of melanoma generally have a prognosis much worse than the more common types of melanomas.[4,21,50] The survival rates vary a good deal from clinic to clinic but are under 50% for plantar and palmar lesions. In most clinics, the figures for subungual melanomas are little better.[50] Figures from the SMU, however, suggest that patients with subungual melanomas may have a much better survival rate than patients with melanomas on the palms or soles (83% 5-year survival rate compared to 42%, respectively). The numbers of patients are small, and the data, therefore, are liable to interpretive error. The reason for poor prognosis in melanoma patients with palm and sole lesions seems to be delay in diagnosis.

MITOTIC ACTIVITY

Some published reports ascribe independence in prognostic significance to mitotic activity, while others do not. One of the reasons for lack of unanimity is that microscopes vary a good deal in the area of their high-power fields (hpf); consequently, the 5 hpf recommended by the 1972 committee that met in Sydney[40] would in some cases be more than 1 mm², and in others, less. The members of the recent workshop that met in October 1982 to make recommendations on nomenclature and classification agreed that mitoses should be counted in an area of 1 mm² in that part of the histologic section in which they were most numerous.

In general, thick tumors have more mitoses than thin tumors, and NM have more mitotic activity than SSM.[43] Mitotic activity should be recorded in the pathologist's report to the surgeon, as it may give some idea of the aggressiveness of the tumor.

REGRESSION

While partial regression seems to have no significant effect on survival rates, it is probably important in some individual patients. Consequently, regression should be recorded as either active or inactive. When the fibrosis and residual inflammation associated with a regressed melanoma extend to the reticular zone, it means that the melanoma was probably much thicker before the regression process began. The pathologist should therefore make an estimate as to how thick the melanoma might have been prior to regression. This would be helpful information for the surgeon.

LYMPHOCYTIC REACTION

Lymphocytes are usually present in aggregates of moderate size at the periphery of melanomas and also in smaller discrete aggregates beneath the invading front. As the melanoma invades more and more deeply, the lymphocytic infiltrates beneath the invading front diminish in size, while those at the periphery remain the same.[46] Because the degrees of lymphocytic response at the margins and the invading tumor front frequently vary, they should be recorded separately. Whether the diminishing lymphocytic response is caused by greater invasiveness or whether the deeper invasion is caused by the diminishing lymphocytic response is unknown.

Some pathologists attach little significance to the presence of lymphocytes, whereas others have found that the prognosis is distinctly better when the lymphocytic infiltrate is heavy than when it is sparse. However, there is no unanimity in the method of recording lymphocyte infiltration. Since the degree of lymphocytic infiltrate beneath the invading front is inversely proportional to the thickness of the lesion, it can be assumed that the size of the lymphocytic infiltrate is not an independent variable and not an essential feature of the pathologist's report.[46]

PIGMENT

Tumors that clinically are fairly deeply pigmented may appear under the microscope to have very little pigment. This is because of the fact that very fine pigment may not appear in the form of granules but rather as stainable cytoplasm. While the presence of pigment can assist the pathologist in arriving at the correct diagnosis, it plays no part in assisting the surgeon's decisions concerning management of the patient. This is because the degree of pigmentation seems to be inversely dependent on thickness and has no independent significance in survival.[45]

CELL TYPE

Every pathologist has a different way of recording cell type. A melanoma may consist entirely of one cell type, or it may have one or more clones of other cells. The most common cell types are epithelioid, epithelioid nevuslike, spindle cell, spindle nevuslike, and balloon cells. Epithelioid nevuslike cells are derived from cells resembling ordinary epithelioid cells; therefore, some pathologists record the cell type as mixed. At present, there is no standardized way of recording cell types of melanomas, and many pathologists record the predominant cell type only. Spindle nevuslike cells are uncommon and should, perhaps, be included with epithelioid nevuslike under the general heading "nevuslike."

In Australia, it has been shown that melanomas consisting predominantly of nevuslike epithelioid cells are associated with a better prognosis than melanomas of other cell types.[45] The fact that many melanomas are multiclonal may be of relevance in spontaneous regression, which in the majority of cases is only partial. Different clones may have different antigenic structures. Balloon cells are the result of altered organelles, and though there is no reported series of melanoma in which these cells predominate, the general impression is that balloon cell transformation does not confer any special properties on the tumor. Metastases, too, can be entirely or partially composed of balloon cells.

VASCULAR INVASION

The recognition of vascular invasion is difficult, and very frequently shrinkage of tissues during processing creates clefts in the collagen of the reticular dermis that simulate lymphatic vessels and lymphatic permeation. The presence of melanoma cells in blood vessels or lymphatics does not mean that metastases invariably occur, but when there is incontrovertible evidence of invasion of vessels, the prognosis is usually adversely affected.[32] Unequivocal vascular invasion is uncommon. Little[33] recorded it in 0.7% of cases, Larsen and Grude[32] in 5.8%, while others report up to 37%.[25]

ASSOCIATED NEVI

Junctional or compound nevi of childhood type are not usually associated with melanoma, but dysplastic junctional nevi form the adjacent component in 40% of SSM. In a survey from Sydney,[37] intradermal nevi were associated in routine section with 35% of SSM, 25% of NM, and 4% of LMM. Ackerman and Su,[1] by step-sectioning, found intradermal nevi in 50% of SSM. The presence or absence of an associated nevus does not have any significant effect on survival, but should be reported because nevi may be important in histogenesis.

SOLAR DEGENERATION

The effects of solar radiation are much more readily recognized clinically than histologically. Any melanocytic lesion associated with severe solor elastosis should be suspected of being LMM. Frequently, a flat pigmented lesion is called LMM because it is flat or lentiginous. Melanoma with an adjacent lentiginous component without solar degeneration of the skin occurs on glabrous skin of the palms, soles, and subungual regions. There are other features that differentiate these melanomas from LMM, but the absence of solar effects is the most important.

McGovern and associates[44] showed that it was not solar degeneration *per se* that was responsible for the good prognosis enjoyed by patients with LMM, since those patients with either SSM or NM lesions of the head or neck that displayed solar degeneration had a poorer prognosis than those patients whose lesions were not accompanied by solar degeneration.

THE PATHOLOGIST'S REPORT

The report of the pathologist to the clinician does not need to contain all the histologic information available. The clinician needs to know certain basic facts in order to plan his management of the case and to assess prognosis. Features he wishes to know for other purposes can always be obtained from the pathologist, who should record all histologic features that could possibly lead to a better understanding of the biological nature of melanoma. The following are basic facts of importance to the clinician.

MACROSCOPIC FEATURES

The specimen should be measured and its depth recorded, whether to deep fascia or only to subcutaneous fat. This is of importance for identification purposes. The size of the lesion, its shape, contours, color, and closeness to the margin of resection must be recorded, and a drawing of the specimen or a Polaroid photograph should be made with the sites marked where the blocks of tissue were taken.

HISTOLOGIC FEATURES

The depth of invading tumor must be assessed both by measurement of *tumor thickness* and determination of *microanatomical level*. In addition to the presence or absence of *ulceration,* its extent should be measured if possible. The *growth pattern* must be reported and the number of *mitoses* per mm^2 counted where they are most numerous. The diagnosis of *active regression* can be made by recognizing degenerating melanoma cells in the lymphocytic infiltrate. For the diagnosis of *past regression,* there must be evidence of cell dropout and fibrosis. It is desirable to identify either *lymphatic* or *blood vessel invasion.*

The pathologist may include several other histologic features in addition to those required by the surgeon. In the case of SSM, it is worth recording whether the *adjacent component* is melanoma *in situ* or a remnant of a precursor dysplastic nevus. If more than one *type of cell* is present, the predominant one should be noted. Additional features include the *pigment content* of the lesion, the disposition and relative size of *lymphocytic infiltration,* and the presence of an *associated intradermal nevus* or *solar elastosis.*

HISTOLOGIC DIAGNOSIS OF MELANOMA

METHODS

The clinical diagnosis of melanoma can be quite difficult at times, and lesions suspicious of melanoma can prove to be benign. For this reason, a tissue diagnosis is essential before embarking on extensive surgery. An adequate clinical history must be given to the pathologist, who should, if possible, have examined the lesion prior to surgery. The specimen to establish the diagnosis can be obtained by simple excision or by incisional biopsy (see Chap. 6). There is some controversy about using incisional or punch biopsies. Those in favor of these methods claim to have no problems resulting from them, while those who oppose them point out that the deepest part of the lesion may not be in the specimen. Furthermore, they fear implantations that may not be removed in the subsequent surgery. In very extensive lesions, however, incisional biopsies may be the more appropriate method. Whichever is used, care should be taken to include the full thickness of the skin down to the subcutaneous fat to ensure that the deepest part of the lesion is included in the biopsy. Curette and shave biopsies are contraindicated, even for lesions that are only suspicious. The diagnosis may then be made on frozen section, or the specimen can be processed by the standard method of paraffin section.

Frozen section

Frozen section is the method preferred by some surgeons, but only very experienced pathologists should attempt it. In frozen sections, the distinction between keratinocytes and melanocytes is not always easy, and in about 4% of cases, paraffin sections must be awaited.[34,39] False-positive diagnoses are rare, but when they do occur, the lesions are usually compound nevi or combined nevi, as in the case of a dysplastic junctional nevus combined with a cellular blue nevus, for example. False-negative diagnosis is more common than false-positive diagnosis owing to the difficulty in frozen section of distinguishing between melanocytes and keratinocytes. Very small specimens should not be submitted to frozen section, as the entire lesion may be lost in trimming the block, or there may be an inadequate portion of the lesion remaining for paraffin sections.

Fixation

The best routine fixative is buffered 10% formalin for 18 to 24 hours. The fixation process can be enhanced by using other fixatives instead, such as B-5 or Bouin's fixatives. These fixatives enhance nuclear details and can be used to better demonstrate melanosomes by electron microscopy.

Staining

The hematoxylin and eosin stain is the mainstay in making the histologic diagnosis of melanoma. A high quality of staining is necessary if pigment is to be recognized and mitoses are to be counted. The most useful method of separating atypical fibroxanthoma and malignant fibroxanthoma (malignant histiocytoma) from melanoma is by reticulin staining. These tumors have reticulin patterns of atypical mesenchymal type in which there is reticulin surrounding every individual cell. Reticulin staining may also define the intact basement membrane of the epidermis, though this is not invariable. Reticulin can also separate long-standing intradermal nevi from melanoma, the former having a mesenchymal reticulin pattern and the latter having a carcinoma pattern with reticulin surrounding groups of cells. When no pigment can be seen with hematoxylin and eosin staining, the Fontana-Masson silver stain may reveal pigment or pigment precursors. More often, however, it is not helpful. With the periodic acid Schiff stain, melanocytes often have a weakly positive reaction.

Electron microscopy

Electron microscopy is not usually helpful in the diagnosis of primary melanoma. Its main role is to establish a metastatic lesion of unknown primary site as being of melanocytic origin. This is based on the identification of melanosomes in tumor cells. These are usually rare in a melanotic lesion, but in the SMU experience they can always be found in some of the cells. In melanoma, one can usually find single and packaged melanosomes in the cytoplasm of the cells as well as different stages of differentiation of the melanosomes (Fig. 3-13). These premelanosome stages are usually disorganized and may vary from one cell to another. By themselves, they are not diagnostic for melanoma and cannot be used alone as a diagnostic criterion of malignancy.

THE DIFFICULT DIAGNOSIS
Nonmelanocytic lesions

Atypical fibroxanthomas occur on solar-damaged skin of the elderly. From the pathologist's point of view, this is the most difficult of lesions to distinguish from melanoma. Frequently, the cells of this tumor appear to be coming from the basal layer of the epidermis; as with reticulin stains, the basement membrane may appear disrupted. The diagnostic feature is that every cell is enclosed by argyrophilic fibers.

Malignant fibrous histiocytoma is similar to atypical fibroxanthoma. It occurs in the skin of covered regions as well as exposed areas. However, patients with this type of neoplasm are usually in their fourth or fifth decade. Histologic difficulties in diagnosis are the same as for atypical fibroxanthoma, and the

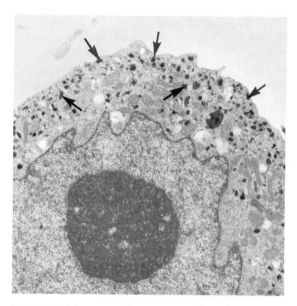

FIG. 3–13 Ultrastructural examination of a melanoma by electron microscopy showing typical melanomosomes in the cytoplasm (*arrows*) that can distinguish melanoma from other malignant tumors. (Balch CM et al: Cutaneous Melanoma. In Hardy JM (ed): Textbook of Surgery: Basic Principles and Practice, p 304. Philadelphia, J B Lippincott, 1983

means of recognition are also by use of reticulin stains. In both types of lesion, electron microscopy should indicate the histiocytic nature of the tumor.

Squamous cell carcinoma can simulate melanoma. By electron microscopy, tonofibrils should be demonstrable, and by polarization fine birefringence should be visible. This may also occur in histiocytic lesions, but the birefringence is coarser.

Pigmented basal cell carcinomas, particularly those of hamartomatous type, may be associated with melanocytes. Phagocytes ingest the pigment and usually aggregate within the lesion. The key to diagnosis when there is no palisade layer is the presence of a fine collagenous stroma surrounding the mass or masses of tumor similar to that surrounding hair follicles. Again, electron microscopy, if available, can be helpful.

Pigmented Bowen's disease may present difficulties to the clinician, but it should be readily diagnosed by the pathologist.

Malignant eccrine acrospiroma is not a very common tumor. If ductule formation or squamous foci are present, this tumor should not be misdiagnosed as amelanotic melanoma. The electron microscope should demonstrate intracytoplasmic ductule formations if none can be found with light microscopy.

Invasion of the epidermis by the cells of *mycosis*

fungoides may simulate SSM. However, recognition of mycosis cells in the dermal infiltrate and their similarity to the epidermotropic cells should enable the correct diagnosis to be made.

Extramammary Paget's disease can occur in carcinoma of apocrine sweat glands or, more rarely, in mucinous carcinoma of the anal canal. The Paget cells have a relatively large cytoplasmic volume, and mucin stains are useful in arriving at the correct diagnosis.

Lichenoid keratosis can be mistaken for a regressing melanocytic lesion, especially as the patient often gives a history of having had a pigmented lesion at the site. Furthermore, these lesions are not always on exposed areas. They are usually single, and histologically have a remarkable resemblance to lichen planus.

Pigmented seborrheic keratosis is commonly biopsied or excised as a possible melanocytic lesion. It very rarely presents problems histologically.

A *Merkel cell tumor* is very rare. Histologically,

it has the appearance of a uniform tumor of small cells often growing from the basal region of the epidermis so that it simulates melanoma. Electron microscopy is helpful; it demonstrates secretory granules.

Benign melanocytic lesions

Pathologists are sometimes perplexed because an otherwise benign lesion has mitoses, bizarre cells, or an unexpected amount of pigment. These are not criteria of malignancy. The lesions that present the greatest perplexity to pathologists, even those of considerable experience, are Spitz nevi, regressing nevi, cellular blue nevi, and nevi within lymph nodes.

The *Spitz nevus* is one of the most common lesions that the pathologist may have difficulty in diagnosing. Seldom, however, does the clinician have any doubt about the benign nature of the lesion (Fig. 3-14*A*). Originally, these lesions were defined

FIG. 3–14 (*A*) Typical Spitz nevus. It is raised and pink with regular, circular periphery. (*B*) Photomicrograph of Spitz nevus (not that in *A*). The cells are a mixture of spindle and epithelioid with a tendency to fasciculation. Lymph-filled vesicles are present in the epidermis, and melanocytes are floating in them.

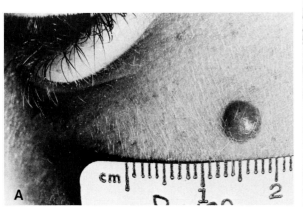

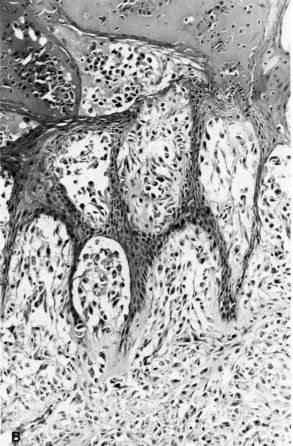

as benign by Sophie Spitz,[57] who called them juvenile melanomas. In a more recent study of Weedon and Little[59] on 211 patients with Spitz nevus in Queensland, 60% of lesions were amelanotic, 30% had moderate pigmentation, and 10% had heavy pigmentation. In children, they are more inclined to be unpigmented and usually have the appearance of a pink, domed lesion about 5 mm in diameter. They may be composed of spindle cells or epithelioid cells, or a mixture of the two. When spindle cells are present, they are usually in fascicles (Fig. 3-14B). There are usually ectasia of superficial vessels and edema, sometimes with vesicle formation.

When the margins of a Spitz nevus end abruptly or are in the form of junctional clusters, the lesion is benign. If there is pagetoid invasion of the epidermis extending peripherally beyond the margin of the tumor, the lesion is a melanoma. Spitz tumors can occur at any age but are most frequently encountered in the first two decades of life. The older the patient, the more carefully the lesion must be examined, as some melanomas simulate Spitz nevi. For a correct diagnosis, the cellular pattern and the margins of the lesion are the most helpful features.[39]

A *regressing nevus,* usually a compound nevus, often has a depigmented halo, which is reassuring to the clinician but not to the pathologist. Regressing nevi frequently have very atypical cells in their junctional components that can be mistaken for melanoma. A regressing nevus, at full activity, has the general pattern, apart from the presence of melanotic cells, of lichen planus (Fig. 3-15). It can be identified by the cluster pattern of the junctional cells and the fact that the intradermal cells, which are

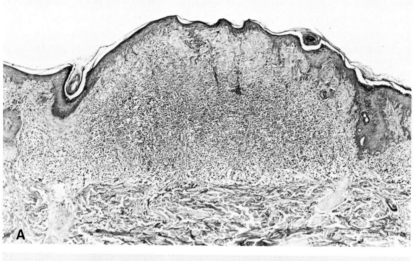

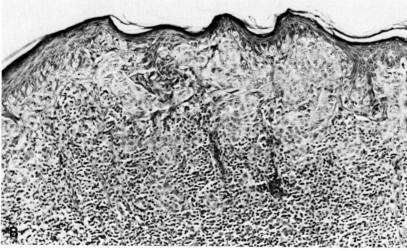

FIG. 3–15 (A) Low-power view to show the resemblance of regressing nevi to lichen planus. The inflammatory infiltrate has a well-demarcated lower border, and the overlying epidermis has lost some of its basophilia. (B) In this case of the resemblance of lichen planus to regressing nevi, the cells of the junctional component are rather pale. They are larger than those of the usual halo nevus. Disintegrating nevus cells can be identified among the lymphocytes.

obviously nevus cells, are also degenerating. When a melanoma associated with an intradermal nevus is regressing, the nevus cells are not involved in the regression. If there are too few surviving cells for recognition of the lesion as a nevus undergoing regression, the patient should be examined for other regressing nevi.

Cellular blue nevi[54] should be assessed as any other spindle cell tumor. Pleomorphism with prominent mitotic activity usually means malignancy. Others with marked cellularity of uniform short spindle cells are benign. The latter sometimes have rounded masses of pale cells with no pigment production that conform to Masson's neuronevus.[48] These may be thought to be malignant because nerves are sometimes involved, although whether these are being invaded or are contributing to the tumor is usually difficult to determine. Occasionally in young patients, cellular blue nevi, usually composed of coarse spindle cells, can metastasize to regional lymph nodes without further spread. In general, malignant blue nevi are rare, and so dissemination from what was diagnosed as a cellular blue nevus in most cases means a misdiagnosis. A partially regressed melanoma in which surviving neoplastic cells have multiplied to form a nodule may be thought to be a cellular blue nevus.

Occasionally, a nevus dating back to childhood *becomes darker* without any alteration in size or irregularity of its shape and is histologically found to be an intradermal nevus with a clone of deeply pigmented cells. This is essentially a benign nevus. More significant, however, is the lesion with an irregular outline often 5 mm or more in diameter in which there is some variegation in color. This lesion commonly has a long-standing intradermal neval component and a more recent junctional component of the dysplastic neval type. The alteration in color is probably a result of the recent development of dysplastic proliferation of junctional melanocytes overlying a pre-existent intradermal nevus. In some cases, it may result from the development of melanoma *in situ* in a dysplastic nevus, while in others it is caused by extension of a preexistent dysplastic nevus. Recent darkening of a nevus is an indication for excision and histologic assessment.

The importance of *lesions of odd clinical appearance* is recognizing those that are benign; this can only be done histologically. Lesions such as a junctional nevus or a dysplastic nevus combined with a blue nevus can be puzzling to both the clinician and the pathologist.

Recurrent nevi can be a problem. If an intradermal nevus has been incompletely excised, it can recur with a junctional component where none previously existed.[31] Compound nevi that have been completely excised, as far as it is possible to determine, can also recur.[39] This can be particularly disturbing when the lesion is a spindle cell (non-Spitz) nevus. However, the pathologist can be confident of the benign nature of recurrences if any atypia is confined to the epidermal region and if the junctional component ends abruptly and does not extend peripherally in a pagetoid fashion. Nevertheless, recurrence after excision of a dysplastic nevus is quite likely to be melanoma.

Miscellaneous difficulties

Melanoma in children before puberty has a mortality rate of about 60%.[39] Fortunately, it is rare, and some use its rarity as a diagnostic criterion. However, melanoma in children is similar to melanoma in adults, and the same diagnostic criteria apply.

Melanomas with no junctional component may present a problem. The differential diagnosis among metastatic melanoma, a partially regressed melanoma, or malignant blue nevus has been described earlier.

Some melanomas differentiate into *nevuslike cells*. When there is an associated intradermal nevus as well, it is often difficult to determine where melanoma ends and where nevus begins. Even when there is no associated intradermal nevus, the diagnosis can be difficult. Long-standing intradermal nevi have a dense reticulin pattern with almost every cell surrounded by reticulin. Melanoma cells, however, have a pattern more like that of a carcinoma in which reticulin surrounds groups of cells. Spitz nevi have a similar pattern to that of melanoma.

Ordinary intradermal *nevus cells* may occasionally be found in *lymph nodes*.[35] When they are found in the lymph nodes of a patient with melanoma who has had an elective dissection of regional lymph nodes, they can be disquieting. However, recognition that the nevus cells are in trabeculae or in the capsule and not in sinuses, should allay any suspicions of metastasis. Similarly, blue nevi with abundant pigment occur in lymph nodes, and this is probably the reason for the cellular nevus, which apparently metastasizes only to the regional lymph nodes and no further—the patient has two blue nevi, one in the skin and the other in a lymph node.

At present, it is impossible to predict which melanomas are going to metastasize; however, reasonable estimates can be made on the basis of statistical probabilities. Most melanomas metastasize to the regional lymph nodes. It has been shown that patients with *micrometastases in lymph nodes* have al-

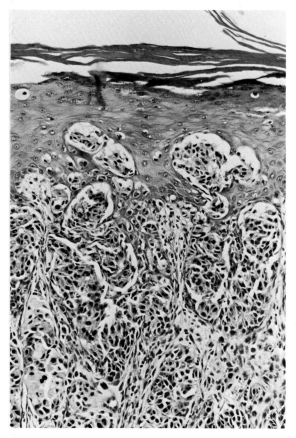

FIG. 3–16 One of many cutaneous metastases in a woman aged 37 years who had a primary growth on the skin of her leg. The melanoma cells have pushed into the epidermis, simulating a primary growth.

most as good a prognosis as clinical stage I patients with no demonstrable involvement of lymph nodes.[7,17] It must be remembered, however, that the absence of metastatic tumor in routine histologic sections does not mean that no metastases exist in the lymph nodes. The pathologist examines only a minute fraction of each block of tissue, since the examination of multiple serial sections is usually not performed. The number of positive lymph nodes correlates directly with mortality (see Chap. 19). The pathologist should therefore block each lymph node in its entirety; or if that is not possible, representative samples of each, so that he can determine how many nodes are involved.

There are two situations in which melanoma *metastasizes to skin*. One is intransit metastases between the site of the original excision and the site of lymph node dissection. The other is in areas so remote from the site of the primary growth that the lesion cannot be the result of direct lymphatic extension. As already mentioned, cutaneous metastases have a tendency to be situated in the upper dermis, where they can simulate new primary growths both clinically and histologically (Fig. 3-16).

Melanoma can metastasize to any organ or tissue, but there are two sites that present clinical problems. In a series from the Royal Prince Alfred Hospital, 25% of all metastatic tumors in patients presenting as primary *intracranial tumors* were melanoma.* Melanoma also has an affinity for the upper *small intestine* (Fig. 3-17), where fungating masses

*Unpublished observation

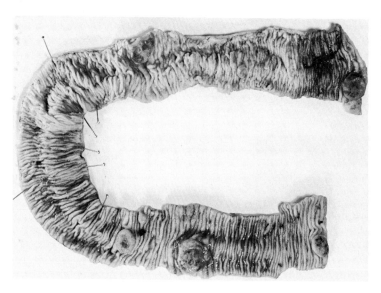

FIG. 3–17 Jejunum of man, aged 37 years, who had had a melanoma removed from his shoulder 7 years previously. He presented with melena. Jejunum has six polypoid metastases.

may cause obstruction. The reason for this predilection is unknown. These tumors may be amelanotic and may resemble large cell lymphoma. Lymphoma of the jejunum occurs in patients with either overt or subclinical adult celiac disease and is usually multiple. In such cases, there is typical villous atrophy of the intestinal mucosa. If electron microscopy is available, melanosomes should be demonstrable in a melanoma metastasis.

Metastatic melanoma with no obvious primary growth is a constantly recurring problem. When the neoplasm is amelanotic, Fontana-Masson stains and electron microscopy should demonstrate its melanocytic origin. The pathologist has to elucidate its nature, so that the clinician can search for the site of the regressed primary growth. If present, it should be excised and examined for surviving melanoma cells.

CONCLUSIONS

For the best results, there must be a good working arrangement between the clinician and the pathologist. The clinician must be familiar with the various histologic features of melanoma and their prognostic significance in order to plan the appropriate management of the case.

REFERENCES

1. Ackerman AB, Su WPD: The histology of cutaneous malignant melanoma. In Kopf AW, Bart RS, Rodriguez-Sains RS, Ackerman AB (eds): Malignant Melanoma, p 25. New York, Masson, 1979
2. Allen AC: A reorientation on the histogenesis and clinical significance of cutaneous nevi and melanomas. Cancer 2:28, 1949
3. Anderson DE: Clinical characteristics of the genetic variety of cutaneous melanoma in man. Cancer 28:721, 1971
4. Arrington JH III, Reed RJ, Ichinose H, Krementz ET: Plantar lentiginous melanoma: A distinctive variant of human cutaneous malignant melanoma. Am J Surg Pathol 1:131, 1977
5. Balch CM, Murad TM, Soong S–j, Ingalls AL, Halpern NB, Maddox WA: A multifactorial analysis of melanoma: Prognostic histopathological features comparing Clark's and Breslow's staging methods. Ann Surg 188:732, 1978
6. Balch CM, Murad TM, Soong S–j, Ingalls AL, Richards PC, Maddox WA: Tumor thickness as a guide to surgical management of clinical stage I melanoma patients. Cancer 43:883, 1979
7. Balch CM, Soong S–j, Murad TM, Ingalls AL, Maddox WA: A multifactorial analysis of melanoma. III. Prognostic factors in melanoma patients with lymph node metastases (stage II). Ann Surg 193:377, 1981
8. Balch CM, Wilkerson JA, Murad TM, Soong S–j, Ingalls, AL, Maddox WA: The prognostic significance of ulceration of cutaneous melanoma. Cancer 45:3012, 1980
9. Becker SW: Dermatological investigations of melanin pigmentation. In Miner RW, Gordon M (eds): The Biology of Melanomas, Vol IV, p 82. Special Publications of the New York Academy of Sciences, 1948
10. Breslow A: Thickness, cross-sectional areas and depth of invasion in the prognosis of cutaneous melanoma. Ann Surg 172:902, 1970
11. Chung AF, Woodruff JM, Lewis JL Jr: Malignant melanoma of the vulva: A report of 44 cases. Obstet Gynecol 45:638, 1975
12. Clark WH Jr: A classification of malignant melanoma in man correlated with histogenesis and biologic behavior. In Montagna W, Hu F (eds): Advances in Biology of the Skin, Vol. 8, The Pigmentary System, p 621. London, Pergamon Press, 1967
13. Clark WH Jr, Ainsworth AM, Bernardino EA, Yang C, Mihm MC Jr, Reed RJ: The developmental biology of primary human malignant melanomas. Semin Oncol 2:83, 1975
14. Clark WH Jr, Mihm MC Jr: Lentigo maligna and lentigo-maligna melanoma. Am J Pathol 55:39, 1969
15. Clark WH Jr, Reimer RR, Greene M, Ainsworth AM, Mastrangelo MJ: Origin of familial malignant melanomas from heritable melanocytic lesions: "The B-K mole syndrome." Arch Dermatol 114:732, 1978
16. Conley J, Lattes R, Orr W: Desmoplastic malignant melanomas (a rare variant of spindle cell melanoma). Cancer 28:914, 1971
17. Day CL Jr, Sober AJ, Lew RA, Mihm MC Jr, Fitzpatrick TB, Kopf AW, Harris MN, Gumport SL, Raker JW, Malt RA, Golomb FM, Cosimi AB, Wood WC, Casson P, Lopransi S, Gorstein F, Postel A: Malignant melanoma patients with positive nodes and relatively good prognoses: Microstaging retains prognostic significance in clinical stage I melanoma patients with metastases to regional nodes. Cancer 47:955, 1981
18. Elder DE, Goldman LI, Goldman SC, Greene MH, Clark WH Jr: Dysplastic nevus syndrome: A phenotypic association of sporadic cutaneous melanoma. Cancer 46:1787, 1980
19. Elder DE, Greene MH, Bondi EE, Clark WH Jr: Acquired melanocytic nevi and melanoma: The dysplastic nevus syndrome. In Ackerman AB (ed): Pathology of Malignant Melanoma, p 185. New York, Masson, 1981
20. Eldh J, Boeryd B, Peterson L: Prognostic factors in cutaneous malignant melanoma in stage I: A clinical, morphological and multivariate analysis. Scand J Plast Reconstr Surg 12:243, 1978

21. Feibleman CE, Stoll H, Maize JC: Melanoma of the palm, sole and nailbed: Clinicopathologic study. Cancer 46:2492, 1980

22. Ferrone S, Natali PG, Cavaliere R, Bigotti A, Nicotra MR, Russo C, Ng AK, Giacomini P: Antigenic heterogeneity of surgically removed primary and autologous metastatic human melanoma lesions. J Immunol 130:1462, 1983

23. Greeley PW, Middleton AG, Curtin JW: Incidence of malignancy in giant pigmented nevi. Plast Reconstr Surg 36:26, 1965

24. Gromet MA, Epstein WL, Blois MS: The regressing thin malignant melanoma: A distinctive lesion with metastatic potential. Cancer 42:2282, 1978

25. Hornstein OP, Weidner F: Untersuchungen zur prognostischen Bedeutung der "Stromareaktion" beim malignen Melanom. I. Vascularisation und Prognose. Virchows Arch [Pathol Anat] 359:67, 1973

26. Hutchinson J: Melanosis often not black: Melanotic whitlow. Br Med J 1:491, 1886

27. Hutchinson J: Senile freckles. Arch Surg 3:319, 1892

28. Jones RE Jr, Cash ME, Ackerman AB: Malignant melanomas mistaken histologically for junctional nevi. In Ackerman AB (ed): Pathology of Malignant Melanoma, p. 93. New York, Masson, 1981

29. Kaplan EN: The risk of malignancy in large congenital nevi. Plast Reconstr Surg 53:421, 1974

30. Kopf AW, Bart RS, Hennessy P: Congenital nevocytic nevi and malignant melanomas. J Am Acad Dermotol 1:123, 1979

31. Kornberg R, Ackerman AB: Pseudomelanoma: Recurrent melanocytic nevus following partial surgical removal. Arch Dermatol 111:1588, 1975

32. Larsen TE, Grude TH: A retrospective histological study of 669 cases of primary cutaneous malignant melanoma in clinical stage I. IV. The relation of cross-sectional profile, level of invasion, ulceration and vascular invasion to tumour type and prognosis. Acta Pathol Microbiol Immune Scand [A] 87:131, 1979

33. Little JH: Histology and prognosis in cutaneous malignant melanoma. In McCarthy WH (ed): Melanoma and Skin Cancer, p 107. Sydney, Blight, 1972

34. Little JH, Davis NC: Frozen section diagnosis of suspected malignant melanoma of the skin. Cancer 34:1163, 1974

35. McCarthy SW, Palmer AA, Bale PM, Hurst E: Naevus cells in lymph nodes. Pathology 6:351, 1974

36. McGovern VJ: Melanoblastoma in Australia. In Della Porta G, Mühlbock O (eds): Structure and Control of the Melanocyte, p 312. Heidelberg, Springer-Verlag, 1966

37. McGovern VJ: Melanoma: Growth patterns, multiplicity and regression. In McCarthy WH (ed): Melanoma and Skin Cancer, p 95. Sydney, Blight, 1972

38. McGovern VJ: Malignant melanoma: Clinical and Histological Diagnosis, p 131. New York, Wiley, 1976

39. McGovern VJ: Melanoma: Histological Diagnosis and Prognosis. New York, Raven Press, 1982

40. McGovern VJ, Mihm MC Jr, Bailly C, Booth JC, Clark WH Jr, Cochran AJ, Hardy EG, Hicks JD, Levene A, Lewis MG, Little JH, Milton GW: The classification of malignant melanoma and its histologic reporting. Cancer 32:1446, 1973

41. McGovern VJ, Shaw HM, Milton GW: Prognosis in patients with thin malignant melanoma: Influence of regression. Histopathology 7:673, 1983

42. McGovern VJ, Shaw HM, Milton GW: Histogenesis of malignant melanoma with an adjacent component of the superficial spreading type. Pathology (in press)

43. McGovern VJ, Shaw HM, Milton GW, Farago GA: Prognostic significance of the histological features of malignant melanoma. Histopathology 3:385, 1979

44. McGovern VJ, Shaw HM, Milton GW, Farago GA: Is malignant melanoma arising in a Hutchinson's melanotic freckle a separate disease entity? Histopathology 4:235, 1980

45. McGovern VJ, Shaw HM, Milton GW, Farago GA: Cell type and pigment content as prognostic indicators in cutaneous malignant melanoma. In Ackerman AB (ed): Pathology of Malignant Melanoma, p 327. New York, Masson, 1981

46. McGovern VJ, Shaw HM, Milton GW, Farago GA: Lymphocytic infiltration and survival in malignant melanoma. In Ackerman AB (ed): Pathology of Malignant Melanoma, p 341. New York, Masson, 1981

47. McGovern VJ, Shaw HM, Milton GW, McCarthy WH: Ulceration and prognosis in cutaneous malignant melanoma. Histopathology 6:399, 1982

48. Masson P: Neuro-nevi "bleu." Arch De Vecchi Anat Patol 14:1, 1950

49. Mehnert JH, Heard JL: Staging of malignant melanomas by depth of invasion: A proposed index to prognosis. Am J Surg 110:168, 1965

50. Patterson RH, Helwig EB: Subungual malignant melanoma: A clinical-pathologic study. Cancer 46:2074, 1980

51. Reed RJ: Acral lentiginous melanoma. In New Concepts in Surgical Pathology of the Skin, p 89. New York, Wiley, 1976

52. Reed WB, Becker SW Sr, Becker SW Jr, Nickel WR: Giant pigmented nevi, melanoma, and leptomeningeal melanocytosis: A clinical and histopathological study. Arch Dermatol 91:100, 1965

53. Reimer RR, Clark WH Jr, Greene MH, Ainsworth AM, Fraumeni JF Jr: Precursor lesions in familial melanoma: A new genetic preneoplastic syndrome. JAMA 239:744, 1978

54. Rodriguez HA, Ackerman LV: Cellular blue nevus: Clinicopathologic study of forty-five cases. Cancer 21:393, 1968

55. Sagebiel RW: Histopathology of borderline and early malignant melanomas. Am J Surg Pathol 3:543, 1979

56. Smith JL Jr, Stehlin JS Jr: Spontaneous regression of primary malignant melanomas with regional metastases. Cancer 18:1399, 1965

57. Spitz S: Melanomas of childhood. Am J Pathol 24:591, 1948

58. Wallace DC, Exton LA, McLeod GRC: Genetic factor in malignant melanoma. Cancer 27:1262, 1971

59. Weedon D, Little JH: Spindle and epithelioid cell nevi in children and adults. A review of 211 cases of the Spitz nevus. Cancer 40:217, 1977

ALFRED S. KETCHAM
CHARLES M. BALCH

Classification and Staging Systems
4

THE NEED FOR STAGING SYSTEMS

Uniform classification and staging of cancer must be recognized as the first basic requirement to ensure the most reliable treatment comparisons. The dilemma in establishing a reproducible and uniformly acceptable melanoma classification and staging system has led to great confusion, particularly as it relates to comparing treatment results. Many institutional and cooperative group trials involving melanoma treatments have failed to demonstrate unanimity in therapy results despite seemingly uniform treatment approaches. A uniform quality control of all treatment modalities involved in any clinical investigation must be maintained to avoid spurious interpretation of results, so as to account for variations on the part of the different surgeons, pathologists, radiotherapists, or medical oncologists involved in delivering patient care. In a recent adjuvant therapy study for melanoma conducted by a major cooperative group, 20% of the patients were judged to have inadequate or inappropriate surgery in a retrospective review.[1] While differences in results among institutions could be explained by both surgeon and patient idiosyncrasies, the basic question of whether identical or similar disease entities are being compared stage for stage is often overlooked. If disease characteristics differ between patients or between studies, valid comparisons cannot be made and the reasons for failing to obtain similar results are more easily explained. Other phenomena such as genetic, physiologic, and immunologic variations between patients are recognized as uncontrolled variables in staging systems at the present time.

A staging system for melanoma must also be comprehensive enough to encompass all manifestations of disease at the time of primary tumor presentation. In addition, one must be able to describe accurately and document in a succinct manner the extent of recurrent or metastatic disease and quantitate the variable responses to treatment.

There are numerous staging systems that are now being used for melanoma, but none has gained worldwide acceptance. It is imperative, therefore, for melanoma investigators to identify clearly the staging system they are using. This chapter reviews the most common staging systems in use today and their limitations, and describes the new staging system for melanoma adopted by the American Joint Committee on Cancer.[2]

CURRENT STAGING SYSTEMS

ORIGINAL THREE-STAGE SYSTEM

The original, and most widely used, system involves three stages (Table 4-1).[6,9] It is simple and easy to recall but, unfortunately, does not include such important disease criteria as tumor thickness, which allow for more accurate staging. A slight modification of this staging system delineates patients with local recurrences, satellites, and intransit metastases (Table 4-2).[5] However, these latter terms have different meanings among clinicians and pathologists. A major limitation of this system is that 85% or more of melanoma patients diagnosed now have clinically localized disease (stage I), as shown in Figure 4-1. This is particularly true for melanomas diagnosed in the 1980s, when the proportion of stage I melanomas is even higher. This disproportionate number of patients in one stage defeats the purpose of a classification system designed to categorize metastatic risk.

M. D. ANDERSON STAGING SYSTEM

Less popular has been a four-stage system used by the M. D. Anderson Hospital.[10] Stage I refers only to the primary or multiple primary tumor situation;

TABLE 4–1
ORIGINAL CLINICOPATHOLOGIC STAGING OF MELANOMA

Stage	Criteria
I	Localized primary melanoma
IA	Localized recurrence (local satellites)
II	Metastases to regional lymph nodes or intransit metastases
III	Disseminated melanoma

TABLE 4–2
MODIFICATION OF ORIGINAL CLINICOPATHOLOGIC STAGING OF MELANOMA

Local
Primary lesion alone
Primary and satellites within a 5-cm radius of the primary
Local recurrence within a 5-cm radius of a resected primary
Metastases located more than 5 cm from the primary site but within the primary lymphatic drainage

Regional nodal disease

Disseminated disease

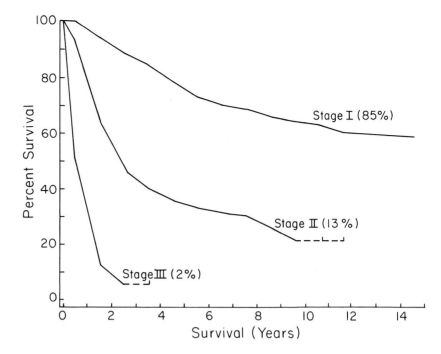

FIG. 4–1 Fifteen-year survival results for over 4000 melanoma patients treated at UAB and SMU, subgrouped by the most commonly used three-stage system. The distribution of patients is shown in parentheses. Note that 85% of the patients were grouped into one stage with clinically localized disease (stage I). In this figure and in Figure 4-2, survival curves are drawn as *solid lines* to the point of longest survival before death from disease; the continued *broken lines* indicate the survival duration of patients remaining alive.

stage II represents local recurrence or local satellite disease; stage III indicates regional metastatic spread with or without intransit, local, regional, or satellite disease; stage IV indicates distant metastatic disease (Table 4-3). This staging system also does not include microstaging criteria, and nearly all patients would be grouped under stage I, while only a minuscule number of patients would fit into stage II.

TABLE 4–3
STAGING FOR MELANOMA–M. D. ANDERSON HOSPITAL

Stage	Criteria
I	Primary melanoma only
	IA: Intact primary melanoma
	IB: Primary melanoma, locally excised
	IC: Multiple primary melanomas
II	Local recurrence of metastases
	(All disease within 3 cm of primary site)
III	Regional metastases
	IIIA: Tissues excluding nodes
	IIIB: Node(s)
	IIIAB: Skin, etc., plus node(s)
IV	Distant metastases
	IVA: Cutaneous metastases only
	IVB: Any visceral metastases

INTERNATIONAL UNION AGAINST CANCER (UICC) STAGING SYSTEM

In 1978, the UICC used two new modalities to stage melanoma more accurately: level of invasion[4] and tumor thickness.[3] Their published staging recommendations[7] are listed in Table 4-4. This staging system used TNM criteria, but most patients were still grouped in stage I (localized disease) and the definition of juxtaregional lymph node spread of intransit metastases (stage III) involved only a few patients.

TABLE 4–4
STAGING FOR MELANOMA—UICC, 1978

Stage	Criteria
IA	Tumor invading the papillary dermis but not invading the reticular dermis (levels II and III) and ≤ 1.50 mm in thickness
IB	Tumor invading the reticular dermis or the subcutaneous tissue (levels IV or V) and ≥ 1.51 mm in thickness
II	Regional lymph node spread
III	Juxtaregional lymph node spread
IV	Distant metastasis

NEW STAGING SYSTEM ADOPTED BY THE AMERICAN JOINT COMMITTEE ON CANCER*

THE NEED FOR A NEW STAGING SYSTEM

Many investigators have developed a staging system that satisfactorily serves their needs. To ask institutions with a long experience in treating melanoma patients to change their staging system is difficult, but mandatory. Separate systems of staging and classification of cancer are often tailored to the particular treatment modalities being used at that institution. For example, some use a staging system that separately defines satellitosis, because their investigators are studying isolated limb perfusion as treatment for this entity. At most institutions, however, this entity comprises a small fraction of their patient population.

A staging system loses its value when almost all the patients are grouped into one stage, as they are in the current three-stage system that is most popular (see Fig. 4-1). Moreover, melanoma is one of the few types of cancer in which only three stages are used for classification. Most other cancers have a four-stage classification in which the first two stages delineate patients mainly on the basis of the primary tumor size, of which breast and head and neck cancers are two examples. Finally, an important reason to have a uniform staging system that is broadly applicable is that different centers throughout the world can better exchange information about diagnosis and treatment results.

The American Joint Committee on Cancer has worked for over 10 years to develop uniform staging systems for all cancer types. In its extensive retrospective studies of melanoma, many factors influencing treatment results were identified. These included age, sex, ulceration, lesion location and size, and the presence of regional satellites or intransit or metastatic disease. Many microscopic characteristics involving cell differentiation, mitotic activity, and vascular invasion have been shown to correlate with survival results. Which characteristics are the most reliable for accurate staging and which are most appropriate to both the practicing clinician as well as

*Members of the Melanoma Subcommittee of the American Joint Committee on Cancer were Drs. Alfred Ketcham (Chairman), Charles M. Balch, William M. Christopherson, Wallace H. Clark, Thomas B. Fitzpatrick, Edward T. Krementz, and Charles McBride.

the investigator studying the biology of this disease are still being examined.

The subsequent material in this chapter is a compilation of years of retrospective and prospective trials involving several thousand patients. A four-stage system is proposed.[2,8] Basically, this system divides patients with clinically localized melanomas into two groups according to microstaging criteria, with the result that the metastatic risk categories are more evenly grouped among four stages (Fig. 4-2). While this proposed staging and classification system may have its weaknesses and fails to identify certain criteria that some investigators claim to be significant, it appears to be usable and interpretable by all. It should serve as a useful and practical classification for all clinicians treating melanoma.

RULES FOR CLASSIFICATION

Clinical–diagnostic staging

The following careful clinical examination is essential: inspection for tumor size, ulceration, and nodularity; inspection of the surrounding skin and subcutaneous tissue for satellites and intransit metastases leading toward the regional lymph node-bearing areas and other suspicious skin lesions; and palpation of the regional nodes. Chest x-ray films and hemograms are required, and blood chemistry profiles are encouraged. Other radiographic and radioisotopic procedures are optional, depending on clinical presentation. A clinical–diagnostic staging classification has not been developed for cutaneous melanoma; however, clinical observations may contribute in a meaningful way to postsurgical resection–pathologic staging.

Postsurgical resection–pathologic staging

Evaluation of the entire primary tumor is always advised, and, rather than just a wedge or punch biopsy, the entire specimen should be examined for accurate classification. Regional nodes should be meticulously evaluated if made available with the specimen and recorded as the number of positive lymph nodes found with the total number of lymph nodes removed (*e.g.,* N1, 3/21).

Retreatment staging

Any recurrence or metastatic lesion should be biopsied for confirmation if possible. An appropriate metastatic workup is advised.

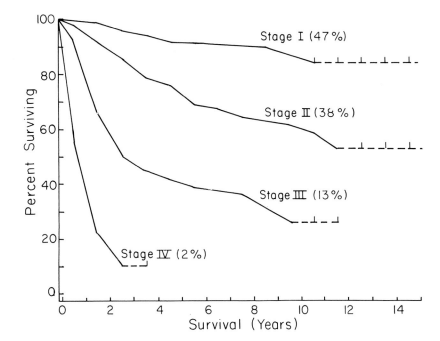

FIG. 4–2 Fifteen-year survival results for the same melanoma patients described in Figure 4-1, but subgrouped according to the new four-stage system proposed by the American Joint Commission on Cancer.[2] The distribution of patients is shown in *parentheses*. Note that the patients with clinically localized melanoma (stage I by the original three-stage system) have now been divided into two stages according to tumor thickness and level of invasion (newly designated stages I and II).

TNM CRITERIA

Primary tumor (T)

Both the level of invasion and the maximum measured thickness determine the T classification and should be recorded. The definitions are listed in Figure 4-3A. While both of these parameters are important prognostic factors, it is well documented that thickness is a relatively more accurate and reproducible criterion than the level of invasion. Therefore, when the level of invasion and the thickness measurement do not match the categories of T classification, the thickness measurement should take precedence in assigning a T status (*i.e.,* a 0.6-mm, level III lesion is T1, a 2-mm, level III lesion is T3).

Satellite lesions or nodules within 2 cm of the primary tumor are included in the T classification, and the primary tumor is automatically considered T4, regardless of the primary tumor level of invasion or thickness. Satellite lesions or subcutaneous nodules at a greater distance from the primary tumor but not beyond the site of primary lymph node drainage are considered intransit metastases and are listed under N categories.

Nodal and distant metastases

These definitions are listed in Figure 4-3A.

Recurrent tumor (r)

The development of local recurrence at the site of the previous surgery calls for specific recognition when staging by using the prefix "r" (rTNM).

New primary tumor

A new or second primary melanoma or the simultaneous presentation of more than one primary melanoma is to be staged with the specific identification of this unusual second primary phenomenon. The detailed pathology interpretation justifying the diagnosis of a second melanoma rather than metastatic disease will determine the staging and specific identification of this clinical circumstance.

STAGE GROUPING OF TNM

The stage grouping proposed by the American Joint Committee on Cancer comprises four stages (Table 4-5). Stages I and II consist of patients with clinically localized disease subdivided into A and B according to the microstaging (thickness and level). Stage III patients have nodal metastases in a single lymph node basin, while stage IV patients have one of the following: (1) distant metastases, (2) nodal metastases involving two or more lymph node basins (*e.g.,* bilateral axillary nodal metastases), (3) ≥5 intransit

(*Text continues on page 62*)

Data Form for Cancer Staging

Patient identification
Name _____
Address _____
Hospital or clinic number _____
Age _____ Sex _____ Race _____

Institutional identification
Hospital or clinic _____
Address _____

Oncology Record

Anatomic site of cancer _____
Chronology of classification*   [ ] Clinical-diagnostic (cTNM)
                                 [ ] Surgical-evaluative (sTNM)
Date of classification _____

Histologic type† _____ Grade (G) _____
[ ] Postsurgical resection–pathologic (pTNM)
[ ] Retreatment (rTNM)   [ ] Autopsy (aTNM)

Definitions: TNM Classification

Primary Tumor (T)

[ ] TX No evidence of primary tumor (unknown primary or primary tumor removed and not histologically examined)

[ ] T0 Atypical melanocytic hyperplasia (Clark Level I); not a malignant lesion

[ ] T1 Invasion of papillary dermis (Level II) or 0.75-mm thickness or less

[ ] T2 Invasion of the papillary–reticular-dermal interface (Level III) or 0.76- to 1.5-mm thickness

[ ] T3 Invasion of the reticular dermis (Level IV) or 1.51- to 4.0-mm thickness

[ ] T4 Invasion of subcutaneous tissue (Level V) or 4.1 mm or more in thickness or satellite(s) within 2 cm of any primary melanoma

Nodal Involvement (N)

[ ] NX Minimum requirements to assess the regional nodes cannot be met.

[ ] N0 No regional lymph node involvement

[ ] N1 Involvement of only one regional lymph node station; node(s) movable and not over 5 cm in diameter or negative regional lymph nodes and the presence of less than five in-transit metastases beyond 2 cm from primary site

[ ] N2 Any one of the following: (1) involvement of more than one regional lymph node station; (2) regional node(s) over 5 cm in diameter or fixed; (3) five or more in-transit metastases or any in-transit metastases beyond 2 cm from primary site with regional lymph node involvement

Distant Metastasis (M)

[ ] MX Minimum requirements to assess the presence of distant metastasis cannot be met.

[ ] M0 No known distant metastasis

[ ] M1 Involvement of skin or subcutaneous tissue beyond the site of primary lymph node drainage
        Specify _____

[ ] M2 Visceral metastasis (spread to any distant site other than skin or subcutaneous tissues)
        Specify _____

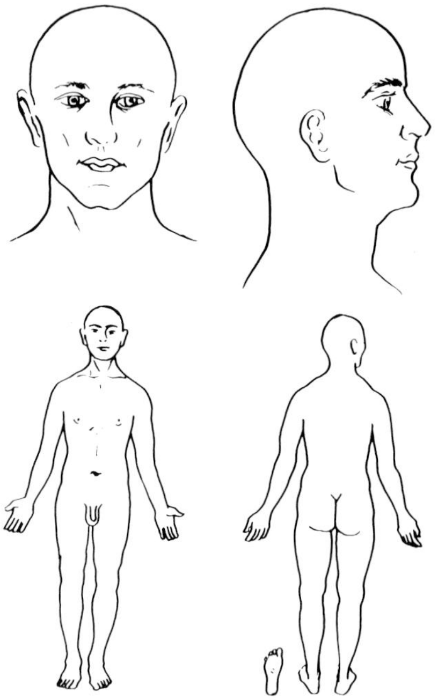

Type of Lesion

[ ] Lentigo maligna   [ ] Radial spreading
[ ] Nodular   [ ] Acral lentiginous
                             [ ] Unclassified

Fig. 4-3A

Indicate on diagrams primary tumor and regional nodes involved.

Depth of Invasion
[ ] Level I (not a melanoma and further characterization is not necessary)
[ ] Level II   [ ] Level IV
[ ] Level III   [ ] Level V
Other description _____
Maximal thickness (mm) _____
Site of primary lesion (check diagram)

_____

Extent of primary lesion (include all pigmentation)

_____

Size in greatest diameter _____ . cm

Characteristics

[ ] Ulceration
[ ] Other _____

Examination by _____ M.D.
Date _____

Stage Grouping

[ ] Stage IA   T1, N0, M0
[ ] Stage IB   T2, N0, M0
[ ] Stage IIA   T3, N0, M0
[ ] Stage IIB   T4, N0, M0
[ ] Stage III   Any T, N1, M0
[ ] Stage IV   Any T, N2, M0
                 Any T, any N, M1 or M2

Staging Procedures

A variety of procedures and special studies may be employed in the process of staging a given tumor. Both the clinical usefulness and cost efficiency must be considered. The following suggestions are made for staging of malignant melanoma:

Essential for staging

1. Complete physical examination
2. Pathologic study of surgically removed material, including depth of invasion and thickness of primary tumor
3. Chest roentgenogram
4. Known residual tumor at primary site if present

May be useful for staging or patient management

1. Multichemistry screen
2. Gallium scan
3. Bone scan
4. Liver–spleen scan
5. CT scans
6. Brain scans
7. Performance status (Karnofsky or ECOG)

Primary Tumor (T)

Both the depth of invasion and the maximum measured thickness determine the T-classification and should be recorded. When the depth of invasion and the thickness do not match the categories of T-classification, whichever of the two is greatest should take precedence.

Regional Nodes (N)

The regional nodes are related to the region of the body in which the tumor is located; such first station nodes are as follows:

1. For head and face: preauricular, cervical
2. For neck and upper chest wall: cervical (anterior–posterior), supraclavicular, axillary
3. For chest wall, anterior and posterior, and arms above elbow: axillary
4. For hands and upper extremities below the elbow: epitrochlear or axillary
5. For the abdominal wall, anterior and posterior, and lower extremities above the knee: femoral inguinal nodes (groin)
6. For the feet and below the knees: popliteal or femoral inguinal nodes (groin)

Histopathology

Types of malignant melanoma: lentigo maligna (Hutchinson's) with adjacent intraepidermal component of radial spreading type (superficial spreading), without adjacent intraepidermal component (nodular), and unclassified.

Both the depth of invasion (Clark) and the thickness of the tumor (Breslow) have been shown to have prognostic significance and both parameters should be reported by the pathologist.

Five levels of the skin have been designated for identification of depth of invasion:

[ ] Level I (epidermis to epidermal–dermal interface). Lesions involving only the epidermis have been designated level I. These lesions are considered to be "atypical melanocytic hyperplasia" and are not included in the staging of malignant melanoma, *for they do not represent a malignant lesion.*
[ ] Level II (papillary dermis). Invasion of the papillary dermis does not reach the papillary–reticular dermal interface.
[ ] Level III (papillary–reticular dermis interface). Invasion involves the full thickness of, fills, and expands the papillary dermis; it abuts upon but does not penetrate the reticular dermis.
[ ] Level IV (reticular dermis). Invasion occurs into the reticular dermis but not into the subcutaneous tissue.
[ ] Level V (subcutaneous tissue). Invasion moves through the reticular dermis into the subcutaneous tissue.

Histologic Grade

[ ] G1   Well differentiated
[ ] G2   Moderately well differentiated
[ ] G3–G4   Poorly to very poorly differentiated

Postsurgical Resection–Pathologic Residual Tumor (R)

Does not enter into staging but may be a factor in deciding further treatment

[ ] R0   No residual tumor
[ ] R1   Microscopic residual tumor
[ ] R2   Macroscopic residual tumor
         Specify _____

Performance Status of Host (H)

Several systems for recording a patient's activity and symptoms are in use and are more or less equivalent as follows:

AJCC	Performance	ECOG Scale	Karnofsky Scale (%)
[ ] H0	Normal activity	0	90–100
[ ] H1	Symptomatic but ambulatory; cares for self	1	70–80
[ ] H2	Ambulatory more than 50% of time; occasionally needs assistance	2	50–60
[ ] H3	Ambulatory 50% or less of time; nursing care needed	3	30–40
[ ] H4	Bedridden; may need hospitalization	4	10–20

Fig. 4-3B

FIG. 4–3 (*A, B*) Standardized forms published by the American Joint Committee on Cancer showing groupings into four stages and definitions for classification. (Beahrs OH, Myers MH: Manual for Staging of Cancer, p 117. American Joint Committee on Cancer. Philadelphia, JB Lippincott, 1983)

**TABLE 4–5
STAGING FOR MELANOMA—AMERICAN JOINT
COMMITTEE ON CANCER**

Stage	Criteria
IA	Localized melanoma ≤0.75 mm or level II* (T1, N0, M0).
IB	Localized melanoma 0.76 mm to 1.5 mm or level III* (T2, N0, M0).
IIA	Localized melanoma 1.5 mm to 4 mm or level IV* (T3, N0, M0).
IIB	Localized melanoma >4 mm or level V* (T4, N0, M0).
III	Limited nodal metastases involving only one regional lymph node basin, or <5 intransit metastases but without nodal metastases (any T, N1, M0).
IV	Advanced regional metastases (any T, N2, M0) or any patient with distant metastases (any T, any N, M1 or M2).

*When the thickness and level of invasion criteria do not coincide within a T classification, thickness should take precedence.

metastases, or (4) nodal metastases over 5 cm in diameter or fixed. The prognosis for these latter patients with advanced regional disease is considered to be the same as those patients with distant metastases.

RESULTS OF STAGE GROUPING

The four-stage system described above delineates distinct prognostic groups of patients that are more evenly divided than any previous staging system. Survival curves and distribution of 4000 patients into the four stages are shown in Figure 4-2 for the combined Sydney Melanoma Unit and University of Alabama in Birmingham series.

OTHER CRITERIA

The operational definitions for the staging and classification of melanoma recommended by the American Joint Committee on Cancer are shown in Figure 4-3B.

DATA COLLECTION FORMS FOR CANCER STAGING

Data staging forms are used to document accurately the information needed for cancer staging (see Fig. 4-3A and B). It is recommended that these forms be available wherever patients might be evaluated, whether in the doctor's office, the hospital emergency room, hospital admitting room, or the hospital bed area. Because of the relative infrequency with which melanoma patients may be admitted to most hospitals, it is mandatory that the data forms include definitions and descriptions of

TNM classification and staging procedures. The inclusion of such material allows for immediate referral and provides more accurate completion of the data form checklist.

SUMMARY

In spite of certain understandable reservations related to host–tumor variables, the sponsoring organizations of the American Joint Committee on Cancer have all agreed to recommend the material that has served to complete this chapter. Through the cooperation of the American Cancer Society, National Cancer Institute, College of American Pathologists, the American College of Physicians, American College of Radiologists, and the American College of Surgeons, a manual for staging and its recommended data collection and checkoff forms are available from the offices of the American College of Surgeons, 55 East Erie Street, Chicago, Illinois 60611.

REFERENCES

1. Balch CM, Durant JR, Bartolucci AA, and The Southeastern Cancer Study Group: The impact of surgical quality control in multi-institutional group trials involving adjuvant cancer treatments. Ann Surg 198:164, 1983
2. Beahrs OH, Myers MH: Manual for Staging of Cancer, p 117, American Joint Committee on Cancer. Philadelphia, JB Lippincott, 1983
3. Breslow A: Thickness, cross-sectional areas and depth of invasion in the prognosis of cutaneous melanoma. Ann Surg 172:902, 1970
4. Clark WH Jr, Ainsworth AM, Bernardino EA, Yang CH, Mihm MC Jr, Reed RJ: The developmental biology of primary human malignant melanomas. Semin Oncol 2:83, 1975
5. DeVita VT Jr, Hellman S, Rosenberg SA: Cancer: Principles and Practice of Oncology, p 1138. Philadelphia, JB Lippincott, 1982
6. Goldsmith HS: Melanoma: An overview. CA—A Cancer Journal for Clinicians 29:194, 1979
7. International Union Against Cancer: TNM Classification of Malignant Melanoma, 2nd ed. Geneva, Switzerland, International Union Against Cancer, 1978
8. Ketcham AS, Christopherson WO: A staging system for malignant melanoma. World J Surg 3:271, 1979
9. McNeer G, DasGupta T: Prognosis in malignant melanoma. Surgery 56:512, 1964
10. Smith JL: Histopathology and biologic behavior of melanoma. In Neoplasms of the Skin and Malignant Melanomas, p 293. Chicago, Year Book Medical Publishers, 1976

ARTHUR W. BODDIE, JR.
CHARLES M. MCBRIDE

Melanoma in Childhood and Adolescence

5

Though most authorities now agree that true childhood and adolescent melanomas do not differ in metastatic potential from their adult counterparts,[6,29,32] separate consideration of melanomas arising in these age groups is justified by continued difficulty in distinguishing them from the Spitz nevus. In addition, they have some distinctive clinical features, such as the tendency to arise in giant hairy nevi and in the leptomeninges or to develop in association with other conditions such as xeroderma pigmentosum or familial melanoma.[2,6,15]

INCIDENCE

Childhood melanoma is defined as melanoma occurring in prepubescent children with the upper age limit at 12 to 14 years of age.[3,14,32] The rare cases of maternal melanoma metastatic to the newborn are also included by many investigators.[14,29,32] Adolescent and young adult melanomas include those developing from puberty through 20 years of age.[3]

Prior to 1953, there were approximately 102 cases of childhood melanoma reported in the medical literature.[16] When the Spitz nevus was defined in 1948 as an entity that may closely mimic the histopathologic appearance of childhood melanoma, a reevaluation and reclassification of many of these

earlier cases was made,[17,25,28,30] and the number of verified cases in 1966 was estimated at only 45.[16] Subsequent publication of two large series has expanded this total considerably.[3,25] Allen and Spitz[1] and Myhre[19] estimated the incidence as between 0.3% and 0.4% of tumor registry cases.

With the onset of adolescence, the reported frequency of melanoma increases sharply (Fig. 5-1).[3,25] This increase roughly parallels the time course of development of benign nevi that peaks at 15 years of age in boys and at 20 to 29 years of age in women.[20]

RISK FACTORS

Despite the rarity of these lesions in the general population, certain groups of patients appear to be at higher risk for development of melanomas at an early age. These include patients born to mothers with melanomas,[14,29] so-called "congenital" melanomas,[14,29] patients having giant hairy nevi,[3,10,14,29] and those with xeroderma pigmentosum.[3] Patients from a family with a history of melanoma are reported to have a higher risk of developing melanoma during adolescence.[2,33] Since the above high-risk groups account for 16% to 40% of reported cases of prepubertal melanoma,[3,6,14,16,25] special attention will be given to their clinical features.

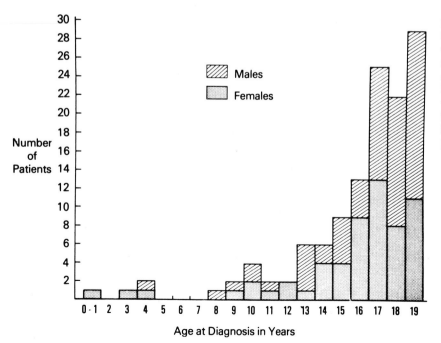

FIG. 5–1 Age incidence of malignant melanomas in children and young adults shows sharp increase in numbers around puberty. (Boddie AW Jr, Smith JL Jr, McBride CM: Malignant melanoma in children and young adults: Effect of diagnostic criteria on staging and end results. South Med J 71:1074, 1978. Reprinted by permission.)

CONGENITAL MELANOMA

Melanoma is capable of metastasizing to the placenta in gravid women with the disease,[31] and rare but well-documented instances of transplacental metastases have been reported.[14,29,32] In most reported instances, the mothers have had widespread dissemination of melanoma[14,29,32] at the time of delivery. In instances where infants have developed clinical metastases, presumably a state of immunologic tolerance has been induced, and the majority have died within days to months of delivery.[14,29,32] Placental metastases without subsequent development of melanoma in the child have also been reported.[31] This may suggest that metastases have occurred at a later stage of gestation after the fetus has developed immunocompetence. At least one unsuccessful attempt has been made to transfer immunity passively from child to mother by exchange transfusion.[31]

GIANT HAIRY NEVI

Congenital pigmented nevi are present in approximately 2.5% of neonates.[22] Giant pigmented nevi are a subtype of congenital nevi and constitute about one tenth of the total cases seen in specialty centers.[18] Giant pigmented nevi have been defined by Greeley as "lesions that cover an area greater than 144 square inches . . . or smaller lesions that involve an entire orbit or the major portion of the face and hand."[9] For those giant pigmented nevi that are "of large size relative to the patient," some authors have used the term *garment* nevi, and, depending on actual location, even more picturesque terms have been applied: *bathing trunk nevus, shoulder stole nevus, coat sleeve nevus,* or *stocking nevus.*[18,34]

Despite differences in size, giant hairy nevi share many histologic features with smaller congenital nevi, and both are histologically distinct from acquired nevi. The histologic features of these lesions have been well characterized by Mark and colleagues[18] and include: (1) nevus cells present in the lower two thirds of the reticular dermis in almost all cases, and into the subcutaneous layers in more than half of cases; (2) nevus cells disposed between collagen bundles singly or in Indian files; (3) nevus cells commonly involving appendages, nerves, and vessels in the lower two thirds of the reticular dermis or subcutaneous tissue.

A variety of cell types may be found in the giant hairy nevus, including the nevus cell, Schwann-type cells, dermal melanocytes, and spindle and epithelioid cells similar to those seen in benign juvenile melanoma (Spitz nevus).[34] In the large series of giant hairy nevi reported by Reed and co-workers, 40 of 55 lesions (73%) were "nevocytic," while the remaining 15 were "neuroidial."[27]

The incidence of malignancy developing in giant pigmented nevi has varied from 2% to 42% in reported series.[10] An example is shown in Figure 5-2. In the collected review of 360 patients, the overall incidence of melanoma was 14%.[10] Conversely, in series of well-documented childhood melanomas, 16% to 40% have been estimated to arise in congenital or giant hairy cell nevi.[3,6,14,16,25]

The risk of developing melanoma in these large lesions has been related to the number of melanocytes contained within them, as well as to increased potential for malignant degeneration of the cells they contain. In this regard, it is notable that some authors regard any congenital nevus, regardless of

FIG. 5–2 Cutaneous melanoma arising in a giant hairy nevus in a young girl.

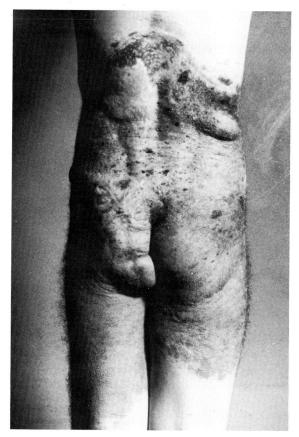

size, as at increased risk for malignant degeneration.[10,24] The risk of developing a malignancy in a giant hairy nevus is greatest during childhood, where 60% of related tumors develop, but extends also into adolescence (10%) and into adult life (30%).[10] Since a benign giant hairy nevus may contain a variety of cell types, several histologic types of tumors may develop in these lesions, including melanomas, neurogenic tumors, and malignant blue nevi.[10]

Because of the significant risk of malignancy associated with giant hairy nevi, prophylactic excision, in stages if necessary for larger lesions, has been recommended. A policy of observing these lesions and treating them expectantly may not suffice, since many patients who go on to develop melanoma will die of metastases. For example, 5 of 7 patients with melanomas arising from a giant hairy nevus died of metastases in the Stanford series.[10]

XERODERMA PIGMENTOSUM

Xeroderma pigmentosum is a chronic progressive disease inherited as an autosomal recessive trait[15] that is often regarded as a skin disorder. However, Lynch has emphasized that it is really a multisystem disease with associated ocular, central nervous system (CNS), hematologic, and endocrinologic aspects.[15] Tumor development in this disorder is felt to be the result of actinic damage, superimposed on deficiencies in repair of DNA.[7] These patients are prone to development of a variety of skin tumors: basal cell cancers, squamous cell cancers, and melanomas.[15] Melanomas develop in 3% of these patients, a rate that is roughly 1000 times that of the general population. They are sometimes multiple.[3,15] In the M. D. Anderson series of adolescent melanomas, 2 of 110 arose in patients with xeroderma pigmentosum.[3]

FAMILIAL MELANOMA

Genetic factors do not appear to play a strong role in the development of melanoma, since overall only 3% to 6% of melanoma patients give a history of other family members with the disease.[15] Patients from melanoma families who develop melanoma do, however, tend to do so at an earlier age.[2] In a study of 106 familial and 2128 nonfamilial cases at the M. D. Anderson Hospital (Fig. 5-3), there is a much sharper rise in the percentage of familial patients developing the disease between 10 and 20

years of age than in nonfamilial cases.[2] In a series of 110 adolescent melanomas reported from the M. D. Anderson Hospital, two arose in patients with a family history of melanoma.[3]

CHILDHOOD AND ADOLESCENT MELANOMA

PROBLEM OF THE SPITZ NEVUS

In the cases of childhood and adolescent melanoma that are not associated with some predisposing condition, the difficulty of diagnosing and treating the disease is greatly complicated by its histologic resemblance to the much more commonly occurring Spitz nevus. The difficulty of distinguishing benign moles and melanomas in young patients was reported as early as 1910 by Darier and Civatte.[8] The distinction was best defined by Spitz's description in 1948 of the "juvenile melanoma"[30] as a benign lesion with certain histologic similarities to melanoma. Other pathologists have criticized the ambiguity of using the term *juvenile melanoma,* with its connotation of malignancy, for a benign lesion. A variety of other names has since been applied, with the designations *Spitz tumor* or *spindle and epithelioid cell nevus* currently favored by most authors.[23] In a large series of 211 cases, the clinical features of these lesions were characterized as typically small (2 mm–17 mm in diameter), variously flat to hemispherical, and infrequently ulcerated.[35] The majority of these lesions are single, but diffuse as well as regionally grouped cases have been reported.[4,5,13] Spitz nevi are typically reddish rather than black,[26] but neither color nor other morphologic features reliably distinguish these lesions from melanomas.[26]

Spitz believed that the "presence of giant cells" was the principal histologic feature distinguishing these tumors from true melanomas, but added that giant cells were found in only about "one half" of cases.[30] Subsequent authors have attempted to delineate further the differences between Spitz nevi and true melanomas leading to a rapid proliferation of diagnostic criteria. The historical aspects of the criteria used by various authorities have been well documented in a review by Paniago-Pereira and co-workers.[23] Further pathologic descriptions are found in Chapter 3.

The proliferation of criteria is itself testimony to the continued difficulty in consistently distinguishing these lesions. Okun,[21] for example, has recently reported three cases that had respectively

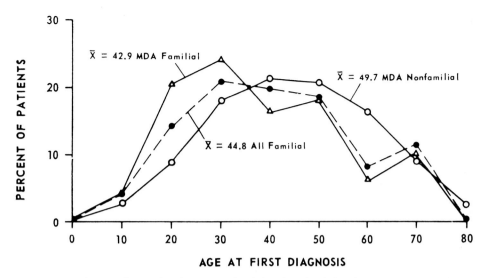

FIG. 5–3 Distribution of age at first diagnosis in familial and nonfamilial melanoma patients. (Anderson DE: Clinical characteristics of the genetic variety of cutaneous melanoma in man. Cancer 28:721, 1971)

"eight . . . five . . . and six . . ." criteria that were considered important in confirming the diagnosis of spindle-epithelioid nevus by Paniago-Pereira.[23] Subsequent clinical behavior confirmed that all three of these lesions were true melanomas. Cytologic features (cellular atypia, pleomorphism, frequency of mitosis, and degree of organization) figure prominently in the distinction, although a clear separation may not be possible in all cases.[3,11,23,25,26,30] The most balanced view would appear to be that, while pathologic distinction between these lesions is possible in a significant percentage of cases, there are also a fair number of cases that still fall into a diagnostic gray zone.[12,21,23,30]

"TRUE" CHILDHOOD MELANOMAS

In most reported series, 16% to 40% of true childhood melanomas develop in association with some unusual predisposing condition such as giant hairy nevi or leptomeningeal melanomas.[3,6,14,16,25] Patients with predisposing skin lesions exhibit symptomatology similar to that seen with adult melanomas: morphologic or color changes (usually occurring over a period of a few months), bleeding, ulceration, crusting, and, less frequently, itching.[3,6,11,14,16,25,26] Patients with primary CNS melanomas developing in conjunction with leptomeningeal melanosis present with a variety of neurologic symptoms, depending on the actual site of the tumor.[10] The remaining childhood melanomas develop in proximity to some small, previously innocuous skin lesion, which may or may not have been labeled a nevus.[25] In the M. D. Anderson series[13] of 15 childhood melanomas, only one was asymptomatic. Of the remaining 14, size change was the main symptom in seven; bleeding, in three; color change and subcutaneous mass, in two each.[3] In this series, 41% of the patients with prepubertal melanomas were boys and 59% were girls.[3] Forty-one percent of the lesions arose in limbs, 35% in the head and neck, and 23% on the trunk.[3]

When a melanoma occurred in an adolescent patient, the association with preexisting conditions was less strong. Probably less than 3% to 4% have definite predisposing conditions such as xeroderma pigmentosum or familial melanoma.[3,25] Presenting signs and symptoms of the 110 adolescent patients with melanomas seen at the M. D. Anderson Hospital and Tumor Institute are listed in Table 5-1. Changes in size and color or bleeding were most common.[3] Only six lesions were asymptomatic. Fifty-four percent arose in boys and 46% in girls. Truncal primaries accounted for 38% of lesions, followed by limb (30%), head and neck (24%), and undetermined site (7%).[3]

In contrast to the situation in adults, there is an impression by some that tumor thickness has less prognostic significance for melanomas in this age group.[3,14] However, to some degree this may still be due to difficulty in distinguishing childhood melanomas from Spitz nevi, which may also invade deep

TABLE 5–1
PRESENTING SIGNS AND SYMPTOMS OF ADOLESCENT MELANOMAS TREATED AT THE M. D. ANDERSON HOSPITAL AND TUMOR INSTITUTE

Sign or Symptom	Frequency*
Change in size	55%
Bleeding	35%
Change in color	23%
Itching in the mole	15%
No symptoms	7%
Enlarged nodes	7%
Subcutaneous metastases	6%
Pain in the mole	4%
Distant metastases	2%
Scab formation	1%
Drainage	1%

*86 of 110 patients had recorded information.

structures such as the dermis, subcutaneous tissue, nerves, and hair follicles.[18,23,35]

TREATMENT

The treatment of melanomas, even in adult patients, remains controversial, and there are presently ongoing discussions regarding what constitutes adequate wide excision for superficial primary melanomas, which patients (if any) should have elective node dissection, the role of perfusion in invasive extremity melanomas, and the roles of adjuvant immunotherapy and chemotherapy. When the diagnostic uncertainty that underlies stage I childhood and adolescent melanomas is added to these controversies, the result has been that therapy is often begun relatively late in the course of the disease and is often inconsistent. In general, the treatment recommendations are the same as those for adults (see Chapters 6, 7, 8, 13). An appropriate excision of the primary melanoma is essential, the width of the margins being dependent on the location and thickness of the melanoma (Fig. 5-4).

In the collected series of childhood melanomas from Memorial Sloan–Kettering (12 cases), the University of Texas System Cancer Center M. D. Anderson Hospital (15 cases), Mayo Clinic (5 cases), and the Christie Hospital and Holt Radium Institute (11 cases), there were 43 cases of childhood melanoma.[3,14,16,25] In 25 of these 43 cases (58%), delay in diagnosis, inadequate primary therapy, or presentation in advanced stage occurred. Of these 25 patients, 17 have died despite subsequent attempts at salvage, a 5-year mortality rate of 68%. Of the remaining 18 cases, 17 were judged to have been diagnosed early and treated adequately (wide excision ± regional node dissection, regional perfusion, and so

FIG. 5–4 Malignant melanoma of scalp just before primary excision and repair with rotation flap, showing hair growth and surface ulceration. (*B*) Skin graft defect after wide excision of primary melanoma. (Keall J et al: Malignant melanoma in childhood. Br J Plast Surg 34:340, 1981)

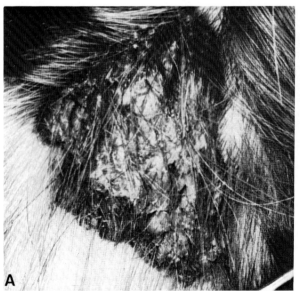
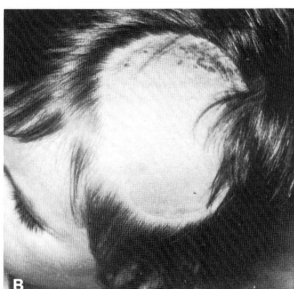

forth). In one case, insufficient information was available to determine the adequacy of treatment or initial stage. Nine of these 17 patients (53%) are alive 5 years from diagnosis.

Since 16% to 40% of childhood and adolescent melanomas arise in association with congenital nevi or xeroderma pigmentosum,[3,6,14,16,25] a high degree of suspicion is warranted when children with these conditions develop symptoms related to pigmented skin lesions. All congenital nevi should be removed prophylactically where feasible; and for giant nevi, staged resection may be necessary.[10] In many children, however, data are based on historical reviews and thus may not allow distinction between true congenital nevi and acquired nevi developing in the first year of life.[10] Since the great majority of melanomas are symptomatic,[3] any such moles should be biopsied and examined pathologically. Because of the low risk of melanoma in the general childhood population,[1,19] prophylactic removal of asymptomatic noncongenital moles is unwarranted.

SUMMARY

True childhood melanomas are rare, but approximately 50% of patients have some predisposing conditions such as congenital nevi (particularly giant hairy nevi) and xeroderma pigmentosum that should raise the index of suspicion. Melanomas occurring in adolescence arise in conjunction with other diseases much less frequently. In the majority of instances, both childhood and adolescent melanomas are symptomatic. Hence, congenital nevi should probably be removed prophylactically, and any symptomatic pigmented lesion in a child or adolescent should be biopsied and examined pathologically. In both childhood and adolescence, there is continued difficulty in distinguishing true melanomas from Spitz nevi. These difficulties may delay treatment or may result in suboptimal therapy that adversely affects the outcome of the disease in a significant percentage of cases. With correct initial diagnosis and treatment, the results of retrospective data analysis show that about 50% can be cured.

REFERENCES

1. Allen AC, Spitz S: Malignant melanoma: A clinicopathological analysis of the criteria for diagnosis and prognosis. Cancer 6:1, 1953
2. Anderson DE: Clinical characteristics of the genetic variety of cutaneous melanoma in man. Cancer 28:721, 1971
3. Boddie AW Jr, Smith JL Jr, McBride CM: Malignant melanoma in children and young adults: Effect of diagnostic criteria on staging and end results. South Med J 71:1074, 1978
4. Burket JM: Multiple benign juvenile melanoma. Arch Dermatol 115:229, 1979
5. Capetanakis J: Juvenile melanoma disseminatum. Br J Dermatol 92:207, 1975
6. Clark WH Jr, Ainsworth AM, Bernardino EA, Yang CH, Mihm MC Jr, Reed RJ: The developmental biology of primary human malignant melanomas. Semin Oncol 2:83, 1975
7. Cleaver JE: Defective repair replication of DNA in xeroderma pigmentosum. Nature 218:652, 1968
8. Darier J, Civatte J: Naevus ou naevo-carcinome chez un nourisson. Bull Soc Trane Dermatol Syph 21:61, 1910
9. Greeley PW, Middleton AG, Curtin JW: Incidence of malignancy in giant pigmented nevi. Plast Reconstr Surg 36:26, 1965
10. Kaplan EN: The risk of malignancy in large congenital nevi. Plast Reconstr Surg 53:421, 1974
11. Keall J, McElwain TJ, Wallace AF: Malignant melanoma in childhood. Br J Plast Surg 34:340, 1981
12. Kernen JA, Ackerman LV: Spindle cell nevi and epithelioid cell nevi (so-called juvenile melanomas) in children and adults: A clinicopathological study of 27 cases. Cancer 13:612, 1960
13. Krakowski A, Tur E, Brenner S: Multiple agminated juvenile melanoma: A case with a sunburn history, and a review. Dermatologica 163:270, 1981
14. Lerman RI, Murray D, O'Hara JM, Booher RJ, Foote FW Jr: Malignant melanoma of childhood: A clinicopathologic study and a report of 12 cases. Cancer 25:436, 1970
15. Lynch HT: Skin, heredity and cancer. Cancer 24:277, 1969
16. McWhorter HE, Woolner LB: Pigmented nevi, juvenile melanomas, and malignant melanomas in children. Cancer 7:564, 1954
17. Malec E, Lagerlof B: Malignant melanoma of the skin in children registered in the Swedish Cancer Registry during 1959–1971. Scand J Plast Reconstr Surg 11:125, 1977
18. Mark GJ, Mihm MC Jr, Liteplo MG, Reed RJ, Clark WH Jr: Congenital melanocytic nevi of the small and garment type. Hum Pathol 4:395, 1973
19. Myhre E: Malignant melanomas in children. Acta Pathol Microbiol Scand (A) 59:184, 1963
20. Nicholls EM: Development and elimination of pigmented moles, and the anatomical distribution of primary malignant melanoma. Cancer 32:191, 1973
21. Okun MR: Melanoma resembling spindle and epithelioid cell nevus: Report of three cases. Arch Dermatol 115:1416, 1979

22. Pack GT, Davis J: The pigmented mole. Postgrad Med 27:370, 1960
23. Paniago-Pereira C, Maize JC, Ackerman AB: Nevus of large spindle and/or epithelioid cells (Spitz's nevus). Arch Dermatol 114:1811, 1978
24. Pers M: Naevus pigmentosus giganticus. Ugeskr Laeger 125:613, 1963
25. Pratt CB, Palmer MK, Thatcher N, Crowther D: Malignant melanoma in children and adolescents. Cancer 47:392, 1981
26. Reed RJ, Ichinose H, Clark WH Jr, Mihm MC Jr: Common and uncommon melanocytic nevi and borderline melanomas. Semin Oncol 2:119, 1975
27. Reed WB, Becker SW Sr, Becker SW Jr, Nickel WR: Giant pigmented nevi, melanoma, and leptomeningeal melanocytosis: A clinical and histopathological study. Arch Dermatol 91:100, 1965
28. Saksela E, Rintala A: Misdiagnosis of prepubertal malignant melanoma: Reclassification of a cancer registry material. Cancer 22:1308, 1968
29. Skov-Jensen T, Hastrup J, Lambrethsen E: Malignant melanoma in children. Cancer 19:620, 1966
30. Spitz S: Melanomas of childhood. Am J Pathol 24:591, 1948
31. Stephenson HE Jr, Terry CW, Lukens JN, Shively JA, Busby WE, Stoeckle HE, Esterly JA: Immunologic factors in human melanoma "metastatic" to products of gestation (with exchange transfusion of infant to mother). Surgery 69:515, 1971
32. Trozak DJ, Rowland WD, Hu F: Metastatic malignant melanoma in prepubertal children. Pediatrics 55:191, 1975
33. Wallace DC, Exton LA, McLeod GRC: Genetic factor in malignant melanoma. Cancer 27:1262, 1971
34. Walton RG: Pigmented nevi. Pediatr Clin North Am 18:897, 1971
35. Weedon D, Little JH: Spindle and epithelioid cell nevi in children and adults: A review of 211 cases of the Spitz nevus. Cancer 40:217, 1977

MARSHALL M. URIST
CHARLES M. BALCH
GERALD W. MILTON

Surgical Management of the Primary Melanoma

6

INDICATIONS AND TECHNIQUES OF BIOPSY

INDICATIONS AND TIMING

Any pigmented lesion with clinical characteristics suspicious of melanoma should be biopsied; such a lesion should not simply be observed to see if it changes further. This policy applies especially to any cutaneous lesion that undergoes a *change* in its size, color, shape, or outline (see Chap. 2 for details). A biopsy is also justified if a patient is concerned about the possibility of malignancy and cannot be reasonably assured that the lesion is benign.

It is preferable to refer the patient with a highly suspicious lesion directly to the surgeon who will be responsible for the definitive treatment. This is particularly true for large lesions (*i.e.*, >1.5 cm), since it offers several advantages to the surgeon, who can then (1) better assess the lesion clinically, (2) minimize the time between the biopsy and the surgery, (3) plan the direction of the biopsy incision with the definitive surgery, and (4) process the entire lesion so as to maximize the diagnostic reliability and microstaging. As an alternative, the physician taking the biopsy should supply a photograph of the lesion to the surgeon. Significant problems in planning treatment arise with an inadequate or poorly oriented specimen. Whoever undertakes the biopsy should ensure that reliable and complete information is obtained.

The biopsy is either excisional or incisional. Whichever technique is used, it must be a full thickness biopsy into the subcutaneous tissue to permit microstaging of the lesion (for thickness and level of invasion). Shave or curette biopsies are absolutely contraindicated for lesions suspected of being melanomas.

There is some debate about the timing of the biopsy in relation to the definitive surgical excision of the primary melanoma (*i.e.*, immediate surgery versus delayed surgery after biopsy). Some experienced surgeons prefer to excise a suspicious lesion, obtain a frozen section biopsy, and then proceed immediately with further surgery if the lesion is malignant.[22,31,37] However, frozen section biopsies should be performed only by pathologists who routinely and frequently use this approach in the diagnosis and microstaging of melanoma. Alternatively, a suspicious lesion is excised and, if it proves malignant, the scar is re-excised as an elective procedure as soon as possible, usually within a week after the biopsy. This two-step approach gives the surgeon more time to plan definitive treatment.[18,21,33] The Sydney Melanoma Unit (SMU) uses either of the above methods, the choice often being determined by the patient's situation. The Surgical Oncology Unit at the University of Alabama in Birmingham (UAB) generally uses the latter two-step approach. Although there is a theoretical risk that manipulation of the tumor at the time of biopsy may increase the risk of local and distant spread, there is, in fact, no convincing evidence that a delay of even 1 to 6 weeks jeopardizes the outcome of the treatment.[15,17,19,22]

EXCISIONAL BIOPSIES

An excisional biopsy is indicated for a suspicious lesion that is not large (*i.e.*, <1.5 cm in diameter) and is situated so that the amount of skin excised is not critical (*e.g.*, on the trunk). The lesion should be excised with an elliptical incision, including a narrow margin (2 mm) of normal-appearing skin. Taking slightly larger margins (*e.g.*, 1 cm) of skin may be insufficient for a malignant lesion and excessive for a benign one (Fig. 6-1).

FIG. 6–1 The width of this biopsy excision on the chest was improper because it removed an excessive amount of skin and extended deep to the pectoralis fascia. The intent was to diagnose and treat the melanoma simultaneously, but the margins of excision were insufficient, and a wider reexcision of the biopsy site than ordinarily would have been necessary was required.

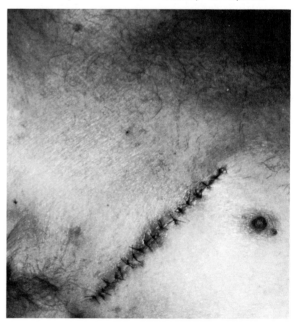

The direction of the biopsy incision is important, since a biopsy that is not oriented properly may necessitate a skin graft when an elliptical incision and primary closure might have been possible. Furthermore, it is important to remove the entire biopsy site (which is potentially contaminated by melanoma cells) completely and orient the incision to remove the surrounding lymphatics. The dermatologist, surgeon, or physician performing the biopsy should therefore orient the biopsy incision so that it can be re-excised with optimal skin margins and yet with minimal skin loss (Fig. 6-2). The excisional biopsy technique is illustrated in Figure 6-3.

INCISIONAL BIOPSIES

Incisional biopsies should be performed when the amount of skin removed is critical (*e.g.*, face, hands, or feet). They may also be indicated for large lesions, when a complete excision itself would be a formidable procedure. An incisional biopsy can be made with a scalpel, but a punch biopsy is preferred at UAB (Fig. 6-4). A 6-mm (or 4-mm) punch biopsy can be used to take a full-thickness core of skin and subcutaneous tissues from the most raised or irregular area of the lesion. It should not be taken at the periphery of the lesion unless there are areas of raised nodularity at this location.

FIG. 6–2   (*A*) The orientation of this biopsy was incorrect. It required an excision with split-thickness skin grafting rather than an elliptical incision and primary skin closure. Skin grafting requires longer hospitalization, costs more, and leads to more morbidity. Furthermore, less of the surrounding lymphatics draining the melanoma site can be incorporated. (*B*) A correct orientation of the biopsy site. The definitive excision parallels the lymphatic drainage and also permits a generous elliptical excision with primary skin closure after the skin edges are mobilized. Note that the incision is oriented slightly toward the medial aspect of the arm, along the lines of lymphatic drainage. In general, the biopsy incision should point toward the first basin of regional lymph node drainage and be oriented so that the entire biopsy site can be reexcised with a minimum of skin loss.

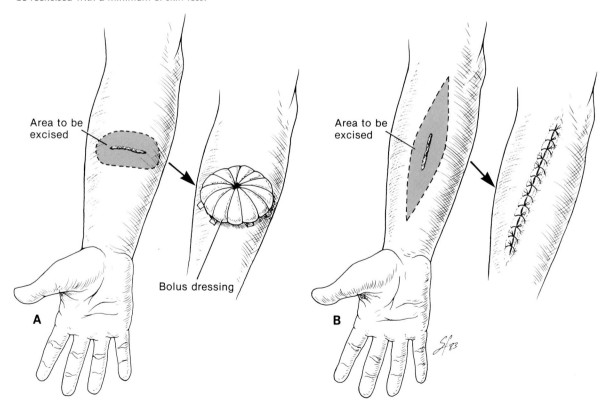

Area to be excised

Bolus dressing

A

Area to be excised

B

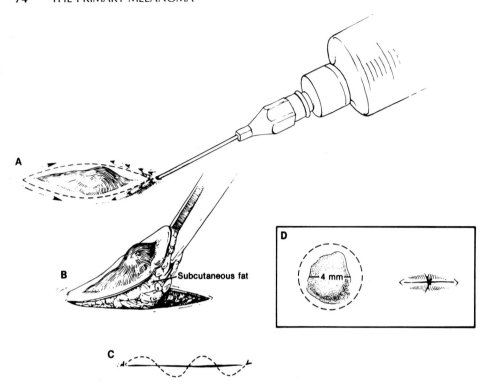

FIG. 6–3 Technique of excisional biopsy for melanoma. (*A*) The suspicious lesion is infiltrated with local anesthetic (bupivacaine hydrochloride [Marcaine] is preferred) elliptically around but not into the lesion itself. (*B*) The entire lesion is excised with a narrow rim (1–2 mm) of normal-appearing skin around it, including the underlying subcutaneous fat. Care is taken to avoid crushing the specimen with forceps. (*C*) The incision is closed after hemostasis is completed. This can be performed with simple interrupted nylon sutures (4–0 or 5–0). At UAB, the preferred technique is to approximate the subcutaneous tissues and then close the skin with an absorbable subcuticular suture such as polydioxanone suture (PDS) or polyglycolic acid (Dexon). (*D*) An alternative approach for small lesions. An excision with a 6-mm punch is an inexpensive and expedient office procedure. The lesion is completely excised with the punch biopsy instrument, and the skin edges are closed with a single 4–0 nylon suture.

EXCISIONAL VERSUS INCISIONAL BIOPSIES

There has been considerable debate about whether incisional biopsies are safe or whether all patients should have a total excision of the lesion to establish the diagnosis of melanoma.[3,14,18,21,42,44,45]

An excisional biopsy has the following advantages over an incisional biopsy: (1) if the lesion proves benign, the excision constitutes treatment; (2) if the diagnosis of malignancy is equivocal, the pathologist can examine the entire lesion; and (3) with an excisional biopsy, there is theoretically less risk of causing a local recurrence or dissemination of the disease. This last point, however, is still under debate.

Some retrospective studies have implied that patients undergoing incisional biopsies had a worse survival rate.[22,42] However, the comparisons of the biopsy methods were probably not valid, since there was, no doubt, selection bias in choosing the biopsy technique (larger or thicker lesions were more likely to have incisional biopsies), and the differences in survival rates could have resulted from imbalances in other prognostic factors that were not controlled or accounted for.

In the UAB experience, incisional biopsies using a 4-mm or 6-mm punch are often used, and no decrease in survival rates or increase in local recurrence rates has been observed using this procedure during the past 5 years. Moreover, an incisional biopsy is a simple, expedient office procedure and, if taken properly, provides representative tissue. Just as important, such an approach is more cost effective than inpatient biopsies, especially those taken

FIG. 6–4 Technique of punch biopsy. (*A*) The suspicious lesion is anesthetized around (but not within) the tumor. A 6-mm (or sometimes a 4-mm) punch biopsy is then placed over the most raised portion of the tumor, and a core of tissue is taken by rotating the punch in a circular fashion. (*B*) The base of the core biopsy is then amputated with a fine-tipped scissors. Care is taken to avoid crushing the specimen. (*C*) Cross-sectional drawing illustrating the proper depth of the biopsy to the underlying subcutaneous tissue so that the histologic diagnosis can be made and microstaging performed. The punch biopsy specimen usually (but not always) provides representative microstaging information when the most raised portion of the lesion is incorporated in the specimen. (*D*) An incisional biopsy should be performed for large lesions or in certain locations where the amount of skin removed is critical (e.g., face, hands, or feet). The biopsy can be obtained with a simple wedge incision using a scalpel or with a punch.

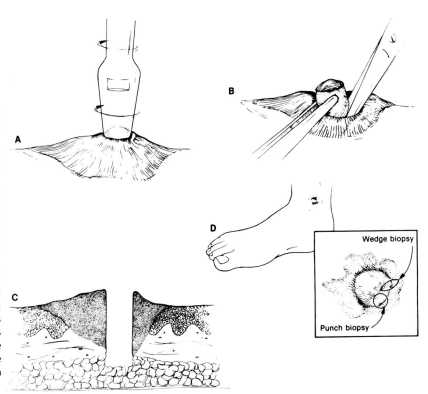

under general anesthesia. Others have similarly found no increased risk with such an approach.[3,25]

BIOPSIES OF SUBUNGUAL LESIONS

Differential diagnoses of subungual pigmented lesions are described in Chapter 2. For any suspicious subungual lesions, surgical removal of the nail and an incisional biopsy is necessary. Punch biopsies of the nail matrix are generally inadequate for diagnosis. A digital block can be performed, and either the entire nail bed or a window can then be excised. If the tumor has broken through the nail bed, a simple incisional biopsy will suffice. Thickness is not known to be a prognostic factor in subungual melanoma, and therefore full-thickness or excisional biopsies are unnecessary.

APPROPRIATE SURGICAL MARGINS FOR EXCISING MELANOMAS

Local control of a primary melanoma consists of a wide excision of the tumor or biopsy site with a margin of normal-appearing skin. Until recently,

the routine surgical approach was to excise all primary melanomas with a 3-cm to 5-cm margin and apply a split-thickness skin graft to the defect. However, it has become increasingly clear that the risk of local recurrence correlates more with the tumor thickness than with the margins of surgical excision.[4,9,13,14,34] It therefore seems more rational to excise melanomas using surgical margins that vary according to tumor thickness, since this factor correlates best with the risk for local recurrence (Tables 6-1 and 6-2).

The earliest lesion is a melanoma *in situ*. This is a noninvasive tumor that does not metastasize but is

TABLE 6–1
RECOMMENDED SKIN MARGINS FOR EXCISING MELANOMAS OF DIFFERENT TYPES

Type	Margins (cm)*
In situ	1
<1 mm	1–2
≥1 mm	3
Lentigo maligna melanomas (all types)	1

*For anatomical sites where these margins cannot be used, the widest practical margin of excision is acceptable.

TABLE 6–2
LOCAL RECURRENCE RATES IN PATIENT SUBGROUPS WITH STAGE I MELANOMA FROM THE UAB AND SMU DATA

Prognostic Category	Total Number of Patients	Calculated Incidence After 5-Year Follow-up
Tumor Thickness		
<0.76 mm	708	0.4±0.2%
0.76 mm–1.49 mm	721	2.1±0.7%
1.5 mm–3.99 mm	907	6.4±1.1%
≥4 mm	291	13.2±3.2%
Ulceration		
Absent	1733	1.9±0.4%
Present	537	11.5±1.9%
Growth Pattern		
Nodular	858	5.6±0.9%
Superficial spreading	1680	2.5±0.4%
Lentigo maligna	95	2.1±1.5%
Major Anatomical Site		
Trunk	1215	1.2±0.4%
Lower extremity	1099	4.7±0.7%
Upper extremity	545	1.6±0.7%
Head and neck	586	4.4±0.9%
Anatomical Subsite		
Foot	107	11.6±4%
Hand	25	11.1±10.5%
Face	251	5.7±1.6%
Scalp	71	5.6±2.7%
Ear	65	5.3±3%
Leg	978	4.7±0.8%
Abdomen	48	4.2±4.1%
Neck	146	1.9±1.4%
Arm	486	1.5±0.6%
Chest	306	1.3±0.6%
Shoulder	170	1.2±0.8%
Back	758	1.1±0.5%

capable of recurring locally.[24] Although the natural history of these noninvasive lesions is not completely understood, there is a risk of local recurrence (either as an *in situ* melanoma or an invasive melanoma) if they are not re-excised after biopsy. It is therefore recommended that the biopsy site of an *in situ* melanoma be excised, usually with a 0.5-cm to 1-cm margin of skin.

For thin melanomas (measuring <0.76 mm in thickness), there is only a minimum risk of a local recurrence in all reported patient series.[3,4,6,9,14,46,48] This is true despite wide variations in margins of excision. In other words, survival is not influenced by the size of the resection margins. This does not mean that re-excision is unnecessary, but that the minimum "safe" margin has not been established in any scientific study. At the present time, a wide

excision consisting of a 1-cm to 2-cm minimum margin of skin is recommended by many melanoma surgeons.[4,6,14,48] This can be performed as a generous elliptical excision and a primary skin closure. In a recent study of 936 patients with melanomas <1 mm thick, there was not a single local recurrence, despite the fact that 61% of patients had conservative margins (≤2 cm) of excision.* For intermediate and thick melanomas (*i.e.,* those >0.76 mm in thickness), a 3-cm margin is usually employed because of an increasing risk of local recurrence and satellitosis (*i.e.,* metastases less than 5 cm from the primary melanoma). This risk may exceed 10% to 20% for those melanomas over 4 mm in thickness.[4,14,46] Since lentigo maligna melanomas have a low risk for recurrence and generally occur on the face, they can be safely excised with a 1-cm margin of excision.

Melanomas located on the hands, feet, and face generally do not lend themselves to a wide surgical excision because of their anatomical location. In these circumstances, the surgeon must use his judgment to excise the lesion as widely as possible within the anatomical constraints of surrounding structures. It is interesting to note that, in our practice, the policy for surgical resection has always been to excise head and neck melanomas with a narrow margin, and only recently has this policy been adopted for trunk melanomas with a thickness <1 mm (Fig. 6–5). Over the years, there has been no increased risk of local recurrences for patients with trunk melanomas despite the use of more conservative margins; those with head and neck melanomas have had about the same incidence of local recurrence despite the conservative excisions required by their anatomical location.

SHOULD THE FASCIA BE EXCISED?

The rationale for incorporating the fascia is to interpose a barrier between the surgical boundary and the melanoma. This is a theoretical consideration and may not be essential for melanomas in many locations unless the lesion is deeply invasive or there is little subcutaneous fat in the perilesional area.

In general, the underlying fascia is incorporated

*Balch CM, Milton GW: Unpublished observations from the Sydney Melanoma Unit data, 1983

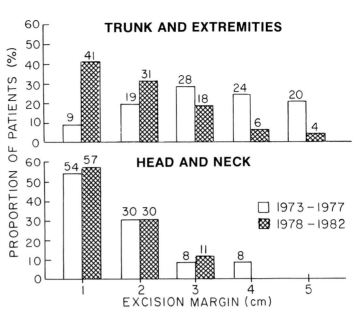

FIG. 6–5 Patterns of surgical treatment for primary melanoma at SMU during two periods. Between 1973 and 1977, the majority of melanomas (72%) arising on the trunk and extremities were excised with a 3- to 5-cm surgical margin. During a more recent period (1978 to 1982), the majority (72%) were excised with more conservative margins of 1 to 2 cm. Melanomas arising in the head and neck area have always been treated with conservative surgical margins because of their anatomical location. The incidence of local recurrences in these two anatomical areas is very similar (after matching for tumor thickness), despite the differences in the surgical treatment for head and neck melanomas dictated by the anatomical location. Moreover, there has been no increase in local recurrence rates from trunk melanomas as more conservative excision margins were adapted.

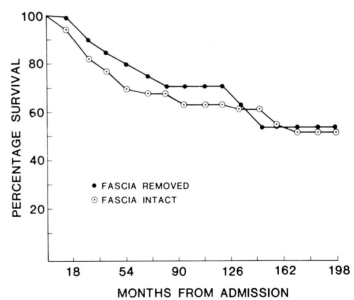

FIG. 6–6 Comparison of fascial removal (107 patients) or fascia left intact (95 patients) for melanoma of the trunk and proximal limbs. All patients underwent wide excision without lymph node dissection at the M.D. Anderson Hospital and Tumor Institute. There was no significant difference in survival between these two groups, nor were there any differences in the incidence of local or regional recurrences. (Kenady DE, Brown BW, McBride CM: Excision of underlying fascia with a primary malignant melanoma. Surgery 92:615, 1982)

into the surgical resection, especially for thicker melanomas (*i.e.*, >1 mm). The evidence documenting the need for a subfascial dissection is sparse, although Olsen[36] has suggested that excision of the deep fascia may actually increase the risk for metastatic disease. A more recent study by Kenady and colleagues[26] showed no difference in patients who had a subfascial excision compared to those who did

not, both in terms of local recurrence and overall survival rates (Fig. 6-6).

The following additional points should be made with regard to fascial excision. First, the deep fascia proper exists only on the limbs and the neck. On the trunk, the broad flat muscles have a layer of perimysium that has fibrous filaments between the larger muscle bundles, and this may be thickened in places to form part of the muscular origin. The lymphatics pass to the draining nodes in the subcutaneous fat *superficial* to the perimysium. Excision of these lymphatics without cutting into them can be accomplished if the perimysium is dissected off the muscles, where possible, as a layer with the subcutaneous fat. Second, there are places on the limb where the deep fascia forms part of a muscle origin (*e.g.*, over the upper part of the tibialis anterior) or part of a muscle insertion (*e.g.*, iliotibial tract for the tensor fascia lata), or blends with the periosteum of a bone (*e.g.*, on the anteromedial aspect of the tibia). In all these situations, an excision of the deep fascia increases the morbidity of the operation, so the fascia is better left intact. The excision should leave a thin layer of areolar tissue to permit a split-thickness skin graft to take successfully. The lymphatics in the limb pass toward the draining nodes *superficial* to the deep fascia, so that excision of the fascia helps to guarantee their ablation. Excision of the fascia, therefore, may make the operation simpler but does not affect the incidence of local recurrence or intransit metastases.

TECHNIQUE OF SURGICAL EXCISION

ELLIPTICAL INCISIONS

A standard elliptical incision is most commonly employed to excise melanomas. With generous skin flaps, even large defects can be mobilized for primary skin closure. The technique is shown in Figure 6-7. To achieve adequate skin for closure, the long axis or length of the incision should be three to four times the width of the incision. After excision of the specimen and mobilization of the flaps, the incision is closed with interrupted subcutaneous sutures, and the skin approximated with either nylon sutures or a subcuticular closure with a suitable absorbable suture, such as PDS or Dexon.

Cassileth and colleagues[10] performed an important psychological study on 176 patients regarding the emotional impact of the scar after primary melanoma excision. Interestingly, the length of the scar did not affect the cosmetic impact, but the degree of surgical indentation or depression had a

FIG. 6–7 Technique of excising a primary melanoma with an elliptical excision and primary skin closure. (*A*) The surgical margin consists of a 3 cm radius of normal-appearing skin surrounding the biopsy site or the lateral margin of the intact melanoma. The long axis of the incision should be three to four times the width of the incision. After the melanoma is excised, skin flaps are raised in a plane above the deep fascia for a sufficient distance to close the skin edges without undue tension. The most extensive area of mobilization is near the center of the flaps, and it often is necessary to mobilize the skin flaps for a distance twice that of the excised skin margin. Skin flaps can be closed primarily in two layers by approximating the subcutaneous tissues and deep dermis in one layer with a second layer to approximate the skin with either a standard suture technique or subcuticular skin closure. It is often necessary to place a suction drain in the surgical wound. (*B*) Cross-section of the excision site. A skin margin of 3 cm from the tumor is shown. Flaps of gradually increasing thickness are raised for an additional 1 cm to 2 cm to remove any surrounding subdermal lymphatics. Excising the fascia is optional.

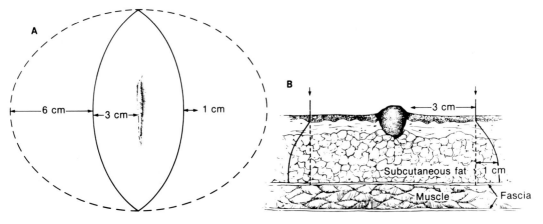

highly negative effect (p < 0.0001). Those patients whose scar was the same size as was expected from preoperative discussions were more accepting of the outcome cosmetically, but over two thirds of the patients indicated that their scars were actually larger than they anticipated. Women were more distressed than men about the outcome, especially for scars located on exposed surfaces of the body. These observations suggested that primary skin closures, rather than skin grafts, have important psychological benefits for patients, and that physicians can assist postoperative emotional adjustments by giving patients accurate information about the expected appearance of their scars.[10] Photographs of other patients with similar scars might be helpful in this regard.

FLAPS

Another means of avoiding a skin graft for covering a defect is to use skin flaps.[1,20] A rotational advancement flap is especially well suited for melanomas involving the face and neck, where the cosmetic result is more important than at other sites (Fig. 6-8).[20] At UAB, this approach is commonly used for closing surgical defects that are not otherwise amenable to primary closure with an elliptical excision. Such a flap provides better padding over bony prominences (*e.g.*, scapula) and a superior cosmetic effect compared to a skin graft (Fig. 6-9).

SKIN GRAFT TECHNIQUES

For larger defects, a split-thickness skin graft may be required, except on the face, where small defects may be covered with a full-thickness graft using skin from behind the ear or the supraclavicular fossa. Donor skin can be taken with a Reese (Padgett) dermatome, a Weck (or Humby) knife, or a Brown dermatome, with dermatome settings usually at 0.14 inches (0.36 mm) (Fig. 6-10). The Reese technique[43] for obtaining donor skin is shown in Figure 6-11.

The skin graft is usually taken from skin over the anterolateral thigh or the lateral shoulder. It is important *not* to take donor skin from a site of po-

FIG. 6–8 Technique of closing a defect with rotational advancement flap. *(A)* A melanoma located over the right scapula is excised with a circumferential margin of skin. The *shaded tip* medial to this area is also excised to shape the flap. *(B)* The flap is mobilized down to its base (take care to avoid its blood supply coming from the axilla) and then rotated into a position in the central part of the defect. *(C)* The skin edges surrounding the defect are mobilized sufficiently to close the wound without undue tension.

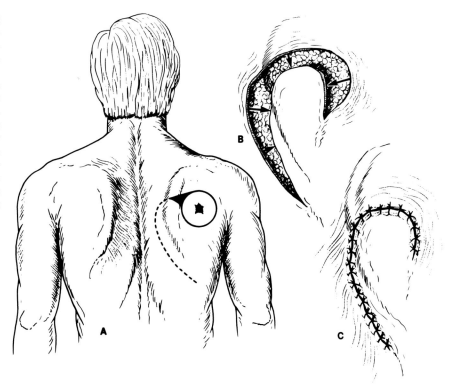

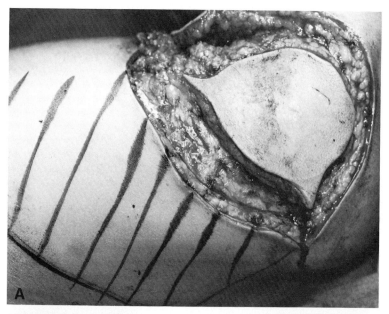

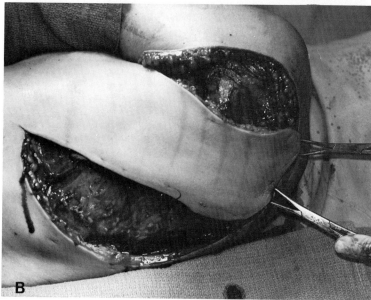

FIG. 6–9 Rotational flap technique for a melanoma located over the scapula. *(A)* The melanoma biopsy site was excised with a 3-cm margin of skin. The skin tips were included with the specimen to fashion the skin flap *(cross-hatched area)* later used to cover the defect. *(B)* The large skin flap was mobilized and moved into a central position over the defect. The skin and subcutaneous tissues over the shoulder and back were then mobilized extensively. *(C)* After skin mobilization, the flap was sewn to the skin edges. In this case, the incision was closed with multiple segments of running absorbable 3–0 suture (PDS) and a 4–0 subcuticular absorbable suture. Suction catheters were placed in the wound *(upper lefthand corner)*. The drainage subsided after a few days. The patient had an uneventful postoperative course and an excellent functional and cosmetic result.

tential intransit metastases, such as the ipsilateral thigh for a melanoma of the foot. The incised skin edges, beveled peripherally as the melanoma is excised, are then sewn to the underlying muscle or fascia using horizontal stent sutures.[35] The donor skin is then placed on the recipient site after absolute hemostasis is obtained.

In some cases, it may be necessary to mesh the graft to increase the amount of tissue it can cover. However, this will result in a less suitable cosmetic appearance. A meshed graft may be preferable for covering a large defect on the back, especially over the scapula, since it is difficult to provide adequate immobility.

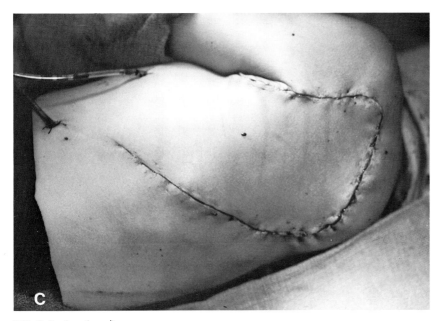

FIG. 6–9   (continued)

FIG. 6–10   Different instruments used for obtaining split-thickness skin grafts. (A) Brown dermatome, (B) Reese dermatome, (C) Humby knife. The Reese (Padgett) dermatome is preferred at UAB, while the Humby knife is preferred at SMU.

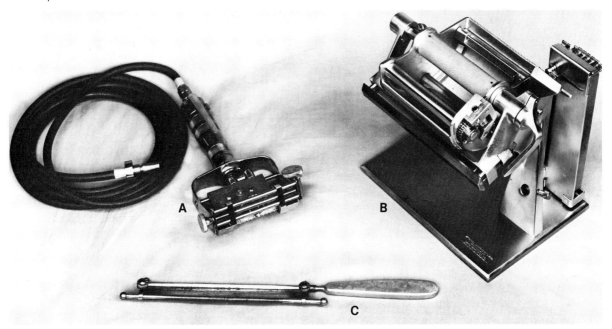

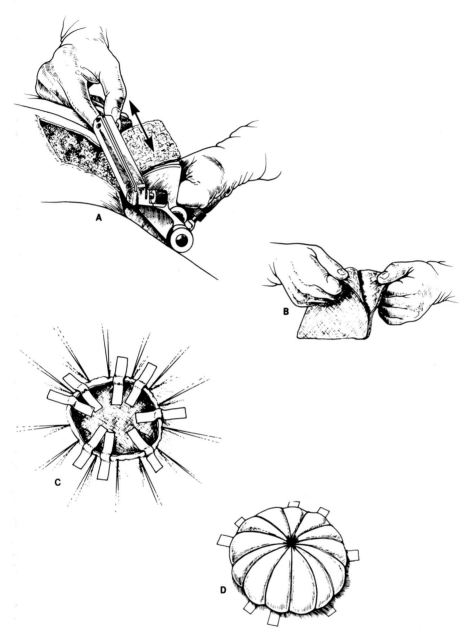

FIG. 6–11 The Reese technique for skin grafting. *(A)* The dermatome is applied to the skin and the blade moved sideways to split the skin (usually with a 0.14-in thickness). It is sometimes helpful for the first assistant to apply two straight hemostats alongside the dermatome as the graft is being taken to avoid taking extra divits of skin. *(B)* The tape is split to separate the two rubber backings. *(C)* The skin graft and the flexible rubber backing is fashioned to the defect and then placed in the defect (skin side down). The edges of the rubber backing are then steristripped to the skin edges. In some cases, it is necessary to partially close the defect with horizontal stent sutures of 3–0 silk. *(D)* A standard stent bolus dressing is then applied to maximize donor skin apposition to the recipient site. For extremity lesions, a posterior mold splint is used to further immobilize the graft site. The Reese technique gives a better texture, color, and cosmetic appearance of the skin graft compared to a freehand-sewn technique. For further details, see reference 43.

Recipient site management

The skin graft is attached to the edges of the recipient site with continuous plain catgut suture, staples, or Steri-strips and covered with a bolus dressing (see Fig. 6-11). The most common cause of graft failure is hemorrhage beneath the graft, which indicates inadequate operative hemostasis. Immobilization of the skin is also of utmost importance. Failure of a major part of the graft to take should be a rare event when the graft can be well supported and the limb temporarily immobilized for several days. A stent dressing using gauze pledgets and acrylon will provide steady downward pressure and help in immobilization (see Fig. 6-11). Grafts on distal extremities should be further immobilized with splints. Bed rest and elevation of the extremity for 24 hours or longer may help decrease edema, maximize immobilization, and increase the chances of a successful take.

The dressings over the recipient site are carefully removed on the fifth postoperative day, although they can be removed earlier if infection or hemorrhage is suspected. For lesions on the back, the dressing may be inspected earlier (*e.g.,* 48 hours postoperatively) to be sure that there is no appreciable hemorrhage beneath the graft. If hemorrhage has occurred, the graft should be removed, the recipient site washed clean of clot, and the graft replaced. The graft should be left exposed to air, during which time the patient may sit up with his back exposed. Dressings are later applied. Using this technique, a considerable number of grafts that might otherwise fail will take satisfactorily.

Stent sutures that have been used to immobilize the skin edges around the recipient site are generally left in place for up to 2 weeks before they are removed. A xeroform and gauze dressing is replaced over the graft and changed daily. The graft can be left open after the seventh to ninth postoperative day.

Donor site management

The donor site is covered with xeroform, scarlet red dressing, or Opsite. Opsite coverage is preferred at UAB, since it markedly decreases the burning sensation associated with other types of dressings. A pressure dressing can be made with crepe bandage supported by an outer layer of Elastoplast. The Opsite or xeroform is left in place for 14 to 21 days, by which time the donor site should be healing well. Fluid collections beneath the Opsite can be aspirated or drained through a small incision. This new method of dressing has facilitated the management of the donor site for the staff and is better for the patient because the donor site is virtually pain-free. When xeroform is used for coverage, the donor site is exposed to air on the first postoperative day, and a heat lamp is used to dry it. Mineral oil may be applied several times a day afterward to minimize crusting. Postoperatively, the patient should avoid getting the xeroform wet for at least 2 weeks. Both the xeroform and the Opsite will come off by themselves when new skin has grown beneath them. Scarlet red dressings can also be used, but they cause staining of clothing and linen.

Antibiotics

When skin grafts are employed, antibiotics are used. At UAB they are started the night before surgery and continued for 5 days. A cephalosporin (*e.g.,* 500 mg tid) is preferred. At the SMU, the patient is given a single intramuscular injection of penicillin (1 g) at the time the preoperative premedication is administered.

SPECIAL SITES

Fingers and toes

A melanoma located on the skin of a distal digit or beneath the fingernail must be removed by a digital amputation. When such a biopsy-confirmed lesion is located on the fingers (especially the thumb), it is important to save as much of the digit as possible to maximize function. This depends on the extensiveness of the lesion (*e.g.,* some have significant nail-bed or paronychial involvement) and the location of its proximal border. In general, an amputation of a digit is performed proximal to the interphalangeal joint of the thumb (Fig. 6-12) and the distal interphalangeal joint for the fingers, as long as the lesions are small and confined to the nail bed. The excision should include a border of normal-appearing skin of at least 1 cm from the edge of the tumor. This approach of partial amputation retains the maximum function of the digit and is especially important for the thumb (Fig. 6-13).

An amputation of the entire finger or thumb (as a ray amputation) is recommended for more extensive lesions, especially those with satellites. Papachristou and Fortner[39] found that the incidence of local recurrence was 22% or greater for conservative amputations, but 0% for amputations at the metacarpal–phalangeal joint. In the UAB experience, there have been no local recurrences in any patients with a more conservative amputation of the digit.

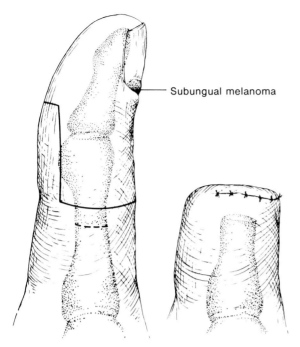

FIG. 6–12 Amputation of the thumb for a subungual melanoma. The skin level of amputation is just beneath the distal interphalangeal joint, with a flap on the volar side to be used as a full-thickness skin covering on the tip. The metacarpal bone is amputated at a level below the skin incision.

FIG. 6–13 Postoperative patient with an amputation of a distal thumb for subungual melanoma. The patient has an excellent functional and cosmetic result.

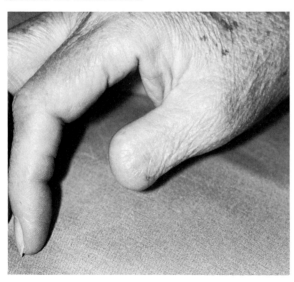

For melanomas located on a toe, an amputation of the entire digit at the metatarsal–phalangeal joint is indicated, and this generally does not cause any significant morbidity. Subungual melanomas, especially those involving the toes, are more frequently associated with local recurrences, intransit metastases, and nodal metastases.[38,39] Elective lymph node dissection is recommended for clinical stage I patients with subungual melanomas. Good results have also been obtained with isolated limb perfusion (see Chap. 10).

Sole of the foot

Melanomas on the plantar surface often involve a sizable defect in a weight-bearing area. If possible, a portion of the heel or ball of the plantar surface should be retained to bear the greatest burden of pressure. Where possible, the deep fascia over the extensor tendons should be preserved as a base for the skin coverage. Generally, these defects are covered with a split-thickness skin graft, and satisfactory results have been obtained at UAB and at the SMU. Woltering and associates[55] reported similar findings. Occasionally, muscle transposition flaps may be used to cover the heel,[5] but this is usually not necessary. Isolated limb perfusion may be of value, especially for large and thick lesions.[28] Amputations of the foot are rarely indicated.

Ear

In an excellent study of 102 patients with melanoma of the external ear, Byers and colleagues[8] recommend less than total amputation of the ear, especially if the patient needs the upper portion of the ear to support spectacles. An ear prosthesis adds to the cosmetic rehabilitation.

For a small suspicious lesion of the helix, the preferred initial procedure for diagnosis is excisional biopsy followed by a wedge re-excision if the diagnosis of melanoma is confirmed (Fig. 6-14). A partial amputation may be necessary for larger lesions. A total amputation of the ear is restricted to patients with widespread local disease or those with recurrence after partial amputation.

In the M. D. Anderson Hospital experience, the local recurrence rate was 8% and the overall incidence of metastatic nodes was 42%.[8] The most common sites of drainage were (1) the periauricular nodes (pre- and retroauricular), (2) the parotid nodes, and (3) the upper neck or jugulodigastric nodes. Their data suggested a benefit of elective lymphadenectomy in selected patients (see also

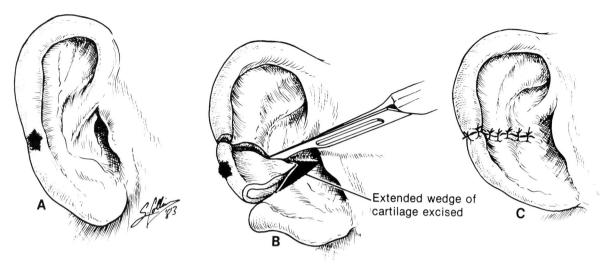

FIG. 6–14   Technique of wedge excision for a melanoma on the outer helix of the ear. It is important to carry the incision down to the inner helix of the ear and to include a wedge of the cartilage to the external auditory canal to mobilize fully the ear for closure.

Chap. 7). This consisted of a modified cervical dissection plus the excision of the periparotid nodes. Storm has also emphasized the importance of excising the parotid nodes for melanomas involving the ear.[51]

Female breast

There is some controversy as to whether melanomas overlying the breast should be treated by a wide excision of the skin and subcutaneous tissue or by a total mastectomy.[2,23,29,47] In the experience at UAB and at the SMU, such lesions could safely be treated as any other cutaneous melanoma, with skin margins determined by the tumor thickness and other criteria as described earlier in this chapter. Others have also had excellent results with this approach.[40,47]

LOCAL RECURRENCES AND THEIR MANAGEMENT

A local recurrence is defined as any tumor that occurs within 5 cm of the scar of a previously excised melanoma.* This definition is important in analyz-

*Lesions that recur after a biopsy *only* are considered as inadequate surgery and not as local recurrences for the purpose of this discussion.

ing the risk factors involved and the influence of the surgical margins of excision for the primary melanoma. Local recurrences should be considered as retained extensions of the primary tumor. They are distinct from satellites and intransit metastases that are intralymphatic in origin and occur between the primary tumor site and the regional lymph nodes. The definitions of these entities are a little arbitrary, especially since they may occur concomitantly. For example, when multiple intransit metastases occur and some are near but not within the scar, these are not defined as a local recurrence but as part of the intransit metastases. The width of the surgical margin around the primary melanoma probably does not influence the risk of intransit metastases, although pathologic properties of the primary melanoma probably do (*e.g.,* a thick, ulcerative melanoma).

RISK FACTORS

In general, the highest risk for local recurrence involves melanomas that have metastasized or those with poor prognostic features. An analysis of local recurrences from the UAB and SMU data (see Table 6-2) demonstrated that stage I patients with the highest risk had melanomas with any of the following features: (1) thickness ≥ 4 mm (13% incidence), (2) ulceration (11.5% incidence), or (3) location on the foot, hand, scalp, or face (5%–12% incidence). Reports from other institutions concluded that patients with the highest risk include those with (1) nodal metastases[30,32,46]; (2) primary melanomas on the sole, scalp, and subungual area[11,39,49]; and (3) thick or ulcerative melanomas.[4,9,14,46,48]

INFLUENCE OF SURGICAL MARGINS

Surprisingly, there are no data to prove that the width of surgical margins has any influence on the risk for local recurrence. That is, it has not been proved that a very wide excision of a melanoma offers some extra measure of protection compared to a narrower excision. These questions are now part of an important and legitimate scientific debate, which several prospective randomized clinical trials are addressing (see below).

The overall risk for local recurrence is extremely low, being 3.2% in collected series involving 3520 patients (Table 6-3). When the data were further subgrouped, the stage I patients who were at risk for developing local recurrences had thicker and more ulcerative melanomas (see Table

6-2). Local recurrences usually develop within 5 years after primary melanoma excision (Fig. 6-15), but sometimes as late as 10 years.[7,34]

Stage I patients with a minimal risk for local recurrence were those with melanomas <1 mm in thickness and *not* located on the scalp, sole, or subungual areas. In collected series of 1515 patients with melanomas ≤1 mm thick, only 2 patients (0.1%) had a documented local recurrence, and both of them had a wide excision of their original melanoma (Table 6-4). Regressing lesions were not included, because their thickness might be underestimated. About 40% of these patients had a relatively narrow margin of excision (<2 cm). This does not imply that the margins of surgical excision are meaningless; indeed, the risk of local recurrence is 60% to 70% of those patients with a biopsy alone or curettage.[11,32] Furthermore, the risk of metastatic disease in this patient group is higher in patients with very narrow excisions.[48] It appears quite clear, however, that the margins for surgical excision for thin melanomas (<1 mm in thickness) in favorable sites can be scaled down to 1 cm to 2 cm without increasing the risk for local recurrence.

TABLE 6–3
LOCAL RECURRENCE RATES FOR PRIMARY MELANOMA

Series	Reference Number	Number of Patients	Local Recurrence Rate
All Sites			
Balch	4	287	3%
Pitt	41	509	6%
Cascinelli	9	593	4%
Kenady	26	202	4%
Elder	14	109	0%
Das Gupta	12	269	3%
Bagley	3	103	6%
Roses	47	658	1%
Veronesi	54	395	2%
		3520	3.2%
Specific Sites			
Ear			
Byers	8	102	8%
Urist	53	66	5%
Subungual			
Papachristou	39	52	22%
Lower leg			
Lewis	30	83	3%
Scalp			
Close	11	125	31%
Urist	53	71	6%
Trunk			
Sugarbaker	52	418	3%

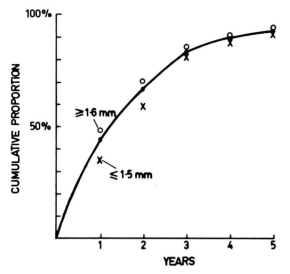

FIG. 6–15 The cumulative proportion of patients who develop a local recurrence (scar or intransit metastases). *Open circles* represent lesions thicker than 1.6 mm, while the *X* represents lesions < 1.5 mm thick. More than 80% of local recurrences occurred within 3 years, and 90% did so within 5 years. The thicker tumors recurred more quickly than the thinner tumors.

MANAGEMENT

Comparative studies of treatment alternatives have not been performed for local recurrences. There are at least three options: (1) surgical excision, (2) isolated limb perfusion with regional chemotherapy and hyperthermia, and (3) irradiation therapy. A single local recurrence, especially in a patient with a previously excised melanoma having favorable prognostic features, can probably be excised with a generous surgical margin and no further treatment. On the other hand, patients with multiple recurrences (either simultaneous or sequential) or who have poor prognostic features of the primary melanoma (*e.g.,* tumors >4 mm in thickness, especially with ulceration) might be considered for isolated limb perfusion, because the risk of additional recurrences and intransit metastases is substantially increased (see Chap. 10). In patients in whom surgical excision is not feasible, such as those in whom lesions have recurred on multiple occasions, irradiation therapy using electrons and a rapid-fraction technique might be considered (see Chap. 15). An amputation (partial or complete) may occasionally be necessary for extensive or deeply infiltrative lesions involving the foot or the hand.

There is a paucity of data about treatment results. Local recurrences imply a poor prognosis and are usually the first sign of metastases, since most patients subsequently develop metastatic disease, both in the UAB and SMU experience and in published reports.[16,46] In the former series, there were 95 patients with a local recurrence (most of whom were referred for treatment of this condition). The median survival was 3 years with a 10-year survival rate of 20% (Fig. 6-16). In two other small series, the outcome was slightly worse, with a median survival ranging from 10 to 26 months after surgical treatment.[16,46] There is some suggestion that isolated limb perfusion is optimal treatment when local recurrence is located on the extremities, since about 25% to 50% of patients treated with regional perfusion are alive 5 to 10 years later.[27,28,49,50]

TABLE 6–4
LOCAL RECURRENCE RATE FOR MELANOMAS <1 MM THICK

Series	Reference Number	Number of Patients	Margins <2 cm	Local Recurrence Rate
All Sites				
Bagley	(3)	33	58%	3%*
Balch	(4)	36	22%	0%
Breslow	(6)	62	56%	0%
Cascinelli	(9)	98	20%	1%*
Elder	(14)	43	37%	0%
Roses	(46)	307	—	0%
Milton	†	936	61%	0%
		1822	42%	0.1%

*>3-cm excision
†Milton GW, Balch CM: Unpublished observations from the Sydney Melanoma Unit data, 1983

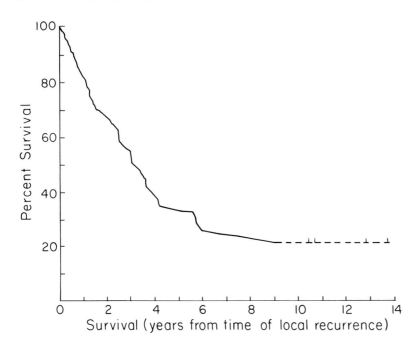

FIG. 6–16 Survival rate for 95 patients treated at UAB or the SMU with a local recurrence as the first site of relapse (calculated from the onset of the local recurrence).

REFERENCES

1. Ariel IM: Tridimensional resection of primary malignant melanoma. Surg Gynecol Obstet 139:601, 1974
2. Ariel IM, Caron AS: Diagnosis and treatment of malignant melanoma arising from the skin of the female breast. Am J Surg 124:384, 1972
3. Bagley FH, Cady B, Lee A, Legg MA: Changes in clinical presentation and management of malignant melanoma. Cancer 47:2126, 1981
4. Balch CM, Murad TM, Soong S-j, Ingalls AL, Richards PC, Maddox WA: Tumor thickness as a guide to surgical management of clinical stage I melanoma patients. Cancer 43:883, 1979
5. Bostwick J III: Reconstruction of the heel pad by muscle transposition and split skin graft. Surg Gynecol Obstet 143:973, 1976
6. Breslow A, Macht SD: Optimal size of resection margin for thin cutaneous melanoma. Surg Gynecol Obstet 145:691, 1977
7. Briele HA, Beattie CW, Ronan SG, Chaudhuri PK, Das Gupta TK: Late recurrence of cutaneous melanoma. Arch Surg 118:800, 1983
8. Byers RM, Smith JL, Russell N, Rosenberg V: Malignant melanoma of the external ear: Review of 102 cases. Am J Surg 140:518, 1980
9. Cascinelli N, van der Esch EP, Breslow A, Morabito A, Bufalino R: Stage I melanoma of the skin: The problem of resection margins. Eur J Cancer 16:1079, 1980
10. Cassileth BR, Lusk EJ, Tenaglia AN: Patients' perceptions of the cosmetic impact of melanoma resection. Plast Reconstr Surg 71:73, 1983
11. Close LG, Goepfert H, Ballantyne AJ, Jesse RH: Malignant melanoma of the scalp. Laryngoscope 89:1189, 1979
12. Das Gupta TK: Results of treatment of 269 patients with primary cutaneous melanoma: A five-year prospective study. Ann Surg 186:201, 1977
13. Day CL Jr, Mihm MC Jr, Sober AJ, Fitzpatrick TB, Malt RA: Narrower margins for clinical stage I malignant melanoma. N Engl J Med 306:479, 1982
14. Elder DE, Guerry D IV, Heiberger RM, LaRossa D, Goldman LI, Clark WH Jr, Thompson CJ, Matozzo I, Van Horn M: Optimal resection margin for cutaneous malignant melanoma. Plast Reconstr Surg 71:66, 1983
15. Eldh J: Excisional biopsy and delayed wide excision versus primary wide excision of malignant melanoma. Scand J Plast Reconstr Surg 13:341, 1979
16. Elias EG, Didolkar MS, Goel IP, Formeister JF, Valenzuela LA, Pickren JL, Moore RH: A clinicopathologic study of prognostic factors in cutaneous malignant melanoma. Surg Gynecol Obstet 144:327, 1977
17. Epstein E: Effect of biopsy on the prognosis of melanoma. J Surg Oncol 3:251, 1971
18. Epstein E, Bragg K: Curability of melanoma: A 25-year retrospective study. Cancer 46:818, 1980
19. Epstein E, Bragg K, Linden G: Biopsy and prognosis of malignant melanoma. JAMA 208:1369, 1969

20. Frokiaer E, Kiil J, Sogaard H: The use of skin flaps in the treatment of malignant melanomas in the head and neck region. Scand J Plast Reconstr Surg 16:157, 1982

21. Harris MH, Gumport SL: Total excisional biopsy for primary malignant melanoma. JAMA 226:354, 1973

22. Ironside P, Pitt TTE, Rank BK: Malignant melanoma: Some aspects of pathology and prognosis. Aust NZ J Surg 47:70, 1977

23. Jochimsen PR, Pearlman NW, Lawton RL, Platz CE: Melanoma of skin of the breast: Therapeutic considerations based on six cases. Surgery 81:583, 1977

24. Jones RE Jr, Cash ME, Ackerman AB: Malignant melanomas mistaken histologically for junctional nevi. In Ackerman AB (ed): Pathology of Malignant Melanoma, p 93. New York, Masson, 1981

25. Jones WM, Williams WJ, Roberts MM, Davies K: Malignant melanoma of the skin: Prognostic value of clinical features and the role of treatment in 111 cases. Br J Cancer 22:437, 1968

26. Kenady DE, Brown BW, McBride CM: Excision of underlying fascia with a primary malignant melanoma: Effect on recurrence and survival rates. Surgery 92:615, 1982

27. Krementz ET, Carter RD, Sutherland CM, Campbell M: The use of regional chemotherapy in the management of malignant melanoma. World J Surg 3:289, 1979

28. Krementz ET, Reed RJ, Coleman WP III, Sutherland CM, Carter RD, Campbell M: Acral lentiginous melanoma: A clinicopathologic entity. Ann Surg 195:632, 1982

29. Lee YN, Sparks FC, Morton DL: Primary melanoma of skin of the breast region. Ann Surg 185:17, 1977

30. Lewis MH, Hill JT, Leopold JG, Hughes LE: Guidelines for management of malignant melanoma of the lower limb—based on a study of long-term behaviour. Clin Oncol 8:341, 1982

31. Little JH, Davis NC: Frozen section diagnosis of suspected malignant melanoma of the skin. Cancer 34:1163, 1974

32. McNeer G, Cantin J: Local failure in the treatment of melanoma. Am J Roentgenol 99:791, 1967

33. Mattsson W, Gynning I, Hogeman K-E, Jacobsson S, Linell F: A retrospective study of 304 cases of malignant melanoma in Malmo 1952–71. Scand J Plast Reconstr Surg 10:189, 1976

34. Milton GW, Shaw HM, Farago GA, McCarthy WH: Tumour thickness and the site and time of first recurrence in cutaneous malignant melanoma (stage I). Br J Surg 67:543, 1980

35. Neifeld JP, Chretien PB: An improved technique of excision and skin grafting for primary malignant melanomas. Surg Gynecol Obstet 142:584, 1976

36. Olsen G: Removal of fascia—cause of more frequent metastases of malignant melanomas of the skin to regional lymph nodes? Cancer 17:1159, 1964

37. Olsen G: The malignant melanoma of the skin. Acta Chir Scand (Suppl) 365:91, 1966

38. Pack GT, Oropeza R: Subungual melanoma. Surg Gynecol Obstet 124:571, 1967

39. Papachristou DN, Fortner JG: Melanoma arising under the nail. J Surg Oncol 21:219, 1982

40. Papachristou DN, Kinne DW, Rosen PP, Ashikari R, Fortner JG: Cutaneous melanoma of the breast. Surgery 85:322, 1979

41. Pitt TTE: Aspects of surgical treatment for malignant melanoma: The place of biopsy and wide excision. Aust NZ J Surg 47:757, 1977

42. Rampen FHJ, Van Houten WA, Hop WCJ: Incisional procedures and prognosis in malignant melanoma. Clin Exp Dermatol 5:313, 1980

43. Reese JD: Dermatape: A new method for the management of split skin grafts. J Plast Reconstn Surg 1:98, 1946

44. Roses DF: Proper biopsy of a lesion suspected of being a malignant melanoma. Am J Dermatopathol 4:475, 1982

45. Roses DF, Ackerman AB, Harris MN, Weinhouse GR, Gumport SL: Assessment of biopsy techniques and histopathologic interpretations of primary cutaneous malignant melanoma. Ann Surg 189:294, 1979

46. Roses DF, Harris MN, Rigel D, Carrey Z, Friedman R, Kopf AW: Local and in-transit metastases following definitive excision for primary cutaneous malignant melanoma. Ann Surg 198:65, 1983

47. Roses DF, Harris MN, Stern JS, Gumport SL: Cutaneous melanoma of the breast. Ann Surg 189:112, 1979

48. Schmoeckel C, Bockelbrink A, Bockelbrink H, Braun-Falco O: Low- and high-risk malignant melanoma. III. Prognostic significance of the resection margin. Eur J Cancer Clin Oncol 19:237, 1983

49. Schraffordt Koops H, Beekhuis H, Oldhoff J, Oosterhuis JW, van der Ploeg E, Vermey A: Local recurrence and survival in patients with (Clark level IV/V and over 1.5 mm. thickness) stage I malignant melanoma of the extremities after regional perfusion. Cancer 48:1952, 1981

50. Shingleton WW, Seigler HF, Stocks LH, Downs RW Jr: Management of recurrent melanoma of the extremity. Cancer 35:574, 1975

51. Storm FK, Eilber FR, Sparks FC, Morton DL: A prospective study of parotid metastases from head and neck cancer. Am J Surg 134:115, 1977

52. Sugarbaker EV, McBride CM: Melanoma of the trunk: The results of surgical excision and anatomic guidelines for predicting nodal metastasis. Surgery 80:22, 1976

53. Urist MM, Balch CM, Soong S-j, Milton GW, Shaw HM, McGovern VJ, Murad TM, McCarthy WH, Maddox WA: Head and neck melanoma in 536 clinical stage I patients: A prognostic factors analysis and results of surgical treatment. Ann Surg, [in press]

54. Veronesi U, Adamus J, Bandiera DC, Brennhovd
IO, Caceres E, Cascinelli N, Claudio F, Ikonopisov
RL, Javorskj VV, Kirov S, Kulakowski A, Lacour J,
Lejeune F, Mechl Z, Morabito A, Rodé I, Sergeev S,
van Slooten E, Szczygiel K, Trapeznikov NN, Wagner RI: Inefficacy of immediate node dissection in
stage I melanoma of the limbs. N Engl J Med 297:627,
1977
55. Woltering EA, Thorpe WP, Reed JK Jr, Rosenberg
SA: Split thickness skin grafting of the plantar surface
of the foot after wide excision of neoplasms of the
skin. Surg Gynecol Obstet 149:229, 1979

Part II
Regional Metastases

CHARLES M. BALCH
MARSHALL M. URIST
WILLIAM A. MADDOX
GERALD W. MILTON
WILLIAM H. McCARTHY

Management of Regional Metastatic Melanoma

7

Regional metastases are the most common presentation of metastatic melanoma. The physician managing melanoma must be vigilant in making the diagnosis and instituting prompt treatment because some patients can be cured. Moreover, effective palliation can be afforded even to those who are not curable.

There are two forms of regional metastases: lymph node metastases and intransit metastases. The usual treatment for clinically detectable metastatic melanoma in regional lymph nodes is surgical excision. This chapter therefore focuses on the important guidelines and technical details of regional lymphadenectomy and the perioperative management. Intransit metastases are usually a vexing problem, since it is often difficult to obtain complete local disease control because of widespread intralymphatic and nodal disease than at first may be clinically apparent. The management of intransit metastases is described in this chapter as well. The controversy regarding elective lymph node dissection for suspected microscopic (or occult) nodal metastases is described in Chapter 8.

DIAGNOSIS OF NODAL METASTASES

A lymph node containing metastatic melanoma has some distinctive characteristics that differ from other causes of lymphadenopathy. Lymph nodes containing metastatic melanoma are generally firmer, more rubbery, and nontender when compared to inflammatory nodes, which are usually softer, more resilient, and tender. Often, there is evidence of infection or injury that would account for benign causes of adenopathy. Nodes invaded by melanoma do not always continue to grow inexorably after they have been diagnosed. They may actually stabilize or shrink during the days or weeks after detection, leading to a false sense of security. Sooner or later, however, nodal enlargement continues. One explanation for this observation is hemorrhage, which may occur in or around a metastasis so that the nodal dimensions fluctuate as the hematoma is absorbed. It should be emphasized that some normal regional nodes are palpable in thin people (especially if the patient has had a previous biopsy), while others may appear as "shotty" nodes that have persisted for months or years.

Any adenopathy suspected of harboring metastatic disease should be investigated. If the index of suspicion for metastatic disease is low, the node may be followed by frequent examination until a diagnosis can be made. In some instances, either fine needle or open biopsy is warranted if the examination is equivocal or close follow-up is not possible. Patient assistance is extremely helpful in the assessment of size changes. If the index of suspicion for metastases by clinical examination is high, especially if the adenopathy is within the draining area of a primary melanoma, definitive surgical treatment is recommended without a biopsy. This policy is recommended to avoid disrupting fascial planes during biopsy, with the potential consequence of seeding tumor cells into the wound.

GENERAL PRINCIPLES OF LYMPHADENECTOMY

1. The surgeon must thoroughly understand the anatomy of the lymph nodes in each area of the body and should incorporate into the surgical specimen all the draining nodes at risk for metastatic melanoma. The treatise by Haagensen and colleagues is particularly enlightening in regard to lymphatic anatomy and its implications in cancer.[29] A cutaneous lymphatic scan may be helpful in identifying ambiguous lymphatic drainage from melanomas located on the trunk or head and neck area (see Chap. 9).

2. It is important to emphasize that lymph nodes are broadly distributed and that many are located outside the major draining basins. We have excised metastatic melanoma in unusual sites, such as over the scapula, along the iliac crest, along the saphenous vein in the midthigh, and alongside the posterior axillary line. It is interesting to note that melanomas rarely metastasize to the popliteal and epitrochlear lymph nodes from lesions distal to these sites.[18,29] Epitrochlear nodal metastases may occur with some frequency from primary melanomas located on the anterior and medial aspect of the forearm or sometimes from subungual melanomas (Fig. 7-1).[60,61] Popliteal nodal metastases have been reported from melanomas situated over the heel or medial malleolus.[29]

3. Incontinuity resection of the primary melanoma and radical lymph node dissection are performed together wherever feasible rather than as two separate procedures. This approach incorporates the lymphatics between the primary melanoma site and the regional lymph nodes into the specimen (Fig. 7-2). The theoretical reason for an incontinuity dissection is to remove any intransit

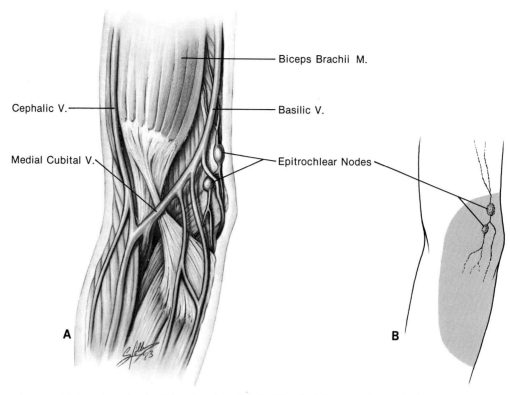

FIG. 7–1 *(A)* Location of epitrochlear lymph nodes. *(B)* The shaded area indicates the locations of melanomas that may metastasize to epitrochlear nodes. Epitrochlear nodal metastases can also occur with subungual melanomas (adapted from Smith TJ, et al: Epitrochlear node involvement of melanoma of the upper extremity. Cancer 51:756, 1983)

FIG. 7–2 Incontinuity lymph node dissection. This surgical specimen incorporated the skin around a primary melanoma arising on the back, the axillary lymph nodes, and the fatty and lymphatic tissue between them.

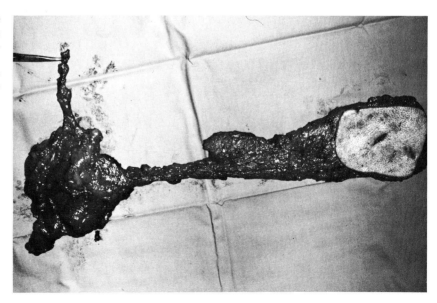

disease trapped in major lymphatic trunks or in regional nodes at the periphery of the primary nodal basin. This is particularly, but not exclusively, true for trunk melanomas. It is not uncommon to encounter patients with recurrent nodal metastases at the periphery of the operative field or intransit metastases that might have been avoided had an incontinuity dissection been performed.[26] While this approach becomes impractical in certain anatomical areas (*e.g.,* distal extremities), it can be performed with relatively little additional morbidity or operating time for melanomas located on the trunk and proximal extremities. If a regional lymph node dissection is indicated for a melanoma located distal to the elbow or knee, the two areas are excised as two separate procedures under the same anesthesia (*i.e.,* wide excision of the primary and a discontinuity lymphadenectomy).

4. Skip involvement of lymph nodes is infrequent. When it happens, the first nodes in the line of drainage from the primary tumor are bypassed, and the next group of more proximal nodes are involved. For example, a primary tumor located on the leg may occasionally bypass the inguinal lymph nodes and involve the iliac or hypogastric lymph nodes.[17,25] It is rare that a melanoma metastasizing from the arm to the supraclavicular nodes will bypass the axillary lymph nodes.

5. A partial or incomplete lymph node dissection is generally not acceptable. More than two thirds of patients with nodal metastases will have more than one or other additional metastatic nodes elsewhere in the regional nodal basin.[4]

6. The incision providing access to the underlying regional nodes should be correctly placed to minimize the risk of dividing lymphatic vessels that could contain malignant cells. By injecting patients with methylene blue dye, it has been demonstrated that divided lymphatics may weep lymph into the wound for some hours during and after surgery. Wound irrigation with cytostatic agents at the conclusion of the operation will probably not decrease the risk of wound recurrence because of delayed postoperative lymphatic drainage into the wound.

7. Skin flaps from a lymph node dissection should be made relatively thin, especially in areas that might contain intralymphatic metastases. This can be achieved by holding the knife aslant to the skin, away from the cancer-containing tissue. Undercutting the flap away from the main excision also has a cosmetic advantage, because the wound edge slopes toward the skin graft rather than making an abrupt step. By contrast, the part of the incision that does not involve lymphatic drainage from the primary melanoma can be thicker (*e.g.,* the superior flap of an axillary node dissection for a melanoma located on the back).

8. The goals of lymph node dissection must be clearly defined. They include any one or a combination of the following: (1) curative intent, (2) local disease control (*i.e.,* palliation), or (3) staging. Each type of regional lymph node dissection has its own set of acceptable risks in different patient settings based on such parameters as age and general health. For example, some patients with bulky nodal metastases may be cured by surgical excision, so it is imperative for the surgeon to perform a thorough operation. A palliative lymph node dissection may be indicated in patients with large, symptomatic metastases even if other distant metastases are present. In such a setting, removal of the metastatic nodes may be beneficial as long as the distant metastases are not an immediate threat to life. Staging to determine the presence or absence of metastatic disease in the regional lymph nodes will assume increased importance as adjuvant chemotherapy or immunotherapy becomes available for high-risk patients with nodal metastases. At present, however, currently available forms of adjuvant treatment are not of proven benefit (see Chap. 11).

9. About one fourth of patients will experience wound-related, short-term complications after lymphadenectomy; however, these rarely result in long-term functional deficits.[68] In an analysis of 204 regional node dissections performed at the University of Alabama in Birmingham (UAB), the most frequent short-term complications were seromas (22%), temporary nerve dysfunction or pain (14%), and wound infections (6%) (Table 7-1). Wound complications extended the mean hospital stay by 0.6 to 4.8 days (Table 7-2). Residual lymphedema of the leg was measurable in 26% of groin dissection patients after 6 months or longer, but most of the edema was confined to the thigh. Only 8% of patients had significant functional deficit from lymphedema. The risk of developing at least one complication for all patients was increased for obese patients (p = .05) and increasing age (p = .01) (Table 7-3). These risk factors should be considered when evaluating melanoma patients for regional lymph node dissection.

TABLE 7–1
SURGICAL MORBIDITY AFTER REGIONAL LYMPH NODE DISSECTION IN PATIENTS TREATED AT THE UNIVERSITY OF ALABAMA IN BIRMINGHAM

	Regional Lymph Node Dissections	Cervical Lymph Nodes	Axillary Lymph Nodes	Inguinal Lymph Nodes
Number of Patients	204	48	98	58
Hospital Stay				
Mean	9.6 days	10 days	9.5 days	9.4 days
Median	8 days	8 days	8 days	9 days
Range	5–36 days	6–24 days	8–36 days	5–23 days
Wound Catheter Suction				
Mean	6.4 days	6 days	6.6 days	6.3 days
Median	6 days	6 days	6 days	6 days
Range	3–24 days	3–10 days	3–13 days	2–20 days
Short-term Complications				
Wound infection	6%	4%	7%	5%
Seroma	22%	10%	27%	23%
Nerve dysfunction/pain	14%	19%	22%	0%
Hemorrhage	1%	2%	1%	0%
Skin slough	3%	10%	0%	2%
Long-term Complications				
Edema	8%	0%	1%	26%
Functional deficit	8%	7%	9%	8%
Pain	6%	6%	6%	5%
Unrelated Major Complications	6%	10%	3%	9%

TABLE 7–2
HOSPITAL STAY (DAYS) AT THE UNIVERSITY OF ALABAMA IN BIRMINGHAM AFTER REGIONAL LYMPHADENECTOMY

	No Complications	Wound Complication	Major Hospital Complication
All (204)	(N = 138)	(N = 56)	(N = 13)
Mean	9	10.2	16.3
Median	8	9	17
Cervical Node Dissection			
(48)	(N = 38)	(N = 10)	(N = 5)
Mean	9.3	14.1	15.2
Median	8	9.5	13
Axillary Node Dissection			
(98)	(N = 67)	(N = 31)	(N = 3)
Mean	9.1	9.7	20.7
Median	8	8	
Inguinal Node Dissection			
(58)	(N = 41)	(N = 17)	(N = 5)
Mean	7.8	9.9	15.4
Median	7	9	17

TABLE 7–3
PROBABILITY OF NOT DEVELOPING AT LEAST ONE WOUND COMPLICATION*

Node Dissection	Increasing Age	Weight Over 75th Percentile	Metastatic Lymph Nodes	Women
Cervical	0.90	0.03	0.24	0.50
Axillary	0.04	0.18	0.26	0.17
Inguinal	0.01	0.81	0.38	0.38
All sites	0.01	0.05	0.92	0.76

*Seroma, infection, nerve dysfunction/pain, hemorrhage, skin slough.

PREOPERATIVE MANAGEMENT

Lymphadenectomy is a major operative procedure. Therefore, each patient should have the usual preoperative evaluation, especially for cardiac, pulmonary, renal, and liver function. Since infection is one of the most common complications after lymphadenectomy, special care is taken to minimize this risk. Patients are not shaved until immediately before the operation, rather than the day prior to surgery, in order to minimize the risk of superficial skin infections and folliculitis. Patients are asked to scrub the operative site with antiseptic soap on several occasions during the 24 hours prior to surgery. Finally, antibiotics are administered on call to the operating room for all patients undergoing skin graft. This may consist of penicillin (1 g IM) or a cephalosporin (1 g). Some surgeons use antibiotics more liberally for axillary and inguinal lymph node dissections, even when a skin graft is not employed.

Patients undergoing inguinal or iliac node dissections should have the involved leg measured for an elastic stocking prior to surgery so that it can be worn as soon as possible after the operation.

ILIOINGUINAL NODE DISSECTION

RATIONALE

There are two contiguous node-bearing basins in this area that might contain metastatic melanoma. The first is composed of the femoral nodes that are located within the femoral triangle. Adjacent inguinal nodes are found along the saphenous vein inferiorly, adjacent to the pubis, and over the lower portion of the external oblique aponeurosis superiorly (Fig. 7-3A). The second nodal basin is composed of the iliac lymph nodes. These also include the obturator nodes and the node of Cloquet at the iliofemoral junction (Fig. 7-3).

In patients with demonstrable nodal metastases, a combined dissection of the iliac and femoral lymph nodes is recommended. This is because 25% to 50% of patients with femoral node metastases will have iliac nodal involvement as well.[19,23] There is some controversy concerning the benefit of iliac lymph node dissection. Some surgeons have stated that patients cannot be cured if their nodal metastases extend above the inguinal ligament and that a combined ilioinguinal lymph node dissection is associated with a higher risk of leg edema and wound complications compared to excision of the inguinal nodes alone.[44] Other surgeons have demonstrated that some patients with iliac nodal metastases can either be cured or demonstrate prolonged survival

(with a 9% to 20% 5-year survival) with iliac lymph node dissection, particularly those patients with microscopic metastases in the inguinal nodes.[19,23,25] Excision of the obturator lymph nodes is important, because they can also be involved with metastases.[30,35]

Bilateral groin dissections are performed only in the unfortunate few patients who have demonstrable metastases in both of these areas. For patients with clinically normal nodes, recommendations for bilateral elective regional node dissection (RND) are made more strictly because of the increased morbidity of the operation, especially edema of both legs and the genitalia.

A groin dissection is sometimes associated with wound complications, including infection, seroma, and flap necrosis.[9,32,68] Careful attention to aseptic procedures and operative technique will minimize these risks. Some of these wound complications can be minimized by excising the skin over the femoral triangle and closing the defect with a split-thickness skin graft. The reason for this is that the main blood supply to the skin overlying the femoral triangle comes from a series of small anterior branches of the femoral artery. These small arteries pass directly through the cluster of femoral lymph nodes. Any complete excision of these nodes divides most, if not all, of these vessels. It follows that the vitality of the skin close to the incision and for a distance of up to 10 cm below the inguinal ligament may be impaired no matter where the incision for lymphadenectomy is placed. The reduced blood supply to the skin may result in either slow wound healing or complete breakdown of this part of the wound, particularly in older persons.

The deep lymph vessels in the groin can be shown by dye injections to lie adjacent to the adventitia of the femoral artery and vein. This differs from the position of major axillary lymph trunks, which lie in the axillary fat away from the vessels. Some of the smaller deep lymph nodes in the groin lie between the femoral artery and vein. Higher up in the iliac region, there may also be both lymph nodes and lymphatic vessels between and behind the major blood vessels. Dissection along the artery and vein must therefore include the adventitia to incorporate these lymphatics and lymph nodes.

TECHNIQUE OF INGUINAL (SUPERFICIAL) LYMPHADENECTOMY

The surgical technique employed at both the University of Alabama in Birmingham (UAB) and the Sydney Melanoma Unit (SMU) is quite similar.

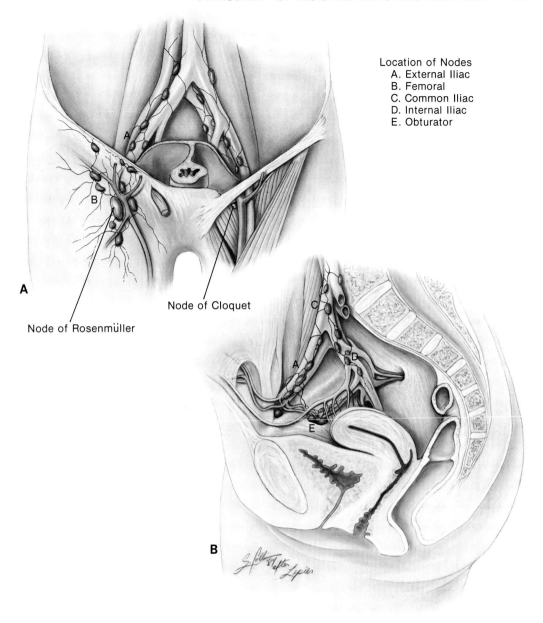

Location of Nodes
A. External Iliac
B. Femoral
C. Common Iliac
D. Internal Iliac
E. Obturator

Node of Cloquet

Node of Rosenmüller

FIG. 7–3   *(A)* Lymphatic anatomy of the inguinal area demonstrating the superficial and deep lymphatic chain. The node of Rosenmüller, which lies at the confluence of the saphenous and femoral veins, is frequently involved when metastases are present. Note that lymph nodes are also present over the external oblique aponeurosis and along the saphenous vein. The node of Cloquet lies at the transition between the superficial and deep inguinal nodes. It is located beneath the inguinal ligament in the femoral canal. *(B)* The iliac nodes include those on the common and superficial iliac vessels and the obturator nodes. It is important to excise the obturator nodes as part of the iliac nodal dissection, since they may contain metastatic disease.

This approach has been previously described by other surgeons as well.[16,29,32,35,48]

---

1. Anesthesia
   a. General or epidural anesthesia is used for most patients, depending on the surgical and anesthetic risks, as well as patient preference.
   b. If an epidural anesthetic is administered, the catheter may be left in place for up to 2 days postoperatively. This approach provides good anesthesia intraoperatively and postoperatively. The epidural anesthesia during surgery is usually supplemented with general anesthetic.
2. Position and draping
   a. The patient is placed in a supine position with the leg abducted. A Foley catheter is used routinely at the SMU and is retained until the first dressing change (usually 5 to 6 days postoperatively). At UAB, the Foley catheter is optional and is retained for only 6 to 24 hours after surgery in these patients when required.
   b. The abdomen, groin, perineum, and upper leg are prepped circumferentially to the ankles and draped with sterile sheets.
   c. Skin markers can be used to outline the incision as well as the anterior superior iliac spine (ASIS), the pubic tubercle, the line of the inguinal ligament, and the line of spread from the site of the primary to the central region of the inguinal lymph nodes (*i.e.,* a point within the femoral triangle about 3 cm below the inguinal ligament).
3. Incision and flap formation
   a. The options for incisions are shown in Figure 7-4. The basic incision in most patients is triangulated to incorporate an island of skin over the femoral triangle. An alternative incision is a gentle reverse "S" that is used if a skin graft is not planned.
   b. Perimeters of soft-tissue dissection vary according to the primary site of the melanoma. For melanomas located on the leg, it is important to excise the major lymph channels and saphenous lymph nodes in the upper thigh. This is because recurrences can develop distal to a more limited groin dissection. At the SMU, the surgical incision extends inferiorly to include the major lymph trunks down to about 8 cm above the knee.[48] A 4-cm band of skin and slightly wider amount of subcutaneous tissues underlying and surrounding the saphenous vein are incorporated in the specimen (Fig. 7-4B).

   For melanomas located on the trunk, the dissection does not have to proceed further inferiorly than the femoral triangle. However, it is important to incorporate the major lymphatics and lymph nodes along the lower abdominal wall.
   c. The incision should be made through the dermis and not into the underlying fat. Adair breast clamps, skin hooks, or rake retractors are used to retract the skin upward on tension.
   d. With the surgeon's left hand on a surgical gauze, the subcutaneous tissues are sharply retracted downward so as to identify a deeper plane of dissection.
   e. The superior flap is made to the external oblique aponeurosis 8 cm to 12 cm above the inguinal ligament. The fatty and lymphatic tissues are then swept down over the external oblique aponeurosis and the cord structures until the inguinal ligament is reached.
   f. The medial flap is then made, working toward the *medial* border of the adductor longus muscle (Fig. 7-4D). It is easier to start in the superior aspect of this flap by dissecting the fatty tissue off the pubic symphysis, for the origin of the adductor muscle is just beneath this. As the dissection proceeds inferiorly, the fascia of the adductor muscle is excised to the point where it traverses beneath the sartorius muscle. At the inferior aspect of the medial flap, the saphenous vein is clamped, divided, and ligated.
   g. The lateral flap is then made. In this step, the surgeon must hold the Adair clips or retractors upward with his hand, while the first assistant strongly retracts the subcutaneous tissues downward to identify the appropriate tissue planes. The perimeter of this flap is the *lateral* border of the sartorius muscle. This is best identified by starting at the superior aspect of the flap at the ASIS and working inferiorly from this point. The origin of the sartorius muscle is identified, and the dissection proceeds inferiorly to the lowermost portion of the femoral triangle.
   h. An alternative is a gentle reverse "S" incision that does not require a skin graft (Fig. 7-4C)[30,32] However, there is greater tension on this wound, and the central portion of the femoral area has been devascularized. The risk of sloughing of the skin edges is greater

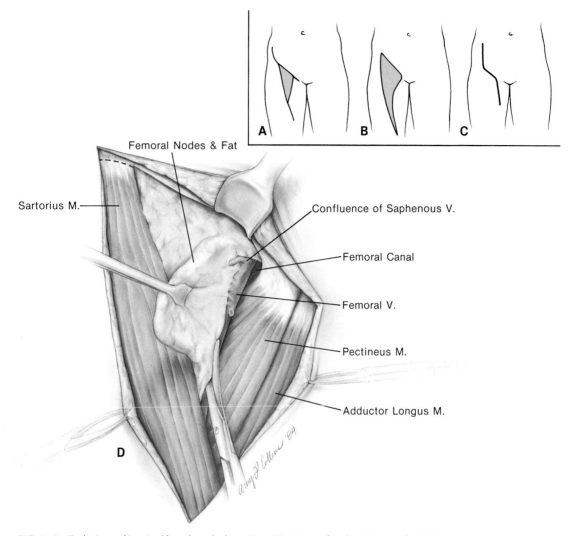

FIG. 7–4 Technique of inguinal lymph node dissection. *(A)* A triangulated incision used at UAB removes the island of skin overlying the femoral triangle. *(B)* The incision preferred at the SMU includes a more generous amount of skin overlying the saphenous vein. This incision is used particularly for melanomas arising on the extremity. *(C)* An alternative incision that avoids a skin graft but is associated with an increased risk of wound breakdown. It may be considered for younger patients. *(D)* Medial dissection of the fatty and lymphatic tissue overlying the femoral triangle. This has been excised off the adductor longus muscle until the femoral vein is exposed. The dissection then proceeds superiorly along the femoral vein. The saphenous vein is transected at the confluence of the femoral vein. Dissection then continues beneath the inguinal ligament to remove the node of Cloquet.

than that for the triangulated incision described above, particularly in older patients. On the other hand, this incision does not require a skin graft and may be used safely in younger patients.

4. Soft-tissue dissection
  a. The specimen is dissected in a subfascial plane, working toward the femoral vessels and nerve.
  b. The superior tissue has been dissected off the external oblique aponeurosis to a point just below the inguinal ligament. The pectineus fascia is incised, taking care to avoid injury to the underlying femoral vessels. This fas-

cial incision begins immediately beneath the pubic symphysis and extends over the vessels, the femoral nerve, and the sartorius muscle up to its attachment to the ASIS.

c. Laterally, the specimen is dissected off the sartorius muscle in a subfascial plane, working toward the femoral nerve. The fascia is again incised as the medial border of the sartorius muscle is reached. The main trunk of the femoral nerve should be identified at this point, as it emerges below the inguinal ligament and is located deep to the fascia iliaca. The specimen is dissected superficial to the nerve until the femoral artery is encountered.

d. The sheath overlying the femoral artery is incised along its entire length from the inguinal ligament superiorly to the inferiormost aspect of the incision. Beginning inferiorly, the artery is skeletonized (using scissors or a knife) beneath the adventitia. The anterior half of the femoral artery is then skeletonized. Branches coursing anteriorly are divided and ligated. The medial aspect of the femoral vein sheath is also incised at this point.

e. The medial soft-tissue dissection is then performed in a subfascial plane over the adductor longus and pectineal muscles (see Fig. 7-4D). The overlying fascia must again be incised adjacent to the femoral vein. At this point, the specimen is dissected off the femoral vein in a subadventitial plane, working from the inferiormost aspect of this vein toward the inguinal ligament. As the confluence of the saphenous vein and the femoral vein is approached, care must be taken to dissect off all investing connective tissue around the proximal saphenous vein at the fossa ovalis. It is this point, where the Rosenmüller's node lies, that is a frequent site of nodal metastases. A clamp is placed across the saphenous vein, leaving enough distance for the stump to be ligated without impinging on the lumen of the femoral vein. The saphenous vein is then transected and the stump doubly ligated.

f. The specimen is now attached only by the soft tissue superior and medial to the proximal femoral vein. The dissection is then continued superiorly beneath the inguinal ligaments so as to remove the node of Cloquet, which is located in the femoral canal just medial to the vein (see Fig. 7-3B). After the node is identified, a hemostat is clamped across the fatty tissue just above the node. The specimen is then transected, marked for orientation, and sent for pathologic examination.

5. Transposition of the sartorius muscle

a. This procedure is necessary in all patients to cover the femoral vessels. It protects them from drying in case any wound breakdown should occur postoperatively that would otherwise expose the femoral vessels.

b. The upper part of the sartorius muscle is dissected from its surrounding connective tissue and is freed up to its origin on the anterior iliac spine (Fig. 7-5). It is then divided through the fascia at its origin, since the fascial end will hold sutures more securely to the inguinal ligament when transposed.

c. The sartorius muscle is held up while the dissection proceeds inferiorly, sacrificing the upper branches of the vessels and nerves. The muscle is mobilized sufficiently to be transposed over the femoral vessels without undue tension.

d. The stump of the muscle is sutured to the external oblique aponeurosis, using transverse mattress sutures of 2–0 silk (Fig. 7-6). The muscle is also loosely approximated to the abductor longus muscle medially and the quadriceps fascia laterally, using interrupted sutures.

6. Closure of the incision

a. Using the standard technique at UAB, the wound is ready to be closed. Using the variation described from the SMU, the inguinal ligament had previously been detached from the ASIS. At the time of closure, the inguinal ligament is not reattached to the ASIS but closed onto the fascia overlying the iliacus muscle. The muscular part of the incision at its lateral extent is first closed by sewing the upper part of the muscles to the stump left on the iliac crest. A finger is then passed under the iliac fascia and the femoral nerve is felt as a tight cord on a plane behind the fascia (and deep to the femoral artery). The nerve can be protected by the surgeon's finger, while the free border of the inguinal ligament is sewn to the iliac fascia over the femoral nerve with a continuous nonabsorbable suture.

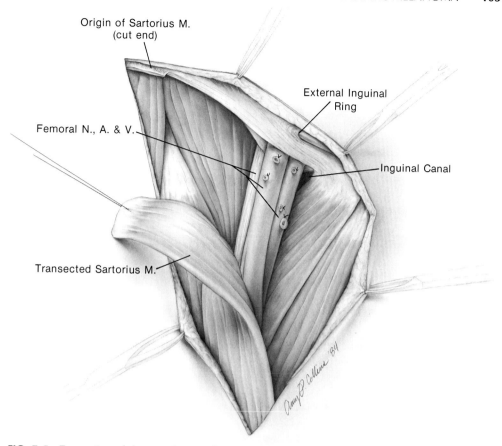

Origin of Sartorius M.
(cut end)

External Inguinal
Ring

Femoral N., A. & V.

Inguinal Canal

Transected Sartorius M.

FIG. 7–5 Transection of the sartorius muscle at its origin on the anterior superior iliac spine. It is important to incise the muscle directly off the bone to preserve the fascial end, which holds sutures better. The muscle is then dissected free of surrounding tissues and transposed over the femoral vessels and nerves.

b. The medial end of the inguinal ligament is sewn to the periosteum of the superior ramus of the pubic bone or to the pectineus fascia. Nonabsorbable sutures should be used to approximate the medial aspect of the inguinal ligament to the underlying muscular fascia, but they should be tied down gently so they will not obstruct the femoral vein.

c. Two suction catheters are placed in the inferior aspect of the wound. The first is brought through the lateral flap and courses superiorly to the ASIS. The other is brought through the medial flap and courses upward to the pubic ramus. They should not cross beneath the suture line because there is an increased risk of air leaks. The use of suction drains at the SMU is optional.

d. Each apex of the triangulated incision is closed, using interrupted vertical mattress sutures (silk or nylon) or absorbable, synthetic subcuticular sutures so as to leave a triangulated defect with the transposed sartorius muscle at its base.

e. Skin sutures of 3–0 silk are then placed circumferentially around the triangulated defect, using horizontal mattress sutures 1 cm apart and 0.5 cm away from the skin edge (see Fig. 7-6). The ends are left long as stent sutures.

f. A split-thickness skin graft from the opposite thigh is taken from a donor site. It is used to cover the defect over the transposed sartorius muscle. A standard stent dressing is applied as described in Chapter 6.

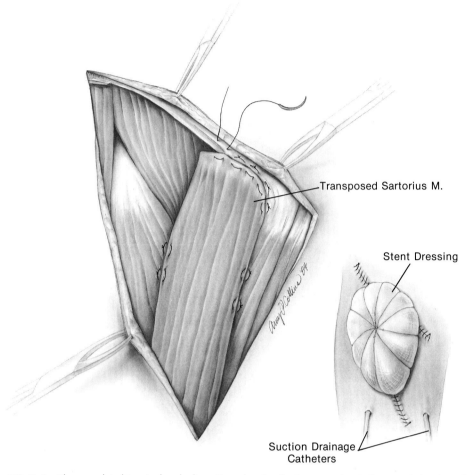

Transposed Sartorius M.

Stent Dressing

Suction Drainage
Catheters

FIG. 7–6 The completed inguinal node dissection, showing the transposed sartorius muscle in place. It is sutured to the external oblique aponeurosis with interrupted nonabsorbable horizontal mattress sutures. Suction catheters are then placed in the lateral and medial aspects of the wound and the incision is closed. (Inset) When a skin graft is used to cover the triangulated defect overlying the transposed sartorius muscle, a standard stent bolus dressing is applied.

TECHNIQUE OF ILIAC (DEEP) LYMPHADENECTOMY

1. At UAB, the incision is made through the external oblique aponeurosis. The internal oblique and the transversus abdominis muscle are split in the direction of their fibers. The incision is continued to include the lateral sheath of the rectus abdominis muscle.
2. At the SMU, access to the iliac lymph nodes is achieved by detaching the lateral end of the inguinal ligament from the ASIS and dividing the abdominal muscles about 3 cm above and parallel to the iliac crest and the inguinal ligament. The incision must be placed far enough away from the internal inguinal ring so that the oblique musculature can be easily approximated without narrowing the internal ring.
3. The deep circumflex artery and vein are identified and ligated where they lie between the internal oblique and transversus muscles.
4. As the inguinal ligament is reflected upward and the peritoneum lifted off the iliac fossa, the inferior epigastric vessels are identified, passing upward and medially from the point where the femoral arterial pulsations can be felt. The vas deferens (or the round ligament) will be seen at this stage, and should be preserved, as should the testicular vessels that lift off the iliac fossa with the peritoneum.

5. The retroperitoneal fat is encountered and the peritoneum swept upward with the hand or with a sponge-stick to expose the underlying iliac vessels. Two large retractors are used to hold the peritoneal contents off the pelvic brim.

6. Dissection around the external iliac vessels is usually performed with sharp instruments up to the level of the ureter, crossing the bifurcation of the common iliac artery, or higher if clinically detectable nodes are involved along the iliac vessels.

7. Beginning at the inguinal ligament inferiorly, the lymph nodes are dissected off the artery and vein, working within the vessel sheath. Small vessels and lymphatics at the perimeter of the excision should be ligated, cauterized, or clipped to avoid hemorrhage or lymphoceles. The dissection then continues superiorly up to the common iliac vessels.

8. The pelvic dissection is facilitated by reflecting the peritoneum medially with broad retractors and then working downward, using the fingers as blunt dissectors. The advantage of this method is that the obturator nerve is very close to the major lymph nodes and can be felt as a taut cord that moves away from the side wall of the pelvis. If this part of the dissection is performed with a sharp instrument, there is some danger of damaging the nerve.

9. As soon as the specimen containing the lymph nodes is lifted upward in one unit with the external iliac nodes, abdominal packs are placed firmly in the pelvis and left until the operation is complete, by which time any bleeding will have stopped.

10. At UAB, the peritoneum is opened for palpation of the abdominal contents for metastases, especially in patients with large or multiple nodal metastases. Such a policy has been advocated by others as well.[14,17] The peritoneum is incised sufficiently for the surgeon's hand to enter the peritoneal cavity. The periaortic lymph nodes are then palpated as are the liver and intestine. If any of these areas is suspected of harboring metastatic disease, consideration should be given to a separate midline laparotomy incision to confirm the diagnosis. After the abdominal exploration, the peritoneum is reapproximated with figure-of-eight 3–0 silk sutures. The incision in the abdominal wall is then closed in layers.

11. Closure of the skin and the use of drains are described above.

POSTOPERATIVE MANAGEMENT

1. If suction drains are used, they are generally removed by the sixth to eighth postoperative day, or earlier if the wound drainage is less than 40 ml per day.

2. Patients are encouraged to ambulate as soon as they are able. At UAB, this usually occurs on the night of surgery or the first postoperative day. At the SMU, mobilization is not encouraged until after 48 hours.

3. Elastic stockings or wrappings should be used whenever the patient is ambulating. If the patient has been measured for a custom-fitted stocking preoperatively, this should be used as soon as it becomes available. Otherwise, elastic wrappings or size-fitted elastic stockings should be used.

4. At UAB, diuretics are often started after the first postoperative week (hydrochlorothiazide, 50 mg per day) and continued for 6 months. Appropriate potassium replacement is advised. This is not used at the SMU unless there is some evidence of leg edema.

5. Patients should be advised to elevate their legs above their chests routinely for 5 to 10 minutes three times a day for at least the first few months after surgery, or whenever they have leg edema.

COMPLICATIONS AND THEIR MANAGEMENT

In an analysis of 58 patients who underwent inguinal dissections at UAB, the short-term complications were relatively infrequent and of short duration (Table 7-1).[68] The complications included wound infection in 5%, seroma in 23%, and skin slough in 2%. None of the patients had significant hemorrhage or nerve dysfunction. Leg edema was a frequent long-term complication (in 26%), but this was largely confined to the thigh, and only 8% of patients had edema of the lower leg. Pain (5%) and functional deficit (8%) were uncommon. Only one patient (2%) had persistent severe edema. The occurrence of a wound complication extended hospitalization by an average of 2.1 days (Table 7-2). Increasing age was the major risk factor for the development of one or more wound complications (Table 7-3).

Seroma occurred in 23% of patients despite the use of Hemovac suction catheters. However, it is generally straightforward to treat with simple incision and drainage. The wound is dressed and packed several times a day. It can usually be cared for at home by the patient, his family, or a visiting home nurse. Significant problems with wound healing (such as severe wound edge necrosis requiring regrafting) have been infrequent (about 5%).

These results are better than those reported in some other series. This may be due in part to the use of a skin graft to cover the femoral triangle. It is also important to trim the wound edges prior to closure if their blood supply appears tenuous. These wound complications should be avoided if possible, especially infection, because the risk of leg edema increases significantly with a wound abscess or cellulitis.[33]

If the lymphadenectomy has been performed thoroughly and no skin is excised, there is a danger of slow wound healing and sloughing in the upper part of the thigh wound. If the wound looks pink after surgery, wound healing is likely to be slower than normal. The skin sutures should be left in up to 2 weeks longer. If the wound edges become quite inflamed, the sutures should be removed and replaced immediately with Steristrips. These should be left in place for at least 1 week. If the wound slough is not deep, it is best to excise the necrotic edges rather than wait for the wound to separate. Once excised, the development of healthy granulation tissue can be encouraged by frequent dressing changes (using hypochlorite or saline soak dressings). The wound can either be left to heal by secondary intention or covered with small split-thickness skin grafts.

Residual edema can be a debilitating sequel of inguinal node dissection. This complication mainly occurs when the primary melanoma is on the leg and is less frequent when it is located on the lower trunk.[37] Three series have now shown a decreased incidence of leg edema after groin dissection as a result of using preventative measures that included perioperative antibiotics, elastic stockings, leg elevation exercises, and diuretics.[32,37,68] Vigorous prophylactic measures are important because it is difficult to reverse the progression of edema. The patients in one series who followed this prophylactic regimen had a markedly lower incidence of leg edema than those who did not (7% versus 46%, $p < 0.004$).[37]

Edema was objectively documented in 26% of the patients treated at UAB who were evaluated 6 months or later after a superficial groin dissection.[68] The edema was usually confined to the thigh and had little cosmetic or functional consequence. Only 4 patients (8%) reported a deficit requiring a change

in life-style or occupation as a result of swelling and decreased range of motion of the extremity. Risk-factor analysis for this long-term complication did not show any significant association with age, weight, lymph node status, or sex.[68] This incidence of measurable lymphedema (21% to 26%) was similar to that observed by Holmes and colleagues[32] and by Karakousis and colleagues.[37] Earlier studies reported a higher rate of edema, particularly when both inguinal and iliac nodes were excised or when prophylactic measures to prevent lymphedema were not used.[9,30,33,44,53]

One late-occurring complication in a lymphedematous limb is a streptococcal lymphangitis, which is characterized by the rapid development of a red, tender, swollen limb associated with fever, rigors, and malaise. This condition develops in a few hours and causes considerable morbidity. The organisms are almost always sensitive to penicillin, and the condition of both the patient and his limb improve within 24 hours of its administration. The danger of relapse is considerable unless the penicillin is maintained for a long period after the resolution of all signs of inflammation. A recommended approach is to give the patient 1 g of penicillin orally every 6 hours until the inflammation or the general symptoms have resolved, then every 8 hours for 2 months. If the condition recurs, oral penicillin may have to be continued for as long as 4 months. It is important to sustain the antibiotic treatment, since each episode of inflammation appears to result in increased scarring around the lymphatics, which leads to more troublesome edema.

Lymph fistula in the groin is not a common complication but is more frequent following excisional biopsy of a single lymph node in the groin. This can usually be treated by suction drainage or by pressure and immobilization. However, complete immobilization of the leg in an air splint will diminish the flow of lymph, and adequate pressure over the wound area will close the leaking lymphatics. Some degree of perseverance and ingenuity is required to provide adequate pressure to the wound, but it can be achieved by gauze pads firmly bound to the groin with an elastic adhesive bandage.

The occurrence of clinically detectable deep venous thrombosis (DVT) was very infrequent (<5%) in the UAB and SMU series. In one study, 44 patients with venograms were used to assess DVT, and the incidence rate was only 13.6%.[2] The occurrence of DVT was not lowered with prophylactic minidose heparinization.

AXILLARY LYMPH NODE DISSECTION

RATIONALE

The most important feature of this operation is the completeness of the dissection, including the level III lymph nodes medial to the pectoralis minor muscle (Fig. 7-7). It is tragic when a patient presents with a recurrence of the apical axilla, because these nodes should have been excised with the original operation. A partial axillary node dissection has no place in the management of melanoma. There is little additional morbidity or operative time involved in a complete axillary node dissection.

At the SMU, complete axillary node dissection is accomplished by transecting the pectoralis major muscle. At UAB, the level III nodes are approached by adducting the arm over the chest wall to facilitate retraction of the pectoralis muscles to the maximum degree.

The surgeon should remember that metastatic nodes may be present at the perimeters of a traditional axillary node dissection. Lymph nodes that might be missed include those along the posterior axillary line, the lower chest wall, and along the long thoracic nerve (Fig. 7-7).

SURGICAL TECHNIQUE

The following outline describes the surgical technique used at UAB and the SMU. Other surgeons have described and illustrated similar approaches.[13,29,31,73]

FIG. 7–7 Lymphatic anatomy of the axilla demonstrating three subgroups of axillary lymph nodes. The highest axillary nodes (level III) medial to the pectoralis minor muscle should be included in a radical axillary lymph node dissection.

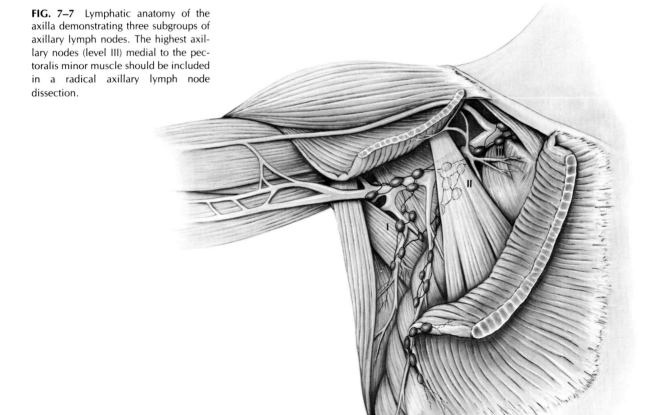

1. Anesthesia

   A general anesthetic is required.

2. Position and draping

   a. The patient is placed in a supine position with the ipsilateral arm placed on an arm board. It is helpful to have a folded sheet placed under the scapula so that the latissimus dorsi muscle is off the operating table.

   b. The chest, shoulder, axilla, and arm (to the upper forearm) are prepped.

   c. It is desirable to move the arm during the operation so the hand and forearm are draped in a half sheet or a stockinette up to the elbow so that it can be manipulated during the operation (Fig. 7-8A).

3. Incisions

   A transverse incision is made over the fourth rib beginning at a point just lateral to the midclavicular line and extending transversly into the axilla to the posterior axillary line (Fig. 7-8A). An alternative incision can be made vertically along the anterior axillary line that curves superiorly along the pectoralis insertion to the humerus.

4. Skin flap formation

   a. Towels are placed along the incision and clipped to the skin edges with Adair breast clips placed about 2 cm apart. Alternatively, skin hooks or rake retractors can be used.

   b. The superior flap is raised first. The clamps or rakes are held on tension and in a perpendicular direction. Using the scalpel tip, the dermal–subcutaneous junction is incised for a distance of approximately 0.5 cm. The belly of the scalpel blade is then used to develop a relatively thin flap within the subcutaneous tissue. It is important to raise the flaps with a fairly uniform (or gradually increasing) thickness. The surgeon's opposite hand should be used to apply strong counteraction on the soft tissues in order to facilitate the dissection and to identify the appropriate tissue planes better.

   c. The superior perimeter of the dissection is the incised fascia overlying the pectoralis muscle near its insertion onto the humerus; the medial perimeter of the dissection is the pectoralis fascia approximately at the midclavicular line. The inferior perimeter is located approximately at the level of the sixth rib, where the posterior perimeter is the leading edge of the latissimus dorsi muscle.

   d. In general, the surgeon dissects the specimen from the pectoralis major muscle along the chest wall and then superiorly up the latissimus dorsi muscle. As the dissection proceeds in a cephalad direction along the leading edge of the latissimus dorsi muscle, the tendinous insertion is reached. Approximately 1 cm to 2 cm cephalad from this is the axillary vein. Continued careful dissection with the knife is used to incise the axillary vein fascia. The blunt end of the knife handle is then used to sweep tissues overlying the anterior surface of the axillary vein in a medial direction for about 1 cm.

   e. The fatty and lymphatic tissue overlying the pectoralis major muscle anteriorly is dissected in a subfascial plane over the leading edge of the muscle and then on its underneath surface until the pectoralis minor muscle is encountered.

   f. A large retractor is used to lift up the pectoralis major muscle and expose the interpectoral groove.

   g. The dissection continues along the undersurface of the pectoralis major muscle and then on to the anterior surface of the pectoralis minor muscle. At this point, it is important to identify the medial pectoral nerve as it emerges either through or just medial to the pectoralis minor muscle (Fig. 7-8A). This nerve must be preserved, or the pectoralis major muscle will atrophy.[50] The dissection proceeds superficial and lateral to this nerve and then continues over the anterior surface of the pectoralis minor muscle.

   h. The specimen is now dissected off the lateral edge of the pectoralis minor muscle and through the deep axillary fascia (the character of the fat changes as this fascia is incised).

   i. At this point, attention is shifted to the lateral aspect of the coracobrachialis muscle. The fascia overlying the muscle is incised in a medial and inferior direction along the coracobrachialis muscle until the coracoid process is reached.

5. Dissection of the upper axillary lymph nodes

   a. There are several approaches to the upper axillary lymph nodes (Fig. 7-8). These include (1) adducting the arm over the chest and sharp retraction of the pectoralis muscles in an upward direction, (2) the Patey procedure to in-

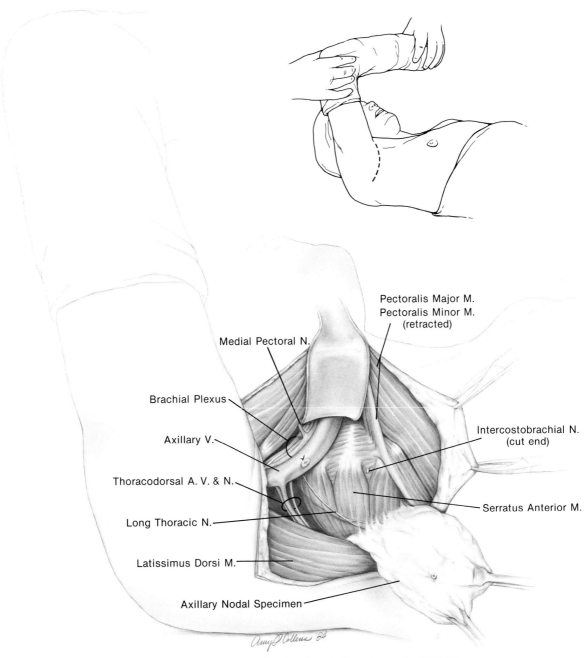

FIG. 7–8   Access to the upper axilla. *(A)* Technique of axillary lymph node dissection used at UAB. The inset shows the arm draped so that it can be brought over the chest wall during the operation. This facilitates retraction of the pectoralis major and minor muscles upward to reveal the upper axillary contents. It is important to avoid injury to the medial pectoral nerve, whose anatomical variations are described in reference 50.

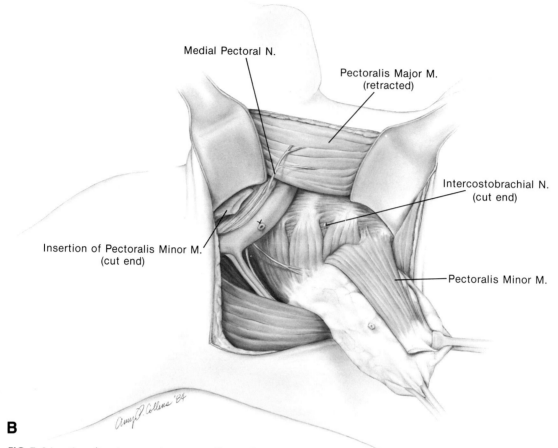

Medial Pectoral N.

Pectoralis Major M.
(retracted)

Intercostobrachial N.
(cut end)

Insertion of Pectoralis Minor M.
(cut end)

Pectoralis Minor M.

B

FIG. 7–8 (*continued*).   Access to the upper axilla. *(B)* The Patey procedure to excise the pectoralis minor muscle as part of the axillary dissection.

corporate the pectoralis minor muscle as part of the dissection, and (3) taking down the pectoralis muscle at its insertion of the humerus.

b. The upper axillary node dissection should be sufficiently complete so that the surgeon can demonstrate to an assistant the thoracic outlet beneath the clavicle and the subclavius muscle as it courses over the axillary vein.

c. At the SMU, the pectoral head of the insertion of the pectoralis major muscle is detached from the humerus and that part of the muscle is folded anteriorly, toward the opposite side, as if opening a book. Harris and colleagues have described a similar approach.[31] The insertion of the muscle is identified at the interpectoral groove between the clavicular and sternal head of the pectoralis major muscle.

The cleft between the two parts of the muscle is divided sharply.

The medial pectoral nerve passes through the pectoralis minor muscle and is accompanied by branches of the thoracoacromial artery, the trunk of which passes anteriorly and proximal to the upper border of the pectoralis minor muscle. The coracoid process is identified, and the short head of the pectoralis minor muscle is transected sharply off the coracoid process (Fig. 7-8C). The dissection begins at the apex of the axilla and then proceeds laterally to incorporate the lower axillary nodes as described below.

At the conclusion of the operation, the head of the pectoralis major muscle is repaired by attaching the tendon of the sternal head of that

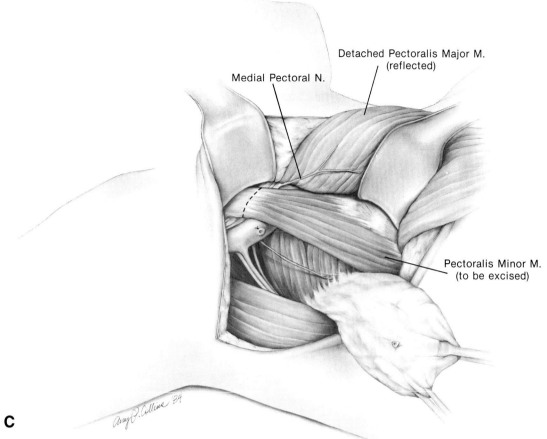

Medial Pectoral N.

Detached Pectoralis Major M.
(reflected)

Pectoralis Minor M.
(to be excised)

C

FIG. 7–8 (continued).   Access to the upper axilla. (C) Detachment of the pectoralis major muscle from its insertion on the humerus to facilitate exposure of the axilla. The pectoralis minor muscle is excised as well. The pectoralis major muscle is sutured back together with nonabsorbable suture at the completion of the operation.

muscle to either the humeral stump of the muscle or to the intact insertion of the clavicular head as close as possible to the bicipital groove of the humerus.

d. At UAB, the upper axilla is approached by adducting the arm over the chest (Fig. 7-8A) and retracting the pectoralis muscles upward. Alternatively, the level III lymph nodes can be dissected free by entering the clavipectoral groove and retracting the clavicular and sternal heads of the pectoralis muscle with retractors. The level III nodes are then dissected free from the axillary vein, the Halsted's ligament, and other surrounding tissues. They are dissected medially to the level of the pectoralis minor muscle.

The patient's arm has been brought over the chest in extreme abduction and internal rotation. The first assistant holds or steadies the arm while the second assistant sharply retracts the pectoralis muscles upward with a large retractor. This maneuver opens the axilla and greatly facilitates the axillary dissection.

e. The Patey modification of the axillary dissection is used to remove the pectoralis minor muscle from the coracoid process and its origin on the chest wall (Fig. 7-8B). This maneuver facilitates exposure of the level III lymph nodes. It should be especially considered if the patient is large or if there are grossly involved lymph nodes in this area.

6. Dissection of the lower axillary nodes

a. The fatty and lymphatic tissue are dissected downward over the brachial plexus and axillary artery, beginning at the coracoid process, until the axillary vein is exposed on its anterior surface.

b. Starting at the apex of the axilla, all the fatty and lymphatic tissues anterior and inferior to the axillary vein are now divided. As hemostats are applied to branches of the axillary vessels coursing into the specimen, they are handed to the first assistant. It is important that the first assistant gently palm the hemostats as a unit for two reasons: (1) they serve as retractors to hold the axillary vein up during the inferior and posterior aspect of the dissection around the vein, and (2) too much manipulation of the hemostats may avulse the clamped branches of the axillary vein.

c. The second assistant holds the pectoralis muscles upward with a Richardson retractor to expose the axillary vein underneath the pectoralis minor muscle (Fig. 7-8A). A Kelly clamp is used to strip all the fatty and lymphatic tissues surrounding the axillary vein, reaching as far underneath the pectoralis minor muscle as possible. If any of the lymph nodes in this area appear to be grossly involved with metastatic disease, it is probably best to take down the pectoralis minor muscle from its insertion on the coracoid process to facilitate exposure and remove all level III lymph nodes (Fig. 7-8B). The apex of the specimen is then tagged with a #3 metal marker for specimen orientation for the pathologist.

d. Using the knife, the fatty and lymphatic tissue is dissected from the inferior and posterior aspect of the axillary vein through its entire course. The dissection should continue until the thoracodorsal vessels are identified. These enter the axillary vessels more posteriorly and inferiorly than do the other venous branches.

e. The long thoracic and the thoracodorsal nerves are then identified and held with Allis clamps. The long thoracic nerve lies in a groove right alongside the chest wall superficial to the investing fascia of the serratus anterior muscle. It can be gently pinched to verify its innervation with the serratus anterior muscle. The thoracodorsal nerve courses medially and adjacent to the thoracodorsal vessels. It is similarly retracted with an Allis clamp.

f. The fatty tissue between the two nerves (marked by the Allis clamps) is separated from the underlying subscapularis muscle, using a long hemostat. The fatty tissue between the nerves is then clamped just inferior and posterior to the axillary vein. Another clamp is placed just inferior to this, and the tissues between the two clamps are divided. The inferior clamp is then pulled down sharply so as to strip the fatty tissue off the underlying subscapularis muscle.

7. Chest wall dissection

a. The specimen is then removed from the lateral chest wall by dissecting just superficial to the long thoracic nerve.

b. The intercostobrachial nerve will be identified as it comes off the chest wall and courses directly into the specimen (Fig. 7-8A). It must be sacrificed.

c. The specimen is finally swept off the leading edge of the latissimus dorsi muscle and the serratus anterior muscle until the entire specimen is removed and sent to pathology.

d. The level II lymph nodes (those behind the pectoralis minor muscle) are marked with a #2 metal tag, while the level I axillary nodes alongside the chest wall are marked with a #1 tag for the pathologist (see Fig. 7-7).

8 Wound closure

a. The wound is irrigated with saline and inspected to be sure that hemostasis is complete.

b. Two suction catheter drains are placed percutaneously through the inferior flap. One catheter courses anteriorly over the pectoralis muscle, while the other courses into the depths of the axilla.

c. The skin is closed with vertical mattress sutures of nylon. These should remain in place for 10 to 14 days. Alternatively, the skin can be approximated with a subcuticular closure, using a synthetic absorbable suture.

POSTOPERATIVE MANAGEMENT

The postoperative management of these patients is straightforward. Wound catheter suction drainage is continued until the output is less than 40 ml per day. By the sixth to eighth day, the suction catheters are removed regardless of the drainage, for they would otherwise act as a potential source of infection. If there is any subsequent collection of serum, a simple counterincision is made at the most dependent area of drainage to relieve the seroma. The wound is then packed open and treated on an outpatient basis until it heals by secondary intention. Alternatively, the seroma can be treated by needle aspiration and repeated as necessary.

Mobilization of the arm is not encouraged during the first 7 to 10 days after surgery. Early exercise can actually have a deleterious effect on wound healing and on the amount of lymphatic drainage.[42] Gradually over the ensuing 1 to 4 weeks, mobilization of the arm is encouraged with active exercises. These may include (1) standing next to a wall and abducting the arm against it, (2) pulley exercises, or (3) sports activities that encourage full motion of the arm, such as swimming or golf.

COMPLICATIONS AND THEIR MANAGEMENT

The complication rate for axillary node dissection is low, the most frequent being a wound seroma.[13,31,68] In a series of 98 radical axillary dissections in melanoma patients treated at UAB,[68] wound-related complications included infections (7%), seroma (27%), nerve dysfunction or pain (22%), and hemorrhage (1%) (see Table 7-1). Wound-related complications extended the average hospitalization by less than 1 day (see Table 7-2). Long-term complications included arm edema (1%), pain at the operative site (6%), and functional deficit (9%). Analysis of risk factors showed that increasing age and obesity were significantly associated with wound complications (Table 7-3).

The management of other wound complications and seromas is similar to that described above for inguinal node dissections.

CERVICAL NODE DISSECTION

RATIONALE

Metastases to lymph nodes from primary melanomas in the head and neck area via lymphatics are fairly predictable (Fig. 7-9). Melanomas occurring anterior to the pinna of the ear generally produce nodal metastases to the parotid, submandibular, submental, upper jugular, and posterior triangle (spinal accessory, transverse cervical) lymph nodes. Lesions occurring inferior to the lateral commissure of the lip will spread to cervical lymph nodes rather than parotid nodes. Melanomas occurring on the scalp posterior to the pinna of the ear usually spread to occipital, postauricular, posterior triangle, or jugular chain nodes.

Radical neck dissection is recommended when nodal metastases are clinically evident. A modified neck dissection or a radical neck dissection can be employed when elective lymphadenectomy is being considered in patients in whom the cervical nodes are at high risk for harboring occult nodal metastases (see Chap. 8).

TECHNIQUE OF RADICAL NECK DISSECTION

Since the first systematic description of the radical neck dissection by George Crile, Sr., in 1906,[15] many authors have published alternative techniques for the same operation.[3,5,7,46] The following description of the radical neck dissection is based on these fundamental techniques.

1. Position

The patient is positioned supine, with the contralateral arm placed on an arm board. The vertex of the head is placed at the end of the table, with the patient slightly nearer the operative side of the table. A folded sheet is placed beneath the shoulders to extend the neck. The head is draped with two small sheets of heavy fabric that are placed beneath the head against the superior aspect of the shoulders. The top sheet is wrapped across the ear and eyebrow on the contralateral side and above the ear on the operated side. This drape is clipped firmly to carry the weight of the anesthesia apparatus that will be brought out over the forehead. Small sheets are placed along the head and over the shoulder and chest on each side. Another sheet is placed across the chest below the clavicles. The first assistant stands across from the surgeon, and the second assistant stands at the head of the table, with airway tubes passing between them to the anesthesia apparatus.

3. Incisions

A number of different incisions may be used according to the location of the primary melanoma and the necessary skin to be sacrificed (Fig. 7-10). If the primary lesion is outside the neck, an incision from the mastoid process to the clavicle with an anterior extension for the development of flaps will suffice.

4. Skin-flap formation

a. After the skin incision is made down to the underlying platysma muscle, skin flaps are developed below to the platysma muscle superiorly to the horizontal ramus of the mandible and tail of the parotid gland. At the SMU, the flaps are sometimes infiltrated with

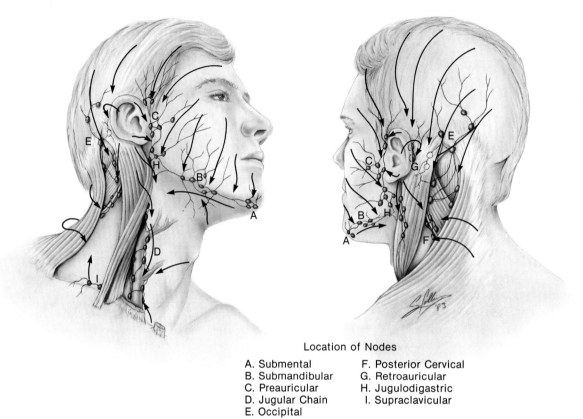

Location of Nodes

A. Submental   F. Posterior Cervical
B. Submandibular   G. Retroauricular
C. Preauricular   H. Jugulodigastric
D. Jugular Chain   I. Supraclavicular
E. Occipital

FIG. 7–9 Lymphatic anatomy for the head and neck area. Melanomas arising on the face, forehead, and anterior scalp generally drain to the parotid lymph nodes as well as to the cervical nodes. Melanomas arising from the posterior scalp and neck may metastasize first to the occipital and posterior cervical nodes. Melanomas arising from the ear may metastasize to the preauricular, parotid, or retroauricular lymph nodes.

a vasopressin solution (5 IU/ml in 20 ml of normal saline). This is injected just beneath the platysma muscle and into the supra- and retroclavicular part of the posterior triangle. This maneuver can facilitate the dissection and decrease blood loss.

b. The external maxillary artery is identified after dividing the platysma muscle at this point. The mandibularis branch of the facial nerve can be identified passing over this artery; it is retracted upward with the artery to protect it from injury. The medial skin flap is similarly developed to the anterior belly of the omohyoid muscle and the strap muscles. Flaps are developed inferiorly to the clavicle and laterally to a line extending from the mastoid process to the anterior border of the trapezius muscle in the posterior neck.

5. Dissection of the cervical nodes

a. Just lateral to the clavicular insertion of the sternomastoid muscle, the external jugular vein and the posterior belly of the omohyoid muscle are identified and divided (Fig. 7-11). The contents of the supraclavicular fossa are then raised until the brachial plexus is identified, with the phrenic nerve traversing downward on the anterior scalene muscle. The contents of the posterior triangle of the neck are dissected upward and medially. The transverse cervical artery and vein are divided, with the spinal accessory nerve at its entrance into the trapezius muscle. Care is taken not to sacrifice small motor nerves to the levator scapula and scalene muscles. The contents of the posterior triangle are further dissected up to the level of the inferior cervical plexus.

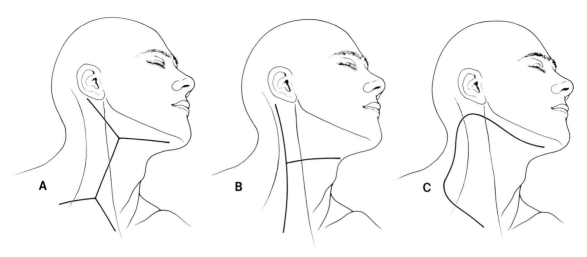

FIG. 7–10 Incisions used at UAB and SMU for radical or modified radical neck dissections. *(A)* The double ''Y'' incision. *(B)* The half ''H'' incision. *(C)* The Schobinger incision.

b. The sternal and clavicular insertions of the sternomastoid muscle are divided. The carotid sheath over the jugular vein in the inferior neck is incised and, using a blunt clamp, the sheath is dissected away from the vein medially. The sternohyoid muscle is retracted medially, and the vein is further dissected out on each side. Before division of the vein, it is prudent to identify the vagus nerve and common carotid artery. The vein is then divided between clamps and ligated.

c. Better exposure of the major structures in the lower neck is easily afforded by dividing the branches of the ansa hypoglossi as they enter the strap muscles. The carotid sheath can then be dissected off the common carotid and vagus nerves in a superior direction.

d. The dissection of the area between the carotid artery and the phrenic nerve in the lower neck is critical, since the thyrocervical trunk arises from the subclavian artery in this area and the thoracic duct on the left side or a major lymphatic duct on the right side may be encountered. After identification of the thyrocervical trunk, the transverse cervical branch is divided, leaving the inferior thyroid artery intact. When the thoracic duct is seen, it is best left unmolested. However, if it obstructs proper dissection, it can be sacrificed.

e. At this point, all major structures at the base of the neck that are to be sacrificed have been divided (Fig. 7-11). The contents of the neck are then dissected superiorly, sacrificing the trunks of the cervical plexus. Care is taken to identify and preserve the sympathetic nerve located posterior to the carotid sheath. The anterior belly of the omohyoid muscle is followed up to the hyoid bone, where it is detached. A small amount of areolar tissue just above the hyoid bone is incised to identify the anterior belly of the digastric muscle. This dissection is continued upward to the carotid bifurcation and beyond where the hypoglossal nerve is identified, passing across the external carotid artery. The ansa hypoglossi nerve can be severed at its takeoff from the main hypoglossal nerve trunk. Posteriorly, the origin of the sternomastoid muscles is detached from the skin of the neck.

f. The loose tissue external to the superior thyroid artery, hypoglossal nerve, and digastric tendon is dissected. Care is taken to avoid the superior laryngeal nerve, artery, and vein traversing posterior to the external carotid artery.

g. The posterior dissection is carried upward, just beyond the prominent transverse process of the second cervical vertebra. The digastric muscle is identified just lateral to this and medial to the mastoid process.

h. The dissected neck contents are reflected downward and the tail of parotid is then divided between the angle of the mandible and the tip of the mastoid process, avoiding the

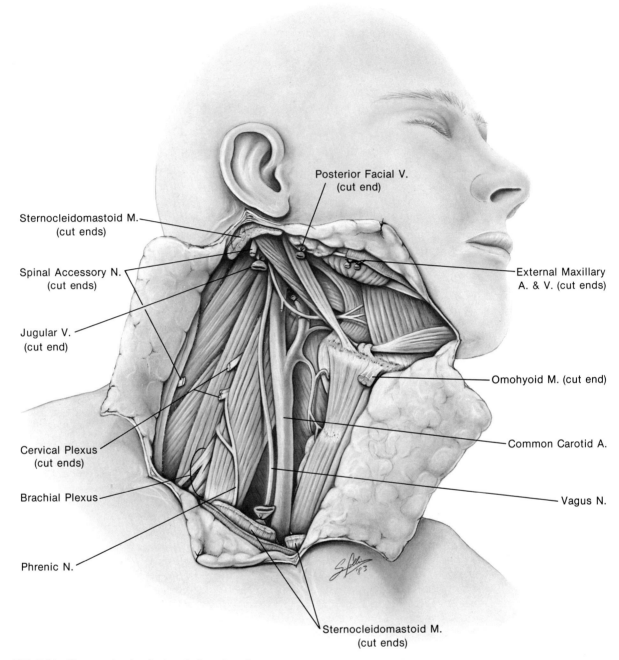

Posterior Facial V.
(cut end)

Sternocleidomastoid M.
(cut ends)

Spinal Accessory N.
(cut ends)

Jugular V.
(cut end)

External Maxillary
A. & V. (cut ends)

Cervical Plexus
(cut ends)

Omohyoid M. (cut end)

Brachial Plexus

Common Carotid A.

Vagus N.

Phrenic N.

Sternocleidomastoid M.
(cut ends)

FIG. 7-11   The completed radical neck dissection, demonstrating important anatomical landmarks.

mandibular branch of the seventh nerve. Superficial temporal vessels are encountered as the tail of parotid is divided. These are divided and ligated. The medial side of the sternomastoid muscle is then followed up to the mastoid process and transected. The posterior

belly of the digastric muscle arises immediately beneath and is retracted upward.

i. Dissection of the upper end of the jugular vein is begun from its lateral side. The occipital artery passes anterior to the vein and is divided. Using smooth-tipped scissors, the loose tissue on the lateral surface of the jugular vein is divided. The approach to the jugular vein from the medial side is just external to the hypoglossal and vagus nerves. Once the jugular vein is cleared of the node-bearing and areolar tissue, it is divided between right-angle clamps and ligated. The dissection below the digastric muscle is concluded by dividing the occipital artery at its origin from the external carotid artery and division of veins traversing between the digastric muscle and the hypoglossal nerve.

j. The submandibular triangle dissection may also include the submental nodes, depending on their actual or potential involvement with metastatic disease. The node-bearing tissue over the digastric muscle and mylohyoid muscles is reflected laterally, dividing the branches of the mylohyoid nerve and vessels. The lateral edge of the mylohyoid muscle is retracted medially, exposing the lingual nerve. Its parasympathetic branch to the submaxillary ganglion is divided. The hypoglossal nerve is identified inferiorly in this area, and the submaxillary duct between the two nerves is divided. The contents of the submaxillary triangle are reflected laterally to the external maxillary artery, which is divided just above the digastric tendon to complete the dissection.

6. Wound closure
   a. The wound is irrigated with saline and hemostasis is completed. Another search is made for any lymph draining from thoracic duct injury on the left side area or lymphatic duct on the right side. The anesthetist can hold the lungs in an expanded position for 10 seconds to increase intrathoracic pressure and help identify any leakage.
   b. Two suction catheters are placed through the inferior flap—one medial and one lateral. The wound is closed, using a continuous subcutaneous absorbable suture and a continuous vertical mattress suture with 4–0 nylon to approximate the skin. Alternatively, the skin can be closed in a subcuticular fashion, using a synthetic, absorbable suture.

MODIFIED NECK DISSECTION

While there has never been a comparative study of modified versus radical neck dissection for melanoma, many surgeons have now adopted the modi-

fied approach because of favorable results in patients with squamous cell carcinoma. This operation is generally reserved for patients undergoing elective neck dissection. Several variations of a basic technique have been described.[8,10,11,34,41,65] Compared to the radical neck dissection described above, the only differences in the operative procedure are the sparing of the spinal accessory nerve and the sternomastoid muscle (Fig. 7-12). To facilitate this, it is necessary to incise the fascia over the sternomastoid muscle and dissect the muscle and spinal accessory nerve free of node-bearing areas. The nerve is usually identified along the medial border of the trapezius muscle at the junction of the middle and upper third of it. The upper jugular chain nodes are not excised as cleanly in a nerve-sparing procedure; therefore, this operation should not be performed when there is suspected metastatic disease in this area.

There are two advantages to this approach. First, there is better shoulder function and no shoulder drop. Second, the cosmetic result is better (Fig. 7-13). Studies evaluating the functional results of modified neck dissection have shown a good cosmetic result, although 30% do not retain full spinal accessory nerve function.[57]

OCCIPITAL PLUS POSTERIOR NECK DISSECTION

The technique for dissection of the occipital and posterior neck lymph nodes incorporates the same principles used in the radical neck dissection. The technique described in this section is similar to that described by other surgeons as well.[24,70]

1. Incision
   The incision is structured to facilitate excision of a primary tumor in continuity with intervening lymphatics to the base of the neck. The incision from the primary tumor site should be extended to allow removal of postauricular and occipital lymphatics from the pinna of the ear to the midline of the posterior neck. This is usually 3 cm to 4 cm posterior to the mastoid process and extends inferiorly to the midclavicle. A horizontal extension toward the hyoid bone may be necessary for adequate exposure.

2. Skin-flap formation
   a. Skin flaps at the occipital level are developed posteriorly to the midline and laterally to the pinna of the ear and mastoid process.
   b. At the neck level, the posterior flap is reflected posteriorly well off the trapezius muscle to the

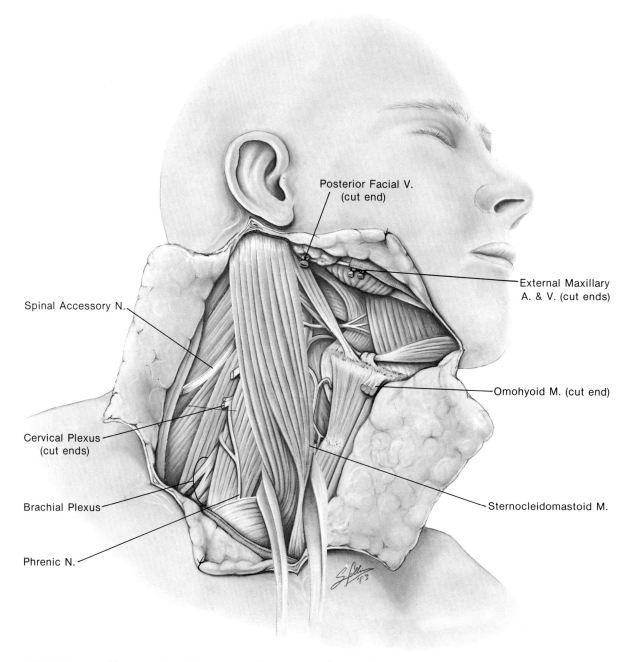

Posterior Facial V.
(cut end)

Spinal Accessory N.

External Maxillary
A. & V. (cut ends)

Omohyoid M. (cut end)

Cervical Plexus
(cut ends)

Brachial Plexus

Sternocleidomastoid M.

Phrenic N.

FIG. 7–12 A modified radical neck dissection. In this operation, the spinal accessory nerve and the sternomastoid muscle are spared. This operation is considered for patients undergoing elective node dissections.

clavicle and medial to the sternohyoid muscle and posterior belly of the digastric muscle.
3. Dissection of the scalp and posterior neck

The plan of dissection is to sacrifice the sternomastoid muscle, spinal accessory nerve, and jugular vein and portions of the trapezius muscle and splenius capitus muscle (Fig. 7-14). The submandibular triangle lymph nodes are not dissected unless there is evidence of metastatic involvement.
a. The dissection begins superiorly at the site of the primary tumor with a minimum of 3 cm

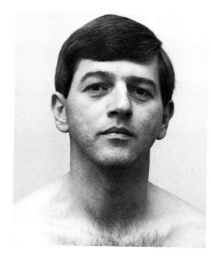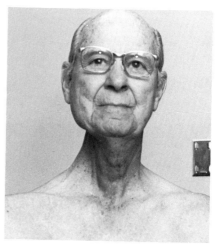

FIG. 7–13 Postoperative results of (*Left*) A modified neck dissection and (*Right*) A classic radical neck dissection. The modified neck dissection achieves a better cosmetic result and there is less functional disability of shoulder motion.

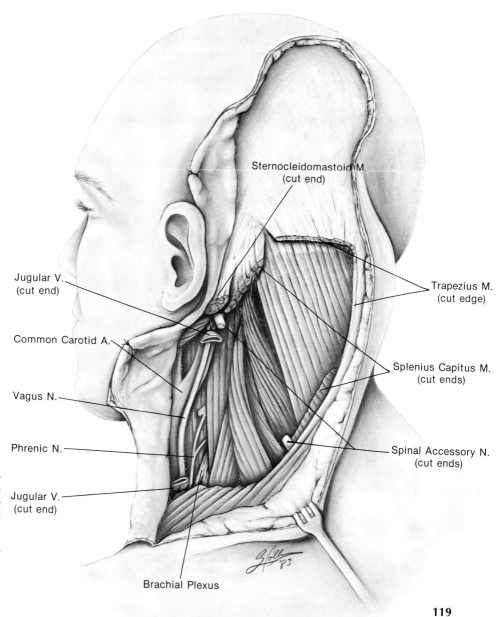

Sternocleidomastoid M. (cut end)

Jugular V. (cut end)

Trapezius M. (cut edge)

Common Carotid A.

Vagus N.

Splenius Capitus M. (cut ends)

Phrenic N.

Spinal Accessory N. (cut ends)

FIG. 7–14 A completed occipital and posterior neck dissection. A melanoma of the scalp has been widely excised and regional nodes have been removed as an incontinuity dissection. The upper portion of the trapezius muscle is included with the specimen.

Jugular V. (cut end)

Brachial Plexus

119

of skin removed in all directions. For scalp melanomas, the periosteum of the skull is left intact. The dissection continues medially and laterally as the occipital and postauricular nodal areas are approached to encompass the subcutaneous tissue and underlying fascia from the midline posteriorly to the pinna of the ear. As the origin of the trapezius muscle and splenius capitus muscles is approached, the muscles are detached from the skull and reflected downward with their underlying lymphatics, making the base of the dissection on the semispinalis capitus muscle. About 4 cm of the trapezius muscle is taken down to its insertion and reflected anteriorly.

b. The remainder of the operation involving the neck is exactly the same as was described for the radical neck dissection (see Technique of Radical Neck Dissection, above).

POSTOPERATIVE MANAGEMENT

Patients are encouraged to be out of bed within a few hours following recovery from anesthesia. Elevating the head of the bed or sitting in a chair lessens the degree of edema about the neck and pharynx. This is important to avoid aspiration and pulmonary infection. There is relatively little postoperative pain, and only mild analgesics are usually required.

Wound catheter drainage gradually reduces to less than 40 ml per day by the fifth or sixth day, and the drains are removed. Should further serum collection occur in the supraclavicular area, the wound can be reopened, and healing usually progresses without further complication.

COMPLICATIONS AND THEIR MANAGEMENT

A review of complications after radical neck dissection for melanoma revealed that short-term complications (seroma, pain, skin slough) were relatively common [10% to 19%]. Long-term problems (neck pain and functional deficit) occurred in only 6% to 7% of patients.[68]

A chylous leak can occur even when great care is used to detect any leak prior to closing the neck wound. If the leak is less than 50 ml daily, it will usually stop within 7 to 10 days. If the leak is greater, the lower end of the wound is usually opened without anesthesia. With good light and suction, the chylous leak area can be identified. It is most commonly situated behind the carotid artery

and vagus nerve, where the duct emerges from the mediastinum. The lymphatics are oversewn with 5–0 silk, using nearby tissue to hold the suture and tamponade the leaking area. It is seldom possible to clamp the leaking lymphatic vessel and apply a tie successfully. A nonoperative approach sometimes used at the SMU is to place the patient on a strict fruit diet to reduce the lymph flow and drainage.

PAROTID LYMPH NODE DISSECTION

RATIONALE

Parotid lymph node metastases may be extraglandular or intraglandular. The most common extraglandular metastases are located in the preauricular nodes and the nodes located about the tail of parotid. Intraglandular nodes are within the substance of the parotid gland and are usually located superficial to the seventh cranial nerve.

Melanomas arising on the scalp or face, anterior to the pinna of the ear, and superior to the commissure of the lip are at risk to metastasize to parotid lymph nodes (see Fig. 7-9).[64] This parotid chain of nodes is contiguous with the cervical nodes; for this reason, it is generally advisable to combine neck dissection with parotid lymph node dissection when parotid nodes are involved with metastatic melanoma. The exception to this rule might be a tumor arising immediately over the parotid gland requiring wide local removal of the tumor, thus necessitating parotid dissection to avoid injury to the seventh cranial nerve in an effort to contain the primary tumor. Details of the surgical technique have been published.[6,45,71]

SURGICAL TECHNIQUE

1. Anesthesia
   a. General anesthetic is required, using a flexible anode endotracheal tube.
   b. Position and draping are similar to the techniques described for radical neck dissection (see Technique of Radical Neck Dissection, 1, above).
2. Incisions

   The incisions may vary according to the size of the parotid mass or the location of the primary melanoma in the area. The most cosmetically desirable incision is placed in the skin crease just anterior to the tragus and is extended down along the pinna to the earlobe, then behind the earlobe to the mastoid process, and finally in an inferior direction to below the angle of the mandible in the skin lines to a point 1 cm or 2 cm anterior to the angle of the mandible (Fig. 7-15).

3. Skin-flap formation
   a. The skin over the parotid gland is reflected anteriorly off the parotid fascia. This flap is raised to a point anterior to the parotid gland where branches of the seventh nerve can frequently be seen as they emerge from the gland over the masseter muscle. If additional exposure is needed, the upper end of the incision can be extended in a transverse direction just below the zygomatic arch.

FIG. 7–15 Anatomical landmarks after completion of a superficial parotidectomy. This operation is generally performed in conjunction with a radical neck dissection, especially when the primary melanoma arises on the face, ear, or anterior scalp and there are metastases either in the parotid or the cervical nodes. (*Inset*) Incision used for a parotid dissection, commonly used for parotidectomy.

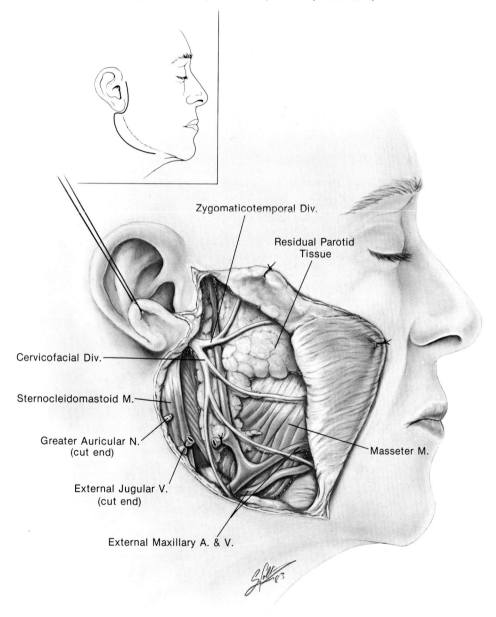

Zygomaticotemporal Div.

Residual Parotid Tissue

Cervicofacial Div.

Sternocleidomastoid M.

Greater Auricular N. (cut end)

External Jugular V. (cut end)

Masseter M.

External Maxillary A. & V.

b. The external auditory canal cartilage is best exposed by blunt dissection just anterior to the cartilage. The dissection is extended by spreading with scissors over the surface of the cartilage. This maneuver of dissecting in juxtaposition to the cartilage avoids potential injury to the seventh nerve.

c. The skin over the mastoid process is then reflected posteriorly for a short distance. The fascia over the sternomastoid muscle and mastoid process is incised and reflected anteriorly off the muscle. The greater auricular nerve is identified as it courses over the upper end of the sternomastoid muscle, and is sacrificed.

4. Parotid dissection

a. The posterior edge of the parotid gland is reflected anteriorly. The fascia overlying the upper end of the sternomastoid muscle is reflected in an anterior direction with the blunt end of the scissors until the parotid parenchyma is encountered.

b. The seventh cranial nerve is now identified by placing a straight hemostat anterior to the mastoid process at a point halfway between the external auditory canal cartilage and the tip of the mastoid process. The tip of the hemostat should lie about 2 cm deep to the external surface and at a right angle to the head. This point is also identified at a level just superior to the attachment of the sternocleidomastoid muscle on the mastoid process. The tissues are then spread in an anterior–posterior direction. With the first clamp held in place, the parotid tissue is gently pushed forward with another hemostat until the major trunk of the seventh nerve is identified. Positive identification is confirmed by tracing the main trunk to the major bifurcation of the nerve (Fig. 7-15).

c. The nerve is maintained in view with a small retractor on the gland. The parotid gland is spread away from the nerve with small forceps and scissors. The tissues exterior to the nerve are incised so that the parotid gland, with its node-bearing tissue, is excised superficial to the seventh nerve, working in an anterior direction.

d. Sacrifice of the seventh nerve branches is necessary at times, but only when metastatic disease is intimately adherent or in close proximity to the nerve. Any amount of nerve that can be left intact will increase the possibility of nerve function recovery. A nerve graft should be considered if the proximal and distal segments can be saved. If the total gland must be removed, the nerve trunks can be maneuvered in such a manner as to allow a total parotidectomy without sacrificing the nerve. This technique is followed until the entire gland is removed with the lymph nodes about the tail, which are external to the posterior belly of the digastric muscle.

5. Wound closure

a. The wound can be irrigated with saline, and hemostasis is completed. The skin flap is returned to its original position.

b. A suction catheter is placed percutaneously into the wound and the incision is closed.

COMPLICATIONS

Complications after parotidectomy are uncommon when the principles outlined above are followed. The incidence of facial nerve injury is proportional to the extent of dissection and the type and amount of tumor.[20,54,72] For elective dissection of parotid tumors in general, temporary paralysis of the facial nerve is reported to occur in 10% to 20% of patients and permanent paralysis in 1% to 3%. When recognized at operation, facial nerve injury should· be repaired by primary anastomosis or nerve grafting from the contralateral greater auricular nerve. Seromas and salivary fistulas are uncommon, and are usually self-limited. Gustatory sweating (Frey's syndrome) occurs more often than is generally reported but presents problems in only about 5% of patients.[54]

MANAGEMENT OF INTRANSIT METASTASES

DIAGNOSIS

Intransit metastases are located between the primary melanoma and the first major regional nodal basin. They probably originate from melanoma cells trapped in lymphatics. Although they may occur in deeper lymphatics, intransit metastases are usually observed as either subcutaneous or intracutaneous metastases (satellitosis).

Patients with a recurrence in the skin or subcutaneous tissue may present with painless nodules that appear as shotty lumps pushing against the surface. They are usually small (*i.e.,* <0.5 cm) and have a bluish coloration; the larger ones may ulcerate through the overlying epidermis (Fig. 7-16). It is best to examine the skin for intracutaneous metastases under a bright light and by gentle palpation over the skin for flat nodules. Satellites may be single or multiple and are generally slightly raised nodules that may or may not be pigmented (Fig. 7-17). Many patients with satellites or subcutaneous metastases will have regional lymph node metastases as well.

Occasionally, these metastases may have the appearance of a primary (nodular) melanoma or a

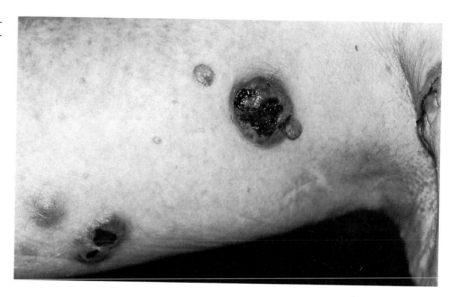

FIG. 7–16 Intransit metastases involving the upper arm with breakdown of the overlying epidermis.

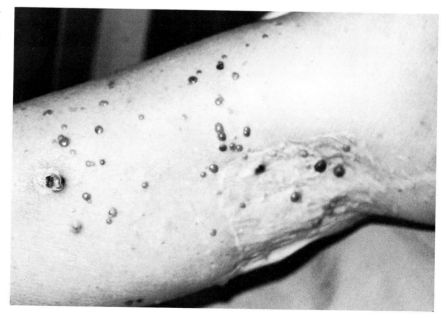

FIG. 7–17 Multiple intracutaneous metastases involving the leg. This condition is sometimes termed "satellitosis."

basal cell carcinoma. A biopsy is necessary to distinguish between these entities. Untreated recurrences in scars or skin usually grow and ulcerate; they may become secondarily infected, leading to a major problem of local wound care.

There have been suggestions in the literature that intransit metastases are related to lymphedema of an extremity after lymphadenectomy,[36,44,49,61] or intralymphatic entrapment after lymphadenectomy.[22,28,61] The evidence for any of these potential etiologies is tenuous. Several reports do not substantiate these potential causes.[1,40,55,59,69] In the UAB and SMU experience, the risk of intransit metastases is almost the same for those who have a wide local excision alone and is not related to whether or not a regional lymph node dissection is performed. Patients at increased risk for intransit metastases are those with thick, ulcerative melanomas or any patient with lymph node metastases.[36,44,47,55]

Intransit metastases can have a heterogenous set of clinical presentations, each with its own implication for survival. These include the number and location of metastases and the presence of regional node metastases. Those patients with few intransit metastases have a better prognosis than those with multiple lesions. In the Tulane Medical Center series, patients with four or fewer lesions had a better outcome than those with five or more lesions.[66] This parameter has thus been incorporated into the new staging system promulgated by the American Joint Committee on Cancer (see Chap. 4). Intransit metastases located within the skin have a better prognosis than those in subcutaneous tissues.[63] Regional nodal metastases occur in about two thirds of these patients and, if present, are associated with a lower survival rate.[63,67]

The reported incidence of intransit metastases is variable. This is partly owing to different definitions of this entity, the referral patterns of the reporting institution, and the proportion of patients with high-risk melanomas. Those centers that practice isolated limb perfusion report a substantially higher incidence of intransit metastases than those that do not. The actual incidence is probably 2% in most current surgical practices,[55] including our own. The reported incidence of 10% to 20% in some series reported in the 1960s and early 1970s[25,44,49,61] probably results from the fact that the majority of melanomas diagnosed at that time were thicker, more ulcerated, and associated with a higher risk for nodal metastases than the average melanoma diagnosed in the 1980s.

TREATMENT OPTIONS

The treatment is not well standardized. It depends primarily on the number and location of these lesions in the integument, the site where they are located, the presence of metastases elsewhere, the risk of the treatment, and whether previous metastases have been treated successfully. It seems clear that aggressive local treatment is more effective than presently available systemic treatment. The treatment options include the following:

1. *Surgery.* This approach may be considered for one or a few lesions. Even with multiple lesions, excision of larger metastases (*i.e.,* greater than 2 cm) may prevent or relieve symptoms. Usually, a regional lymph node dissection is performed in these patients (if not done previously), since there is a substantial risk of nodal metastases. Amputation of an extremity is rarely indicated, and then only when other treatments have failed and the patient is quite symptomatic.

2. *Isolated limb perfusion.* This is probably the treatment of choice for most patients with intransit metastases involving an extremity (see Chap. 10 for details). Sometimes dramatic results can occur, as illustrated in Figures 7-18 and 7-19, both in terms of local disease control and prolongation of life.

3. *Regional chemotherapy infusion.* Intra-arterial infusion of DTIC or cis-platinum can reduce tumor burden in occasional patients.[12,21,56] It may be considered for extremity lesions if isolated limb perfusion has previously failed, or if it is unavailable. Partial response rates of 40% to 50% have been reported, but the duration of the responses was short.

    A new and novel approach for metastastic melanoma involving an extremity is the use of regional chemotherapy with Adriamycin in a limb in which circulation is temporarily occluded for 5 minutes with a proximal tourniquet.[38] Good results have been obtained in some patients in preliminary studies, especially if grossly detectable tumor can be excised, but the local toxicity is high.

4. *Radiation therapy.* This can be an effective means of controlling intransit metastases and is used especially for multiple lesions involving the trunk or head and neck area. Radiation therapy is sometimes recommended as adjuvant treatment

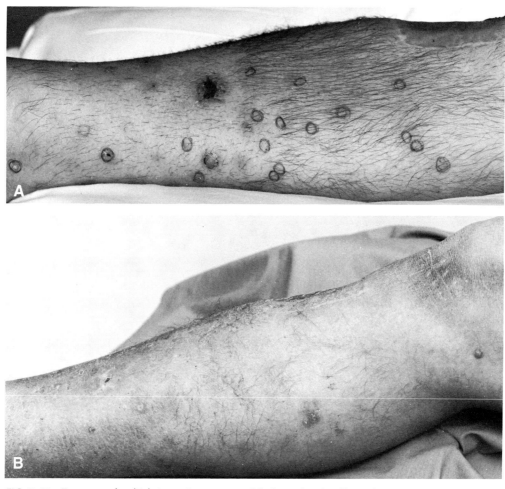

FIG. 7–18 Treatment of multiple intransit metastases of the leg with isolated hyperthermic limb perfusion at UAB. *(A)* Pretreatment photograph showing numerous subcutaneous and cutaneous nodules of the lower leg. *(B)* Three months later, there was complete regression of all lesions. The patient has remained in remission for one year.

for the anatomical region where solitary intransit metastases occurred sequentially on repeated occasions. The dose schedules are described in Chapter 14. Some centers have reported success in combining radiation therapy with hyperthermia for treating these lesions.[39,43,52]

5. *Intralesional immunotherapy.* Some of the first successful treatments using nonspecific immunotherapy were for intransit metastases. It has been administered as intralesional injections using a variety of agents, including BCG, vaccinia virus, DNCB, or other agents.[36,51,58] An example of a successful treatment is shown in Figure 7-20.

6. *Cryotherapy.* This may be considered in occasional patients, especially when other treatments have failed, or in elderly patients where the risk of operative intervention is high (Fig. 7-21). It is particularly effective if the metastases arise within or just below the epithelium.

7. *Systemic chemotherapy.* In most instances, systemic DTIC chemotherapy (alone or in combination) offers little success for controlling intransit metastases. Nevertheless, tumor growth can be temporarily arrested in an occasional patient, but usually for only a few months. It may be considered for multiple lesions, especially if

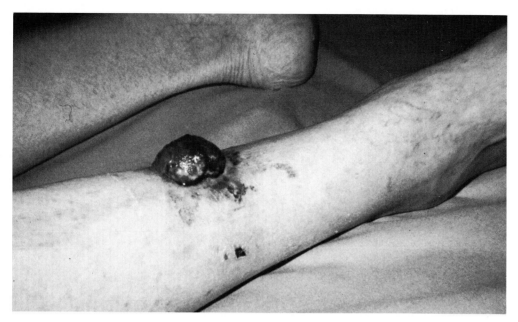

FIG. 7–19   This 78-year-old woman presented at UAB with a 17 mm polypoid melanoma of right lower leg. Within six months, she developed three subcutaneous intransit metastases of the thigh, each within a 4-week period. She underwent hyperthermic limb perfusion and still has no evidence of metastatic disease five years after treatment for multiple intransit metastases.

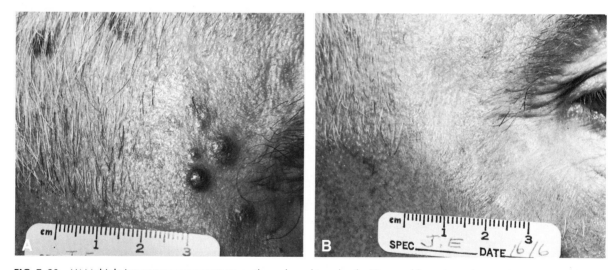

FIG. 7–20   (A) Multiple intracutaneous metastases on the scalp and temple of a 58-year-old man treated at SMU. The patient was treated with multiple vaccinia inoculations into each tumor at one session under a short general anesthetic. (B) Thirteen months later, the tumors had completely disappeared. The patient died one year thereafter from a cerebral metastatic melanoma.

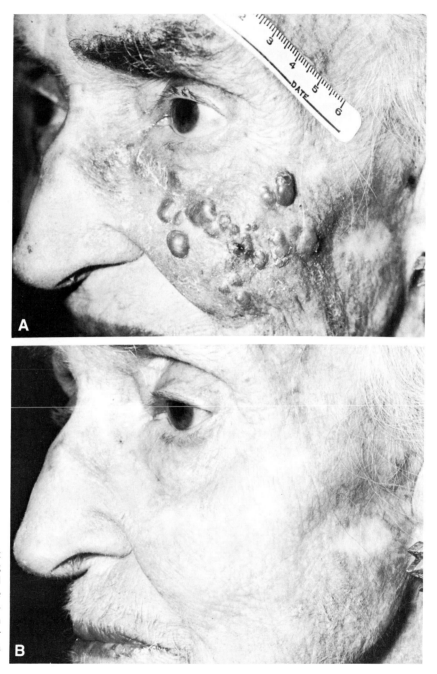

FIG. 7–21 *(A)* Extensive intransit metastases of a melanoma involving the left cheek of an 85-year-old woman treated at SMU. These were treated by weekly cryotherapy sessions. *(B)* The same patient, seven months later. Twelve months after the first treatment, she died from a cerebral hemorrhage.

symptomatic and if some of the other treatment alternatives described above cannot be used or have previously failed.

In summary, the treatment approach for intransit metastases must be individualized, but some form of aggressive regional treatment is best. The long-term results of treatment are not good in most series, since the majority of patients eventually develop systemic metastases. The median survival rate ranges from 19 months to 42 months.[22,27,36,55,58]

The best long-term results occur in patients treated with regional chemotherapy and hyper-

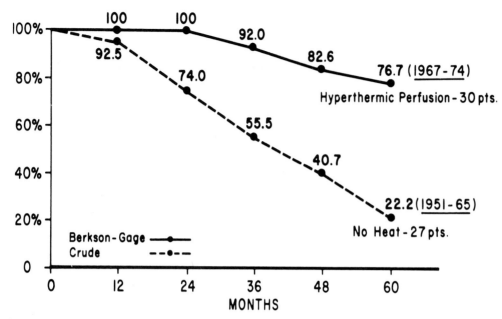

FIG. 7–22   Retrospective comparison of survival rates for patients with intransit metastases treated with and without hyperthermic limb perfusion (Stehlin JS Jr, et al: Results of hyperthermic perfusion for melanoma of the extremities. *Surg Gynec Obstet* 140:339, 1975).

thermia, using the isolated limb perfusion technique. There is a paucity of comparative data, except for a retrospective comparison by Stehlin and colleagues (Fig. 7-22).[62] One of the best series was reported by Krementz and colleagues, who obtained a 28% 15-year survival in 161 patients with intransit metastases treated by isolated limb perfusion, 54% of whom also had nodal metastases (see Chap. 10). These excellent results warrant a strong recommendation for limb perfusion as the treatment of choice for intransit metastases involving the extremities.

REFERENCES

1. Ames FC, Sugarbaker EV, Ballantyne AJ: Analysis of survival and disease control in stage I melanoma of the head and neck. Am J Surg 132:484, 1976
2. Arbeit JM, Lowry SF, Line BR, Jones DC, Brennan MF: Deep venous thromboembolism in patients undergoing inguinal lymph node dissection for melanoma. Ann Surg 194:648, 1981
3. Bakamjian VY, Miller SH, Poole AG: A technique for radical dissection of the neck. Surg Gynecol Obstet 144:419, 1977
4. Balch CM, Soong S–j, Murad TM, Ingalls AL, Maddox WA: A multifactorial analysis of melanoma. III. Prognostic factors in melanoma patients with lymph node metastases (stage II). Ann Surg 194:377, 1981
5. Beahrs OH: Surgical anatomy and technique of radical neck dissection. Surg Clin North Am 57:663, 1977
6. Beahrs OH, Adson MA: The surgical anatomy and techniques of parotidectomy. Am J Surg 95:885, 1958
7. Beahrs OH, Gossel JD, Hollinshead WH: Technique and surgical anatomy of radical neck dissection. Am J Surg 90:490, 1955
8. Becker GD, Parell GJ: Technique of preserving the spinal accessory nerve during radical neck dissection. Laryngoscope 89:827, 1979
9. Bland KI, Klamer TW, Polk HC Jr, Knutson CO: Isolated regional lymph node dissection: Morbidity, mortality and economic considerations. Ann Surg 193:372, 1981
10. Bocca E, Pagnataro O: A conservative technique in radical neck dissection. Ann Otol Rhinol Laryngol 76:975, 1967
11. Calearo CV, Teatini G: Functional neck dissection: Anatomical grounds, surgical technique, clinical observations. Ann Otol Rhinol Laryngol 92:215, 1983
12. Calvo DB III, Patt YZ, Wallace S, Chuang VP, Benjamin RS, Pritchard JD, Hersh EM, Bodey GP, Mavligit GM: Phase I-II trial of percutaneous intra-arterial cis-diamminedichloro platinum (II) for regionally confined malignancy. Cancer 45:1278, 1980
13. Chretien PB, Ketcham AS, Hoye RC, Sample WF: Axillary dissection with preservation of the pectoralis major muscle. Ann Surg 173:554, 1971

14. Cohen MH, Schour L, Felix EL, Bernstein AD, Chretien PB, Rosenberg SA, Ketcham AS: Staging laparotomy in the treatment of metastatic melanoma of the lower extremities. Ann Surg 182:710, 1975

15. Crile GW: Excision of cancer of the head and neck, with special reference to the plan of dissection based upon 132 operations. JAMA 47:1780, 1906

16. Das Gupta TK: Radical groin dissection. Surg Gynecol Obstet 129:1275, 1969

17. Das Gupta TK: Results of treatment of 269 patients with primary cutaneous melanoma: A five-year prospective study. Ann Surg 186:201, 1977

18. Das Gupta T, McNeer G: The incidence of metastasis to accessible lymph nodes from melanoma of the trunk and extremities—its therapeutic significance. Cancer 17:897, 1964

19. Dasmahapatra KS, Karakousis CP: Therapeutic groin dissection in malignant melanoma. Surg Gynecol Obstet 156:21, 1983

20. Dunn EJ, Kent T, Hines J, Cohn I Jr: Parotid neoplasms: A report of 250 cases and review of the literature. Ann Surg 184:500, 1976

21. Einhorn LH, McBride CM, Luce JK, Caoili E, Gottlieb JA: Intra-arterial infusion therapy with 5-(3,3-dimethyl-1-triazeno) imidazone-4-carboxamide (NSC-45388) for malignant melanoma. Cancer 32:749, 1973

22. Elias EG, Didolkar MS, Goel IP, Formeister JF, Valenzuela LA, Pickren JL, Moore RH: A clinicopathologic study of prognostic factors in cutaneous malignant melanoma. Surg Gynecol Obstet 144:327, 1977

23. Finck SJ, Giuliano AE, Mann BD, Morton DL: Results of ilioinguinal dissection for stage II melanoma. Ann Surg 196:180, 1982

24. Fisher SR, Cole TB, Seigler HF: Application of posterior neck dissection in treating malignant melanoma of the posterior scalp. Laryngoscope 93:760, 1983

25. Fortner JG, Booher RJ, Pack GT: Results of groin dissection for malignant melanoma in 220 patients. Surgery 55:485, 1964

26. Fortner JG, Schottenfeld D, Maclean BJ: En bloc resection of primary melanoma with regional lymph node dissection. Arch Surg 110:674, 1975

27. Fortner JG, Strong EW, Mulcare RJ, Schottenfeld D, Maclean BJ: The surgical treatment of recurrent melanoma. Surg Clin North Am 54:865, 1974

28. Goldsmith HS, Shah JP, Kim D-H: Prognostic significance of lymph node dissection in the treatment of malignant melanoma. Cancer 26:606, 1970

29. Haagensen CD, Feind CR, Herter FP, Slanetz CA Jr, Weinberg JA (eds): The Lymphatics in Cancer. Philadelphia, WB Saunders, 1972

30. Harris MN, Gumport SL, Berman IR, Bernard RW: Ilioinguinal lymph node dissection for melanoma. Surg Gynecol Obstet 136:33, 1973

31. Harris MN, Gumport SL, Maiwandi H: Axillary lymph node dissection for melanoma. Surg Gynecol Obstet 135:936, 1972

32. Holmes EC, Moseley HS, Morton DL, Clark W, Robinson D, Urist MM: A rational approach to the surgical management of melanoma. Ann Surg 186:481, 1977

33. James JH: Lymphoedema following ilio-inguinal lymph node dissection. Scand J Plast Reconstr Surg 16:167, 1982

34. Jesse RH, Ballantyne AJ, Larson D: Radical or modified neck dissection: A therapeutic dilemma. Am J. Surg 136:516, 1978

35. Karakousis CP: Ilioinguinal lymph node dissection. Am J Surg 141:299, 1981

36. Karakousis CP, Choe KJ, Holyoke ED: Biologic behavior and treatment of intransit metastasis of melanoma. Surg Gynecol Obstet 150:29, 1980

37. Karakousis CP, Heiser MA, Moore RH: Lymphedema after groin dissection. Am J Surg 145:205, 1983

38. Karakousis CP, Rao U, Holtermann OA, Kanter PM, Holyoke ED: Tourniquet infusion chemotherapy in extremities with malignant lesions. Surg Gynecol Obstet 149:481, 1979

39. Kim JH, Hahn EW, Ahmed SA: Combination hyperthermia and radiation therapy for malignant melanoma. Cancer 50:478, 1982

40. Lee Y-TN: Diagnosis, treatment and prognosis of early melanoma: The importance of depth of microinvasion. Ann Surg 191:87, 1980

41. Lingeman RE, Helmus C, Stephens R, Ulm J: Neck dissection: Radical or conservative. Ann Otol Rhinol Laryngol 86:737, 1977

42. Lotze MT, Duncan MA, Gerber LH, Woltering EA, Rosenberg SA: Early versus delayed shoulder motion following axillary dissection: A randomized prospective study. Ann Surg 193:288, 1981

43. Luk KH, Francis ME, Perez CA, Johnson RJ: Radiation therapy and hyperthermia in the treatment of superficial lesions: Preliminary analysis: Treatment efficacy, and reactions of skin, tissues subcutaneous. Radiation Therapy Oncology Group Phase I-II Protocol 78-06. Am J Clin Oncol (CCT) 6:399, 1983

44. McCarthy JG, Haagensen CD, Herter FP: The role of groin dissection in the management of melanoma of the lower extremity. Ann Surg 179:156, 1974

45. Martin H: Operations for parotid tumors. In Martin H (ed): Surgery of Head and Neck Tumors, pp 321. New York, Hoeber-Harper, 1957

46. Martin HE, Del Balle B, Ehrlich H, Cahan WG: Neck dissection. Cancer 4:441, 1951

47. Milton GW, Shaw HM, Farago GA, McCarthy WH: Tumour thickness and the site and time of first recurrence in cutaneous malignant melanoma (stage I). Br J Surg 67:543, 1980

48. Milton GW, Williams AEJ, Bryant DH: Radical dissection of the inguinal and iliac lymph-nodes for malignant melanoma of the leg. Br J Surg 55:641, 1968

49. Moore GE, Gerner RE: Malignant melanoma. Surg Gynecol Obstet 132:427, 1971

50. Moosman DA: Anatomy of the pectoral nerves and

their preservation in modified mastectomy. Am J Surg 139:883, 1980

51. Morton DL, Eilber FR, Holmes EC, Hunt JS, Ketcham AS, Silverstein MJ, Sparks FC: BCG immunotherapy of malignant melanoma: Summary of a seven-year experience. Ann Surg 180:635, 1974

52. Overgaard J: Fractionated radiation and hyperthermia: Experimental and clinical studies. Cancer· 48:1116, 1981

53. Papachristou D, Fortner JG: Comparison of lymphedema following incontinuity and discontinuity groin dissection. Ann Surg 185:13, 1977

54. Powell ME, Clairmont AA: Complications of parotidectomy. South Med J 76:1109, 1983

55. Roses DF, Harris MN, Rigel D, Carrey Z, Friedman R, Kopf AW: Local and intransit metastases following definitive excision for primary cutaneous malignant melanoma. Ann Surg 198:65, 1983

56. Savlov ED, Hall TC, Oberfield RA: Intra-arterial therapy of melanoma with dimethyl triazeno imidazole carboxamide (NSC-45388). Cancer 28:1161, 1971

57. Schuller DE, Reiches NA, Hamaker RC, Lingeman RE, Weisberger EC, Suen JY, Conley JJ, Kelly DR, Miglets AW: Analysis of disability resulting from treatment including radical neck dissection or modified neck dissection. Head Neck Surg 6:551, 1983

58. Shingleton WW, Seigler HF, Stocks LH, Downs RW Jr: Management of recurrent melanoma of the extremity. Cancer 35:574, 1975

59. Sim FH, Taylor WF, Ivins JC, Pritchard DJ, Soule EH: A prospective randomized study of the efficacy of routine elective lymphadenectomy in management of malignant melanoma: Preliminary results. Cancer 41:948, 1978

60. Smith TJ, Sloan GM, Baker AR: Epitrochlear node involvement in melanoma of the upper extremity. Cancer 51:756, 1983

61. Stehlin JS Jr, Clark RL: Melanoma of the extremities: Experiences with conventional treatment and perfusion in 339 cases. Am J Surg 110:366, 1965

62. Stehlin JS Jr, Giovanella BC, de Ipolyi PD, Muenz LR, Anderson RF: Results of hyperthermic perfusion for melanoma of the extremities. Surg Gynecol Obstet 140:339, 1975

63. Stehlin JS Jr, Smith JL Jr, Jing B, Sherrin D: Melanomas of the extremities complicated by in-transit metastases. Surg Gynecol Obstet 122:3, 1966

64. Storm FK, Eilber FR, Sparks FC, Morton DL: A prospective study of parotid metastases from head and neck cancer. Am J Surg 134:115, 1977

65. Suen JY, Wetmore SJ: Cancers of the neck. In Suen JY, Myers EN (eds): Cancers of the Head and Neck, pp 185. New York, Churchill-Livingston, 1981

66. Sutherland CM, Mather FJ, Krementz ET: Factors influencing survival among patients with regional melanoma treated by regional perfusion. Submitted for publication, 1984

67. Treidman L, McNeer G: Prognosis with local metastasis and recurrence in malignant melanoma. Ann NY Acad Sci 100:123, 1963

68. Urist MM, Maddox WA, Kennedy JE, Balch CM: Patient risk factors and surgical morbidity after regional lymphadenectomy in 204 melanoma patients. Cancer 51:2152, 1983

69. Veronesi U, Adamus J, Bandiera DC, Brennhovd IO, Caceres E, Cascinelli N, Claudio F, Ikonopisov RL, Javorskj VV, Kirov S, Kulakowski A, Lacour J, Lejeune F, Mechl Z, Morabito A, Rodé I, Sergeev S, van Slooten E, Szczygiel K, Trapenznikov NN, Wagner RI: Inefficacy of immediate node dissection in stage I melanoma of the limbs. N Engl J Med 297:627, 1977

70. Wander JV, Chaudhuri PK: Dissection of the posterior part of the neck. Surg Gynecol Obstet 143:97, 1976

71. Woods JE: Parotidectomy: Points of technique for brief and safe operation. Am J Surg 145:678, 1983

72. Woods JE: The facial nerve in parotid malignancy. Am J Surg 146:493, 1983

73. Yonemoto RH, Thompson WC, Byron RL, Riihimaki DU: Complete axillary node dissection with preservation of the pectoralis major muscle. Arch Surg 102:578, 1971

CHARLES M. BALCH
NATALE CASCINELLI
GERALD W. MILTON
FRANKLIN H. SIM

Elective Lymph Node Dissection: Pros and Cons

8

Since the regional lymph nodes are the most common site of metastases, considerable attention has been focused on their management. Surgical excision of these metastatic nodes is the only effective treatment for either cure or local disease control. Some surgeons prefer to excise only clinically demonstrable metastatic nodes. This has been termed a therapeutic or delayed lymph node dissection (LND). Other surgeons choose to excise the nodes even when they appear normal because of the risk of occult or microscopic metastases. This has been termed an elective lymph node dissection (ELND; also called an immediate LND, or a prophylactic LND).

The issue of ELND is probably one of the most important controversies in the management of patients with melanoma. It has been debated for several decades. There is unanimous opinion that not all melanoma patients need an ELND. Therefore, the current debate centers around two issues: (1) Is it possible to accurately identify a subgroup of melanoma patients with a high risk for microscopic regional node metastases? (2) What is the optimal timing of the operation (immediate versus delayed) even if such a high-risk group can be delineated? In this chapter, four experienced surgeons describe their respective positions (and supporting data) for and against ELND.

ELECTIVE LYMPH NODE DISSECTION IS OF BENEFIT IN SELECTED MELANOMA PATIENTS (C. M. BALCH AND G. W. MILTON)

RATIONALE FOR ELECTIVE LYMPH NODE DISSECTION

The potential benefit of ELND is based on a hypothesis that microscopic metastases may disseminate sequentially from the primary melanoma to the regional lymph nodes and then to distant sites. Therefore, survival will be increased if these nodal micrometastases are surgically excised before they progress to distant sites. Conversely, if the surgeon waits until the nodal metastases have progressed to a clinically palpable size, most patients will have distant metastases and, therefore, a lower probability of cure from a regional operation.

Thus, elective lymphadenectomy has the major theoretical advantage of definitive treatment given at a relatively early stage in the natural history of nodal metastases when the tumor burden is gener-

ally less than several million cells (Fig. 8-1*A*). It has the disadvantage that some patients may be subjected to an operation when they do not have metastases in the lymph nodes. Conversely, the advantage of delayed lymphadenectomy is that only patients with demonstrable metastases undergo a major operation. It has a great disadvantage in that treatment is delayed until the metastases are clinically palpable, when the tumor burden is much greater (*i.e.,* many billions of metastatic cells) (Fig. 8-1*B*). As a consequence, the chances for cure are diminished. Thus, by the time regional nodal metastases can be detected clinically, 70% to 85% of the patients will have distant micrometastases from which they will eventually die.[6]

Since the cure rate for a delayed LND is so poor (*i.e.,* 25% survival at 10 years), we advocate immediate excision of regional lymph nodes in selected patients to remove nodal micrometastases before they can disseminate to more distant sites. In this setting, the surgical decisions depend on knowing which prognostic factors can reliably identify those patients at risk for occult metastatic melanoma.

CHOOSING PATIENTS WHO MIGHT BENEFIT FROM ELECTIVE LYMPHADENECTOMY

Before defining risk factors for occult metastatic disease in melanoma patients with clinically normal lymph nodes (clinical stage I), it is important to categorize them biologically into three groups, each with a different surgical treatment approach: (1) those patients with melanoma localized to the primary lesion site; (2) those with local disease plus possible regional node micrometastases; and (3) those with local disease plus distant micrometastases, irrespective of whether they have nodal micrometastases as well. Intuitively, it is not too difficult to design a surgical strategy to excise the primary lesion site widely as the sole procedure in the first instance and to remove regional nodes containing microscopic or occult metastases in the second instance. However, regardless of the surgical treatment at the primary and regional sites, the survival for patients in the third category is dictated by the potentially lethal distant disease. In this instance, the goals of treating the regional nodes are either palliative (for local disease control) or for staging purposes.

To distinguish between these three categories, the use of tumor thickness provides a quantitative estimate of the risk for occult metastatic melanoma at regional and distant sites (Fig. 8-2). In fact, mela-

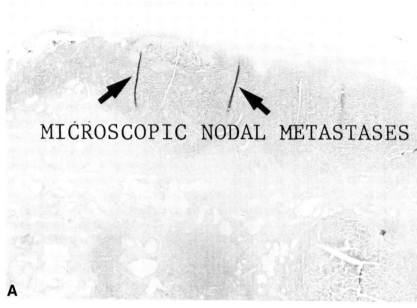

MICROSCOPIC NODAL METASTASES

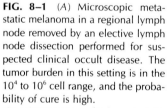

FIG. 8–1 (A) Microscopic metastatic melanoma in a regional lymph node removed by an elective lymph node dissection performed for suspected clinical occult disease. The tumor burden in this setting is in the 10^4 to 10^6 cell range, and the probability of cure is high.
(B) Microscopic multiple metastatic melanoma in regional lymph nodes removed by a therapeutic lymph node dissection for clinically palpable disease. The tumor burden in this setting exceeds 10^9 cells, and the probability of cure is low. (Balch CM, Urist MM: Melanoma: When to suspect metastases—and what to do. Your Patient and Cancer, p 33, June 1983)

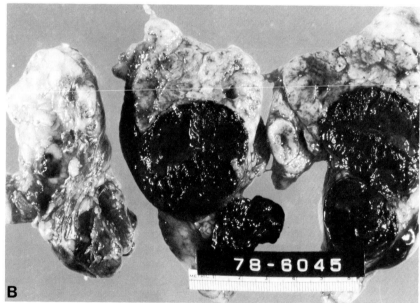

noma thickness is the most important but not the sole guide for selecting patients who might benefit from ELND.[2] The major advantage of using tumor thickness for these surgical decisions is that it can provide a quantitative estimate of the risk for occult metastatic melanoma in both regional and distant sites.[2,3,4,5,7] Thus, *thin melanomas* (<0.76 mm) are associated with localized disease and a 95% or

greater cure rate. An ELND would provide no therapeutic benefit in such patients. *Intermediate thickness melanomas* (0.76 mm–4 mm) have an increasing risk (up to 60%) of harboring occult regional metastases, but have a relatively low risk (less than 20%) of distant metastases (Fig. 8-2). Patients with these lesions might therefore benefit from an ELND.[2,4,5,22,28] *Thick melanomas* (≥ 4 mm) not only

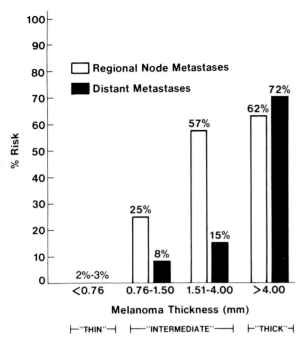

FIG. 8–2 Estimated biologic risk that microscopic metastases will become clinically evident in regional nodes (within 3 years) and at distant sites (within 5 years) for melanomas subgrouped by thickness categories (Balch CM: Surgical management of regional lymph nodes in cutaneous melanoma. J Am Acad Dermatol 3:511, 1980)

tremity melanomas have a more favorable outlook, while those with melanoma on the trunk or head and neck area have a higher risk of microscopic metastatic disease, even with equivalent tumor thicknesses. Extremity melanomas in women have the lowest biologic potential for metastatic melanoma compared to lesions of equivalent thickness on the extremities of men, while patients with melanomas located on the trunk or head and neck areas fare worse regardless of sex.[32] Finally, ulcerative melanomas have a higher risk for micrometastases than their nonulcerated counterparts, even when matched for other prognostic parameters such as tumor thickness.[1,4,20,28]

The growth pattern is also important to consider in this decision-making process. Lentigo maligna melanomas (LMM) have a low biologic risk for metastases (see Chaps. 3 and 19), so an elective node dissection is not recommended in these patients. The data described below and treatment recommendations specifically exclude lentigo maligna melanoma lesions.

A consideration of ELND is made selectively in patients according to the estimated risk of nodal metastases in regional lymph nodes and at distant sites. For women with extremity melanomas, ELND is not usually recommended unless the tumor thickness is at least 1.5 mm or more. Conversely, ELND is recommended more liberally for patients at higher risk, such as men with extremity melanomas or men or women with melanomas located on the trunk or head and neck area. A recommendation for ELND might be considered in these latter patients whose tumor thickness is as low as 1 mm. In patients with melanomas > 4 mm in thickness, the risk for distant microscopic metastases is so high that it negates any potentially curative benefit of a regional operation.

Tumor thickness should not be the sole criterion for making surgical treatment decisions. Other factors, such as the presence or absence of tumor ulceration, the patient's sex and age, the anatomical location of the melanoma, and the operative risk should all be considered when making the decision to perform ELND in any individual patient.

In order to integrate these factors for any individual patient setting, a mathematical model has been developed at UAB to predict the clinical outcome for the patient. This model uses the dominant prognostic factor to estimate the risk of regional and distant micrometastases for any given combination of factors (Table 8-1).

have a high risk of regional node micrometastases (greater than 60%), but also are associated with a high risk (greater than 70%) of occult distant disease at the time of initial presentation.[2,4,5] These patients do poorly, since the distant metastases in most instances negate the benefit of surgically excising the lymph nodes. The goal of treating these nodes is palliative, and the operation might be deferred until nodal metastases become clinically evident. Some surgeons prefer to perform an ELND in these patients as expectant palliation to avoid the probability (about 40%) of a second operation for lymph node metastases. An ELND might also be justified as a staging procedure in patients with thick melanomas to document the pathologic status of the lymph nodes prior to entry into clinical trials involving systemic adjuvant chemotherapy or immunotherapy.

The anatomical site of the melanoma is also an important criterion in predicting the risk for regional node micrometastases. Patients with ex-

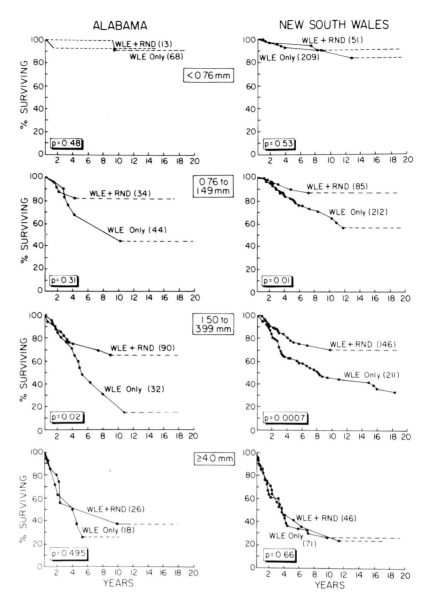

FIG. 8–3 Actuarial survival curves calculated over 20 years for clinical stage I melanoma patients subdivided by thickness subgroups and their initial surgical management (WLE ± ELND). The number of patients in each group is shown in *parenthesis. P* values were calculated for differences between each pair of survival curves. The benefit of ELND was greatest in patients with 1.50 to 3.99-mm-thick lesions. For 0.76 to 1.49-mm melanomas, the differences were significant only for the Australian patients. Note that the survival curves did not begin to diverge significantly until the fifth to eighth postoperative years. Patients with thin melanomas (<0.76 mm) and thick melanomas (≥4.00 mm) did not benefit from an ELND. (Balch CM, et al: A comparison of prognostic factors and surgical results in 1,786 patients with localized (stage I) melanoma treated in Alabama, USA, and New South Wales, Australia. Ann Surg 196:677, 1982).

IDENTIFYING THE REGIONAL LYMPH NODES AT RISK

Melanomas located on the extremity have a fairly predictable lymphatic drainage to the inguinal and axillary regional nodes. Those on the head and neck area are less predictable but usually drain to the ipsilateral cervical nodes. Melanoma located on the anterior scalp, face, and ear have lymphatic drainage to the parotid lymph nodes as well, while those on the posterior scalp can drain to occipital and retro-auricular nodes in addition to the cervical nodes. Lymphatic drainage crossing the midline is not uncommon. The same situation applies to trunk melanomas, when as many as four major nodal basins might be at risk depending on the location of the primary melanoma.

Melanomas located on the trunk and on the head and neck area can therefore have unpredictable lymphatic drainage, making it difficult for the surgeon to decide which nodal basin is at risk for

TABLE 8–1
ESTIMATED RISKS OF REGIONAL AND DISTANT MICROMETASTASES
IN CLINICAL STAGE I MELANOMA PATIENTS

Location of the Primary Melanoma	Risk of Occult Regional Metastases Only*	Risk of Occult Distant Metastases* (± Regional Metastases)
Female Extremity		
<0.76 mm	2%	1%
0.76 mm–1.49 mm	5%–7%	7%–10%
1.50 mm–3.99 mm	7%–19%	10%–24%
≥4.00 mm	0%	48%
Male Extremity		
<0.76 mm	2%	2%
0.76 mm–1.49 mm	22%–24%	22%–24%
1.50 mm–3.99 mm	24%–29%	24%–34%
≥4.00 mm	0%	70%
Female Axial		
<0.76 mm	8%	10%
0.76 mm–1.49 mm	14%–17%	21%–29%
1.50 mm–3.99 mm	17%–21%	29%–41%
≥4.00 mm	0%	60%
Male Axial		
<0.76 mm	9%	14%
0.76 mm–1.49 mm	27%–28%	29%–32%
1.50 mm–3.99 mm	28%–30%	32%–45%
≥4.00 mm	0%	79%

* Estimated risk for microscopic metastases at the time of initial diagnosis in patients with clinically localized cutaneous melanoma based on a mathematical model that did include ulceration as a factor (see Chap. 20 for details).

metastatic disease. In many of these patients, this problem has been surmounted by performing a radionuclide cutaneous scan that can accurately define the location of nodes that are the primary drainage for a melanoma located anywhere on the trunk (see Chap. 9).[21] Figure 8-4 illustrates a patient with lymphatic drainage from a trunk melanoma that was more widespread than predicted. Either all the regional nodes should be removed, or a policy of following multiple nodal sites at risk should be followed. An ELND of two nodal basins (*e.g.,* bilateral axillary dissection) for trunk melanomas may be warranted in very select instances, but removing more than two nodal basins or bilateral cervical dissection as an ELND is never indicated. A bilateral inguinal dissection is usually not performed electively because of its attendant morbidity, especially in edema of the extremities and genitalia.

SURGICAL TECHNIQUE AND COMPLICATIONS

With proper surgical judgment and technique, ELND can be performed in selected patients with minimal morbidity and virtually no mortality.[1,33]

When an ELND of the cervical nodes is planned, with or without the superficial parotid gland and nodes, a modified neck dissection is usually performed. This modified procedure spares the spinal accessory nerve and decreases the morbidity of shoulder function. The sternomastoid muscle, but not the jugular vein, is also spared in most cases. Partial cervical dissections are not generally performed, since it is difficult to define the pathways of nodal drainage to various parts of the neck precisely. When ELND is planned for melanomas located on the arm or upper trunk, a standard radical axillary lymphadenectomy is performed. The postoperative morbidity is extremely low (less than 5%). In patients undergoing ELND for leg or lower trunk melanomas, generally only the femoral nodes are excised (*i.e.,* a superficial inguinal dissection). The iliac nodes are spared to minimize the risk of significant leg edema. However, an iliac node dissection is recommended if there are demonstrable metastases to the femoral nodes at the time of ELND. Using this approach, the long-term operative morbidity is quite low, certainly at an acceptable level in patients with a life-threatening illness.[11,14,16,33] Details of the surgical technique and its complications are described in Chapter 7.

The ELND and the primary melanoma excision are performed under the same general anes-

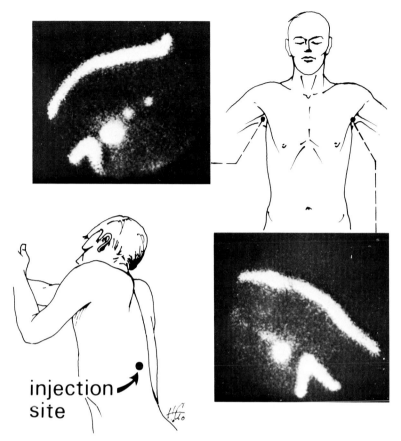

FIG. 8–4 A technetium 99m antimony cutaneous scan of a 3-mm melanoma located at the top of the scapula (8 cm from the midline). The cutaneous scan indicated bidirectional lymphatic drainage to both axillae (*inserts*). Although the patient had no axillary adenopathy, a single metastatic node was found in each axilla at the time of bilateral axillary lymphadenectomy.

thesia. Some surgeons have advocated a 4- to 6-week delay between these two procedures to prevent the trapping of melanoma cells in transit through the intervening lymphatics. The incidence of satellite or intransit metastases is so low (about 2%–5%) that the additional risk and expense of a second hospitalization and anesthesia do not warrant such a two-step approach. Also, it is impossible to predict the transit time in the lymphatics for metastatic melanoma.

RESULTS OF TREATMENT

Results of a prospective but nonrandomized trial involving 1319 patients treated at the SMU have demonstrated an improved survival rate with intermediate thickness melanomas ranging from 0.76 mm to 4 mm (see Fig. 8-3).[4,22] For patients with extremity melanomas, the benefit was greater in men than in women (Fig. 8-5). A similar analysis of 676 patients treated at UAB during the past 25 years also demonstrated a benefit for patients undergoing

ELND who have intermediate thickness melanomas ranging from 1.5 mm to 4 mm (Fig. 8-3).[4,5] Men had the same trends toward an improved survival rate in the 0.76-mm to 1.5-mm range, but this was not statistically significant, largely because the sample size was smaller. Data from the Duke Medical Center and the Memorial Sloan-Kettering Cancer Center also demonstrated an improved survival rate for intermediate thickness melanoma patients who undergo ELND.[28,38]

Patients with melanomas located on axial sites (trunk and head and neck) have a higher risk for metastases than do those patients with extremity melanomas (Table 8-1).[22] There have been no randomized prospective trials addressing ELND for axial melanomas. It is incorrect in our view to extrapolate the data from extremity melanomas and apply it to the treatment of patients with axial melanomas. The results from the UAB and SMU data demonstrate an improved survival rate for all patients with axial melanomas of intermediate thickness (0.76 mm–4 mm). The risk of regional node

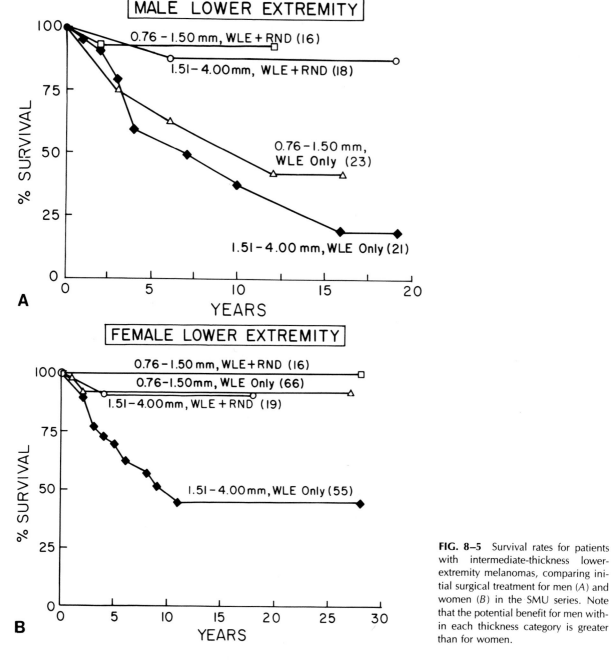

FIG. 8–5 Survival rates for patients with intermediate-thickness lower-extremity melanomas, comparing initial surgical treatment for men (A) and women (B) in the SMU series. Note that the potential benefit for men within each thickness category is greater than for women.

metastases is greater and the benefit of ELND is even more apparent in this patient group than in those with extremity melanomas (Table 8-2).[7,22,32] Hansen and McCarten,[15] in a retrospective analysis of 50 head and neck melanoma patients, also demonstrated an apparent improved survival rate for melanomas exceeding 1.5 mm in thickness.

It is important to emphasize the prolonged follow-up that is necessary in these patients to obtain a complete picture of the surgical results. In the UAB and SMU series, patients were continuing to die from metastatic disease 5 to 10 years after surgery that did not include an ELND. Figure 8-6 shows the conditional probability of dying from

TABLE 8–2
TEN-YEAR SURVIVAL RATES OF CLINICAL STAGE I MELANOMA PATIENTS TREATED AT THE SYDNEY MELANOMA UNIT AND THE UNIVERSITY OF ALABAMA IN BIRMINGHAM

Tumor Thickness	Extremity Melanomas			Trunk and Head and Neck Melanomas		
	WLE Only	WLE and RND	P Value	WLE Only	WLE and RND	P Value
<0.76 mm	94% ± 5% (n = 142)	100% ± 0% (n = 26)	0.230	86% ± 6% (n = 135)	83% ± 8% (n = 38)	0.343
0.76 mm–1.49 mm	74% ± 8% (n = 125)	92% ± 4% (n = 66)	0.042	56% ± 10% (n = 131)	80% ± 7% (n = 51)	0.049
1.50 mm–3.99 mm	54% ± 7% (n = 114)	80% ± 6% (n = 107)	0.005	33% ± 6% (n = 129)	64% ± 7% (n = 129)	0.0008
≥4.0 mm	30% ± 10% (n = 33)	44% ± 13% (n = 34)	0.400	22% ± 9% (n = 56)	26% ± 13% (n = 38)	0.806

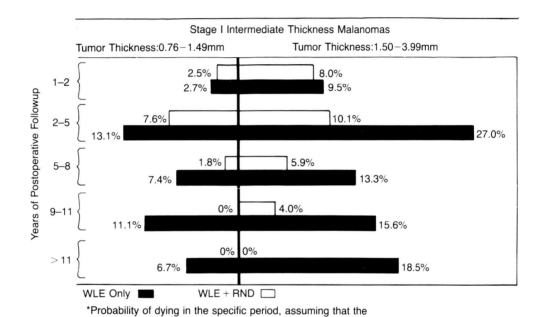

FIG. 8–6 The importance of long-term follow-up in melanoma patients is shown. The conditional probability of dying is shown for varying time periods ranging from 1 to 11 years or more. Patients who had a wide local excision as the initial surgical management for an intermediate-thickness melanoma (0.76 to 3.99 mm) were still at significant risk for dying, even if they were alive after 8 to 11 years. (Balch CM et al: A comparison of prognostic factors and surgical results in 1,786 patients with localized (stage I) melanoma treated in Alabama, USA, and New South Wales, Australia. Ann Surg 196:677, 1982).

disease for the intermediate thickness subgroup when it is subdivided by initial surgical treatment. For example, patients who initially had a wide local excision (WLE) only (*i.e.*, no ELND) and were clinically in remission after 8 years with a 1.5-mm to 3.99-mm melanoma still had a 15.6% risk of dying from metastases within the next 3 years, compared to only a 4% risk if they had had an ELND. Even 11 years after surgery, there was an 18.5% mortality

rate for the WLE group, while none died in the WLE plus ELND group.

OTHER CONSIDERATIONS

Some investigators have argued that the yield of metastatic lymph nodes is quite small in patients undergoing ELND. The proportion of patients with demonstrable metastatic disease who had surgically excised nodes ranges from 10% to 25% in different series.[13,14,31] Within thickness categories, this incidence ranged from less than 5% for melanomas <1.5 mm in thickness to 40% or greater with melanomas exceeding 3 mm in thickness.[3,38] One interpretation of these results is that the majority of patients have no metastatic disease in their nodes and are being overtreated with surgical excision. However, these figures significantly underestimate the actual incidence of nodal metastases, because micrometastases such as that shown in Figure 8-1A may have been present in unsampled areas of the specimen.

It would require multiple sections of each lymph node to be sure micrometastases were not present. A more accurate approach is to analyze the incidence of regional node metastases in a follow-up evaluation of patients treated initially by WLE alone. In a retrospective analysis of patients treated at UAB, those whose melanomas were >1.5 mm thick and who had WLE of their melanomas as their only initial surgical management had a 57% risk that nodal micrometastases would become clinically detectable within 3 years of diagnosis (see Fig. 8-2).[3] This is more than double the incidence of occult nodal metastases found by examining randomly sectioned lymph nodes in the surgical specimen after ELND. This is substantiated in part by the studies of Lane and colleagues[18] and Das Gupta,[11] who examined serial sections of nodes removed electively and found occult metastases in 42%.

Others have argued that ELND might result in entrapment of malignant cells in the lymphatics between the primary lesion site and the nodal basin. While this is indeed a possible risk, the incidence of satellitosis and intransit metastases should be quite low. Although earlier series have reported an incidence exceeding 20%, more recent results have shown a decreased incidence of this condition. In the UAB and SMU experience, the incidence of satellitosis is less than 5% and is not confined to patients undergoing ELND.

Finally, it has been stated that removal of regional lymph nodes may decrease the immunologic response to tumor antigens. Regional immunity has been shown to be important in some animal models,[12] while the opposite conclusion was reached in others. Pendergrast and colleagues, for example, reported that immune sensitization against tumor antigens occurred even if regional nodes were removed.[26] Certainly, decreased regional immunocompetence has not been demonstrated for any human tumor, including melanoma, after lymphadenectomy.

CONCLUSIONS

There is a benefit of ELND in selected patients with cutaneous melanoma of intermediate thickness (0.76 mm–4 mm). This is especially true for 1.5-mm to 4-mm melanomas, but more selectively for 0.76-mm to 1.5-mm lesions when ELND is confined to men with lesions on any anatomical site and women with axial melanomas. Patients with stage I LMM are excluded because of their lower biologic risk for metastases. Realizing that there may be some inherent selection bias in a nonrandomized clinical trial, we are participating in a randomized prospective analysis for intermediate thickness melanomas of all anatomical sites that has been activated by all the cooperative cancer groups in the United States and Canada (see below). The results of this and other trials should settle the debate, but it will take more than 10 years to complete the study and analyze the results.

REBUTTAL (N. CASCINELLI AND F. H. SIM)

Drs. Balch and Milton have outlined very nicely the pros and cons of routine ELND and provide support for their contention that ELND still has a role in patients with stage I melanoma. We agree that it is important to categorize patients biologically. However, studies from the World Health Organization (WHO) Melanoma Group have been unable to identify one or more criteria that accurately predict the pathway of metastatic dissemination (see the next section following Dr. Balch's and Dr. Milton's response). In particular, the tumor thickness does not identify any significant differences that distinguish patterns of metastases to the regional nodes alone versus those to distant sites. These results are in contrast to those described by Drs. Balch and Milton. One explanation might be that the WHO Melanoma Group patients were a uniform population of surgical patients who underwent wide excision alone, while the UAB and SMU patient series contained patients with both elective and delayed lymph node dissection. In other words, they underestimated the numbers of patients who developed simultaneous regional and distant metastases. Details of the WHO Melanoma Group experience are described below. Those patients who had a single metastatic node involved after a delayed (therapeutic) lymphadenectomy had a relatively good prognosis with a 44% 10-year survival rate. In contrast, those patients who had a single metastatic node after an elective lymph node dissection actually had a lower survival, being 28% at 10 years. Thus, there was no survival advantage in this subgroup of patients who underwent ELND.

Drs. Balch and Milton correctly indicate that trunk and head and neck melanomas have a worse prognosis, and they believe that melanomas arising in these anatomical sites may benefit from ELND. There is certainly no definite evidence for addressing the efficacy of ELND in axial melanomas, since no randomized prospective trials have been conducted. Such trials are now under way in two large studies (see the section on new randomized surgical trials, below). In the Mayo Clinic study, 20% of the lesions occurred on the trunk (excluding midline lesions), and there was no demonstrated benefit of ELND in this group as well. Until there is information to the contrary, we suggest a wide excision alone as the primary treatment for axial melanomas. This particularly applies to melanomas arising on the head, since it is quite difficult to accept a radical neck dissection as an elective procedure. Moreover, melanomas arising in the anterior portion of the scalp or the face have to include a superficial parotidectomy as well. Melanomas arising at these sites have ambiguous lymphatic drainage, and it is not possible to perform radionuclide cutaneous scans with any reliability.

The main disadvantage with routine ELND is that many patients will be subjected to unnecessary surgery. Moreover, one must consider the well-known morbidity from lymphadenectomy. While the incidence of intransit metastases has been reported to be as high as 20% following lymphadenectomy, the incidence at the Mayo Clinic is as low as that reported by the UAB and SMU. However, when this does occur, it is a serious problem and is associated with a grave prognosis.

We would also emphasize the need for prolonged follow-up to analyze a complete picture of the surgical results. Contrary to the observations of Drs. Balch and Milton, we have not observed significant differences in ultimate survival rates of patients undergoing WLE alone or with ELND. Thus, for the 43 patients in the WHO Melanoma Group trial who had WLE alone initially, 4 subsequently developed nodal metastases and died between the sixth and eighth year. This compares favorably with the results of 50 patients who underwent ELND, of whom 3 had positive nodes and died between the sixth and seventh year after their surgery. No patients in either treatment group died after 8 years.

As noted by Drs. Balch and Milton, there may be a difficulty in clinical assessment of the regional nodes, and ELND has been advocated in the past as a staging technique. However, in the Mayo study of

110 cases undergoing ELND, microscopy of serial sections revealed involvement in only four instances, and in this study, only 14% of those patients whose lymph nodes were observed subsequently developed regional node metastases (see below).

While the concept of selecting intermediate thickness melanomas for ELND is attractive, we have not been able to confirm this hypothesis in two randomized prospective studies that will be described below. Although the UAB and SMU data stem from a large series of patients that were critically analyzed by modern statistical methods, these data unfortunately have some of the same limitations as other uncontrolled and nonrandomized studies. In our view, the only criterion to decide whether or not to perform ELND is to select patients for this procedure who are unable to be maintained under regular follow-up. We recommend follow-up evaluations for at least 5 years. If the surgeon is uncertain that the patient will follow this plan, ELND may be considered for a melanoma thicker than 2 mm located on any side.

RESPONSE (C. M. BALCH AND G. W. MILTON)

Our statistical approach did take into account the subset of patients with distant plus regional metastases. Thus, the patients who had regional plus distant disease were counted the same as those who had distant metastases alone. The survival curves and incidence rates of nodal metastases were calculated for patients divided into two groups according to the initial surgical management (WLE alone or with ELND). Those patients who initially had WLE alone were followed as a single group, regardless of whether their relapse site was at regional nodes or a distant organ or whether they did not relapse at all. Thus, the statistical analysis was similar to the WHO Melanoma Group, since the surgical treatment groups were comparable.

Our patients who had clinically occult metastatic nodes (clinical stage I, pathologic stage II) had better results than those patients with clinically detectable nodal metastases (clinical stage II, pathologic stage II), even after matching for the number of metastatic nodes (see Chap. 19). It is important to emphasize that patients who may benefit from ELND are not just those with clinically occult nodal metastases, as detected by the pathologist. Those patients who have some nodal microscopic metastases not detectable by routine processing of lymph nodes may actually benefit to an even greater extent than those with pathologically detectable disease.

Thus, the incidence of nodal metastases is underestimated by using the figures from surgical pathology specimens after ELND.

Many comments have been made in the literature regarding the morbidity of ELND. However, in our experience and those of other major melanoma centers, the morbidity of ELND is quite low (see Chap. 7 for details). Moreover, there is some additional morbidity and cost involved in patients at high risk for nodal metastases who are subjected to two separate hospitalizations and operations (*i.e.,* WLE followed by a later lymph node dissection). Cutaneous scans can now be performed for head and neck melanomas with ambiguous drainage as described in Chapter 9. With regard to intransit metastases, the evidence in our patient series shows no correlation with ELND. In other words, patients who have a WLE alone have approximately the same incidence of intransit metastases as those who have an ELND as well.

In our opinion, the Mayo Clinic data on trunk melanomas are too limited to provide meaningful conclusions. There were only 34 patients altogether, only half of whom underwent ELND. Moreover, patients with tumors of all thicknesses were included, when only a subgroup of them would potentially benefit. The UAB and SMU analysis involving 707 patients with trunk and head and neck melanomas is shown in Table 8-2.

Finally, follow-up data of the UAB and SMU patients are different from that described for the WHO Melanoma Group. Patients who underwent WLE alone were still at risk of dying from their disease after 8 years, while those undergoing ELND had a very low rate of relapse after 8 years. This is an important issue because the survival rates were not substantially different in our series for the first 5 years, and the mortality rate in patients thereafter was significant only in the WLE alone group. Hopefully, the randomized clinical trials now in progress will be able to confirm whether this difference is real or only apparent.

DELAYED LYMPH NODE DISSECTION IS ACCEPTABLE TREATMENT IN PATIENTS WITH EXTREMITY MELANOMAS (N. CASCINELLI AND F. H. SIM)

LIMITATIONS OF RETROSPECTIVE STUDIES

Many retrospective studies have been published about ELND for stage I melanoma. The results have been conflicting, with both opponents and pro-

ponents citing considerable evidence to support each side of the issue.[10,13,14,19,23,24,27,30] The problems with retrospective studies and the spurious interpretation of results with selection bias are well known.[8] In fact, much of the enthusiasm for advocating ELND is based on retrospective studies. Several non-randomized but prospective surgical studies have attempted to overcome the disadvantages of retrospective analyses by using multifactorial analysis to examine the surgical results while simultaneously accounting for the influence of other factors. In three large series, patients with lesions of intermediate thickness had improved survival 8 to 10 years after ELND.[4,5,22,28]

Another limitation of analyzing data from patients undergoing ELND is that the results are not strictly comparable to clinical stage II lesions. That is, patients with clinical and pathologic stage II lesions constitute a selected group compared to patients being followed after WLE alone. The latter group may subsequently have surgery for regional metastases, or they may develop simultaneous regional node and distant metastases and not receive surgical treatment.

Because of the difficulty in evaluating treatment in retrospective studies, Ketcham and colleagues[17] stated that prospectively randomized clinical trials are needed to solve this problem: "If truly meaningful results are to be expected, a randomized, well-controlled prospective study that considers the histological criteria as well as the surgical treatment should be undertaken."

METASTASES DO NOT ALWAYS INVOLVE THE REGIONAL LYMPH NODES

The rationale for performing ELND is based on the assumption that melanoma metastasizes sequentially, first in the regional lymph nodes and later at distant sites after hematogenous dissemination. However, there is some evidence that metastatic spread does not always traverse the regional lymph nodes. Data from the WHO Melanoma Group Register showed that 44.3% of patients with stage I lesions (516 of 1164 patients) relapsed within 10 years of treatment; of these, 51% had their first recurrence in the regional lymph nodes, 22% relapsed first at a distant site, while 31% had simultaneous regional node and distant metastases.[9] This analysis was valid because it was comprised of only those patients who had a primary melanoma excision (*i.e.,* no ELND). If one includes patients who underwent ELND, the group of patients who develop regional node and distant metastases simultaneously is underestimated.

PROGNOSTIC FACTORS

A recent WHO Melanoma Group Study was made to identify subgroups of patients who might have a greater risk for regional node metastases.[9,34] Major prognostic factors such as sex, site of primary tumor, maximal tumor thickness, level of invasion, and ulceration were analyzed (Table 8-3). The percentage of men with regional node, distant metastases, or both was greater than that of women. The percentage of patients with regional node, distant metastases, or both was greater for those with ulceration and for those with tumors of increased thick-

ness, although none of the differences were statistically significant. Thus, these criteria identify those patients at risk for metastases but do not predict the site of first recurrence (*i.e.,* regional nodes or some distant site). A cross-tabulation was performed to evaluate the effectiveness of the combined use of ulceration and tumor thickness to predict the site of first recurrence more reliably. However, even this refinement did not delineate these two groups (Table 8-4).

RESULTS OF RANDOMIZED CLINICAL TRIALS INVOLVING ELND

Two prospective trials addressing ELND in stage I melanoma have been performed: an international

TABLE 8–3
DISTRIBUTION OF METASTASES IN 1164 CASES OF MELANOMA FROM THE WHO MELANOMA GROUP REGISTRY

Prognostic Criteria	Number of Patients	Metastases		
		Regional Node	Distant	Simultaneous Nodal and Distant
Sex				
Males	379	30%	21%	17%
Females	785	19%	8%	12%
Site				
Head and neck	250	19%	9%	14%
Extremities	572	22%	6%	13%
Trunk	332	28%	10%	15%
Maximal thickness (mm)				
≤1.5	148	14%	3%	6%
1.51–4.00	240	22%	8%	14%
≥4.01	130	34%	11%	15%
Ulceration				
Present	145	30%	12%	17%
Absent	358	20%	5%	10%

(Cascinelli N, Preda F, Vaglini M, et al: Metastatic spread of stage I melanoma of the skin. Tumori 69:449, 1983)

TABLE 8–4
DISTRIBUTION OF METASTASES FROM 373 CASES OF STAGE I MELANOMA SUBGROUPED BY THICKNESS AND ULCERATION (FROM THE WHO MELANOMA GROUP REGISTRY)

Ulceration	Maximal Thickness (mm)	Number of Patients	Metastases		
			Regional Node	Distant	Simultaneous Nodal Plus Distant
Absent	0.76–1.5	104	10%	11%	6%
	1.51–3.0	158	14%	14%	9%
Present	0.76–1.5	19	16%	11%	5%
	1.51–3.0	92	15%	27%	11%

(Cascinelli N, Preda F, Vaglini M, et al: Metastatic spread of stage I melanoma of the skin. Tumori 69:449, 1983)

cooperative study conducted by the WHO Melanoma Group[35,36,37] and one by surgeons at the Mayo Clinic.[29]

The WHO Melanoma Group study involved 553 patients with stage I primary melanoma in the distal two thirds of the limbs. Of these patients, 286 (52%) were randomized to receive WLE of the primary melanoma and node dissection if regional nodes became clinically detectable and 267 (48%) to receive WLE plus ELND. The two groups were matched according to the major prognostic criteria. No differences in survival were noted between the two groups (Fig. 8-7).

Because subgroups of patients may have benefited from ELND, survival was evaluated according to prognostic criteria: sex (Fig. 8-8), invasion levels III and IV (Fig. 8-9), tumor thickness (Fig. 8-10), and ulceration (Fig. 8-11). No significant survival differences were noted in any of these subgroups.

In 1979, it was reported that patients with intermediate tumor thickness (between 1.5 mm and 4 mm) benefited the most from elective node dissection.[3,5] Because of this finding, a multivariate analysis was performed in a subgroup of 114 melanoma patients from the WHO study with primary tumor thickness between 1.5 mm and 4 mm. Ulceration of the melanoma, as defined by histologic rather than clinical evaluation, was the only factor associated with survival. Other factors did not correlate with survival, including the initial surgical treatment

(WLE with or without ELND), sex, age, and maximal tumor diameter.

Surgeons at the Mayo Clinic conducted a clinical study between 1972 and 1976 in which 171 stage I melanoma patients were randomized into one of three treatment groups: (1) 62 patients had their nodes left intact; (2) 55 had ELND that was delayed 30 to 60 days after the primary melanoma excision; and (3) 54 had ELND concomitantly with the WLE. Patients with lesions of the head and neck and midline trunk were excluded. Characteristics of the patients in these three groups are listed in Table 8-5.

In this study, patients in the subgroup who did not have ELND were older, consisted of more men, and had worse prognostic features (*i.e.,* deeper invasion, thicker lesions, and more nodular lesions) than did the other two subgroups who underwent ELND. Patients in the subgroup with immediate ELND had more primary lesions involving the trunk than did the patients in other subgroups. None of these differences was statistically significant, although patients in the subgroup with intact nodes tended to have an unfavorable prognosis. Six characteristics were analyzed: initial surgical treatment, age, sex, anatomical subsite, tumor thickness, and growth pattern. The only factors that were significantly related to survival were tumor thickness ($p < 0.0001$) and growth pattern ($p = 0.02$).

None of the patients with levels II and III mela-

(*Text continues on page 149*)

FIG. 8–7 Survival of 553 patients with stage I melanoma (WHO Melanoma Group Study Trial #1), analyzed according to treatment. (Veronesi U et al: Delayed regional lymph node dissection in stage I melanoma of the skin of the lower extremities. Cancer 49:2420, 1982)

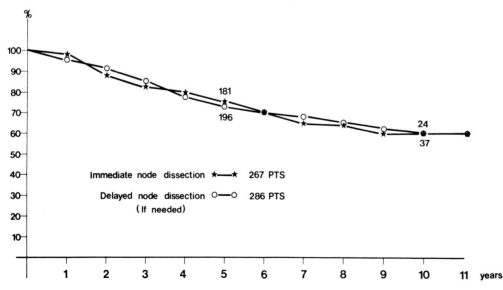

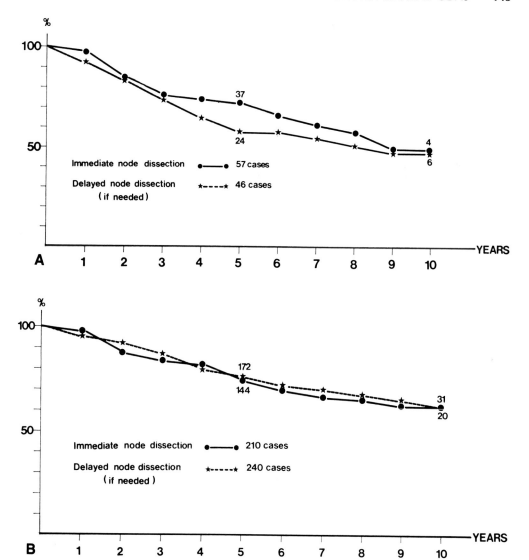

FIG. 8–8   Survival of 553 patients with stage I melanoma (WHO Melanoma Group Study Trial #1), analyzed according to treatment and sex. (*A*) Men. (*B*) Women. (Veronesi U et al: Stage I melanoma of the limbs: Immediate versus delayed node dissection. Tumori 66:373, 1980.)

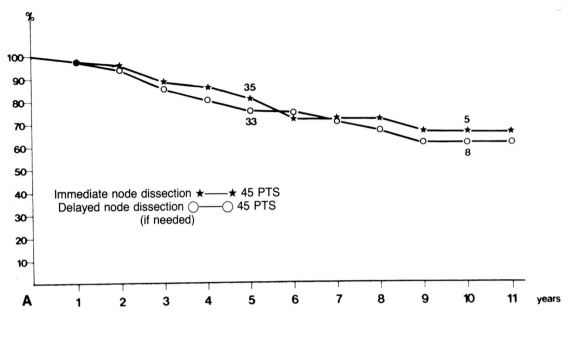

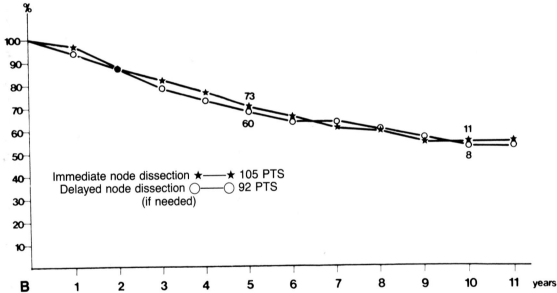

FIG. 8–9. Survival of 287 patients with stage I melanoma (WHO Melanoma Group Study Trial #1), analyzed according to treatment and level of invasion. (A) Level III. (B) Level IV. (Veronesi U et al: Delayed regional lymph node dissection in stage I melanoma of the skin of the lower extremities. Cancer 49:2420, 1982).

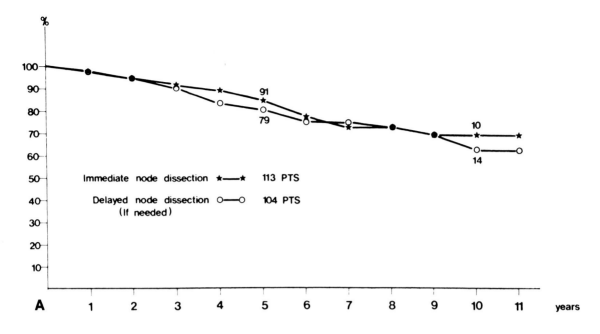

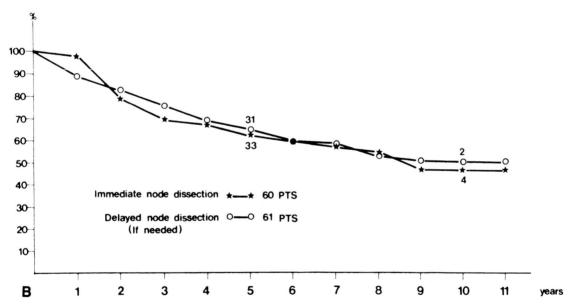

FIG. 8–10 Survival of 338 patients with stage I melanoma (WHO Melanoma Group Study Trial #1), analyzed according to treatment and tumor thickness: (A) <3.5 mm; (B) ≥3.5 mm. (Veronesi U et al: Delayed regional lymph node dissection in stage I melanoma of the skin of the lower extremities. Cancer 49:2420, 1982).

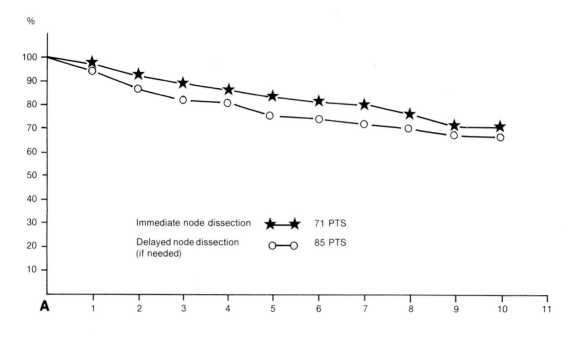

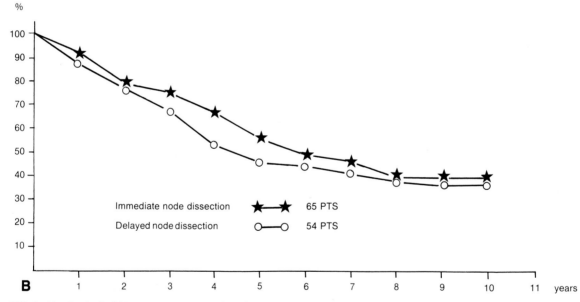

FIG. 8–11 Survival of 275 stage I patients with melanoma (WHO Melanoma Group Study Trial #1), analyzed according to treatment and ulceration. (*A*) Ulceration absent. (*B*) Ulceration present.

TABLE 8–5
PROSPECTIVE RANDOMIZED STUDY ON THE EFFICACY OF ELECTIVE
LYMPHADENECTOMY IN STAGE I MELANOMA: CLINICAL CHARACTERISTICS AND TREATMENT
(MAYO CLINIC, 1971–1976)

Characteristic	Number of Patients	Treatment—excision of nodes		
		None	Delayed	Immediate
Total patients	171	62	55	54
Mean age	171	50 yr	48 yr	46 yr
Males	59	39%	31%	33%
Site				
Distal extremity	83	36%	33%	31%
Proximal extremity	54	37%	33%	30%
Trunk (excluding				
midline)	34	19%	18%	22%
Invasion level				
II	30	23%	37%	40%
III	53	34%	36%	30%
IV	78	37%	32%	31%
V	3	100%	0%	0%
Unknown*	7			
Thickness (mm)				
≤ 0.76	51	25%	43%	31%
0.77–1.50	52	41%	37%	23%
1.51–2.99	28	29%	14%	57%
≥ 3.00	33	28%	17%	15%
Unknown	7			
Growth pattern				
Superficial spreading	105	29%	35%	36%
Nodular	50	42%	32%	26%
Lentigo	4	75%	25%	0%
Other and unknown	12			

* "Unknown" category excluded for determination of percentage.

nomas died, while 20 patients with levels IV and V melanomas died. The overall 5-year survival rate was 77%. In the subgroup of patients with levels IV and V melanomas, the 5-year survival rate was 52% if the thickness was 3 mm or more, while it was 79% for those with melanomas between 1.5 mm and 3 mm thick and more than 90% for those with lesions thinner than 1.5 mm. When data for all levels of invasion were combined, the patients with nodular involvement had a worse prognosis; however, the difference was not significant when the melanoma thickness was taken into account.

Because there was no recurrence of melanoma for levels II or III, only level IV and V lesions were considered in a Cox regression analysis. This analysis indicated that tumor thickness was the other important prognostic factor besides level of invasion when survival was calculated using death rates from melanoma from onset of metastasis (disease-free interval). Furthermore, the data revealed that both the increased thickness and the level of invasion

were important characteristics, and both must be considered.

Thus, although one might have expected a poorer survival in the patients with intact nodes, their survival rates were not significantly different from survival rates of patients in either of the two subgroups who had an ELND.

When overall survival and disease-free survival of the three surgical treatment groups were compared, there were no significant differences. The 5-year survival rate was 85% when the nodes were left intact, 85% when the nodes were removed immediately, and 91% if a delayed elective node dissection was performed. Survival and disease-free survival were significantly related to the thickness of the lesion (Figs. 8-12 and 8-13).

CONCLUSIONS

Both the Mayo Clinic and the WHO Melanoma Group studies indicated no benefit from routine

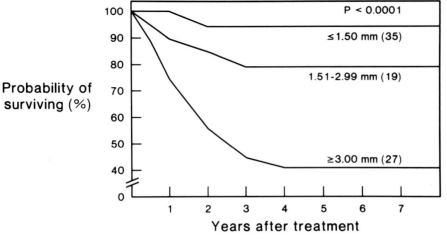

FIG. 8–12 Mayo Clinic randomized prospective study showing disease-free survival for all patients according to lesion thickness (for invasion levels IV and V).

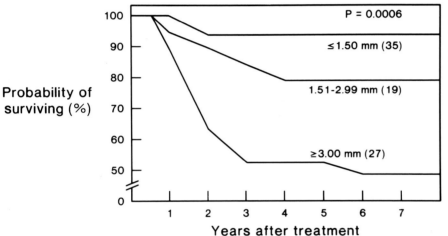

FIG. 8-13 Overall survival to death from melanoma for all patients from the Mayo Clinic study according to lesion thickness (invasion levels IV and V).

ELND for patients with stage I melanoma involving the extremities. After an average follow-up period of 10.4 years in the WHO Melanoma Group series, no differences between the two initial surgical treatments have been noted (WLE ± ELND). These conclusions are made with the proviso that the patients must be checked for nodal metastases every 3 months during the first 3 years after treatment.

Because no randomized studies have been performed involving patients with axial melanomas (trunk and head and neck), the efficacy of ELND for this group is unknown. However, there is no reason to believe that the results observed for melanoma involving the extremity cannot be extrapolated to melanoma of the trunk. This question must be addressed in a randomized clinical trial. Fortunately,

some of the limitations of defining ambiguous lymphatic drainage can now be more precisely defined. A recent study performed at the National Cancer Institute of Milan[25] showed that the site of regional spread is fairly predictable by clinical criteria, but the radionuclide cutaneous scan can more precisely indicate the site of primary drainage (see Chap. 9). For this reason, a randomized clinical trial was recently organized by the WHO Melanoma Group to evaluate the efficacy of ELND in patients with melanoma of the trunk (see the section on randomized surgical trials, below).

There are several reasons why immediate node dissection does not achieve better results than delayed dissection in stage I melanoma involving the extremities. One is that patients with occult nodal metastases have the same prognosis as patients with clinically palpable nodes, as determined by a WHO clinical trial (Fig. 8-14).[37]

Some authors claim that elective node dissection is necessary for staging purposes in order to identify the patients who might require adjuvant treatment. However, the prognosis of patients with stage I melanoma can be assessed by the histologic evaluation of the lesion (see Chap. 19). Moreover, there are presently no randomized trials showing an improvement in survival with adjuvant chemotherapy, immunotherapy, or a combination of the two (see Chap. 11).

There is clearly correlation in the incidence of nodal metastases and increasing thickness of the primary melanoma. This was found in the WHO Melanoma Group study, when the number of subsequent node dissections increased with tumor thickness. Patients with tumors >1.5 mm should therefore be especially closely followed.

Since preliminary analysis of the Mayo Clinic randomized study showed no significant benefit to the patient from immediate or delayed lymphadenectomy for lesions on the trunk and extremities, the current policy is to treat the regional nodes in these areas expectantly and perform a therapeutic dissection at the first clinical suspicion of nodal involvement. This early detection of clinically suspicious nodes may be an important factor in improving the outcome over that for patients who present late and have multiple nodes involved. Twelve of the 62 patients whose nodes were left intact subsequently required therapeutic lymphadenectomy; of this group, six were long-term survivors.

These data indicate that delayed node dissection is as effective as ELND in the control of extremity melanomas. This conclusion was valid regardless of the patient subgroups considered. Elective node dissection might be considered if the patient cannot be examined frequently within the first 3 years after operation. This is especially true in patients with melanomas ≥1.5 mm, when the risk of node metastases developing rapidly is high.

Whether regional lymph node dissection should be part of the primary operation for melanoma has been an area of legitimate concern. These two prospective randomized studies indicate no significant benefit to the patient from ELND for extremity melanomas. This judgment, reinforced by the finding that 103 of 110 patients in one series did not have detectable nodal metastases at ELND, and by the superimposed morbidity and well-known complications of this procedure, suggests that ELND is not indicated in the management of stage I melanoma. Despite these findings, the issue re-

FIG. 8–14   Survival of 118 patients from the WHO Melanoma Group Study comparing occult metastases at ELND ($N_o +$) with palpable metastases after WLE of primary melanoma. There is no difference between the two groups. (Veronesi U et al: Delayed regional lymph node dissection in stage I melanoma of the skin of the lower extremities. Cancer 49:2420, 1982).

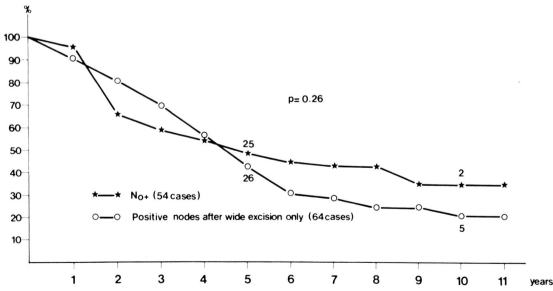

mains unsettled, especially since all anatomical sites of melanoma have not been studied and we cannot rule out a possible benefit in a small subgroup of patients. For these and other reasons, additional randomized prospective studies must be performed that are properly stratified and contain a large number of patients. Only in this way can treatment guidelines that can be agreed on be established.

REBUTTAL (C. M. BALCH AND G. W. MILTON)

The WHO Melanoma Group Trial and the Mayo Clinic Trial are both excellent studies performed by competent investigators. Clearly, not all patients with melanoma benefit from ELND, as demonstrated by these and other studies. However, we believe there are subgroups of patients who might benefit from ELND.

The WHO Melanoma Group was kind enough to share the original data of their surgical trial concerning ELND in stage I patients so that the data could be analyzed independently. They have conducted their analysis in a thorough and open manner and have reported results showing no detectable benefit of ELND. However, there are several aspects of the study that are pertinent to interpreting the results.

First, a multivariate analysis of 205 patients from the WHO Melanoma Group Trial, for whom all pathologic and clinical data were available, showed that tumor thickness and ulceration were the dominant prognostic variables ($p = 0.0006$ and 0.0086, respectively). Neither of these variables was known to be a significant prognostic variable at the time the trial was begun in 1970, so they were not included as stratification criteria. It is interesting to note that the tumor thickness subgroups were fairly equally divided among the two treatment arms; however, there was a marked maldistribution of patients with ulcerative lesions, with more intermediate thickness lesions (1.5 mm–4.9 mm) having ulceration in the ELND group than the WLE alone group (52% versus 19%).

Second, when low-, intermediate-, and high-risk groups were defined by simultaneously accounting for tumor thickness and ulceration (see Fig. 8-15), there was a small subgroup of patients with a 22% improved 10-year survival rate if they had had immediate lymph node dissection (Fig. 8-16). This subgroup of patients with intermediate-risk melanomas comprised less than 20% of the entire study population, and only half of these had had ELND. The potential benefit in this subgroup of

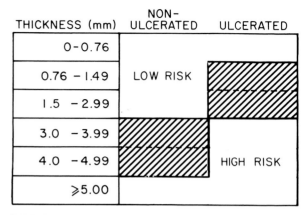

THICKNESS (mm)	NON-ULCERATED	ULCERATED
0 – 0.76		
0.76 – 1.49	LOW RISK	
1.5 – 2.99		
3.0 – 3.99		
4.0 – 4.99		HIGH RISK
⩾ 5.00		

▨▨▨ **INTERMEDIATE RISK**

FIG. 8–15   Three risk groups defined to integrate tumor thickness and ulceration for stage I melanomas involving the extremity. Melanomas with ulceration had a higher risk of metastases than nonulcerated lesions of equivalent thickness.

patients could easily be obscured with analysis of the entire data, especially when the presence of ulceration was not accounted for.

Third, there were some differences in the surgical treatment results when the data were subdivided by the country in which the patients resided. For example, the patients from one country appeared to have had some benefit from immediate node dissection, while patients with similar prognostic characteristics from another country had no benefit. It is possible that this may reflect some genetically determined differences in immunologic responses to melanoma antigens that resulted in different clinical courses of disease among ethnic groups.

Fourth, several participating centers had a high proportion of patients admitted into the study with histologically positive nodes who were clinical stage I (i.e., 25%–30% of all patients). This is three to four times the incidence in our own series as well as those reported elsewhere in the literature (i.e., 6%–8%). This raises the possibility that the clinical staging may not have been uniform from one investigator to another. If this is true, their results may have overestimated the actual proportion of patients with regional or distant metastases, since their patients may have had a higher stage of disease than those reported from UAB and SMU.

Fifth, patients in the WHO Melanoma Group trial who subsequently required a delayed lymph node dissection had only a 15% to 20% 10-year

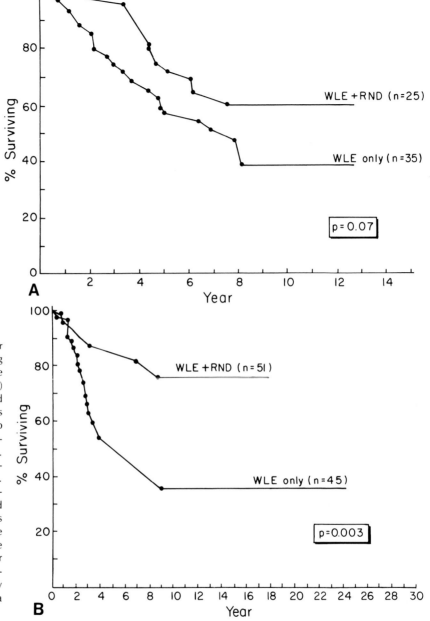

FIG. 8–16 Survival differences for the intermediate risk group comparing (A) initial surgical management in the WHO Melanoma Group Study and (B) the combined series from UAB and SMU. In the small subgroup of patients from the WHO Melanoma Group Trial, there appears to be a trend toward improved survival at 10 years. The P value is of borderline significance, but the sample size is small. These should be regarded as preliminary results that should be confirmed with a larger population of patients with equivalent prognostic factors. The differences in the treatment arms were highly significant in the larger number of patients from UAB and SMU, an observation that lessens the probability that the WHO Melanoma Group data were "false-positive" observations.

survival. This means that almost 75% of these patients had distant microscopic metastases by the time they had clinically evident disease at regional sites, a result that is similar to that of patients with clinical stage II disease at UAB and SMU (Fig. 8-17). We would suggest that immediate lymph node dissection removes these microscopic metasta-

ses trapped in regional lymph nodes before they can disseminate to distant sites.

The UAB and SMU patients with clinically negative but histologically positive nodes had a better survival rate than those with clinically palpable metastases (see Chap. 19, Fig. 19-10). Furthermore, there is clearly a group of patients with microscopic

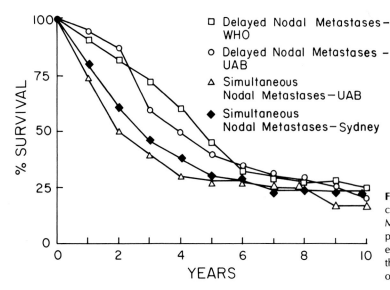

FIG. 8–17 Results of surgical treatment for clinical stage II patients from UAB, SMU, and the WHO Melanoma Group Study Trial. The vast majority of patients with clinically detectable nodal metastases eventually die of metastatic disease, regardless of the clinical setting (*i.e.*, synchronous or metachronous nodal metastases).

disease that is not detected by routine histologic sectioning of the lymph nodes. For example, in the WHO Melanoma Group study, the yield of clinically occult nodal metastases was 21% in patients with melanomas measuring 1.5 mm to 4.9 mm in thickness. However, in patients with equivalent thickness melanomas who had a wide excision alone, 56% subsequently required an LND for nodal metastases. Presumably then, some of the differences in the yield of nodal metastases (21% versus 56%) were because of occult disease in the surgical specimen that was not detected by the pathologist. The latter figure (56%) is more representative of the true risk for nodal metastases in the subgroup of patients with 1.5-mm to 4.9-mm melanomas.

Finally, extremity melanomas, especially in women, have the lowest biologic risk for metastases compared to melanomas located in any other site (see Chap. 19). About 85% of patients in the WHO Melanoma Group trial were women with extremity melanomas. It is not surprising, therefore, that greater differences were not found in such a relatively low-risk population of patients.

The Mayo Clinic surgical trial was also carefully conducted. But it should be pointed out that only a small group of stage I patients in this trial fits into the patient groups we have categorized as being at high risk for regional metastases but low risk for distant metastases at the time of initial diagnosis. Also, this trial did not consider ulceration of the melanoma, either as a stratification criterion or in analyzing treatment results.

In our opinion, there are still legitimate differences in interpreting results that can be resolved only by continuing to study this important question in randomized clinical trials using current stratification criteria and extending these studies to all anatomical sites.

RESPONSE (N. CASCINELLI AND F. H. SIM)

Drs. Balch and Milton's interpretation of the results of the WHO Melanoma Group and the Mayo Clinic trials are of interest, because it indicates how honest and open is the dialogue between serious investigators attempting to address this controversial issue. They correctly point out some of the limitations of the prospective randomized clinical trials that had been designed to answer this controversial question, which has been emotionally debated for decades.

The distribution of ulceration in the WHO Melanoma Group trial was the only one of multiple parameters that was unbalanced. Despite this situation, the analysis of the two treatment modalities is valid because they were allocated at random. The WHO multivariate analysis did not demonstrate any benefit of ELND even when the results were adjusted by ulceration and other prognostic criteria. While ulceration was not evaluated in the Mayo Clinic series, the multifactorial analysis indicated that tumor thickness was the most important prognostic indicator, and the two groups were balanced for this prognostic factor.

The Mayo Clinic study was criticized because it contained a large proportion of low-risk melanomas. However, careful analysis of the 91 patients with level IV and V melanomas measuring more than 1.5 mm in thickness indicated that there was no prognostic disadvantage for those patients who underwent WLE alone in this high-risk subgroup of patients. In the Mayo Clinic analysis of 36 patients with intermediate-thickness lesions, there was no benefit from ELND after 5 years of follow-up. However, the number of patients in this intermediate-thickness group is small, and as emphasized by Drs. Balch and Milton, their survival curves for the two surgical treatment arms did not begin to diverge significantly until after 6 or 7 years of follow-up.

The analysis of the WHO Melanoma Group data from Trial #1 that was performed by Drs. Soong and Balch suggested that a survival difference existed in a small group of patients subgrouped by thickness and ulceration. This may be a "false-positive" result in the range of a 5% alpha error. The potential danger of analyzing extremely small subgroups of patients must be emphasized.

While the differences in treatment results among different countries may be related to genetically determined characteristics, it may also be caused by the relatively limited numbers of patients treated in certain centers. Clinical staging may have been different among the various centers, but this variability should not have biased the results, since the randomization was performed within each center. For this reason, any differences in clinical staging criteria should be weighted to the same degree for each of the treatment arms in the study.

The early clinical detection of suspicious metastatic nodes may be an important factor in improving the outcome of therapeutic lymphadenectomy, compared to the situation in which patients present later in the course of their disease with multiple and large metastatic nodes. In the Mayo Clinic trial, those patients whose lymph nodes were initially left intact and were followed closely, there were 12 patients who later underwent a therapeutic lymphadenectomy, and 6 of these (50%) were alive at 5 years. The WHO Melanoma Group trial also emphasizes the importance of frequent follow-up of these patients.

The 20% 10-year survival rate for patients undergoing therapeutic lymphadenectomy is consistent with that reported in the literature. The hypothesis that removal of microscopic metastases at an earlier stage of disease was not supported by our data.

We certainly agree with Drs. Balch and Milton that there is still no clear consensus regarding optimal treatment and that the role of ELND is an important issue to resolve. We are optimistic that the randomized prospective studies now being conducted on large patient populations will settle this issue and allow the establishment of firm treatment guidelines. In our opinion, there is good evidence that delayed lymph node dissection is as effective as immediate LND in the control of stage I melanoma involving the extremity.

NEW RANDOMIZED SURGICAL TRIALS INVOLVING ELECTIVE LYMPHADENECTOMY

The melanoma patterns of care study described in Chapter 23 clearly demonstrates that there is no standard approach in the United States for selecting patients who should have ELND or those who should not. The available data are still too conflicting, and a clear consensus has not yet been reached. Continued clinical investigations are clearly warranted.

There are now two international cooperative surgical trials that address the efficacy of ELND in selected melanoma patients. One is being conducted under the auspices of the National Cancer Institute in Washington, D.C. (The Intergroup Melanoma Committee), while the second is being confined to trunk melanomas and is being conducted by the WHO Melanoma Group.

The Intergroup Melanoma Protocol includes only those patients who have intermediate-thickness melanomas (1 mm–4 mm) and who have no evidence of metastases in the regional lymph nodes or at distant sites as evidenced by a physical examination and laboratory tests. The four treatment arms for this randomized prospective trial are shown in Table 8-6. All patients with trunk melanomas will have a radionuclide cutaneous scan (as described in Chap. 9), and all nodal basins draining the primary melanoma must be excised if the patient is to be entered onto the study. Patients who have lymphatic drainage to more than two major basins or who have bilateral cervical lymph node drainage are ineligible. Patients will be stratified according to: (1) melanoma thickness (1 mm–2 mm, 2 mm–3 mm, 3 mm–4 mm); (2) location of the primary melanoma (proximal extremity versus trunk, or distal extremity versus head and neck); and (3) ulceration of the epidermis overlying the melanoma on microscopic sections.

TABLE 8–6
PROTOCOL DESIGN USED BY THE INTERGROUP MELANOMA STUDY FOR PATIENTS WITH INTERMEDIATE THICKNESS MELANOMAS (1–4 mm)*

Randomized Treatment Arm	Primary Excision Margin	Elective (Immediate) Lymphadenectomy
1	2 cm[†]	No
2	2 cm[†]	Yes
3	4 cm	No
4	4 cm	Yes

* All the major cooperative groups in the United States and the National Cancer Institute of Canada are participating in the study
[†] Patients with melanomas of the head and distal extremities will all have a 2 cm primary excision and then will be randomized into treatment arm 1 or 2

It is expected that up to 1700 patients will be necessary to complete this trial. Participating institutions include the Cancer and Leukemia Group B, Eastern Cooperative Oncology Group, the National Cancer Institute of Canada, Northern California Oncology Group, North Central Cancer Treatment Group, Southeastern Cancer Study Group, and the Southwest Oncology Group.

A second trial is being conducted by the WHO Melanoma Group in patients with clinically uninvolved regional lymph nodes and whose primary melanoma exceeds 2 mm in thickness and is located on the trunk. The primary tumor must be excised with a 3-cm margin of skin. The lymph node basin to be dissected excludes lesions within 2 cm of the midline (on a vertical axis) or Sappey's line (horizontal axis). A cutaneous scan is recommended but not required. Eligible patients will be randomized to receive either (1) WLE alone plus close follow-up and delayed lymph node dissection if necessary or (2) a WLE plus ELND. Patients will be stratified by the treatment center. All 17 member institutions of the WHO Melanoma Group are eligible to participate in this ongoing trial.

It is likely that the results of these two trials will add significant information about the role (if any) of ELND in selected melanoma patients. The results should be available within the decade. In the meantime, physicians treating melanoma will have to evaluate the currently available information as described in this chapter and make their best judgments about the management of regional lymph nodes in an individual patient setting.

REFERENCES

1. Balch CM: Surgical management of regional lymph nodes in cutaneous melanoma. J Am Acad Dermatol 3:511, 1980

2. Balch CM, Murad TM, Soong S-j, Ingalls AL, Halpern NB, Maddox WA: A multifactorial analysis of melanoma: Prognostic histopathological features comparing Clark's and Breslow's staging methods. Ann Surg 188:732, 1978

3. Balch CM, Murad TM, Soong S-j, Ingalls AL, Richards PC, Maddox WA: Tumor thickness as a guide to surgical management of clinical stage I melanoma patients. Cancer 43:883, 1979

4. Balch CM, Soong S-j, Milton GW, Shaw HM, McGovern VJ, Murad TM, McCarthy WH, Maddox WA: A comparison of prognostic factors and surgical results in 1,786 patients with localized (stage I) melanoma treated in Alabama, USA, and New South Wales, Australia. Ann Surg 196:677, 1982

5. Balch CM, Soong S-j, Murad TM, Ingalls AL, Maddox WA: A multifactorial analysis of melanoma. II. Prognostic factors in patients with stage I (localized) melanoma. Surgery 86:343, 1979

6. Balch CM, Soong S-j, Murad TM, Ingalls AL, Maddox WA: A multifactorial analysis of melanoma. III. Prognostic factors in melanoma patients with lymph node metastases (stage II). Ann Surg 193:377, 1981

7. Balch CM, Urist MM: Melanoma: When to suspect metastases—and what to do. Your Patient and Cancer, p. 33, June 1983

8. Breslow A: Editorial. Surgical pros and cons. Surg Gynecol Obstet 149:731, 1979

9. Cascinelli N, Preda F, Vaglini M, Orefice S, Bufalino R, Morabito A, Nava M, Santinami M: Metastatic spread of stage I melanoma of the skin. Tumori 69:449, 1983

10. Conrad FG: Treatment of malignant melanoma: Wide excision alone vs lymphadenectomy. Arch Surg 104:587, 1972

11. Das Gupta TK: Results of treatment of 269 patients with primary cutaneous melanoma: A five-year prospective study. Ann Surg 186:201, 1977

12. Fisher B, Saffer E, Fisher ER: Studies concerning the regional lymph node in cancer. IV. Tumor inhibition by regional lymph node cells. Cancer 33:631, 1974

13. Goldsmith HS, Shah JP, Kim DH: Prognostic significance of lymph node dissection in the treatment of malignant melanoma. Cancer 26:606, 1970

14. Gumport SL, Harris MN: Results of regional lymph node dissection for melanoma. Ann Surg 179:105, 1974

15. Hansen MG, McCarten AB: Tumor thickness and lymphocytic infiltration in malignant melanoma of the head and neck. Am J Surg 128:557, 1974

16. Holmes EC, Moseley HS, Morton DL, Clark W, Robinson D, Urist MM: A rational approach to the surgical management of melanoma. Ann Surg 186:481, 1977

17. Ketcham AS, Lawrence W Jr, Pilch YH, Rogers CE: Symposium on melanoma. Contemp Surg 2:87, 1973

18. Lane N, Lattes R, Malm J: Clinicopathological correlations in a series of 117 malignant melanomas of the skin of adults. Cancer 11:1025, 1958

19. McCarthy JG, Haagensen CD, Herter FP: The role of groin dissection in the management of melanoma of the lower extremity. Ann Surg 179:156, 1974

20. McGovern VJ, Shaw HM, Milton GW, McCarthy WH: Ulceration and prognosis in cutaneous malignant melanoma. Histopathology 6:399, 1982

21. Meyer CM, Lecklitner ML, Logic JR, Balch CM, Bessey PQ, Tauxe WN: Technetium-99m sulfurcolloid cutaneous lymphoscintigraphy in the management of truncal melanoma. Radiology 131:205, 1979

22. Milton GW, Shaw HM, McCarthy WH, Pearson L, Balch CM, Soong S-j: Prophylactic lymph node dissection in clinical stage I cutaneous malignant melanoma: Results of surgical treatment in 1319 patients. Br J Surg 69:108, 1982

23. Moore GE, Gerner RE: Malignant melanoma. Surg Gynecol Obstet 132:427, 1971

24. Mundth ED, Guralnick EA, Raker JW: Malignant melanoma: A clinical study of 427 cases. Ann Surg 162:15, 1965

25. Nava M, Santinami M, Bajetta E, Marolda R, Vaglini N, Clemente C, Cascinelli N: Il melanoma cutaneo con metastasi ai linfonodi regionali (stadio II): Diagnosi, terapia, prognosi. Arg Onc 3:119, 1982

26. Pendergrast WJ Jr, Soloway MS, Myers GH, Futrell JW: Regional lymphadenectomy and tumor immunity. Surg Gynecol Obstet 142:385, 1976

27. Preston FW, Staley CJ: Controversial aspects of the management of malignant melanoma. Surg Clin North Am 38:183, 1958

28. Reintgen DS, Cox EB, McCarty KS Jr, Vollmer RT, Seigler HF: Efficacy of elective lymph node dissection in patients with intermediate thickness primary melanoma. Ann Surg 198:379, 1983

29. Sim FH, Taylor WF, Ivins JC, Pritchard DJ, Soule EH: A prospective randomized study of the efficacy of routine elective lymphadenectomy in management of malignant melanoma: Preliminary results. Cancer 41:948, 1978

30. Southwick HW, Slaughter DP, Hinkamp JF, Johnson FE: The role of regional node dissection in the treatment of malignant melanoma. Arch Surg 85:63, 1962

31. Sugarbaker EV, McBride CM: Melanoma of the trunk: The results of surgical excision and anatomic guidelines for predicting nodal metastasis. Surgery 80:22, 1976

32. Urist MM, Balch CM, Soong S-j, Milton GW, Shaw HM, McGovern VJ, Murad TM, McCarthy WH, Maddox WA: Head and neck melanoma in 536 clinical stage I patients: A prognostic factors analysis and results of surgical treatment. Ann Surg [in press]

33. Urist MM, Maddox WA, Kennedy JE, Balch CM: Patient risk factors and surgical morbidity after regional lymphadenectomy in 204 melanoma patients. Cancer 51:2152, 1983

34. van der Esch EP, Cascinelli N, Preda F, Morabito A, Bufalino R: Stage I melanoma of the skin: Evaluation of prognosis according to histologic characteristics. Cancer 48:1668, 1981

35. Veronesi U, Adamus J, Bandiera DC, Brennhovd IO, Caceres E, Cascinelli N, Claudio F, Ikonopisov RL, Javorskj VV, Kirov S, Kulakowski A, Lacour J, Lejeune F, Mechl Z, Morabito A, Rodé I, Sergeev S, van Slooten E, Szczygiel K, Trapeznikov NN, Wagner RI: Inefficacy of immediate node dissection in stage I melanoma of the limbs. N Engl J Med 297:627, 1977

36. Veronesi U, Adamus J, Bandiera DC, Brennhovd IO, Caceres E, Cascinelli N, Claudio F, Ikonopisov RL, Javorskj VV, Kirov S, Kulakowski A, Lacour J, Lejeune F, Mechl Z, Morabito A, Rodé I, Sergeev S, van Slooten E, Szczygiel K, Trapeznikov NN, Wagner RI: Stage I melanoma of the limbs: Immediate versus delayed node dissection. Tumori 66:373, 1980

37. Veronesi U, Adams J, Bandiera DC, Brennhovd IO, Caceres E, Cascinelli N, Claudio F, Ikonopisov RL, Javorskj VV, Kirov S, Kulakowski A, Lacour J, Lejeune F, Mechl Z, Morabito A, Rodé I, Sergeev S, van Slooten E, Szczygiel K, Trapeznikov NN, Wagner RI: Delayed regional lymph node dissection in stage I melanoma of the skin of the lower extremities. Cancer 49:2420, 1982

38. Wanebo HJ, Woodruff J, Fortner JG: Malignant melanoma of the extremities: A clinicopathologic study using levels of invasion (microstage). Cancer 35:666, 1975

JOSEPH R. LOGIC
CHARLES M. BALCH

Defining Lymphatic Drainage Patterns with Cutaneous Lymphoscintigraphy

9

Metastatic melanoma most frequently disseminates via lymphatic pathways to the regional lymph nodes. Defining the patterns of lymphatic drainage from a melanoma is therefore important to the clinician. First, it is useful to know which nodal drainage basins are at greatest risk in the pre- and postoperative evaluation of nodal metastases. Second, it provides crucial information about which node-bearing tissues should be removed in patients being considered for elective lymph node dissection. While the lymphatic drainage for extremity melanomas is generally predictable, the pioneer 19th-century studies of Sappey[11] showed that the lymphatic drainage on the trunk was frequently ambiguous. It is difficult, therefore, to determine precisely which lymphatic drainage sites are potentially at risk for most patients with melanomas located on the trunk and also in some areas in the head and neck region.

Cutaneous lymphoscintigraphy represents the only clinically available technique that can accurately identify the lymphatic watershed. This chapter is a review of the experience with this technique at the University of Alabama in Birmingham (UAB) in 71 patients with truncal melanoma. It is a simple, reproducible test that can be implemented in any nuclear medicine department.

HISTORICAL PERSPECTIVE

Nearly 30 years ago, Sherman and Ter-Pogossian[12] documented that interstitially injected radiocolloids were transported via lymphatic pathways to the regional lymph nodes. They used radioactive colloidal gold (^{198}Au) in gelatin solution with a particle size ranging from 50 mμ to 250 mμ in diameter. The radiation emitted from this radiopharmaceutical consisted of penetrating beta particles of 0.9 MeV and gamma rays of 0.41 MeV. ^{198}Au-radiocolloid was subsequently reported by Fee and associates[5] as a useful tracer for the detection of lymphatic drainage sites from melanomas. However, because of the radiation exposure from ^{198}Au, as well as its unfavorable imaging characteristics, alternative agents were sought for lymphoscintigraphy. The liver-scanning agent, technetium-99m (^{99m}Tc)–sulfur colloid, was also shown to be transported via lymphatics to regional nodes following interstitial injection.[6] This agent was subsequently used by the UAB group to study lymphatic drainage of truncal melanomas.[9] Although ^{99m}Tc has optimal imaging qualities for current-generation gamma scintillation cameras, the usual sulfur colloid particle size is large (100 mμ), causing it to migrate somewhat slowly through the lymphatics. As a consequence, the radiopharmaceutical is frequently trapped in the first node of a lymphatic chain so that the full extent of nodal drainage in contiguous areas cannot always be discerned. It should be noted that a sulfur colloid preparation of somewhat smaller particle size is available as an investigational agent and has been used for cutaneous lymphoscintigraphy by Bennett and Lago.[1]

In 1979, a smaller colloid agent, antimony trisulfide, became available as an investigational agent. This colloid, also labeled with ^{99m}Tc (with its optimal imaging properties), has the advantage of being much smaller, with a particle size (3 mμ–12 mμ in diameter) similar to that of ^{198}Au colloid. Antimony radiocolloid is taken up into the lymphatics much more rapidly after intradermal injection than are larger colloids. It frequently identifies not only the entire primary nodal basin but intransit nodes as well. Furthermore, a smaller dose can be used so that the radiation exposure is substantially reduced. During the past 4 years, this investigational drug has been used exclusively at UAB for evaluating lymphatic pathways of truncal melanoma. Extensive studies of lymphatic drainage using ^{99m}Tc–antimony colloid have also been reported to be of value in patients with carcinomas of the breast and prostate.[3,4,7,8,14]

INDICATIONS

Cutaneous lymphoscintigraphy, using ^{99m}Tc-labeled antimony trisulfide colloid, is a diagnostic modality for evaluating any melanoma with possible ambiguous lymphatic drainage. This would include most truncal melanomas. This test is also valuable in patients with potentially bidirectional lymphatic drainage from selected sites on the head and neck as well as the very proximal extremities. Lymphoscintigraphy may also be of value in evaluating vulvar melanomas.

It should be emphasized that maximum information is obtained when the scan is performed prior to or just after biopsy or simple excision. A previous wide excision of the melanoma, especially with node dissection, distorts the true lymphatic pathways of the lesion, fails to identify intransit nodes, and makes it difficult to interpret the results.[1]

TECHNIQUE

Antimony trisulfide colloid is supplied in a sterile, nonpyrogenic kit form.* It is labeled with 500 µCi to 1 mCi of ^{99m}Tc as sodium pertechnetate in a volume of less than 1 ml (Fig. 9-1). When using sulfur colloid, lidocaine is incorporated into the syringe for

*Cadema Medical Products, Inc., Westtown, N.Y.

cutaneous anesthesia, but this is not feasible with the acidic antimony solution. Even though local anesthetic agents cannot be used for the antimony injections, usually only minimal discomfort occurs.

The skin area surrounding the primary lesion is first prepared with 10% povidone-iodine (Betadine). Using a 26-gauge needle, four to six intradermal injections are made circumferentially around the lesion or the biopsy incision. Care must be taken

FIG. 9-1   Preparation of the ^{99m}Tc–antimony trisulfide colloid (Cadema Medical, Inc., Westtown, NY 10998) (A) Inject 500 to 1000 µCi of oxidant and additive-free ^{99m}Tc (*, radioactive) into the vial containing 0.2 ml of 0.5 normal HC1. (B) Add the contents of prepackaged syringe A to the vial. Syringe A contains 0.67 mg antimony as trisulfide. (C) Immerse the vial in boiling water bath (shielded) for 30 minutes to form the colloid. (D) Remove from bath and inject contents of prepackaged syringe B into the vial. Syringe B contains a buffer solution of 24.7 mg dibasic sodium phosphate and 2.7 mg of monobasic sodium phosphate. Cool to room temperature. (E) With aseptic technique and a 26-gauge needle, inject four to six intradermal sites surrounding the lesion, avoiding direct injection into the lesion. After 3 to 4 hours, the patient is ready for imaging with a standard gamma camera equipped with a low-energy, all-purpose, parallel-hole collimator.

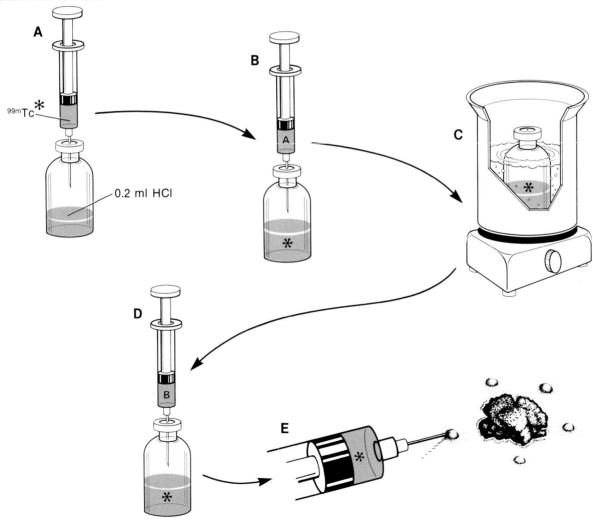

to avoid a deep subcutaneous injection, for such drainage patterns may not mimic the lymphatic basins from a cutaneous melanoma. Care must also be taken not to inject too close to the melanoma to avoid potential disruption of malignant cells. No adverse reactions have been noted in over 71 cutaneous lymphangiograms performed at UAB.

Three to four hours after injection, the patient returns to the nuclear medicine department for imaging studies. The lymphatic regions are imaged, using a 37-photomultiplier tube gamma scintillation camera equipped with an all-purpose, low-energy, parallel-hole collimator and using a 20% window centered over the 140 keV photopeak of ^{99m}Tc. Counts are accumulated for 5 minutes over axillary, inguinal, and cervical lymph node areas and also the perilesional injection site. Occasionally other views, including laterals and obliques, may be of value. It should be emphasized again that lymphatic drainage is altered after a wide excision of a melanoma, especially with regional lymphadenectomy, to the extent that cutaneous lymphoscintigraphy cannot reliably predict lymphatic drainage of such melanomas.[9,10]

RADIATION DOSIMETRY

The radiation burden in cutaneous lymphoscintigraphy is relatively high using ^{198}Au colloid. Not only are there high-energy photons, but also locally destructive particles that contribute to an excessively high absorbed radiation dose at the injection site, which could conceivably cause local tissue necrosis.[2] In contrast, the small dose of ^{99m}Tc used in the UAB studies has no associated local or systemic side-effects, and the radiation burden at the injection site, although not negligible, is entirely within an acceptable range. Residual ^{99m}Tc activity after 24 hours was measured in excised regional lymph nodes immediately after surgery by investigators at UAB and by others.[13] In all cases, radioactivity levels were usually only several μCi of ^{99m}Tc activity/g of tissue. Because of these findings and the clinical value of the studies, the procedure has been approved by the Radioactive Drug Research Committee and the Human Use Committee of UAB for routine use in patients at risk with malignant disease.

FIG. 9–2   Scintigrams recorded from right and left axillary areas (*inserts*). The "scatter" from the primary site (*asterisk*) is seen at the bottom of the image from the right axilla. Note the clearly identified single right axillary node. No activity is visualized in the left axilla. This is concordant drainage of a right anterior chest lesion lateral to the nipple.

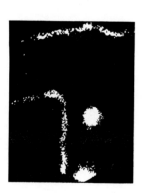
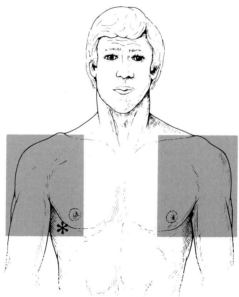
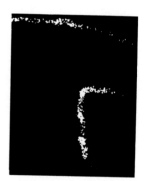

LYMPHOSCINTIGRAPHY FOR TRUNCAL MELANOMAS

Cutaneous lymphoscintigraphy with antimony trisulfide colloid has been performed in 71 consecutive patients with truncal melanoma. Two studies had to be repeated early in our experience, because the first injections of the radiopharmaceutical were too deep into the subcutaneous tissues and there was no directional drainage of the radiolabeled colloid. One patient had no migration of the colloid after two attempts; the reason for this failure was unexplained and this patient was excluded from further analysis.

All patients were studied after biopsy; no previous definitive surgical procedures had been performed.

In 35 patients (50%), the lymphatic watershed was unidirectional (*i.e.,* the ipsilateral axillary or inguinal nodes) (Figs. 9-2 and 9-3). In 3 of these 35 patients, there were lymph nodes adjacent to the melanoma or intransit nodes that were in locations not defined in standard surgical texts. These included lymph nodes over the iliac crest, the scapula, and along the chest wall. Such intransit nodes were not identified with the larger-particle sulfur colloid, a finding also observed by Bennett and Lago.[1]

In the other 35 patients, the lymphatic water-

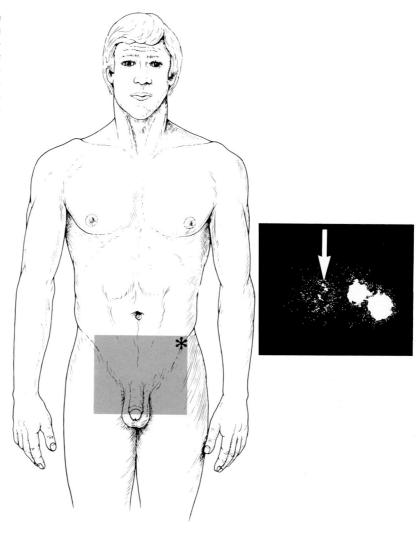

FIG. 9–3 Scintigrams recorded from *insert area*. The lesion was located on the left anterior flank (*asterisk*). The *arrow* identifies activity in the urinary bladder. Two discrete nodes are identified in the left inguinal area. No right-sided nodes are identified. This is concordant drainage to a single lymphatic basin.

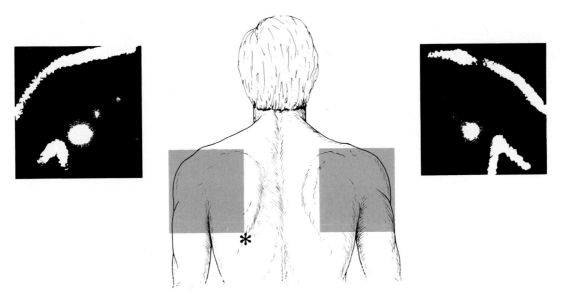

FIG. 9–4 Scintigrams recorded from both axillary areas (*inserts*). The primary lesion was located just below the tip of the left scapula in the midclavicular line (*asterisk*). Note the appearance of bilateral axillary nodal drainage. This is discordant drainage of the posterior chest.

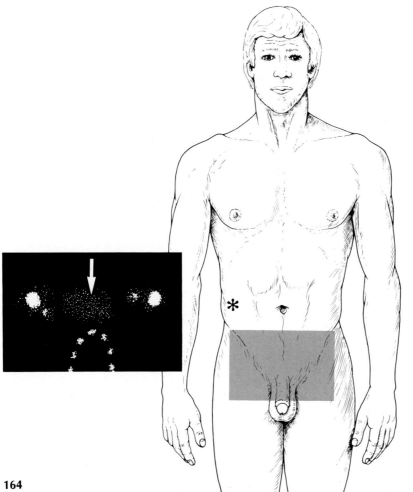

FIG. 9–5 Scintigram recorded from *insert area*. The *arrow* indicates the urinary bladder, and the radioactive rule outlines the inner thighs. The primary lesion was located on the right anterior abdominal wall at the level of the iliac crest (*asterisk*). Note the bilateral inguinal nodal drainage. This is discordant drainage to bilateral inguinal nodes.

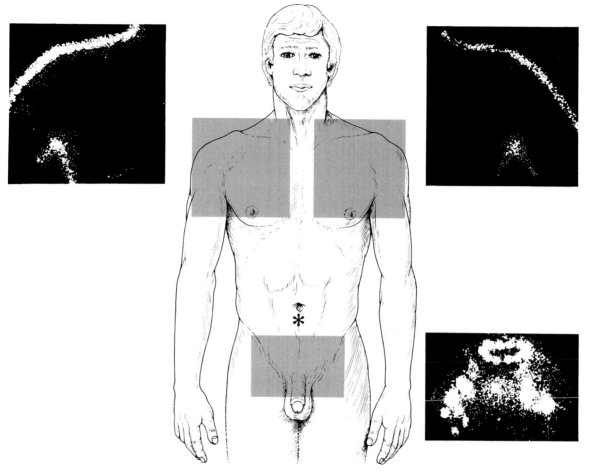

FIG. 9–6 Scintigrams recorded from indicated *insert areas*. The injected lesion is indicated by the injection sites just inferior to the umbilicus (*asterisk*). Note the extensive bilateral inguinal nodal activity. No axillary nodes are identified.

shed for truncal melanoma was multidirectional. In 21 patients, bilateral axillary activity was identified (Fig. 9-4). Bilateral inguinal activity was identified in four patients (Figs. 9-5 and 9-6) while ipsilateral axillary and inguinal nodes were identified in four patients (Fig. 9-7). Three nodal areas were visualized in one patient, and all four nodal areas were visualized in two patients with midline periumbilical lesions (Fig. 9-8). Three patients had ipsilateral axillary and supraclavicular nodes identified. Thus, as in previous studies,[13] about one half of the truncal melanomas in this series had multiple sites of lymphatic drainage. Intransit nodes were identified more frequently when lymphatic drainage was more complex (7 patients).

Thus, at least 26% of those patients with multidirectional lymphatic drainage had melanomas located outside of the anatomical sites that have been repeatedly cited in the literature for bidirectional drainage (*i.e.,* 4 cm from the midline in a vertical plane and 4 cm on either side of Sappey's line in a transverse plane). Indeed, at least 4 patients had melanomas 6 to 8 cm away from these lymphatic watersheds and still had bidirectional drainage. The axillary nodes have an especially broad range of lymphatic drainage in some patients in whom melanomas at the level of the iliac crest drained to the axilla as well as the inguinal nodes. Likewise, melanomas on the upper back can drain to the cervical as well as the axillary nodes. Figure 9-9 shows the areas

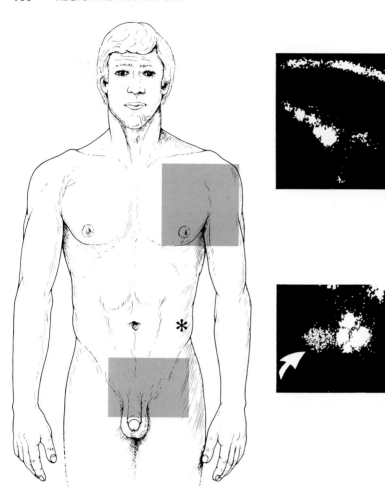

FIG. 9–7 Scintigrams recorded from both *insert areas*. The primary lesion was located on the anterior left flank (*asterisk*). Note left inguinal and left axillary nodal activity.

of the trunk with multidirectional lymphatic drainage in our series.

Not all truncal melanomas have multidirectional drainage, even though they occur on a lymphatic watershed. Indeed, 33% of our patients with a single nodal area of lymphatic drainage occurred in a location where two or more node-bearing areas might have been predicted to be at risk (Fig. 9-10). Some patients with unidirectional drainage, for example, had melanoma localized within 2 cm of the midline or close to Sappey's line. Only the single node-bearing area was excised in these patients, whereas two lymphadenectomies might have been considered using traditional criteria. When mapping the lymphatic drainage for this study, the number of individual variations that were encountered was striking. Some patients had melanomas in precisely the same location on the trunk; one had a uni-

directional lymphatic drainage, while others had bidirectional drainage. These results emphasize the importance of using this simple test when evaluating patients with truncal melanomas.

What is the false-negative rate for cutaneous lymphoscintigraphy? So far in our 6-year experience, not a single patient has developed nodal metastases in a site that was not predicted by lymphoscintigraphy. The opposite event occurred early in our experience, however, when one patient had a 3-mm melanoma located on the lower flank, just above the iliac crest. The scintigram at that time showed lymphatic drainage to the inguinal and axillary lymph nodes. Only a superficial inguinal lymphadenectomy was performed electively; the patient subsequently developed axillary lymph node metastases.

Lymphoscintigraphy has been useful even in patients who do not undergo elective lymphadenec-

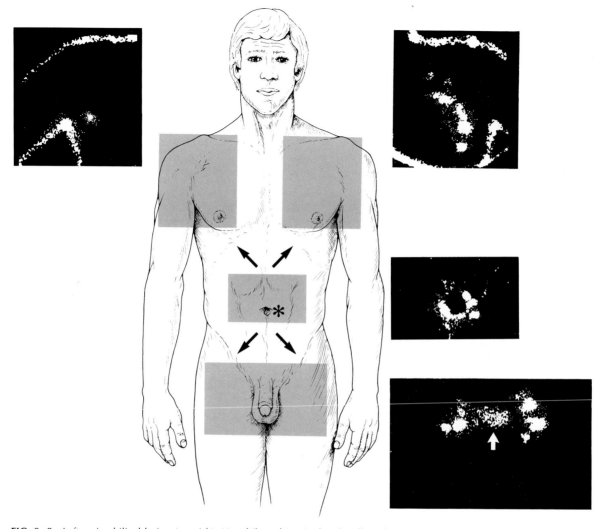

FIG. 9–8 Left periumbilical lesion (*asterisk*). Note bilateral inguinal and axillary drainage sites.

tomy. Thus, patients who subsequently develop subtle lymphadenopathy within the defined lymphatic drainage are more likely to have these nodes removed, while lymphadenopathy in other areas is followed more conservatively unless these are obvious metastases.

LYMPHOSCINTIGRAPHY FOR MELANOMA IN OTHER SITES

Melanomas on the extremities have also been studied in a few patients, but there was no evidence of ambiguous lymphatic drainage. However, melanomas around the shoulder may drain both to the axillary nodes and to the supraclavicular and infraclavicular sites as well. Scalp melanomas can drain either posteriorly to the occipital nodes or anteriorly to the cervical nodes and may have bilateral drainage in some instances (Fig. 9-11). Therefore, lymphoscintigraphy may well prove to be of value not only in melanoma occurring on axial sites but on melanoma in other sites as well. Melanomas located on the neck and shoulder are difficult to scan, because the nodal basin is beneath the injection site. Nevertheless, a few patients with such melanomas will have lymphatic drainage to the axillary nodes that can be observed on lymphoscintigraphy.

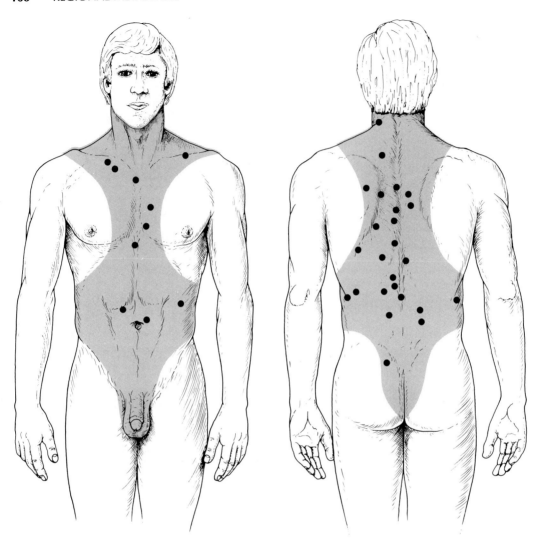

FIG. 9–9 Actual location of 35 trunk melanomas with multidirectional lymphatic drainage (*i.e.*, to 2, 3, or 4 major nodal basins). More than one quarter of these lesions occurred at a site that was predicted to have only unidirectional lymphatic drainage, using standard anatomical text criteria. The *shaded area* represents the locations on the trunk where multidirectional lymphatic drainage might occur in some patients, based on this study.

CONCLUSIONS

Cutaneous lymphoscintigraphy accurately identifies the lymphatic drainage of most melanomas. The procedure using ^{99m}Tc-labeled antimony trisulfide colloid is simple to perform in any nuclear medicine laboratory. The small particle size of this colloid makes it possible to identify multiple nodes in lymphatic chains and intransit nodes, in contrast to ^{99m}Tc–sulfur colloid, which migrates more slowly. The antimony colloid would appear to represent the radiopharmaceutical of choice for lymphoscintigraphy. Dermal lymphatic drainage of an ambiguous nature occurred in over one half of the patients in this series of truncal melanoma. Clearly, cutaneous lymphoscintigraphy is of value for defining

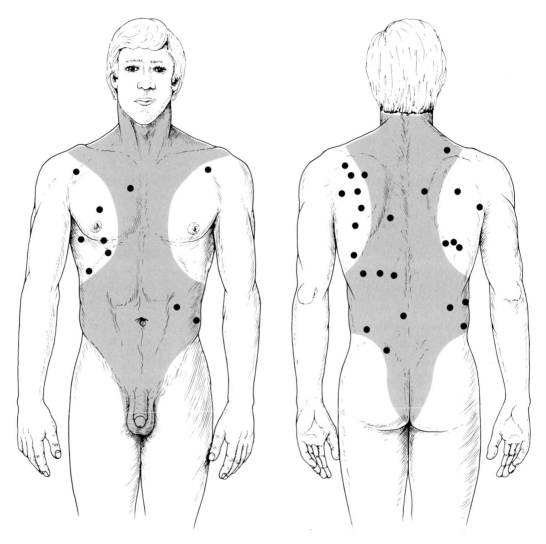

FIG. 9–10 Actual location of another group of 35 trunk melanomas with unidirectional lymphatic drainage to a single nodal basin. More than one third of these lesions occurred in sites where other patients were known to have multidirectional lymphatic drainage (*shaded area*). These data demonstrate the marked individual variation in lymphatic drainage on the trunk and the futility of predicting lymphatic drainage using standard anatomical text criteria.

lymphatic drainage in order to define precisely which nodes are at risk, both for routine follow-up physical examinations and for choosing the appropriate nodal basins to excise in patients selected for elective lymphadenectomy. In *no instance* have nodal metastases developed in an area not predicted by the scintigram. It should be emphasized that lymphoscintigraphy does not identify the presence or ab-

sence of metastases in melanoma. However, metastases in ectopically situated nodes on the lateral chest wall or about the scapula that were not clinically evident have been identified on lymphoscintigraphy. Cutaneous lymphoscintigraphy with ^{99m}Tc–antimony trisulfide colloid thus is a clinically useful technique in the surgical management of melanoma patients.

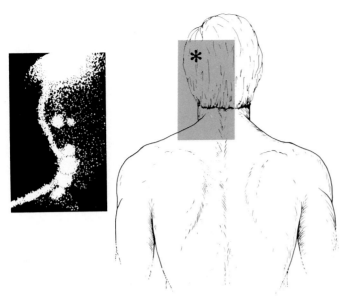

FIG. 9–11 Left posterior parietal melanoma (*asterisk*). Note the exquisite detail of the posterior cervical nodal chain.

REFERENCES

1. Bennett LR, Lago G: Cutaneous lymphoscintigraphy in malignant melanoma. Semin Nucl Med 13:61, 1983
2. Bergqvist L, Strand SE, Persson B, Hafstrom L, Jonsson P: Dosimetry in lymphoscintigraphy of Tc-99m antimony sulfide colloid. J Nucl Med 23:698, 1982
3. Ege GN: Internal mammary lymphoscintigraphy. Radiology 118:101, 1976
4. Ege GN: Internal mammary lymphoscintigraphy: A rational adjunct to the staging and management of breast carcinoma. Clin Radiol 29:453, 1978
5. Fee HJ, Robinson DS, Sample WF, Graham LS, Holmes EC, Morton DL: The determination of lymph shed by colloid gold scanning in patients with malignant melanoma: Preliminary study. Surgery 84:626, 1978
6. Hauser W, Atkins HL, Richards P: Lymph node scanning with ^{99m}Tc-sulfur colloid. Radiology 92:1369, 1969
7. Kaplan WD, Whitmore WF, Gittes RF: Visualization of canine and human prostatic lymph nodes following intraprostatic injection of technetium-99m-antimony sulfide colloid. Invest Radiol 15:34, 1980
8. McIvor J, Massouh H, Blackhouse BM, MacRae KD: Lymphography in prostatic carcinoma: Implications for the diagnosis of metastases. Br J Radiol 53:74, 1980
9. Meyer CM, Lecklitner ML, Logic JR, Balch CM, Bessey PQ, Tauxe WN: Technetium-99m sulfur colloid cutaneous lymphoscintigraphy in the management of truncal melanoma. Radiology 131:205, 1979
10. Rees WV, Robinson DS, Holmes EC, Morton DL: Altered lymphatic drainage following lymphadenectomy. Cancer 45:3045, 1980
11. Sappey MPC: Injection préparation et conservation des vaisseau lymphatiques. Thèse pour le doctorate en médecine, No. 241. Paris, Rignoux Imprimeur de la faculté de Médecine, 1843
12. Sherman AI, Ter-Pogossian M: Lymph node concentration of radioactive colloidal gold following interstitial injection. Cancer 6:1238, 1953
13. Sullivan DC, Croker BP, Harris CC, Deery P, Seigler HF: Lymphoscintigraphy in malignant melanoma: ^{99m}Tc-antimony sulfur colloid. Am J Roentgenol 137:847, 1981
14. Whitmore WF, Blute RD, Kaplan WD, Gittes PF: Radiocolloid scintigraphic mapping of the lymphatic drainage of the prostate. J Urol 124:62, 1980

EDWARD T. KREMENTZ
ROBERT F. RYAN
R. DAVILENE CARTER
CARL M. SUTHERLAND
RICHARD J. REED

Commentary by

H. SCHRAFFORDT KOOPS
J. OLDHOFF
J. W. OOSTERHUIS

Hyperthermic Regional Perfusion for Melanoma of the Limbs

10

In 1957, the Tulane Department of Surgery introduced the use of regional chemotherapy by perfusion for the treatment of cancer.[8,9,36] The method consists of isolating an anatomical region and supplying the area with oxygenated blood extracorporeally. Chemotherapeutic drugs are delivered to the isolated part in concentrations limited only by toxicity to local nerves, blood vessels, and muscles. The procedure has had greatest application in melanoma of the limbs for treatment of intransit metastases. Regional perfusion can achieve excellent control of these metastases and the primary tumor itself, especially when used in combination with surgical excision of the primary or recurrent lesions and with regional lymph node dissection (RLND). In this chapter, the current techniques of limb perfusion at Tulane are described, and the clinical experience for the management of extremity melanomas is reviewed.

OPERATIVE TECHNIQUES

The operative technique for hyperthermic regional perfusion of the upper and lower limbs will be described in such detail that the reader can carry out the procedure. However, a visit to a center where the technique is in frequent use is always advisable, since recent improvements in equipment have greatly facilitated this operation. Notable among these is a disposable oxygenator–heat exchange unit that fits the rotary head pumps used in cardiovascular surgery.

General endotracheal anesthesia is necessary. Spinal anesthesia promotes a peripheral vascular dilatation that is desirable for perfusion, but length of operating time limits its use to occasional lower limb lesions. An indwelling urinary catheter is inserted in order to follow urinary output during the operation and to prevent bladder distention. The patient should be positioned so that a tourniquet can be placed around the base of the limb. For upper limb perfusions, folded sheets are placed beneath the head, back, and shoulder to raise the shoulder about 2 inches off the operating table (Fig. 10-1). An arm board is similarly padded to prevent abduction of the arm and injury to the brachial plexus. For lower limb perfusions, sheets are placed under the sacrum and hips to elevate the buttocks similarly.

Hyperthermic perfusions require a warm environment prior to and during the induction of anesthesia and while the skin is prepped. The operating room temperature should be maintained between

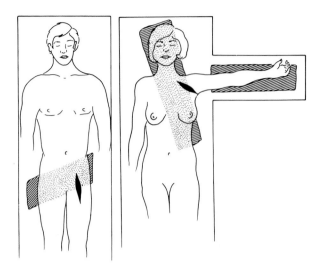

FIG. 10–1 Placement of folded sheets under the buttocks for lower limb perfusions (*A*) and under the shoulder and head for upper limb perfusion (*B*). This permits ease in tourniquet placement, exposes the axilla, and prevents hyperabduction of the arm. (Krementz ET, Campbell M: The role of limb perfusion in the management of malignant melanoma. In Constanzi JJ (ed): Malignant Melanoma 1, p 225. The Hague, Nijhoff, 1983).

22°C and 24°C and the patient placed on a water-circulating blanket set at 41°C. Low body core temperatures (33°C–35°C) increase the pump time required to reach optimal therapeutic limb temperatures by at least 5 to 10 minutes. When perfusion has begun, the operating room temperature may be reduced for the comfort of the operating team after the limb is covered with a heating blanket to keep it warm.

The entire limb is prepped with Betadine scrub and prep, including the axilla, anterior chest, shoulder, and neck for upper limb perfusions and the abdomen, perineum, and hip for lower limb perfusions. For lower extremity perfusions, a sterile towel is taped over the perineum and pelvis so that the external genitalia can be excluded from the operative field. The entire limb is left undraped in the operating field in order to monitor temperatures and blood flow and to perform the required excisional surgery following the perfusion. The hand or foot can be wrapped with sterile drapes if not involved with tumor.

This project was supported in part by the Mel Jacobson Cancer Research Fund, NCI grant number CA 18007 awarded by the National Cancer Institute DHEW, and by the Ladies Auxiliary of the Veterans of Foreign Wars. Dr. Krementz is an American Cancer Society Professor of Clinical Oncology.

PERFUSIONS OF THE ARM

The proximal axillary artery and vein are exposed through an incision extending from the clavicle to the anterior axillary line over the course of the vessels (Fig. 10-2). The pectoralis major muscle is separated in the direction of its fibers, along the cephalic groove; the vessels are exposed; and the pectoralis minor muscle is retracted laterally. It may be divided at its insertion if better exposure is needed. The lymph nodes and fat are removed along the lower surface of the axillary vein and examined pathologically for staging purposes. The lateral axilla is explored by direct palpation. An axillary lymph node dissection can be performed on completion of the perfusion if there are metastatic nodes.

The vessels are secured by placing umbilical tapes about them; these tapes are passed through #14 red rubber tubing as a tourniquet. The patient is heparinized with 150 units heparin/kg body weight. After 2 minutes have elapsed for heparinization, the vessels are occluded, a small longitudinal arteriotomy is made, and the vessel is cannulated distally with a #14 to #16 French catheter. The vein is treated in the same fashion and is cannulated with

a #16 to #18 catheter. The catheters are further secured to the proximal tape to prevent dislodgement during perfusion. The sterile tubing from the pump oxygenator is primed with lactated Ringer's solution and whole blood (at a 2:1 ratio) and is passed to the operator. The lines are clamped, divided, and attached to the perfusion catheters.

Perfusion is then started at flow rates varying from 200 cc to 500 cc per minute, depending on the size of the vessel and the caliber of the catheter used. The arterial flow rate is regulated by the gravity drainage flow from the venous line into the pump-oxygenator. Variations in flow are usually transient, and attempts to compensate for temporary low flows by addition of drugs or fluid are often unsatisfactory. Usually, low flow is the result of improper placement of the catheter or positioning of the tourniquet and can be corrected by proper adjustment. High flow facilitates rapid warming of the limb, which in turn enhances vasodilatation and promotes optimal tumor perfusion. If vasospasm occurs, 30 mg to 60 mg of papaverine may be added to the perfusate in the arterial line.

A tourniquet is applied around the root of the limb; two to three layers of a 4-inch Esmarch rubber

FIG. 10–2 Diagrammatic flow scheme for hyperthermic regional perfusion of the upper limb. (Krementz ET, Campbell M: The role of limb perfusion in the management of malignant melanoma. In Constanzi JJ (ed): Malignant Melanoma 1, p 225. The Hague, Nijhoff, 1983).

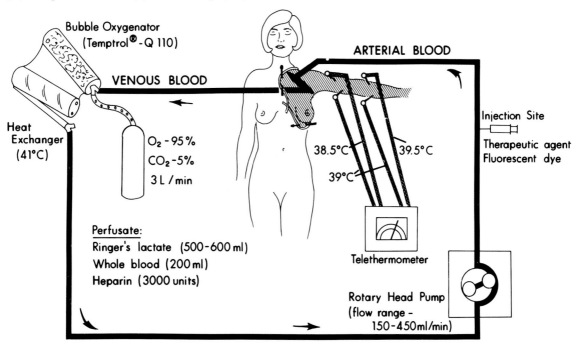

bandage are used. This is anchored posteriorly by large towel clamps placed through the skin and anteriorly by a Steinmann pin placed through the skin and subcutaneous tissue in the midline from the level of the fourth rib superiorly to the sternal notch. A second pin is placed along the course of the eighth rib from the midclavicular line to the anterior axillary line. In women, this is usually placed in the submammary groove. The tourniquet is drawn tight and cross-clamped at a point between the Steinmann pins. The skin may be protected by gauze sponges placed under the clamps.

Complete distribution of the perfusion is confirmed by injecting 2 ml to 3 ml of 10% Fluorescite into the arterial line. With the operating room completely dark, the fluorescein distribution of the arterial flow can be seen readily under a Wood's ultraviolet light. Leaks occurring under the tourniquet can be corrected by readjusting the tourniquet or appropriate padding beneath it. Perfusion of the extremity can be checked and corrected if necessary by repositioning the catheters. Some centers check the loss of perfusate and adequacy of tourniquet exclusion by placing small amounts of radioactive I^{131} in the perfusate and monitoring the isotope counts over the heart or aorta, but at Tulane this has not been found to be necessary.

PERFUSIONS OF THE LEG

In lower limb perfusions, the common femoral vessels are commonly used for treating lesions at the midthigh level or below. Exposure is obtained with an incision over the course of the vessels that extends from just above the inguinal ligament down to the apex of the femoral triangle (Fig. 10-3). Any suspicious nodes are excised and sent for frozen section examination. If the nodes contain metastases, the perfusion approach is altered, and the external iliac vessels are cannulated instead.

For lesions in the upper thigh or groin, perfusion through the external iliac vessels is preferred. These are approached through a lower abdominal wound parallel to the inguinal ligament. The muscles are split in the direction of their fibers, and the vessels are approached through the retroperitoneal space. If nodes are present along the iliac vessels, an attempt is made to cannulate the vessels above the highest positive nodes. If the nodes extend above the external iliac vessels, a common iliac perfusion may be performed by transperitoneal approach. Alternatively, regional chemotherapy may be given by continuous retrograde intra-arterial infusion through a

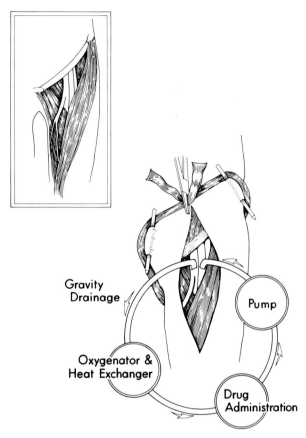

FIG. 10–3 Diagrammatic flow scheme for common femoral perfusion of lower limb with tourniquet in place. *Insert* shows anatomy of femoral triangle.

catheter inserted in the femoral artery with the delivery tip placed in the common iliac artery. Imidizole carboxamide (DTIC) delivered fractionally over a 5-day period provides effective treatment.

For lower limb perfusions, larger catheters are used. The femoral or iliac artery usually takes a #16 or #18 French catheter and the vein, a #18 or #20 catheter (Fig. 10-4). The inferior epigastric vessels are ligated, and the obturator vessels are temporarily occluded to prevent leakage from the perfused limb.

GENERAL PRINCIPLES

Experience has shown that fewer vascular complications follow more proximal placement of the perfusion catheters. Catheter placement and vessel repair are also easier in larger vessels. Finally, higher flow rates that promote optimal tissue oxygenation, higher perfusion pressures, better drug diffusion

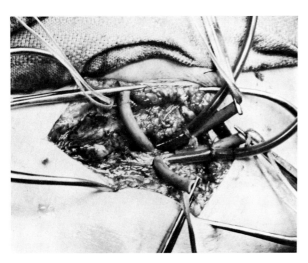

FIG. 10–4 Common femoral cannulization showing placement of catheters, occlusion of vessels with modified Rummel snares, and fixation of catheters to proximal snare before application of tourniquet.

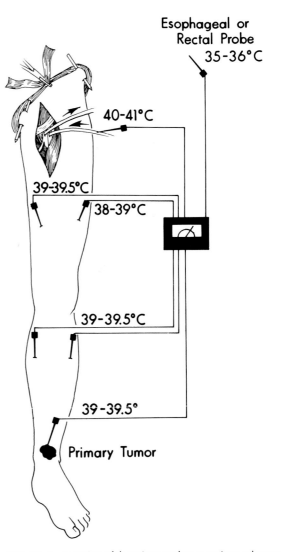

FIG. 10–5 Insertion of thermistor probes at various subcutaneous sites in lower limb extremities to monitor temperatures during hyperthermic perfusion.

into the tissues, and more rapid warming of the limb can be obtained. However, the more proximal the site of the cannulation, the greater the loss of perfusate. The most complete isolation is obtained when perfusing the superficial femoral or the brachial vessels. With axillary or external iliac perfusions, up to half of the drug may be lost during a 60-minute perfusion.

Early in the development of this technique, it was found that complete perfusion of the tumor bed required normothermic perfusate temperatures to avoid vasospasm. In 1967, Cavaliere and colleagues achieved good tumor responses using hyperthermic perfusion alone (40°C–41°C for 4 hours).[5] Later, Stehlin was able to increase tumor destruction by combining chemotherapy with hyperthermia, and currently this is the preferred method.[40] Limb temperatures are monitored by four or more thermistor probes inserted through the skin into the deep subcutaneous tissue (Fig. 10–5). Perfusion is started with the perfusate temperature at 40°C to 41°C, and administration of the drug is begun when the limb temperature reaches 38°C. External heat loss is prevented by wrapping the limb in a sterile water-circulating blanket (such as pediatric size Blanketrol) or sterilized K pads adjusted to the required temperature (Fig. 10–6A and 10–6B). Because of the thermolability of some drugs and increasing chemotherapy reaction in the limb, tissue temperatures should not exceed 40°C. A loss of about 2°C occurs

in the circuit from the femoral artery to the femoral vein.

At the completion of the chemotherapeutic perfusion, a washout is performed in order to remove unbound drug and toxic end products. The rinse is performed by using 300 ml of low molecular weight Dextran, followed by replacement with a similar amount of whole blood infused through the arterial line. The tourniquet is released, the catheters are withdrawn, and the vessels are repaired with running everting sutures of 5–0 Tevdec or Proline. The heparinization is reversed with equal amounts

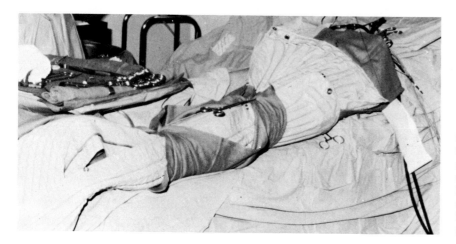

FIG. 10–6 (*Top*) Blanketrol water-circulating blanket wrapped around limb and patient on temperature-controlled water-circulating blanket during course of perfusion. (*Bottom*) Patient undergoing lower limb perfusion with limb wrapped in heating blanket.

of protamine sulfate given slowly into the IV access line over a 5- to 10-minute period. Wound closure, RLND, or excisional surgery of the primary lesion or other lesions are carried out as indicated.

When the RLND is carried out in conjunction with chemotherapeutic perfusion, it is necessary to perform a more conservative dissection with thicker skin flaps to prevent necrosis. In patients who have had a chemotherapeutic perfusion, postoperative bone marrow depression may occur. It is important, therefore, to avoid wound complications such as infection or slough, which can be hazardous, especially when associated with recently repaired blood vessels. Suction drainage catheters are left in the perfusion wounds for several days, and broad-spectrum antibiotics are used routinely during the pre- and postoperative period.

CHEMOTHERAPEUTIC AGENTS

Melphalan (1-phenylalanine mustard or L-PAM) is the drug most widely used for regional perfusion, either alone in adjuvant perfusion, or frequently in combination with other drugs in advanced disease. The intravenous form of melphalan has been used on a worldwide basis since it was formulated in 1954. In the United States, it is still classified as an investigational drug and can be obtained only through the National Cancer Institute for clinical trials. It is a long-acting alkylating agent with low vesicant properties that is poorly soluble in water but readily soluble in ethanol and propylene glycol. It is currently supplied with an acid alcohol solvent and further diluted with buffered propylene glycol. Melphalan was originally selected for melanoma perfusion therapy since phenylalanine, a metabolite of melanin, was thought to carry the attached cytotoxic alkylating radicals into the melanin-producing neoplastic cell. Also, melphalan was found to be effective in the treatment of a mouse melanoma at that time.[25] The melphalan dosage is determined in mg/kg of ideal body weight according to upper and lower limbs and the proportional size of the limb in relation to the total body size. Table 10-1 gives the recommended dose range for drugs commonly used in regional perfusion. Other alkylating agents that have been found useful are triethylenethiophosphoramide (TSPA) and nitrogen mustard (HN$_2$), which are very soluble in water. The latter has strong vesicant properties and is rapidly hydrolized. McBride[26] has reported good results using melphalan, actinomycin D, and HN$_2$ delivered in sequence during perfusion, and this combination has

TABLE 10–1
SAFE RANGE OF DRUG DOSAGES FOR HYPERTHERMIC PERFUSION OF THE LIMBS
(mg/kg BODY WEIGHT, BASED ON LESS OF ACTUAL OR IDEAL WEIGHT)

	Upper Limb		Lower Limb	
Drug	*Range (mg/kg)*	*Maximum Dose (mg)*	*Range (mg/kg)*	*Maximum Dose (mg)*
Single Agents				
Melphalan	0.6–1	60	0.8–1.2	90
Thiotepa	0.6–1	60	0.8–1.2	80
Nitrogen Mustard	0.3–0.6	30	0.4–0.7	40
Multiple Agents				
Melphalan and	0.4–0.7	40	0.5–0.8	55
Thiotepa	0.2–0.3	25	0.4–0.5	35
Melphalan and	0.5–0.8	55	0.7–1.2	70
actinomycin D	0.005–0.008	0.6	0.007–0.012	0.9
Melphalan and	0.5–0.7	45	0.6–0.9	60
nitrogen mustard	0.09–0.14	8	0.11–0.16	10
Melphalan,	0.5–0.7	45	0.6–0.9	60
actinomycin D and	0.006–0.01	0.5	0.008–0.012	0.75
nitrogen mustard	0.07–0.11	8	0.08–0.15	10

also been used at Tulane in recent years for recurrent disease.

The drugs and combinations used in the first perfusion or in subsequent perfusions are shown in Table 10-2. Nitrogen mustard is used most frequently when melphalan has failed to control a lesion or when the patient presents with satellitosis. The combination of melphalan and TSPA is seldom used at present. TSPA can be substituted for melphalan in the same dosages if melphalan is not available.

The duration of perfusion time varies with investigators. It is the Tulane practice to administer the first dose of drug to the perfusate when the limb temperature reaches 38°C and continue perfusing for 45 minutes. Melphalan is injected in aliquots of 15 mg to 20 mg into the arterial line every 3 minutes. Some investigators give the entire dose of melphalan one time but add the drugs into the pump reservoir rather than fractionating it. The more labile HN_2 is given in aliquots of 1 mg to 2 mg in the arterial line every 2 minutes and the perfusion continued for 10 to 15 minutes after the last dose. A large bolus of HN_2 given into the arterial line may cause nerve damage. Actinomycin D is given in 0.1 mg-aliquots every 2 to 3 minutes into the arterial line. The dosage routine for combination of melphalan, actinomycin D, and HN_2 follows the recommendations as described by McBride.[26] The Tulane experience with DTIC, cis-platinum, and Adriamycin for regional chemotherapy has been primarily used as an intra-arterial infusion tech-

TABLE 10–2
DRUGS USED IN 971 PERFUSIONS

Drug	First Perfusion	Subsequent Perfusions
Melphalan	626	53
Melphalan, thiotepa	143	33
Nitrogen mustard	12	43
Melphalan, actinomycin D	6	1
Melphalan, actinomycin D, nitrogen mustard	17	8
Melphalan, nitrogen mustard	14	2
Thiotepa, actinomycin D	2	4
Miscellaneous*	2	5
Totals	822	149

*Epodyl, AB100, cis-platinum, and other combinations.

nique. Pfefferkorn and Dildocher found DTIC effective in perfusion therapy.[34] Adriamycin is precipitated by heparin, which limits its use in perfusion, and cis-platinum in dosages required for perfusion is quite expensive and has not been used routinely.

PERFUSION EXPERIENCE AT TULANE MEDICAL CENTER

CLINICAL MATERIAL

From 1957 to 1981, 822 patients with invasive melanoma of the limbs have received chemotherapeutic perfusion at Tulane. Perfusion is usually performed only once on each patient. Rarely, a second perfusion with a different drug (usually HN_2) may be used to arrest progressive satellitosis.

Single perfusions were performed in 716 patients, while 82 were perfused twice; 17 patients, three times; 5 patients, four times; and 2 patients, five times. Thus, the 822 patients were perfused on 961 occasions.

The staging system developed at the M. D. Anderson Tumor Institute has been used, since it is particularly suited for limb melanoma and separately categorizes satellites. Stage I consists of patients with localized disease only (Table 10-3); stage II disease consists of those with local recurrence or a primary with satellites within 3 cm of the primary; and stage III consists of those with regional disease up to and including the first station nodes. Axillary rather than epitrochlear, or femoral rather than popliteal nodes are considered as first station nodes for upper and lower limbs, respectively. Subgroup A indicates intransit metastases, B indicates nodal involvement, and AB indicates both types. Stage IV includes patients with regional disease and systemic metastases. Patients with positive supraclavicular or iliac nodes are included in stage IV. Table 10-3 lists the 822 patients by stage. The ratio of lower limb/upper limb lesions was 2:1. The female/male ratio was 6:4, and only 6% of the patient population were blacks.

TABLE 10–3
STAGE OF 822 PATIENTS TREATED BY PERFUSION EXCISION FOR MELANOMA OF THE LIMBS (1957–1981)

Stage	Number of Patients
I Localized primary lesion	
Level II	18
Level III–V	336
Total	354
II Metastases within 3 cm of primary	
Primary with adjacent satellites	6
Local recurrence	15
Total	21
III Regional metastases	
A skin/soft tissue (satellites)	74
B regional nodes	127
AB skin/soft tissue and nodes	87
Limb metastases from unknown primary	29
Total	317
IV Systemic metastases	
Positive iliac nodes	39
Extraregional primary	46
Distant disease	45
Total	130

SURGICAL MANAGEMENT POLICIES AND INDICATIONS FOR PERFUSION

Perfusion is recommended as an adjunct to excisional surgery for all stage I melanomas that are level III or ≥0.75 mm thick. For stage II melanomas, perfusion is recommended as an adjunct to wide excision and RLND. For stage IIIA melanomas with limited satellitosis or IIIB with resectable nodes, perfusion is recommended in combination with excisional surgery or node dissection. For IIIA melanomas with more extensive satellitosis or IIIB with nonresectable lymph nodes or nonresectable IIIAB disease, regional perfusion alone may be indicated. In some instances, as when limb metastases or primary melanomas are unresectable, perfusion may be used to render them operable. In stage IV disease, limb perfusion may be used for palliation, to save a functional limb, to relieve pain, to reduce the size of a bulky lesion, or to heal a large ulcerated melanoma.

RESULTS

Figure 10-7 shows the results of regional chemotherapy perfusion alone or in combination with excisional surgery in 775 patients. These data exclude 18 patients with invasive melanoma later classified as level II lesions and 29 patients with regional metastases from an unknown primary. Survival curves were calculated using life-table methods.[10] During this period, only 13 of 822 patients observed for the 21-year period have been lost to follow-up. The difference between survival and disease-free survival at 20 years is remarkably small (Fig. 10-8). Consequently, these results are reported by overall survival only.

All stage I and II patients underwent excisional surgery in addition to perfusion except one patient, a 68-year-old black woman with a large acral lentiginous melanoma of the hand. The patient refused amputation and had a complete remission following perfusion with melphalan and TSPA in 1960 (Fig. 10-9A and B). This patient survived for 15 years without recurrence, dying of other causes in 1975 at 83 years of age.

Until recently, the Tulane treatment policy consisted of widely excising the melanoma with approximately 3 cm to 5 cm or more of normal skin margins and closure of the defect with a split-thickness skin graft. The margins of surgical excision have decreased in recent years and now seldom exceed 3 cm of normal skin. In good prognosis

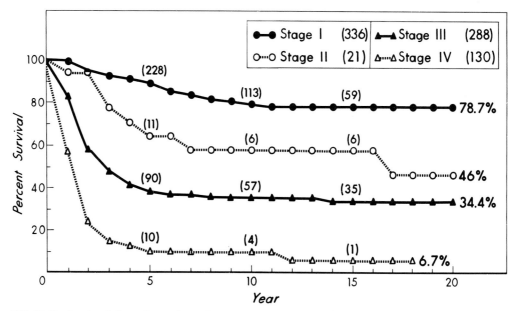

FIG. 10–7   Results of chemotherapy by perfusion in 775 patients according to stage of disease from 1957 to 1981.

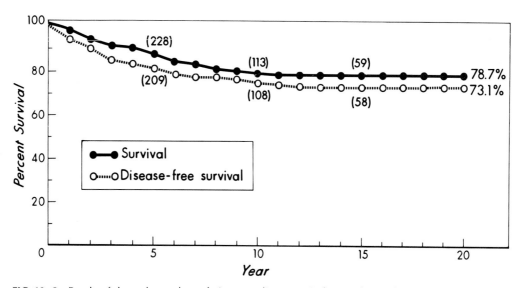

FIG. 10–8   Results of chemotherapy by perfusion according to survival versus disease-free survival in 336 patients with stage I melanoma of the limbs from 1957 to 1981.

patients, primarily those with thin lesions and other favorable indications, the margins are usually even less than 3 cm. Amputations are performed only in toe or finger involvement or in those few cases where bone is involved.

For many years most patients underwent a RLND, the only exceptions being patients judged to have an extremely good prognosis or those who were a poor risk because of extreme obesity, peripheral vascular disease, or acute or chronic infections

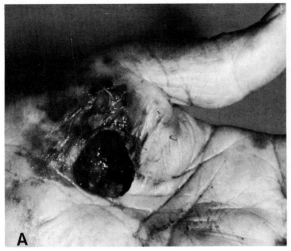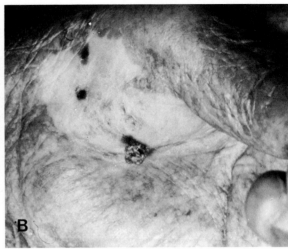

FIG. 10–9 (A) 56-year-old woman treated by chemotherapy by perfusion only. Picture shows a large ALM of the palm of her hand before treatment. (B) The lesion completely regressed over the following 9 months. The patient had no recurrence of metastases and died of hypertensive cardiovascular disease 15 years after perfusion. She suffered slight atrophy of muscles of the hand from chemotherapy.

in the limb. At the present time, RLND is performed more selectively, usually in those patients with poor prognostic signs. However, a node sampling is performed on all patients undergoing perfusion. In upper extremity lesions, the upper axillary nodes (level III) are routinely removed for analysis. In lower limb perfusions, samples are taken of any enlarged or suspicious external iliac nodes or common femoral nodes, depending on which vessels are being perfused. The majority of stage III patients have additional excisional surgery whenever complete removal of all tumor is feasible. In stage IV patients, excisional surgery is carried out only when positive iliac nodes are found coincident to planned dissections for lesser stage disease. In patients who present with metastases to the limb or with bulky or ulcerated lesions, excision or amputation is performed only when the tumor is readily resectable.

Table 10-4 presents the entire experiences according to stage of disease and other prognostic factors with cumulative survival rates at 5, 10, 15, and 20 years.

Stage I melanoma

The results of treatment in melanoma patients with stage I disease of the limb continue to show a difference in survival according to the sex of the patient (see Table 10-4). The 10-year survival differences favored the female patient by 17% (85% compared

to 68%). Patients with upper limb melanomas tended to do better than those with lower limb lesions (7% difference in 10-year survival, but this was not statistically significant). However, stage I patients with melanomas of the foot had the lowest survival compared to the five other subsite categories (upper arm, forearm, hand, thigh, and leg) (Figs. 10-10 and 10-11). Many of these patients have acral lentiginous melanomas of the soles of the feet or subungual melanomas, which have been shown to have a poor prognosis.[22]

When the entire group of 247 patients having RLND was compared to 89 without RLND, the cumulative 10-year survival rate was 77% with RLND, compared to 89% without. These are not significant differences. However, patients who had not undergone RLND did better clinically. It is the Tulane impression that this results from selection, since the decision to include or defer RLND is made by the attending surgeon based on the size; location; histologic characteristics of the primary, such as level and depth; and the patient's risk status (age, general condition, intercurrent disease, and so forth). In most patients, when the RLND was deferred, the patients were judged to have a good prognosis or were a poor operative risk. Another factor is that patients with suspicious nodes, particularly in the femoral area, had their nodes excised for histologic examination. Consequently, any patients found with metastatic nodes were categorized as

TABLE 10–4
RESULTS OF TREATMENT ACCORDING TO STAGE AND CHEMOTHERAPY BY REGIONAL PERFUSION (1958–1981)

Stage/Group	Number of Patients	Cumulative Survival Rates in Years (%)			
		5	10	15	20
I Localized	336	88	80	79	79
Women	219	91	85	84	84
Lower	142	93	85	85	85
With RLND*	102	91	87	87	87
Without RLND	40	97	97	97	97
Upper	77	89	84	80	80
With RLND*	53	88	82	78	78
Without RLND	24	91	91	91	91
Men	117	81	68	68	67
Lower	69	72	56	56	56
With RLND	54	72	57	57	57
Without RLND	15	65	49	—	—
Upper	48	92	84	84	84
With RLND	38	94	84	84	84
Without RLND	10	88	88	88	88
All with RLND	247	87	77	77	77
All without RLND	89	91	89	83	83
All Upper	125	90	84	82	82
All Lower	211	87	77	77	77
II Local Extension or Recurrence	21	64	58	58	45
III Regional	288	39	35	35	35
IIIA Intransit	74	35	28	28	28
No previous diagnosis for metastases	32	23	20	20	20
Previous diagnosis for metastases	42	46	36	36	36
Unresected	41	29	21	21	21
Resected	33	44	39	39	39
IIIB Regional Nodes	127	51	50	48	48
No previous diagnosis Positive at diagnosis	59	33	30	30	30
Single node +	19	47	47	47	47
Multiple node +	40	26	22	22	—
Clinically (+)	34	28	28	28	28
Clinically (−)	25	42	35	35	—
Previous surgery for disease, perfusion, and RLND for relapse	68	55	55	52	52
Single node +	36	72	72	67	67
Multiple node +	32	27	27	27	27
All Single Node +	55	64	64	60	61
All Multiple Node +	72	27	24	24	24
IIIAB Intransit and Nodes	87	31	28	28	28
Resected	47	32	32	32	—
Unresected	40	31	22	22	22
IIIA and B					
Resected	80	41	39	36	36
Unresected	81	30	23	23	23
Primary unknown with regional metastases	29	51	51	51	51
IV Distant	130	10	10	7	—
Iliac nodes	39	18	18	—	—
Primary tumor outside limb	46	9	9	—	—
Systemic	45	6	6	6	—

* Regional lymph node dissection

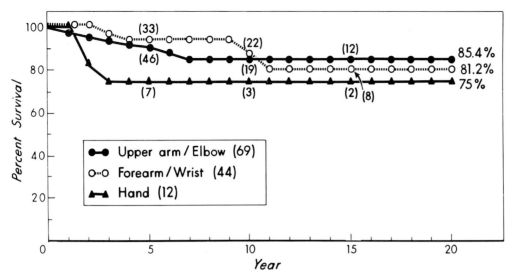

FIG. 10–10 Results of chemotherapy by perfusion of 125 patients with stage I melanoma of upper limbs according to site from 1957 to 1981.

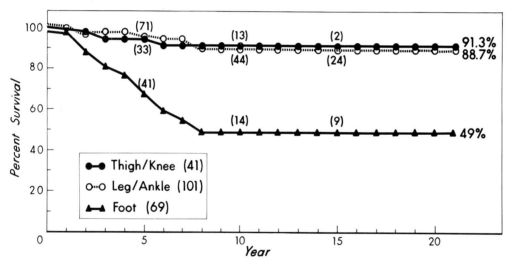

FIG. 10–11 Results of chemotherapy by perfusion in 211 patients with stage I melanoma of lower limbs from 1957 to 1981, according to site.

stage III, while those with negative nodes remaining in stage I may have had some therapeutic benefit from the node sampling.

In 71 stage I limb melanoma patients (21%), a recurrence developed after excision and regional perfusion. Table 10-5 shows the site of first recurrence. Recurrences most frequently occurred on the lower extremities of men (26/71), while the lowest frequency occurred on upper extremities of men

(7/71). Distant metastases alone occurred less frequently in women (6%) than in men (17%).

When this program was begun, the primary melanomas were histologically graded only as invasive or superficial. With the development of microstaging (level and thickness), only patients with level III melanomas or a thickness > 0.75 mm were treated by perfusion. Thus, 18 cases that were originally graded invasive were later classified as level II

TABLE 10–5
SITE OF FIRST RECURRENCE IN 336 SELECTED PATIENTS WITH STAGE I MELANOMAS OF THE LIMBS, FOLLOWING EXCISION AND REGIONAL CHEMOTHERAPY PERFUSION

Anatomical Site of Primary	Number of Patients	Total Recurrence (%)	Regional Only (%)	Regional plus Distant (%)	Distant Only (%)
Men	116	28	8	3	17
Upper Extremity	48	15	2	2	11
Lower Extremity	68	38	12	4	22
Women	220	17	10	1	6
Upper Extremity	77	21	8	1	12
Lower Extremity	143	15	11	1	4
Totals	336	21	9	2	10

TABLE 10–6
INCIDENCE OF RECURRENCE AND DEATH IN 179 PATIENTS FOLLOWING HYPERTHERMIC PERFUSION AND EXCISION OF STAGE I MELANOMA OF THE LIMB ACCORDING TO GROWTH PATTERN AND LEVEL OF INVASION (1970–1981)

Level of Invasion	Number of Patients	Lentigo Maligna*			Superficial Spreading*			Nodular*			Acral Lentiginous*			Unclassified*			Total*		Total Percent of Recurrence
		#	R	D	#	R	D	#	R	D	#	R	D	#	R	D	R	D	
III	82	2	0	0	36	2	0	21	4	3	12	0	0	11	0	0	6	3	7%
IV	86	4	0	0	27	1	1	22	5	3	14	1	1	19	5	4	12	9	14%
V	11							2	2	2	6	5	2	3	0	0	7	4	64%
Totals	179	6	0	0	63	3	1	45	11	8	32	6	3	33	5	4	25	16	
% Recurrence		0%			5%			24%			19%			15%			14%		

*R = Recurrence as of 1/1/83; D = death as of 1/1/83.

TABLE 10–7
SURVIVAL RATES IN 101 PATIENTS WITH STAGE I MELANOMA OF THE LIMBS ACCORDING TO THICKNESS OF PRIMARY TUMOR*

Thickness (mm)	Number of Patients	Cumulative Survival Rate in Years (%)			
		2	5	10	15
0.75–1.4	30	100	100	100	100
1.5–2.9	44	94	94	85	85
3.0–4.9	16	90	57	57	57
≥5	11	80	57	*	*
Total	101				

* No patients observed >6 years.

and are not now included in the survival rates. All these patients remain disease-free, except one patient who had a local recurrence that was controlled by further excision.

Table 10-6 shows the recurrence and death rates in 179 stage I melanoma patients who were followed 2 to 12 years after perfusion and excision. Data on these patients have been available since 1970 and are subgrouped according to the growth pattern and the level of invasion, both criteria that contribute to the prognosis. Lentigo maligna melanoma has a more favorable prognosis but is rarely seen on the limbs, so only 6 patients were included. Superficial spreading melanoma (63 cases) was the most common type and had the best results (5% recurrences) compared to the other growth patterns. The recurrence rates also correlated well with the tumor thickness. Among 101 patients for whom thickness measurements were available, no deaths occurred in patients who had lesions 1.4 mm thick or less and who were followed up to 15 years (Table 10-7). For 3-mm to 4.9-mm thickness melanomas, the 15-year survival rate was lower at 57%. For lesions 5 mm thick or more, there was a 57% 5-year survival, but longer follow-up data are not available. The small number of patients in the various categories decreases the reliability of the observations.

Stage II melanoma

There were only 21 patients with stage II disease. All these patients underwent perfusion, excision, and RLND. The 10-year survival rate was excellent at 57%.

Stage III melanoma

The survival rates for all stage III patients were 35% at 10 years and 34% at 20 years (see Fig. 10-7). The survival rates for regional disease according to substage are shown in Figure 10-12. One hundred and twenty-seven patients with regional node metastases (IIIB) had a survival rate at 10 years of 50% (see Fig. 10-12). Patients with intransit disease or satellitosis (IIIA) had a 10-year survival rate of 28%. An example of the response of a patient with satellitosis to perfusion is seen in Figure 10-13. The group with both intransit and lymph node disease (IIIAB) had a survival rate of 28% at 10 years. Several interesting findings evolve from examination of Table 10-4. First, patients with previously treated intransit metastases did better than those who had no previous treatment when they were referred for perfusion (36% versus 20% 10-year survival). Fur-

ther, those patients who were resected had a better survival than the unresected group (39% versus 21%). The observation that previous treatment correlates with a longer survival is also observed in patients with metastatic lymph nodes. Thus, patients presenting with previously untreated nodal metastases had a lower 10-year survival compared to patients treated at relapse (30% versus 55%). The latter group probably contains more patients with slow-growing, biologically favorable disease. An example of such a patient is seen in Figure 10-14. Patients with a single nodal metastasis had a better 10-year survival than patients with multiple positive nodes (64% versus 24%).

There were 29 patients with unknown primary melanoma who presented with regional metastases (see Table 10-4). These patients were all treated by perfusion and RLND or excision of recurrent lesions; all did extremely well, with a 51% 15-year survival rate.

Stage IV melanoma

There were 130 patients who were treated for distant, or stage IV, disease (see Fig. 10-7). This group consisted of 39 patients with iliac node metastases usually found at the time of treatment for stage III disease, 46 with a melanoma on the trunk or head and neck with metastases to limb or to regional lymph nodes, and 45 with extremity melanomas and systemic disease at the time of perfusion (Table 10-4). These patients were primarily treated for pal-

FIG. 10–12 Results of chemotherapy by perfusion for regional metastases in 288 patients with stage III melanoma of the limb from 1957 to 1981, according to substage.

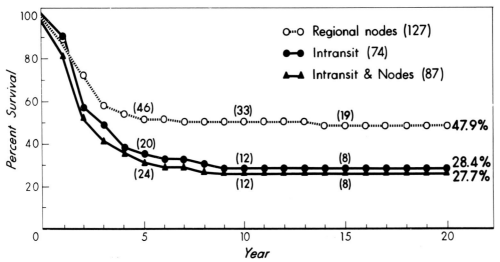

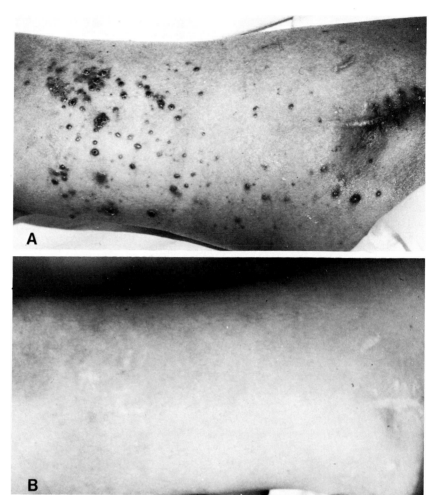

FIG. 10–13 (*A*) A 38-year-old white woman with melanoma of the right ankle that developed during pregnancy. She was treated in 1961 by wide excision and lymph node dissection. Patient developed satellitosis of the thigh in 1962 and was treated with normothermic perfusion with 50 mg of melphalan and 15 mg of triethylenethiophosphoramide (TSPA). (*B*) Her thigh 18 months later. Patient was free of disease for 12 years and then died of carcinoma of the lung.

liation; this was accomplished in a large percentage of cases, since a functional limb was saved, pain was alleviated, or bulky tumors were reduced in size. Those patients with positive iliac nodes had a 5-year survival of 18%. However, there were almost no long-term survivors in this group. The one patient surviving at 10 years did not respond to perfusion but subsequently responded completely to immunotherapy consisting of cross-transplantation and cross-transfusion carried out 3 months following perfusion failure.[21]

Of the 46 patients with stage IV melanoma with a known primary and with metastases to the limbs, 35 had axillary metastases. Following perfusion and RLND when possible, the 5-year survival rate was only 9%. In contrast, those patients with an unknown primary who presented with axillary or groin node metastases had a 51% 5-, 10-, and 15-year survival rate following perfusion and RLND, while the latter group all had apparent disease within the field of treatment. The better survival rate may have been helped by the same autoimmune process that destroyed the original primary tumor. In the 45 patients with systemic disease at the time of palliative limb perfusion, only two patients survived 10 years. Both of these had further treatment for metastases, one having had a resection of a lung metastasis and a solitary metastasis in the femur. This patient remains well 15 years following treatment. The second patient had satellitosis of the leg with multiple distant subcutaneous nodules and liver involvement. The patient had a good response to perfusion locally, and subsequently systemic chemotherapy resulted in a complete remission.

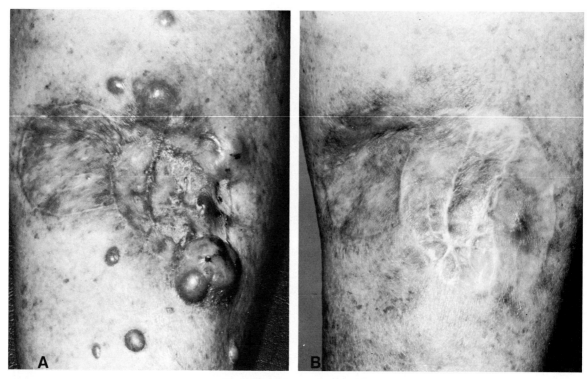

FIG. 10–14 (*A*) A 55-year-old white woman with multiple amelanotic nodules in and around site of previous excision of melanoma of left leg. Patient was first treated in 1975 by wide excision. In 1977 reexcision and lymph node dissection was performed. Further recurrences were treated by immunotherapy (BCG) and multiple courses of systemic chemotherapy with minimal response. In 1978 she was referred for chemotherapy by perfusion. Patient was treated by hyperthermic perfusion with 34 mg of HN_2.(*B*) Twenty months after perfusion all lesions have regressed. Patient is now free of disease, 5 years later.

This patient is free of disease 7 years following treatment.

MORTALITY AND COMPLICATIONS

A high rate of complications might be anticipated with such a complex procedure, especially when combined with extensive surgery, and often being performed in older patients. However, 70% of the 822 patients receiving chemotherapy by regional perfusion had no major complications whatsoever. When complications occurred, they tended to be multiple. Thus, when a patient had a chemotherapeutic dose high enough to produce bone marrow depression with thrombocytopenia and leukopenia, bleeding and infection followed. The same toxic dose may produce a severe local reaction in the limb with edema and vascular damage, thrombosis, or thrombophlebitis. One or more complications oc-

curred in 28% of patients with a single perfusion, but the risk increased to 51% for patients having two or more perfusions.

The introduction of hyperthermia increased the local toxicity significantly and prompted a reduction in drug dose. From 1957 to 1968, 496 perfusions that were normothermic (up to 38°C) were performed; since 1968, 465 perfusions that were hyperthermic (39°C–41°C) were performed. However, local complications did not differ in number or severity between normothermic and hyperthermic periods. Severe bone marrow depression (*i.e.,* leukopenia and thrombocytopenia) was rare with hyperthermic perfusion. All deaths from severe bone marrow depression occurred before 1964, when normothermic temperatures and higher drug doses were used. Increased experience, improvement of isolation techniques, and lower drug doses, as well as the introduction of white cell and thrombocyte transfusions, have resulted in no chemotherapy deaths from perfusion during the last 19 years of our experience.

Three operative deaths occurred in the series because of cardiovascular problems. Another death occurred early in the use of hyperthermia when, inadvertently, excessive temperatures were used that caused tissue necrosis followed by renal failure, massive edema, oliguria, and congestive heart failure.

The most common vascular complication has been thrombophlebitis, which was recognized in 36 patients. However, some cases of thrombophlebitis may escape recognition, particularly when occurring in the axillary veins. Arterial and venous thrombosis occurred in 18 patients, with thrombectomy being required in three patients. Four patients required an amputation because of arterial thrombosis. Careful selection of patients with little or no arterial disease is important. Pulmonary emboli secondary to thrombosis occurred in seven patients. Two of these were treated by vena caval ligation; the remaining five, by anticoagulants.

Sixty patients were judged to have moderate-to-severe chemotherapy reactions, including erythema, edema, and pain. However, in only three cases did these produce residual disability resulting from nerve or muscle damage.

Local chemotherapy reactions were usually self-limited and subsided within several weeks. At the dosages recommended in Table 10-1, severe blistering of the skin or edema requiring fasciotomy did not occur. Other local manifestations of chemotherapeutic reactions, such as temporary loss of nails, drying or slough of the outer skin of palms and soles, inhibition of hair growth on the limb, or transient neuralgia were encountered, but none were disabling and all subsided with appropriate therapy. There have been no instances in which complete scalp hair loss was noted from therapy.

Wound infections are particularly hazardous in the groin and axilla, especially following RLND. Daily Phisohex baths for several days prior to surgery are recommended, as well as prophylactic use of broad-spectrum antibiotics prior to and after operation.

BENEFITS OF PERFUSION

There are several benefits associated with administration of high-dose chemotherapy using hyperthermic oxygenated regional perfusion. Originally, the goal was to increase the chemotherapeutic dose in the isolated area beyond that which could be obtained systemically, as well as to avoid systemic toxicity. However, local tissue toxicity proved to be the dose-limiting factor. As a general rule, the total dose that could be perfused through the lower limb equaled that which could be administered as a single IV systemic dose. The upper limbs could only tolerate lower doses. Nevertheless, experimental studies and clinical trials now demonstrate that the *concentration* of drugs as measured by quantitative isotope determination can be increased from six to ten times that achieved by equal doses given systemically.

The incorporation of a bubble-type oxygenator as part of the extracorporeal circulation produces high tissue-oxygen tensions, with a pO_2 in the range of 400 mm Hg to 500 mm Hg. It has been shown that the increased tissue pO_2 potentiates the effect of alkylating agents on tumor cells by acting as a hypoxic cell sensitizer.[20] This observation has been confirmed by others,[23] and the principle is the same as the use of hyperbaric oxygen to potentiate the effects of irradiation.[15] In addition, the increased pO_2 has a selective tumoricidal effect of its own.[17] The administration of the drug into the arterial system under normal pump pressures and flow rates also ensures thorough perfusion of the tumor with the cytotoxic agent. Potential metastases in the surrounding tissues and regional nodes are perfused with the chemotherapeutic agent.

Hyperthermia has a number of therapeutic effects as well.[16,43] It increases the chemical action of the drug as well as the metabolism of the cells. Hyperthermia produces vascular dilatation so there is more thorough perfusion of all tissues in the isolated system. In 1967, Cavaliere and associates showed that hyperthermic perfusion (40°C–41°C for 4 hours) without tourniquet produced significant tumor response.[5] Later, Stehlin and colleagues[40,41] showed that a combination of chemotherapy and hyperthermia produced better results than those obtained with normothermic perfusions alone. Even though hyperthermia and chemotherapy together increase local toxicity, the Tulane experience is that the combination is more efficacious.

The use of heparin in the extracorporeal circulation is necessary to prevent clotting and allow satisfactory operation of the extracorporeal circuit. Also, it has been shown that heparin acts as an antimetastatic agent, with selective tumoricidal effects of its own.[32]

Lysis of the tumor cells *in situ* by chemotherapy is thought to result in autoimmunization, particularly in immunocompetent patients having intact regional lymph nodes. Clinically, regression of metastases has been observed within the perfusion area long after the chemotherapeutic effects would have occurred. In addition, regression of metastases outside of the perfused area has been observed weeks and months after the perfusions have been performed. Finally, isolation of the perfused area and the washout following perfusion reduce systemic toxicity and therefore minimize depression of the patient's immune system.

DISCUSSION

Surgery remains the most widely applied treatment for primary invasive melanoma. Five-year control of stage I localized invasive melanoma is achieved in approximately 50% to 80% of cases.[1,2,3,12,33] However, when regional metastases are present, the survival rates decline to a range of 15% to 40%.[1,12,33] Intransit metastasis (satellitosis) may occur after radical surgery with RLND for lower limb melanomas. Overall, this averages about 6% but has been reported to occur in up to 20% of cases.[28] For these patients, the 5-year survival rates are low, approximating 10% to 15% following conventional treatment.[12,28] When this study commenced in 1957, the available drugs produced responses in only 5% to 10% of patients.[24] Today, the most effective agent for disseminated disease is DTIC used alone or in combination with other drugs. Objective responses with DTIC may occur in 16% to 30% of patients, with a median survival rate of approximately 3 months.[7] Systemic chemotherapy as an adjunct to surgical excision still has not been proved to add significant benefits.[18,31,35,39,44] Immunotherapy can produce occasional dramatic responses, but it has not been proved reproducibly to be an effective adjuvant treatment.[31,39,44]

With the development of regional chemotherapy by limb perfusion for melanomas, it soon became apparent that objective responses in measurable lesions occurred in more than half of patients. Combination treatment with excisional surgery and regional chemotherapy by perfusion produced 5-year survival rates for all patients with regional disease of 39%, with 15-year survival rates of 35%. These results are not obtainable by conventional surgery. Even the most advanced cases with intransit and regional node metastases have 15-year survival rates of 28% in this series (see Table 10-4).

The improvement in 10-year survival rates using isolated limb perfusion is estimated to be 15% to 20% better than surgical treatment alone for stage I melanoma. The figure of 20% was estimated by comparing the Tulane data with surgical treatment data from the WHO Collaborating Centre for Evaluation of Methods of Diagnosis and Treatment of Melanoma.[45] There were 553 limb melanoma patients entered into the WHO study between 1967 and 1974 who are still under observation. The 288 stage I patients treated at Tulane Medical Center were treated over a longer time period, but in many ways the data are comparable. At 10 years, the overall survival of the WHO study was about 60%, compared to 80% in the Tulane study. In both studies, there was significant survival difference in patients undergoing immediate RLND compared to a delayed RLND if the regional nodes showed clinical evidence of metastases. Level II patients were deleted from the Tulane data set, which had a 2:3 male/female ratio compared to a sex ratio of 1:5 in the WHO Melanoma Group series. Both factors would tend to improve the WHO results compared to the Tulane series. Regional recurrence in the form of satellitosis was reduced to below 5%. Furthermore, excisional surgery combined with regional perfusion has become more conservative, while the surgical treatment alone remains more radical for thicker melanomas.

It has been noted by the Surveillance Epidemiology and End Results (SEER) program that in each 5-year period for the last 30 years, both the incidence and the survival rates of stage I melanoma have increased. The public and the medical profession are more aware of the importance of early diagnosis. Prompt treatment has improved results. Also, better criteria are now established for determining prognosis, and specific therapy tailored for a particular stage has been better defined. It now seems that surgical treatment alone in stage I disease will suffice for level I and II melanomas and some thin level III lesions. For thicker lesions involving a limb, regional perfusion is recommended as the first step in adjuvant therapy. Regional lymph node dissection combined with limb perfusion is recommended for patients with a poor prognosis. Currently the treatment options outlined in Table 10-8 are used by the authors as a guide to therapy for stage I melanoma involving the limbs. It is based on growth pattern, level of invasion, and tumor thickness. These recommendations can be modified by other clinical factors. Most melanomas <0.75 mm thick require a conservative but complete excision.

TABLE 10–8
OUTLINE FOR TREATMENT FOR STAGE I MELANOMA OF LIMBS ACCORDING TO
LEVEL, THICKNESS, AND PATHOLOGIC TYPE

Level of Invasion	Approximate Corresponding Thickness (mm)	Growth Pattern				Usual Excision Margins (cm)
		Lentigo Maligna	Superficial Spreading	Nodular	Acral Lentiginous	
I and II	0.1–0.75	E	E	not seen	E	1–2
III (thin)	0.76–1.4	E	WE and ? perf	WE and perf	WE and perf	1–3
III (thick)	1.5–2.5	WE and ? perf	WE and perf	WE and perf and ? RLND	WE and perf and ? RLND	2–4
IV	2.6–4	WE and perf and ? RLND	WE and perf and ? RLND	WE and perf and RLND	WE, perf, and RLND	2–5
V	>4	WE, perf, and RLND	WE, perf, and RLND	WE, perf, and RLND	WE, perf, and RLND	3–5

Additional Modifying Treatment Factors

	Better prognosis— less radical surgery	Poorer prognosis— more radical surgery
Age	Young	Old
Sex	Female	Male
Site	Proximal	Distal
Growth rate	Slow	Rapid
Ulceration	Absent	Present
Size	Small	Large
Pigmentation	Melanotic	Amelanotic
Lymphocyte infiltrate	Present	Absent

E, Excision (margins 0.5 cm–1.5 cm); WE, wide excision (margins 1.5–5 cm); perf., perfusion; RLND, regional lymph node dissection; ? RLND, regional lymph node dissection is added depending on additional factors.

However, for acral lentiginous melanomas of the feet and hands, RLND is also an important adjunct for thinner lesions, since so many patients otherwise develop delayed lymph node metastases. While limb perfusion results have been extremely gratifying for the thinner melanomas, the added expense of hospital and surgical care may not be cost effective compared to excisional surgery by itself. While many investigators use tumor thickness alone to select treatments, at Tulane additional prognostic characteristics are used in determining therapy.

Results with limb perfusion in stage I melanoma at other treatment centers are summarized in Table 10-9. These results show that consistently high survival rates can be achieved by surgeons skilled in the use of perfusion techniques.

The survival rates of stage I melanoma of the limbs obtained at the University of Alabama Medical Center and the Sydney Melanoma Unit in Australia treated without perfusion[2,3] were compared with the limb perfusion results obtained by Schraffordt Koops and colleagues at their clinic in Groningen, Holland[29,30,37,38] and the Tulane group (Table

10-10). Perfusion as performed by Schraffordt Koops and colleagues used slightly higher drug doses but about the same perfusion temperatures as Tulane did.[37] While slightly better response rates are obtained with higher drug doses, more local reaction occurs, resulting in the need for elective fasciotomy in most cases. Only 101 Tulane patients who had thickness measurements available were used in this comparison (out of the total 380 stage I cases). The small number of patients in the Tulane series with tumors 3 mm to 4.9 mm thick and over 5 mm thick makes the standard error large in these groups. Tulane patients with thinner melanomas did extremely well, with 100% 5-year survival rates for melanomas 0.75 mm to 1.4 mm thick and 94% for 1.5 mm to 2.9 mm melanomas. With the 3 mm to 4.9 mm thickness melanomas, the results obtained by Schraffordt Koops are the best of the four series, with a 91% 5-year survival rate (see Table 10-10). The Alabama and Sydney results seem to indicate that RLND adds to the survival when surgery alone is performed (*i.e.*, without perfusion). With thicker lesions (≥5 mm), the addition of perfusion most

TABLE 10–9
RESULTS OF ADJUVANT CHEMOTHERAPY BY PERFUSION, ALL STAGE I MELANOMAS OF THE LIMBS—COLLECTED SERIES

Author	Reference Number	Year	Number of Patients	Level of Invasion and Thickness	Primary Excision	RLND*	Five-Year Survival Rate (%)	Ten-Year Survival Rate (%)
Sugarbaker	42	1976	199	II–V	WE[†]	14%	88	
Wagner	46	1976	133	Invasive[‡]	—	—	94	
Golomb	13	1976	61	III–V	WE	No	72	
Davis	11	1976	72	II–V	WE	All	90	
Stehlin	41	1977	70	III–V	WE	No	84	
Golomb	14	1979	39	III–V	WE	All	89	
McBride	27	1981	Upper limb, 18	III ≥ 1 mm IV, V	LE[§]	No		78
			Lower limb, 83	III > 1 mm IV, V	LE	No		45
Krementz	19	1983	336	III–V	WE[‖]	247	88	80
			Upper limb, 125				91	84
			Lower limb, 211				87	77

* Regional lymph node dissection
† Wide excision
‡ Large ulcerated primary or single regional node
§ Local excision
‖ one patient treated by perfusion only

TABLE 10–10
COMPARISON OF RESULTS OBTAINED IN STAGE I MELANOMA OF THE LIMBS
BY EXCISION WITH AND WITHOUT RLND[1], WE[2] AND PERFUSION AT FOUR INSTITUTIONS,
OBSERVED 5-YEAR SURVIVAL RATES (±S.E.)*

Thickness (mm)	WE plus Perfusion (Groningen[3])	WE plus RLND (UAB[4] and SMU[5])	WE (UAB and SMU)	WE[7] plus Perfusion (Tulane University[6])
0.75–1.4	—	—	—	100 ± 0
1.5–2.9	86 ± 6	87 ± 9	75 ± 7	94 ± 4
3–4.9	91 ± 5	86 ± 13	51 ± 12	57 ± 20
≥5	67 ± 7	33 ± 29	35 ± 14	57 ± 16

* All figures are percentages
[1] Regional lymph node dissection
[2] Wide excision
[3] University Hospital, Groningen, The Netherlands
[4] University of Alabama Medical Center, University of Alabama in Birmingham, Alabama
[5] University of Sydney and the Sydney Melanoma Unit, Sydney Hospital, Sydney, New South Wales, Australia
[6] Tulane University, New Orleans, Louisiana
[7] Some patients had RLND in addition to WE and Perfusion (numbers not available at this time)

clearly demonstrates an increased survival rate compared to surgical treatment alone (with or without RLND). These comparative results apply only to stage I melanoma. In patients with regional recurrences or with metastatic disease, the benefits of perfusion are even more apparent.

The adjunctive use of regional chemotherapy and hyperthermia by perfusion combined with excisional surgery offers the patient with localized primary melanoma of the limbs an excellent chance for cure. For the patient with regional metastases, limb perfusion offers the most effective treatment for control of disease with limb preservation, while for the patient with distant disease and painful masses or ulceration, it offers an effective regional palliation with salvage of a functional limb.

COMMENTARY ON ISOLATED LIMB PERFUSION PERFORMED AT THE UNIVERSITY OF GRONINGEN, THE NETHERLANDS

H. SCHRAFFORDT KOOPS
J. OLDHOFF
J. W. OOSTERHUIS

In this chapter, Dr. Krementz and his colleagues carefully describe the technique and problems of regional perfusion. It is an honour to comment on this chapter, because one of us (JO) learned the technique in Tulane in 1962. Some 700 perfusions have since been performed in the Department of Surgical Oncology of the Groningen University Hospital, and the operative techniques used in the two departments differ very little. We wish to comment on a few technical details and some of the results at our institution.

INDICATIONS FOR PERFUSION

As at Tulane, the indications for perfusion in clinical stage I patients are made on the basis of microstaging (level and thickness). During the past 5 years, only patients with Clark's level III, IV, or V and a tumor thickness $\geq$ 1.5 mm have been accepted for perfusion.[4] In our opinion, the prognosis in patients with a tumor thickness of 0.75 mm to 1.4 mm is so good and the risk of local recurrence so small that wide excision without perfusion should suffice. Because the risk of local recurrence is so small after regional perfusion, we have now reduced the margin of melanoma excision to about 3 cm, often using a primary closure of the wound without a split-thickness skin graft.

An axillary node dissection is always performed in conjunction with arm perfusion because of the difficulty one would otherwise have examining axillary nodal metastases in perfused patients with an axillary scar. In the past few years, for leg melanomas in stage I patients, the node of Rosenmüller located on the caudal edge of the saphenous hiatus is routinely biopsied at the time of perfusion. If this lymph node contains tumor, a second, femoral, perfusion with inguinal node dissection is performed 6 weeks after the first, iliac, perfusion.[1]

Krementz indicates that patients with a melanoma of the foot have a less favorable prognosis than those with a tumor of the lower leg. Because of this finding, our policy is to give patients with foot melanomas two perfusions at an interval of 6 weeks: the first is an iliac perfusion, while the second is a popliteal perfusion.

In Groningen, perfusion of the leg always involves an iliac perfusion through the external iliac artery and vein. When a parailiac lymph node contains tumor tissue, perfusion is performed only in exceptional cases for palliation.

PERFUSION TECHNIQUES

Until a year ago, we calculated the melphalan dosage on the basis of body weight. Our dosage is conspicuously higher than that at Tulane. For iliac perfusions, a dose of 1 mg to 1.5 mg melphalan per kg body weight was used, while for the upper limbs the dose was 0.5 mg/kg to 0.7 mg/kg. Since January 1982, the melphalan dosage has been calcualted on the basis of the limb volume, as suggested by Wieberdink and colleagues.[5] Prior to surgery, the arm or leg is immersed in water to determine the exact volume. Melphalan is given at a dose of 10 mg/liter perfused tissue. Remarkably, the dosage for an arm perfusion has hardly changed, but it increased substantially for leg perfusions. We now give total doses of 100 mg to 150 mg melphalan and observe the same type and intensity of local toxic reactions in the leg, even though the measured temperature of skin and muscle is maintained at 39°C to 40°C. In the case of satellitosis or a local recurrence, actinomycin D is added to the perfusion fluid (0.006 mg/kg–0.014 mg/kg body weight for arm and leg respectively).[2,3] It is difficult to explain why our patients tolerate a higher melphalan dosage than do Tulane patients. One explanation may be that we inject the cytostatic drugs directly into the oxygenator so that mixing can first occur, whereas at Tulane the drugs are injected into the arterial line to the limb.

The patients at Tulane are heparinized with 150 U heparin/kg body weight at the time of perfusion. We use 3.3 mg/kg body weight—a dosage of heparin at least twice as high. We reverse the heparinization with 50% protamine chloride, avoiding protamine sulfate because we have seen some very severe drops in blood pressure during reversal with this compound. Anticoagulation is started the day after perfusion and continued until the patient walks normally again. We rarely see postoperative thrombophlebitis; only one thrombectomy has been performed in our series of some 700 perfusions, and there have been only a few patients with pulmonary embolism. It seems plausible that the high heparin doses used during perfusion and the postoperative anticoagulant medication have limited thrombophlebitis and thrombosis. We do not routinely give antibiotics either during the preoperative or the postoperative period.

In the past few years, our experimental perfusions in dogs have demonstrated that tissue perfusion during extracorporeal perfusion differs from that in the nonperfused limb. Thus, when the perfusion pressure was reduced below systemic mean arterial pressure, the mean pO_2 values decreased, although the mean flow rates were still above values measured in the intact limb circulation. Adequate tissue oxygenation was maintained only when the perfusion pressure was not lower than 15 mm Hg below systemic mean arterial pressure. Clinical studies have now begun using high perfusion flow rates (up to about 1200 ml/min) in patients. The results suggest that there are fewer local toxic changes with this higher tissue perfusion, and that, consequently, the dosage of cytostatic drugs can possibly be increased. An additional advantage of high flow is that a higher tissue temperature is more quickly attained.

Groningen differs slightly from Tulane in the manner in which the collateral vessels of the skin are occluded with the aid of the Esmarch tourniquet. We insert a Steinmann pin into the head of the humerus to isolate the arm, and into the superior anterior iliac spine to isolate the leg. The rubber bandage is twisted around this pin and the axillary or inguinal skin. In our opinion, the Tulane method gives less perfect isolation because the rubber bandage does not occlude the skin and subcutaneous vessels as well.

RESULTS AND DISCUSSION

Krementz's results in terms of survival, local recurrence, and regional node metastases are excellent. The large numbers of perfused patients make it possible to compare groups of patients with different tumor thickness, sex, site, and other factors.

In Groningen, the results of 132 clinical stage I patients with Clark's level III, IV, or V and a Breslow tumor thickness of 1.5 mm or more were reevaluated in 1983. These patients had a total of 171 perfusions during the period 1965 to 1977, and all patients had a follow-up of 5 years or more. Five patients died from an intercurrent disease, and three (3/132 = 2.3%) had a fatal postoperative complication (two died shortly after the operation from intravascular coagulation, and one died during the postoperative period from a cerebral hemorrhage). Two patients developed a pulmonary embolism long after the operation (7 and 8 months respectively), and one of these was fatal. One female patient died from a second malignant melanoma located on the nonperfused leg 9 years after perfusion of the opposite leg. These nine patients were not included in the reevaluation. In the remaining 123 patients, the 3-year, 5-year, and 10-year crude survival rates were 82%, 78%, and 72% respectively.

The survival of stage I patients was reviewed on the basis of tumor thickness (Table 10-11). It is evident that survival diminishes as tumor thickness increases. The Groningen survival figures are comparable with those of Tulane Medical Center (see Table 10-10). The survival rates for thinner melanomas also corresponded with patients treated by wide local excision and elective lymph node dissection at the University of Alabama in Birmingham and the Sydney Melanoma Unit, Australia. However, it is difficult to compare the sex and site distribution from these figures; both exert a distinct influence on

TABLE 10–11
CRUDE SURVIVAL RATES FOR PATIENTS ACCORDING TO TUMOR THICKNESS

Tumor Thickness	Five-Year Survival	Five- to Seventeen-Year Survival
1.5 mm–1.9 mm	26/29 (90%)	25/29 (86%)
2 mm–2.9 mm	39/42 (93%)	34/42 (81%)
3 mm–3.9 mm	13/17 (76%)	12/17 (71%)
4 mm–4.9 mm	9/14 (64%)	9/14 (64%)
≥5 mm	9/21 (43%)	8/21 (38%)
Total	96/123 (78%)	88/123 (72%)

the prognosis. Local recurrence in the perfused limb was 6.5% in the Groningen patients after a 5-year follow-up; recurrence frequently occurred late. Five local recurrences developed after the first 5-year period, and in one patient a recurrence did not become manifest until after 12 years. In 14 patients (11%) local recurrence was observed during the follow-up period from 5 to 17 years, and in 8 of them the recurrence developed after systemic metastatic spread, which caused their deaths. Of the 6 patients without systemic metastases, 5 are still alive after a follow-up of 14, 22, 48, 55, and 103 months, respectively. In 27 patients (22%) regional node metastases developed during the follow-up. This proved to be an unfavorable prognostic sign, for only 7 (26%) have so far survived.

In our opinion, both the Tulane and the Groningen series demonstrate that survival is improved after isolated limb perfusion using regional chemotherapy and hyperthermia. In an effort to establish whether regional perfusion gives an advantage in terms of local recurrence and survival over conventional surgery, we are now comparing the Groningen perfusion patients with the patients treated at the University of Alabama in Birmingham and at the Sydney Melanoma Unit. Should this comparison fail to reveal any substantial differences, a randomized trial would seem to be the only way to resolve the controversy. Both the WHO and the European Organization for Research and Treatment of Cancer (EORTC) have already made a preliminary design for such a randomized clinical trial.

REFERENCES

1. Ariel IM: Malignant melanoma of the lower extremity. In Ariel IM (ed): Malignant Melanoma, p 413. New York, Appleton-Century-Crofts, 1981
2. Balch CM, Soong S-j, Milton GW, Shaw HM, McGovern VJ, Murad TM, McCarthy WH, Maddox WA: A comparison of prognostic factors and surgical results in 1,786 patients with localized (stage I) melanoma treated in Alabama, USA, and New South Wales, Australia. Ann Surg 196:677, 1982
3. Balch CM, Soong S-j, Milton GW, Shaw HM, McGovern VJ, Murad TM, Maddox WA: Changing trends in cutaneous melanoma over a quarter century in Alabama, USA, and New South Wales, Australia. Cancer 52:1748, 1983
4. Breslow A: Thickness, cross-sectional areas and depth of invasion in the prognosis of cutaneous melanoma. Ann Surg 172:902, 1970
5. Cavaliere R, Ciocatto EC, Giovanella BC, Heidelberger C, Johnson RO, Margottini M, Mondovi B, Moricca G, Rossi-Fanelli A: Selective heat sensitivity of cancer cells: Biochemical and clinical studies. Cancer 20:1351, 1967
6. Clark WH Jr, From L, Bernardino EA, Mihm MC Jr: The histogenesis and biologic behavior of primary human malignant melanomas of the skin. Cancer Res 29:705, 1969
7. Costanzi JJ: The chemotherapy of human malignant melanoma. In Costanzi JJ (ed): Malignant Melanoma 1, p 259. The Hague, Martinus Nijhoff, 1983
8. Creech OJ Jr, Krementz ET, Ryan RF, Reemtsma K, Elliot JL, Winblad JN: Perfusion treatment of patients with cancer. JAMA 171:2069, 1959
9. Creech OJ Jr, Krementz ET, Ryan RF, Winblad JN: Chemotherapy of cancer: Regional perfusion utilizing an extracorporeal circuit. Ann Surg 148:616, 1958
10. Cutler SJ, Ederer F: Maximum utilization of the life table method in analyzing survival. J Chronic Dis 8:699, 1958
11. Davis CD, Ivins JC, Soule EH: Mayo Clinic experience with isolated limb perfusion for invasive malignant melanoma of the extremities. In Pigment Cell, Vol 2, p 379. New York, S. Karger, 1976
12. End Results Section, Biometry Branch, Division of Cancer Cause and Prevention, National Cancer Institute. Cancer Patient Survival. Report Number 5: 1976
13. Golomb FM: Perfusion. In Andrade R, Gumport SL, Popkin GL, Rees TD (eds): Cancer of the Skin: Biology-Diagnosis-Management, Vol II, p 1623. Philadelphia, WB Saunders, 1976
14. Golomb FM, Bromberg J, Dubin N: A controlled study of the survival experience of patients with primary malignant melanoma of the distal extremities treated with adjuvant isolated perfusion. In Jones SE, Salmon SE (eds): Adjuvant Therapy of Cancer, Vol II, p 519. New York, Grune & Stratton, 1979
15. Gray LH, Conger AD, Ebert M, Hornsey S, Scott OAC: The concentration of oxygen dissolved in tissues at the time of irradiation as a factor in radiotherapy. Br J Radiol 26:638, 1953
16. Hahn GM: Interactions of drugs and hyperthermia in vitro and in vivo. In Streffer C (ed): Cancer Therapy by Hyperthermia and Radiation, p 72. Baltimore, Urban & Schwarzenberg, 1978
17. Healy W: The effect of hydrogen peroxide and alkylating agents on sarcoma 37 and Ehrlich ascites tumor in mice. Bull Tulane Med Fac 23:225, 1964
18. Hill GJ II, Moss SE, Golomb FM, Grage TB, Fletcher WS, Minton JP, Krementz ET: DTIC and combination therapy for melanoma. III. DTIC (NSC 45388) surgical adjuvant study COG protocol 7040. Cancer 47:2556, 1981
19. Krementz ET, Campbell M: The role of limb perfusion in the management of malignant melanoma. In

Costanzi JJ (ed): Malignant Melanoma 1, p 225. The Hague, Nijhoff, 1983

20. Krementz ET, Knudson L: The effect of increased oxygen tension on the tumoricidal effect of nitrogen mustard. Surgery 50:266, 1961

21. Krementz ET, Mansell PWA, Hornung MO, Samuels MS, Sutherland CM, Benes EN: Immunotherapy of malignant disease: The use of viable sensitized lymphocytes or transfer factor prepared from sensitized lymphocytes. Cancer 33:394, 1974

22. Krementz ET, Reed RJ, Coleman WP III, Sutherland CM, Carter RD, Campbell M: Acral lentiginous melanoma: A clinicopathologic entity. Ann Surg 195:632, 1982

23. Leather RP, Eckert C: Hyperbaric oxygenation and mechlorethamine effectiveness. Arch Surg 87:144, 1963

24. Luce JK: Chemotherapy of melanoma. Semin Oncol 2:179, 1975

25. Luck JM: Action of p-[Di(2-chloroethyl)]-amino-L-phenylalanine on Harding-Passey mouse melanoma. Science 123:984, 1956

26. McBride CM, McMurtrey MJ, Copeland EM, Hickey RC: Regional chemotherapy by isolation-perfusion. In Murphy GP (ed): International Advances in Surgical Oncology, Vol 1, p 1. New York, Alan R. Liss, 1978

27. McBride CM, Smith JL Jr, Brown BW: Primary malignant melanoma of the limbs: A re-evaluation using microstaging techniques. Cancer 48:1463, 1981

28. McCarthy JG, Haagensen CD, Herter FP: The role of groin dissection in the management of melanoma of the lower extremity. Ann Surg 179:156, 1974

29. Martijn H, Oldhoff J, Schraffordt Koops H: Regional perfusion in the treatment of patients with a locally metastasized malignant melanoma of the limbs. Eur J Cancer 17:471, 1981

30. Martijn H, Oldhoff J, Schraffordt Koops H: Hyperthermic regional perfusion with melphalan and a combination of melphalan and actinomycin D in the treatment of locally metastasized malignant melanomas of the extremities. J Surg Oncol 20:9, 1982

31. Mastrangelo MJ, Bellet RE, Berd D: Postsurgical adjuvant therapy. In Clark WH Jr, Goldman LI, Mastrangelo MJ (eds): Human Malignant Melanoma, p 309. New York, Grune & Stratton, 1979

32. Millar RC, Ketcham AS: The effect of heparin and warfarin on primary and metastatic tumors. J Med Exp Clin 5:23, 1974

33. Milton GW: Malignant Melanoma of the Skin and Mucous Membrane, p 88. London, Churchill Livingstone, 1977

34. Pfefferkorn RO, Dildocher MS: Regional perfusion for melanoma of the extremities. J Extracorporeal Tech 14:475, 1982

35. Quagliana J, Tranum B, Neidhardt J, Gagliano R: Adjuvant chemotherapy with BCNU, Hydrea and DTIC (BHD) with or without immunotherapy (BCG) in high-risk melanoma patients: A SWOG study. Proc Am Soc Clin Oncol 21:399, 1980

36. Ryan CF, Krementz ET, Creech O Jr, Winblad JN, Chamblee W, Cheek H: Selected perfusion of isolated viscera with chemotherapeutic agents using an extracorporeal circuit. Surg Forum 8:158, 1957

37. Schraffordt Koops H, Oldhoff J, van der Ploeg E, Vermey A, Eibergen R: Isolated regional perfusion in the treatment of malignant melanomas of the extremities. Archivum Chirugicum Neerlandicum 17:237, 1975

38. Schraffordt Koops H, Oldhoff J, van der Ploeg E, Vermey A, Eibergen R: Regional perfusion for recurrent malignant melanoma of the extremities. Am J Surg 133:221, 1977

39. Silberman AW, Morton DL: Adjuvant therapy following surgery for primary malignant melanoma. In Costanzi JJ (ed): Malignant Melanoma 1, p 207. The Hague, Nijhoff, 1983

40. Stehlin JS Jr, Giovanella BC, de Ipolyi PD, Muenz LR, Anderson RF: Results of hyperthermic perfusion for melanoma of the extremities. Surg Gynecol Obstet 140:339, 1975

41. Stehlin JS Jr, Giovanella BC, de Ipolyi PD, Muenz LR, Anderson RF, Gutierrez AA: Hyperthermic perfusion of extremities for melanoma and soft tissue sarcomas. In Rossi-Fanelli A, Cavaliere R, Mondoni B, Moricca G (eds): Selective Heat Sensitivity of Cancer Cells, p 171. Berlin, Springer-Verlag, 1977

42. Sugarbaker EV, McBride CM: Survival and regional disease control after isolation-perfusion for invasive stage I melanoma of the extremities. Cancer 37:188, 1976

43. Suit HD, Shwayder M: Hyperthermia: Potential as an anti-tumor agent. Cancer 34:122, 1975

44. Veronesi U, Adamus J, Aubert C, Bajetta E, Beretta G, Bonadonna G, Bufalino R, Cascinelli N, Cocconi G, Durand J, De Marsillac J, Ikonopisov RL, Kiss B, Lejeune F, MacKie R, Madej G, Mulder H, Mechl Z, Milton GW, Morabito A, Peter H, Priario J, Paul E, Rumke P, Sertoli R, Tomin R: A randomized trial of adjuvant chemotherapy and immunotherapy in cutaneous melanoma. N Engl J Med 307:913, 1982

45. Veronesi U, Adamus J, Bandiera DC, Brennhovd IO, Caceres E, Cascinelli N, Claudio F, Ikonopisov RL, Javorskj VV, Kirov S, Kulakowski A, Lacour J, Lejeune F, Mechl Z, Morabito A, Rodé I, Sergeev S, van Slooten E, Szczygiel K, Trapeznikov NN, Wagner RI: Stage I melanoma of the limbs: Immediate versus delayed node dissection. Tumori 66:373, 1980

46. Wagner DE: A retrospective study of regional perfusion for melanoma. Arch Surg 111:410, 1976

COMMENTARY REFERENCES

1. Martijn H, Oldhoff J, Oosterhuis JW, Schraffordt Koops H: Indications for elective groin dissection in

clinical stage I patients with malignant melanoma of the lower extremity treated by hyperthermic regional perfusion. Cancer 52:1526, 1983

2. Martijn H, Oldhoff J, Schraffordt Koops H: Regional perfusion in the treatment of patients with a locally metastasized melanoma of the limbs. Eur J Cancer 17:471, 1981

3. Martijn H, Oldhoff J, Schraffordt Koops H: Hyperthermic regional perfusion with melphalan and a combination of melphalan and Actinomycin-D in the treatment of locally metastasized malignant melanoma of the extremities. J Surg Oncol 20:9, 1982

4. Schraffordt Koops H, Beekhuis H, Oldhoff J, Oosterhuis JW, van der Ploeg E, Vermey A: Local recurrence and survival in patients with (Clark level IV/V and over 1.5 mm thickness) stage I malignant melanoma of the extremities after regional perfusion. Cancer 48:1952, 1981

5. Wieberdink J, Benckhuizen C, Braat RP, van Slooten EA, Olthuis GAA: Dosimetry in isolation perfusion of the limbs by assessment of perfused tissue volume and grading of toxic reactions. Eur J Cancer Clin Oncol 18:905, 1982

CHARLES M. BALCH
PETER HERSEY

Current Status of Adjuvant Therapy

11

Over the past decade, advances in melanoma treatment have evolved largely from a greater knowledge about the natural history of the disease and from more precise definition of prognostic factors as guides to surgical management. Despite the improving cure rate from earlier diagnosis and better surgical treatment, a substantial number of melanoma patients still die of their disease. Because prevention of recurrences following surgery is the next major goal in treatment, attention has been focused on adjuvant treatments such as immunotherapy, chemotherapy, and radiotherapy.

The concept of multimodality therapy is well proven in animal models of human tumors, where the best results were achieved by combining local treatment (*e.g.,* surgery) with systemic treatment (*e.g.,* immunotherapy or chemotherapy). This approach has met with outstanding success for some human cancers, but not for others. Melanoma is one malignant tumor for which results of adjuvant therapy have been disappointing to date. However, recent advances at a conceptual and technical level, especially in immunology, will undoubtedly result in a resurgence of interest in these areas during the coming years. Therefore, considerable emphasis has been given in this chapter to some of the scientific principles relevant to current and future forms of adjuvant immunotherapy. This chapter also reviews some of the principles, rationale, and results of other forms of adjuvant treatment.

CONCEPTS OF ADJUVANT THERAPY

Experimental models of animal tumors have clearly established the principles of adjuvant therapy (as reviewed by Balch and Maddox).[8] When animals were inoculated with a known tumor dose and then randomly allocated to single treatment modalities (*e.g.,* surgery alone) or combination modalities (*e.g.,* surgery plus postoperative chemotherapy), the latter produced clearly superior results.[136,137] Cures were defined as long-term survivals with verification of absence of malignancy by autopsy. Examples of these results in animal model systems are shown in Table 11-1 for surgically treated solid tumors in mice.

These extensive animal investigations have elucidated four fundamental principles that are pertinent to designing treatment strategies for human malignancies: (1) the effectiveness of any given regimen is inversely proportional to tumor burden; (2)

clinically silent micrometastases are generally more susceptible to drug therapy than the larger grossly apparent primary tumor from which they were derived; (3) a drug or combination of agents with activity against moderately advanced tumors is even more active against residual metastatic disease after surgical excision of grossly detectable tumor; (4) a curative treatment of cancer requires complete or nearly complete eradication of cancer cells, because lethal metastases may arise from even a single residual malignant cell.[136,137]

The effectiveness of adjuvant chemotherapy in these experimental studies decreased as (1) the tumor staging advanced before surgery, (2) the interval from surgery to the start of chemotherapy increased, and (3) the drug dose was reduced. Some drugs were marginally effective or ineffective against presurgical total body burden of tumor cells but were curative in some to all mice with metastatic disease if given shortly after surgical removal of the primary tumor.[136] These observations have important and useful application in the design of human studies employing adjuvant therapy.

Surgical treatment is a regional therapy, so it is not curative in those patients harboring occult metastatic disease at distant sites. Additional modalities might be considered for eliminating residual systemic disease in selected patients. Since there is no systemic treatment with proven efficacy, patients should be encouraged to participate in clinical investigational protocols. The decisions to employ systemic adjuvant treatments focus on (1) which patients are at risk for harboring metastatic disease at a microscopic (or occult) level, and (2) which modality should be used.

SELECTION OF PATIENTS

Traditionally, physicians have staged melanoma patients according to their ability to detect metastatic disease clinically. However, a significant number of patients without clinically detectable disease (stage I or II) may harbor literally millions of metastatic melanoma cells that are undetectable by conventional tests (*e.g.,* scans, x-rays films, blood chemistries). Patients at risk for developing metastases from melanoma can be identified only by the prognostic or predictive features involving the tumor or the patient. These are fully discussed in Chapter 19.

Only a minority of stage I patients have a high risk for distant disease. In general, these are patients with melanomas ≥ 4 mm in thickness, especially those with ulceration, or those located at axial

TABLE 11–1
ADJUNCTIVE CHEMOTHERAPEUTIC EXPERIMENTS IN ANIMAL TUMOR MODELS
DONE AT SOUTHERN RESEARCH INSTITUTE*

Tumor	Treatment	Percent "Cures"
Lewis lung carcinoma	Surgery	0
	Me-CCNU	0
	Cyclophosphamide (Cy)	0
	Surgery + Me-CCNU	30–40
	Surgery + Cy	50–90
B16 melanoma	Surgery	0–20
	Me-CCNU	0
	Surgery + Me-CCNU	70
Colon tumor #26	Surgery	20–35
	Me-CCNU	0
	Cy + CCNU-cis	0
	Surgery + Me-CCNU	65
	Surgery + CCNU + Cy	75

*Varying cure rates reflect differences in initial tumor burden and drug doses (Balch CM, Maddox WA: The logic of adjunctive therapy in surgical patients with resectable cancer. South Med J 71:951, 1978)

sites.[9,12,114] Patients with resected nodal metastases have the highest risk for distant micrometastases, estimated at 70% to 80% at many centers.[13,29,46,65,85,158] Conceptually at least, some form of adjuvant therapy should be considered for these patients, since they have such a high risk for distant metastases. The patients actually selected will depend on the clinician's view of what constitutes sufficient risk of recurrence to justify adjuvant therapy and what inconvenience the therapy will have for the patient. For example, if the clinician were to regard a 50% risk of recurrence as unacceptable, patients with melanomas exceeding 3 mm or 4 mm in thickness, especially if located on the trunk or head, or any ulcerated melanoma would be considered for systemic adjuvant therapy. It should be emphasized that these criteria are for identifying patients at sufficient metastatic risk who might be included in adjuvant therapy trials, since no currently available agents are effective enough to recommend as standard treatment.

It is emphasized that the figures quoted above indicate what is expected among large patient groups. Individual patients may behave differently than expected, because additional unidentified factors are important in prognosis. These may include immunologic factors. For example, Thy-1 antigen is expressed on melanoma cells from some primary tumors but only rarely on metastases.[80] This may indicate that absence of Thy-1 on primary tumors may predict those tumors that could metastasize. HLA-DR histocompatibility antigens also show variable expression on melanoma cells and may be important in determining interaction with the immune system.[166] Identification of melanoma cells at various stages of differentiation is now possible using monoclonal antibodies,[89] and classification of melanoma cells on this basis may help to identify tumors with different biologic behavior.

SELECTION OF ADJUVANT THERAPY

A common practice has been to select postoperative adjuvant treatments from those agents with demonstrated efficacy in patients with advanced cancer. This is the reason for using DTIC alone or in combination with other agents in trials of adjuvant therapy for melanoma patients. Response rates with DTIC have been superior to other single agents in advanced melanoma,[36,119] and it has relatively few immunosuppressive effects.[26] It is much more difficult to evaluate immunotherapy agents in patients with advanced disease, since it is unlikely that any currently available immune modulation would have a significant therapeutic effect. Although phase I (i.e., dose schedule) immunotherapy trials might be considered in patients with advanced disease, phase II or III therapeutic trials should be conducted with patients having minimum residual disease. Preferably, these should be patients in whom all detectable metastatic disease has been removed, such as postsurgical stage II patients with documented nodal metastases.

Currently available anticancer drugs and biologic response modifiers (immunotherapy) generally appear to have limited potential against large numbers of tumor cells. That is, a drug's effectiveness against micrometastatic foci may decline when the tumor burden exceeds 10^6 to 10^8 viable tumor cells. It should be emphasized that a tumor comprised of 10^6 cells measures about 1 mm in diameter and that the total residual disease might represent considerably more than this tumor volume. Therefore, if adjuvant treatment modalities are to be employed against a minimum amount of residual disease, they should be initiated as soon after surgery as possible, usually within 2 to 6 weeks postoperatively. The treatment strategy must also use maximum surgical principles, for overly conservative operations might negate the potential benefits of adjuvant therapy. Otherwise, the number of tumor cells left behind after surgery might exceed the number that can be eradicated by drug, immune, or irradiation therapy.

As outlined below, adjuvant trials in melanoma have so far had limited success, but a number of new developments in tumor biology and immunology hold promise for the future. It is imperative that such studies be conducted in a prospective clinical trial setting so that their long-term benefits and risks can be evaluated and the study will receive the maximum support by the medical community. The successful completion of most of these studies requires that all physicians treating melanoma keep up to date about current adjuvant trials being conducted in their geographic areas and encourage their patients to participate in them.

ADJUVANT IMMUNOTHERAPY

RATIONALE

Immunotherapy has been traditionally classified either as active-specific or nonspecific.[22] The use of nonspecific immune-stimulants, such as BCG or *Corynebacterium parvum,* constitute most of the adjuvant immunotherapy trials conducted since the 1960s. The rationale for such studies was twofold. First, it was considered that tumor-associated antigens on melanoma cells induced relatively weak immune responses and that these responses needed only to be augmented by immunotherapy to become effective in controlling tumor growth. A second rationale was that melanoma patients had weakened immune defenses that could be restored by immune stimulants.

Considerable evidence was available to support both contentions. For example, the immunogenicity of melanoma cells was supported by studies showing that immunologic responses to melanoma antigens appeared related to tumor growth.[23,78,83,84,105] Furthermore, the presence of certain antibodies in the serum appeared to have prognostic significance.[79,95] Several studies also showed that both the incidence and the levels of antibody responses to melanoma antigens could be increased by various vaccination procedures.[43,91,93,110,111] However, in some instances these responses were against antigens from fetal calf serum attached to the immunizing cells.[110,111]

Decreased immunocompetence has also been well documented in melanoma patients using a variety of *in vitro* and *in vivo* immunologic assays.[47,59,169] In retrospect, however, it seems probable that the decreased immunocompetence resulted from tumor growth rather than from preexisting immune defects in the host. This was suggested in studies of dinitrochlorobenzene (DNCB) skin testing[29,131] and assays of natural killer (NK) cell activity.[127,148] Defects in the latter assay were apparent in patients with regional lymph node metastases before and after surgical removal of the involved lymph nodes.[76,77] The influence of tumor burden was also shown in responses of patients receiving various forms of immunotherapy, since patients who failed to respond or who showed diminished responses during immunotherapy were those who had early recurrence from their tumor.[42,58,134,150] The skin test response to BCG was also shown to be an important prognostic factor in the survival of patients with high-risk melanomas.[35]

Despite the negative treatment results and the inability to reliably use immunologic monitoring, the prevailing views at the time most adjuvant trials in melanoma were instituted were not illogical, especially since many of the treatments appeared to have been effective against tumor growth in animal models. As discussed below, the extent of their success or failure as surgical adjuvants provided useful information in the design of second generation trials involving adjuvant immunotherapy.

RESULTS
BCG and *Corynebacterium parvum*

Bacillus Calmette-Guerin (BCG) and *Corynebacterium parvum (C. parvum)* were the most frequently used agents in the initial immunotherapy trials (listed in Tables 11-2 and 11-3). The role of BCG in

TABLE 11–2
RANDOMIZED CLINICAL TRIALS INVOLVING NONSPECIFIC IMMUNOTHERAPY

Institution	Reference Number	Number of Patients	Disease Stage	Treatment Evaluated	Results	Comments
Southeastern Cancer Study Group (SEG)	10	260	I	1. *C. parvum* 2. Control	Survival benefit for melanomas >3 mm (p = 0.01)	Only a subset had a benefit; study continuing
Alberta	124	152	I	1. Oral BCG 2. i.d. BCG 3. Control	No difference overall	Significant decrease in local or regional recurrence with BCG (p < 0.01)
UCLA	96	137	I	1. BCG postoperatively 2. BCG preoperatively and BCG postoperatively 3. Control	No difference	
UCSF	145	203	I	1. Levamisole 2. Control	No difference	Trend for increased time to first visceral recurrence with levamisole
UCLA	142	139	II	1. BCG 2. Tumor cell vaccine plus BCG 3. Control	No difference overall	Increased survival after first relapse in BCG patients
Memorial Hospital, New York	125,126	48	II	1. BCG 2. Control	No difference	Low doses of BCG used
Cleveland Clinic	27	36	II	1. Transfer factor 2. Control	No difference	
SEG	12	237	II	1. BCG 2. *C. parvum*	No difference	Slightly better survival and less toxicity with *C. parvum*
Eastern Oncology Group	39	98	I,II	1. BCG 2. Control	No difference	
Yale	2	15	I,II	1. Intralymphatic and i.d. BCG 2. Control	Improved survival for BCG	Pilot study
Pennsylvania State University	102,109	116	I,II	1. BCG 2. *C. parvum*	Significant improvement for *C. parvum* patients in relapse rate and survival for Stage II only	No difference between treatment for stage I, only for stage II

cancer and possible modes of action have been reviewed.[17,98] Several phase II studies were reported in which BCG vaccination in postoperative stage II melanoma patients appeared to prolong the recurrence-free interval.[46,48,65,66] One of these studies used a historical control, while the other used a concurrent control group that was not randomized (Fig. 11-1). More recent results of several large trials showed no statistical benefit from BCG vaccinations as adjuvant to surgery in patients with stage I or II disease.[39,50,124,125,129,142,158] The available evidence

strongly suggests that there is little, if any, effectiveness of BCG in this setting.

Similar comments appear to apply to the use of *C. parvum* as adjuvant therapy. Initial results in melanoma patients appeared promising,[94] but subsequent studies reported no benefit.[7,85] These trials are summarized in Tables 11-2 and 11-3. The few exceptions should be noted. Lipton and colleagues[109] reported that survival was significantly improved in 23 patients with stage II melanoma treated by *C. parvum* compared to 25 patients treated by BCG in

TABLE 11–3
RANDOMIZED CLINICAL TRIALS INVOLVING CHEMOTHERAPY OR COMBINED CHEMOTHERAPY AND IMMUNOTHERAPY (*NONSPECIFIC*)

Institution	Reference Number	Number of Patients	Disease Stage	Treatments Evaluated	Results	Comments
Central Oncology Group	86	174	I, II, III	1. DTIC 2. Control	No benefit	DTIC arm did worse than control
WHO Melanoma Group	158	761	II	1. DTIC 2. BCG (Time) 3. DTIC plus BCG 4. Control	No difference	Patients with 2 or 3 metastatic nodes did better with DTIC plus BCG
National Cancer Institute	50	181	I, II	1. Methyl CCNU 2. BCG 3. BCG plus TCV 4. Control	No difference	Renal toxicity in the methyl CCNU group
Southeastern Cancer Study Group	9	136	II, III	1. C. parvum 2. DTIC plus C. parvum	No difference	No benefit in all subgroups examined
G.I.F., France	115	248	I, II	1. BCG 2. BCG plus CCNU, DTIC, VM26	No difference	Survival after relapse longer with BCG patients
Southeastern Cancer Study Group	128	217	II, III	1. BCNU, Hydrea, DTIC (BHD) 2. BHD plus BCG	BHD alone better than combined	
Massachusetts General Hospital	167	70	I, II	1. DTIC 2. BCG 3. DTIC plus BCG	Combined better than DTIC alone (p < 0.05)	
UCLA	96	66	II	1. DTIC 2. DTIC plus BCG	No difference	Significant DTIC toxicity
Roswell Park Memorial Institute	88	84	I, II	1. DTIC plus Estrocyte 2. BCG 3. Control	No difference	
St. Louis Hospital	15	77	II	1. BCNU, actinomycin plus Vinblastine (BAV) 2. BAV plus BCG plus C. parvum	No difference	
Eastern Oncology Group	39	60	II	1. DTIC 2. DTIC plus BCG	No difference	
Vanderbilt	97	60	I, II	1. BCG plus DTIC 2. BCG plus CCNU	No difference	
Canadian Cooperative Group	129	57	I, II	1. BCG plus DTIC 2. Control	No difference	
EORTC	40	200	I	1. DTIC 2. Levamisole 3. Control	No difference	

a randomized clinical trial. However, a larger study involving 210 stage II patients conducted by the Southeastern Cancer Study Group (SECSG) showed no difference between the two agents[7] (Fig. 11-2). *C. parvum* immunotherapy was found in another SECSG study to have some benefit in stage I melanoma patients whose tumor thickness exceeded 3 mm.[11] These favorable results occurred in only a subgroup of stage I patients and were probably caused by imbalances of prognostic factors, since a subsequent analysis no longer demonstrated any benefit of *C. parvum* (Fig. 11-3).

Several investigators using either BCG or *C. parvum* have noted that the patterns of metastases

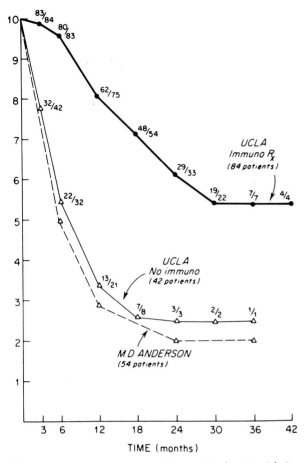

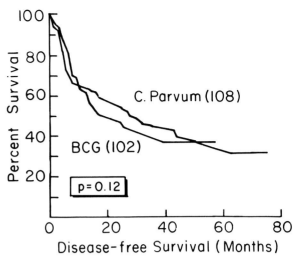

FIG. 11–1 One of the original BCG immunotherapy trials in melanoma was performed by the Division of Oncology, Department of Surgery, UCLA Medical Center. This study appeared to demonstrate an improved survival for BCG-treated stage II patients compared to concurrent, but nonrandomized, controls. It stimulated considerable investigative interest in melanoma immunotherapy studies. A subsequent randomized trial conducted by the same investigators did not appear to confirm these findings, but there were differences in some subgroups of patients, as described in Chapter 26. (Eilber FR, et al: Adjuvant immunotherapy with BCG in treatment of regional lymph node metastases from malignant melanoma. N Engl J Med 294:237, 1976)

FIG. 11–2 A randomized prospective study of 210 stage II melanoma patients (four or fewer metastatic nodes) conducted by the Southeastern Cancer Study Group comparing *Corynebacterium parvum* versus BCG immunotherapy administered every 1 to 2 weeks over 2 years. Survival results were identical for the two vaccines. Subcutaneous injections of *C. parvum* (8 mg/m^2) had less local toxicity compared to BCG given by the Tine technique (one vial). (Balch CM, Bartolucci AA, Presant CA, Durant JR, and the Southeastern Cancer Study Group: Proc Amer Soc Clin Oncol, 1984)

study from Yale Medical Center has yielded encouraging results,[2] but the treatment groups may not have been comparable.[143]

An analysis of these studies showed consistent trends for slightly higher survival rates in patients treated with BCG or *C. parvum* compared to surgical controls. However, this difference did not reach statistical significance in any of the studies. There is probably some benefit to a few patients, but it is not possible to identify prospectively which patients might benefit using either prognostic factors of the tumor or immunologic assessment of the patient. While it is possible that nonspecific immunotherapy is cytostatic and may alter the patterns of metastases, the evidence to date is not conclusive enough to recommend this treatment approach to melanoma patients on a routine basis.

Viral lysates of melanoma cells

One of the methods proposed to increase immune responses to "weak" tumor-associated antigens is to immunize patients with melanoma cells superinfected with nonpathogenic oncolytic viruses. The immune response against the viral antigens associ-

were different compared to controls, and the time from relapse to death was longer in immunotherapy-treated patients.[142] In addition, direct comparisons of *C. parvum* and BCG have demonstrated, in most studies, a trend for higher survival and lower toxicity and a greater ease of administration with *C. parvum* compared to BCG.[11] Another approach has been to administer BCG intralymphatically in selected patients. One pilot

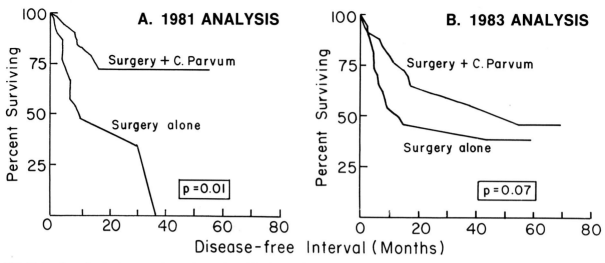

FIG. 11–3 A randomized prospective study conducted by the Southeastern Cancer Study Group of 286 stage I melanoma patients comparing *C. parvum* injections (8 mg/m² SQ every 1 to 2 weeks over 2 years) versus surgical control. There was no survival benefit in a patient with a tumor thickness <3 mm (data not shown). However, there appeared to be an increased survival in *C. Parvum*–treated patients with melanomas ≥3 mm. (*A*) Initial results suggesting an improved survival in subgroup of stage I patients with *C. parvum*. (Balch CM, et al: A randomized prospective clinical trial of adjuvant *C. parvum* immunotherapy in 260 patients with clinically localized melanoma (stage I): Prognostic factors analysis and preliminary results of immunotherapy. Cancer 49:1079, 1982) (*B*) Results obtained 3 years later into the trial showing less potential benefit.

ated with the tumor cell membrane is believed to amplify the immune response to the tumor antigens as well (reviewed by Austin and Boone and by Lindemann).[5,107]

Two viruses appear to be suitable candidates. One is the Newcastle Disease virus (NDV) that is a pathogen in chickens. Studies by Cassel and colleagues[31,32,116] using NDV lysates are encouraging. They have observed only four recurrences (12%) in 32 treated stage II patients after 3 years of follow-up (Fig. 11-4). Recurrences would have been expected in approximately 24 of these patients during this period. Vaccinia virus is also pathogenic for melanoma cells, and vaccination with melanoma cell lysates from cultures infected with this virus were shown to be safe for clinical use.[108,160,161] The results of a multicenter study to evaluate the efficacy of the vaccines in patients with stage II disease will be followed with great interest.

Irradiated or neuraminidase-treated melanoma cells

Vaccination with irradiated allogeneic melanoma cells, either alone or in combination with BCG, has received limited attention. Hedley and colleagues[67]

reported that subcutaneous injection of irradiated melanoma cells with BCG produced no prolongation of disease-free interval in 16 patients with stage II disease compared to 12 patients who received BCG alone. Both groups received chemotherapy with DTIC as well. Fisher and colleagues,[50] in a study of 166 patients, reported that injection of neuraminidase-treated allogeneic melanoma cells with BCG did not appear to have significant effects on the recurrence-free period. In another study by Eilber and colleagues, recurrence rates in the patients treated by irradiated allogeneic melanoma cells were not reduced, although mixed lymphocyte culture (MLC) responses were improved by this therapy.[46,58]

More encouraging results were obtained by Seigler and colleagues at Duke Medical Center in a study that involved over 719 patients and is the largest study of its kind using this treatment approach.[138] Their immunotherapy consisted of subcutaneous injections of neuraminidase-treated allogeneic (and autologous) melanoma cells with BCG. In patients with thicker stage I melanoma, survival rates are better than historical control data from other institutions (Fig. 11-5). Patients with stage II

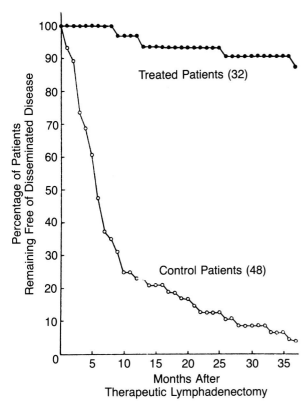

FIG. 11–4 A nonrandomized phase II immunotherapy trial using a Newcastle disease viral oncolysate of allogeneic melanoma cells conducted at Emory University School of Medicine. All treated patients had surgical excision of nodal metastases followed by injections of viral oncolysate over a 37-month period. The concurrent control group of surgical patients had the same stage of disease but were not randomized. (Cassel WA, Murray DR, Phillips HS: A phase II study on the postsurgical management of stage II malignant melanoma with a Newcastle disease virus oncolysate. Cancer 52:856, 1983).

disease had 4-year survivals ranging from 82% to 55% among different subgroups. This compares favorably with an expected 40% survival rate at 4 years.[139] These are excellent results; and as with the preliminary studies of Cassel and colleagues[31] referred to above, they seem unlikely to have occurred by chance. However, the studies have not been confirmed in any randomized (phase III) clinical trial.

Partially purified melanoma antigens

Studies with purified antigen preparations were conducted by Hollinshead and colleagues[87] in 51 patients with stage III melanoma. Eight of 23 patients had a response to immunotherapy alone and 30 of 42

to DTIC plus immunotherapy. These results appear promising and suggest that further evaluation in patients with stage II disease may be warranted.

Levamisole

Following reports that levamisole was of benefit in the treatment of carcinoma of the breast and lung, a randomized trial of levamisole versus placebo was carried out on 180 patients with stage I or II melanoma. A trend for reduction in the time of appearance of visceral metastases was evident at a median follow-up time of 3.5 years, but this was not statistically significant.[144,145] Similar negative results were obtained in a study by the European Organization for Research and Treatment of Cancer (EORTC) in Europe.[40]

Transfer factor

Transfer factor is a dialyzed extract of leukocytes that can enhance delayed hypersensitivity responses in recipients.[103,135] Adjuvant studies with preparations of transfer factor have produced conflicting results. In 100 patients with high-risk stage I melanoma, administration of transfer factor was associated with a significant reduction of recurrence rate and increased survival, compared to concurrent nonrandomized controls.[21] However, in a randomized study of 36 patients with stage II disease, transfer factor did not appear to affect the disease-free interval or significantly prolong survival.[27] Gonzalez and colleagues[60] reported that survival was significantly prolonged in 9 patients treated with transfer factor after removal of melanoma metastases in the lung. Further controlled studies are clearly needed to establish the treatment efficacy of these extracts.

FUTURE DIRECTIONS

The adjuvant studies referred to above, particularly those using bacterial products, suggest that nonspecific stimulation of the immune system by itself is not a rewarding approach. This may be because the original ideas were incorrect or because the immunotherapy (especially with BCG or *C. parvum*) did not achieve the desired effect of correcting abnormalities of the immune system. Information on the latter point is surprisingly limited. Natural killer, antibody-dependent, and lectin-induced cytotoxicity was shown to increase in short-term studies after BCG or *C. parvum* administration[151] and over a longer term during repeated BCG administration in patients with recurrent disease, but not in

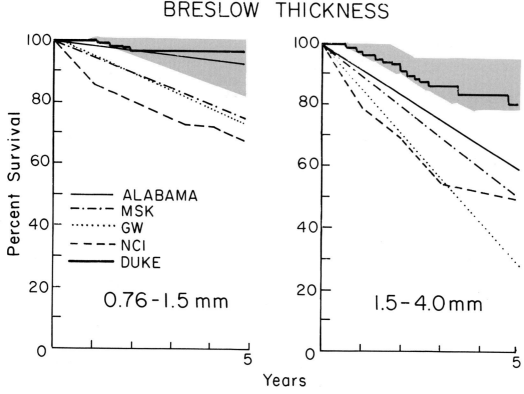

FIG. 11–5 Phase II clinical trial using neuraminidase-treated allogeneic (an autologous) melanoma cells plus BCG conducted by Dr. H.F. Seigler and colleagues in the Department of Surgery, Duke Medical Center. Over 719 patients with stage I and II melanoma have been treated. Results in this figure are both stage I and II patients subgrouped by tumor thickness. The 95% confidence limits are *shaded*. Historical control data were obtained from UAB, Memorial Sloan-Kettering Cancer Institute, George Washington University, and the National Cancer Institute.

those who developed recurrences.[134] In one study, BCG administration did not appear to have any long-term effects on a variety of immune function tests, including NK activity, but was found to depress delayed hypersensitivity skin test responses.[34] Long-term administration of BCG did not appear to affect MLC and lymphocyte mitogenic responses to lectins.[58] Hence, nonspecific immunostimulation with these agents may not have increased immune competence as thought and may have even suppressed some aspects of immune function.

Despite the negative results from many of these clinical studies, considerable information was learned that is now being applied to second generation trials involving adjuvant immunotherapy. A summary of some new treatment strategies is discussed below.

Inhibition of suppressor cell activity

Activation of suppressor cells is one explanation for the failure of immunotherapy to affect tumor growth and to restore immune competence. There is now ample evidence that suppressor cell activity can inhibit tumor-related immunologic responses and thereby promote tumor growth in animal models.[24,52,117] Furthermore, negative regulation by T cells is sufficiently strong to inhibit adoptively transferred effector T cells against tumor cells.[120] Increased suppressor T cell activity associated with tumor growth was demonstrated in patients with stage I and II melanoma.[164] Induction of suppressor cells by sunlight or exposure to ultraviolet light (such as that found in solariums) might also explain the association between solar radiation and the induction of melanoma.[49,74,81] In view of these considerations, it would appear essential that future trials of active immunotherapy should include measures designed to account for and possibly to control suppressor cell activity. It should be emphasized, however, that there are several subpopulations of suppressor lymphocytes and suppressor macrophages that have been defined in humans, each with its own activation requirements and influences on various components of the immune system.[14,153,155]

A more selective approach may be the use of monoclonal antibodies to deplete suppressor cells *in vivo*. In mice, it was shown that antibodies reacting with I-J determinants expressed on suppressor T cells inhibit suppressor cell activity and reduce tumor growth.[62] This approach is not yet possible in humans, as antigens equivalent to those coded by the I-J gene region in mice have not been defined. However, several loci in the DR region (*e.g.*, SB, DR, DC) have been defined in humans that are apparently equivalent to the I-A and I-E regions in mice,[41,157] and it is probably only a matter of time before antigens equivalent to the I-J determinants in mice are identified.

A third approach is the use of pharmacologic agents to inhibit suppressor cells selectively. Levamisole, for example, inhibits suppressor T cell function, with resultant increased antibody production in pokeweed mitogen-stimulated lymphoid cultures.[4,82] Agents that inhibit H_2 histamine receptors, such as cimetidine, may also inhibit suppressor cell activity.[53] The latter agent was shown to prolong survival in tumor-bearing mice[123] and was asssociated with tumor regression in melanoma patients.[152] Whether all suppressor cells have H_2 receptors and whether histamine is involved in antigen-induced suppressor pathways is not yet clear.

Prostaglandins are another category of agents that appear to be involved in suppressor pathways, possibly by inhibiting interleukin-2 (IL-2) production.[33,155] Indomethacin was shown to enhance depressed proliferative responses of lymphocytes from melanoma patients[154,156] and hence may be of value to diminish suppressor cell activity.[45]

A low-dose schedule of cyclophosphamide in mice selectively inhibits suppressor cell activity against cellular immune responses[3] and facilitates tumor rejection in animal models.[133] Information about its selectivity for suppressor cell activity in humans is as yet limited. At certain dose levels of cyclophosphamide, suppressor/cytotoxic cells in the circulation are decreased relative to helper cells,[16] and cellular immune responses are increased.[112] These experimental data suggest that cyclophos-phamide might be useful in controlling suppressor cell activity in humans.

Perhaps one of the most interesting approaches is the use of antibodies against idiotypes on soluble suppressor factors released by suppressor T cells. These factors appear to contain antigen determinants and antigen-binding structures similar to those on T cells. Antibodies against idiotypic determinants on the latter were shown *in vivo* to facilitate rejection of tumors in mice and, when given to non-immune mice, induced immunity against the tumor.[70] Similar priming by anti-idiotypes has been noted in other experimental models.[113] These effects appear ideal as biologic response modifiers and would be a worthwhile goal for future studies in human melanoma.

A number of specific approaches are now being developed to regulate suppressor cell activity. At present, the only agents available are low-dose cyclophosphamide or some of the immunopharmacologic agents that are referred to above. The dose of cyclophosphamide may be hard to regulate in individual patients and have deleterious effects on other aspects of the immune system. It is not known, however, whether the agents referred to will inhibit specific suppressor responses and whether their effects will persist with continued use.

Active-specific immunotherapy with melanoma antigens

The rationale here is to immunize with a melanoma antigen to maintain effective levels of immunity against emergent tumor cell clones. Although many of the nonspecific immunotherapy programs did not appear to influence the natural history of melanoma, some of the most successful treatments reported above[31,88,138] included immunizations with a source of melanoma antigen. Details such as the route of administration, dose, and source of melanoma antigens for such vaccination programs are probably of major importance. For example, the generation and maintenance of tumor immune responses probably require an interaction of the antigen with antigen-presenting cells (APC) such as the epithelium of skin, lymph nodes, or spleen, and possibly in association with DR and HLA antigens compatible with those of the host.[141,168]

The source of melanoma antigen is usually limited to cultured cell lines, since a sufficient amount of autologous melanoma cells are generally not available. It is important that antigens from the cell lines cross-react or are shared with those of an individual patient. Tumor antigens defined by monoclonal antibodies have shown that some tumor-associated antigens may be specific to the individual or only partially cross-reactive with melanoma cells from different patients.[25,28,30,43,44,69,71,92,106,130,140] Heterogeneity of antigens on tumor cells within the tumor itself may also occur.[118]

Ideally, melanoma antigens should be selected on the basis of those known to exist on the patient's own tumor. A few antigens, such as Thy-1 and p97 melanoma antigens, can be identified by immunoperoxidase staining on tissue section.[54,80] Alternatively, a pool of melanoma cells known to express the most common tumor-associated antigens could be used for immunization. The latter approach was adopted by Cassel and colleagues[31] in their studies with NDV melanoma cell lysates. The influence, if any, of alloantigens in such antigen pools has not yet been addressed. Administration of the antigens with viral or bacterial antigens to attract APC and increase local lymphokine release would appear logical.

As a general principle, it appears desirable not to use intact cells, because many melanoma cells release potent immunosuppressive factors, including inhibitors of IL-2 production.[72,75,132,165] This problem may be avoided by vaccination with cell membranes from viral lysates or with antigens purified by various techniques,[87,147] including affinity chromatography of monoclonal antibodies, or production of antigen by DNA cloning techniques (for reviews see Reisfeld and Ferrone).[130] The optimal frequency for induction and maintenance of immunity is yet to be established. For maintenance of specific immunity as distinct from nonspecific immune stimulants, there would appear to be little basis for the frequent and long-term vaccination schedule used in many previous adjuvant studies.

Interleukins and interferons

Recent studies have shown that the generation of cytotoxic T cell responses requires not only antigen recognition events but also interaction with the IL-2 lymphokine.[159] This discovery promises to be an important advance in tumor immunology, since studies in both animal models and human tumors have shown that the addition of IL-2 to lymphocyte tumor cell cultures resulted in the induction of cytotoxic T cell responses to the tumor. These results were confirmed in studies with melanoma cells that otherwise would have been regarded as nonimmunogenic.[63,73] Subsequent studies showed that *in vivo* administration of preparations containing IL-2 is a safe and feasible therapeutic approach.[19] Studies in

mice have shown that IL-2 injections may increase cytotoxic T cell responses against allogeneic tumor cells.[68] These studies therefore hold promise that IL-2 injections will bypass many of the factors that act to inhibit generation of cytotoxic cells in cancer patients. Purification of IL-2 in sufficient quantities for limited clinical studies has been reported,[163] and production by DNA cloning techniques is under study[149] so that the availability of sufficient quantities for more extensive clinical trials can be anticipated.

Interferon can now be produced by DNA cloning procedures.[55,64] This advance has generated an active interest in the potential therapeutic role of interferon in melanoma patients, and several trials using α interferon treatment for advanced melanoma are in progress. Preliminary results suggest that remission rates are comparable to those seen with DTIC (*i.e.*, about 20%). Whether these effects represent direct cytotoxicity on the tumor cells,[38] modulation of host defense mechanisms,[1,57,122] or an as yet unknown mechanism[18] is not clear. If the effects are mediated by actions on the immune system (such as stimulation of NK activity), these results in patients with advanced disease may reflect the limited capacity of the immune system. A more valid assessment of interferon should be performed as an adjuvant treatment in postoperative, high-risk melanoma patients. Such trials are still in the planning stage, so that answers to these questions will not be available for several years. Further studies are also needed to assess the relative efficacy of different interferon preparations and to discover whether combinations of different interferons will enhance their antitumor activity.[51,162]

Other biologic response modifiers

A large number of other immunomodulating agents or biologic response modifiers are under investigation, such as thymic hormones and bacterial products.[6,56] A promising small molecular weight bacterial product, termed Bestatin, appears to increase NK activity, perhaps by effects on IL-2 release.[20] In Japanese studies, Bestatin appeared to produce a significant improvement in the disease-free interval in randomized trials of melanoma patients with stage I and II disease.[90]

A particularly promising area of investigation is the therapeutic use of monoclonal antibodies directed against melanoma antigens (reviewed by Levy and Miller and by Oldham).[104,121] Early trials of monoclonal antibody in experimental animals and humans have indicated its ability to traffic to specific sites and to localize on or around the tumor cells displaying antigens to which the antibody is directed. The evidence of specific targeting of melanoma cells, with preliminary evidence of therapeutic efficacy for monoclonal antibodies and immunoconjugates with drugs, toxins, and isotopes is encouraging.[99,100,101,121,146]

Comment

Previous adjuvant trials of nonspecific immunotherapy, with some exceptions, have yielded disappointing results. This may have been because of their failure to induce specific immunity, to restore immune competence, or to correct imbalances of regulatory cells. Release of immunosuppressive factors from tumors and induction of suppressor cell activity are probably important factors underlying these failures. In view of these conclusions, future trials need to include measures to regulate suppressor cell activity and to immunize with melanoma antigens that cross-react with those of the patient. Viral lysates may provide an immunogenic source of antigen for this purpose and have the added benefit of interferon induction. The role of lymphokines and other pharmacologic agents that may act selectively on the immune system must still be evaluated. Future adjuvant immunotherapy studies will need to account for properties of the tumor cells in individual patients. This includes an assessment of their melanoma antigen expression, DR antigen expression, and the release of soluble factors that may inhibit or regulate immune responses in their vicinity.

Finally, there is an acknowledged need for better criteria for selecting agents suitable for clinical evaluation as adjuvants to surgery. As part of this assessment, it would appear essential that their *in vivo* effects can be monitored for melanoma-specific immune responses, so that modification of the dose and timing of the biologic response modifiers can be based on objective criteria rather than on supposition.

ADJUVANT CHEMOTHERAPY AND CHEMOIMMUNOTHERAPY

RATIONALE

The design of adjuvant chemotherapy trials for melanoma is based on currently available drugs with some activity in patients with distant unresectable disease where response rates can be measured. The most active drug currently used for advanced mela-

noma is dimethyltriazeno imidazole carboxamide (DTIC), usually given in combination with some other drug (see Chap. 14). Because micrometastases grow faster and are more vascularized, they are theoretically more vulnerable to chemotherapy treatment than are larger, clinically apparent tumors.

RESULTS

The results of multiple randomized clinical trials involving DTIC chemotherapy (or combinations of chemotherapy plus immunotherapy) have not shown any benefit compared to a surgical control group of patients who did not receive adjuvant therapy (see Table 11-3). The two largest studies addressing this question were performed by the Central Oncology Group (COG)[86] and the World Health Organization Melanoma Group.[158] Of note in the COG study was the observation that the DTIC-treated patients actually did *worse* than the surgical control group (Fig. 11-6), while there was no difference in the WHO Melanoma Group Study (Fig. 11-7). Several other institutions and cooperative groups have examined other drug combinations with and without immunotherapy as shown in Table 11-3. These studies have also been uniformly negative. For example, a recent study of 146 high-risk melanoma patients conducted by the Southeastern Cancer Study Group showed no benefit whatsoever in those who received DTIC, cyclophosphamide, and *C. parvum* as compared to those who received *C. parvum* immunotherapy alone (Fig. 11-8).[10] The negative results were the same even in subgroups of patients categorized by disease stage, site of metastasis, and sex. A similar comparison of DTIC plus BCG showed no survival benefit compared to BCG alone (see Fig.11-7).[158] Until some new drugs become available with activity in melanoma patients with advanced disease, there is little or no benefit to be gained from administering adjuvant chemotherapy using DTIC alone or in combination for high-risk melanoma patients.

CURRENT AND FUTURE DIRECTIONS

In retrospect, the primary reason why DTIC and other drugs failed to show a benefit in an adjuvant setting is that these drugs have a relatively low activity in melanoma patients with advanced disease. At a cellular level, this lack of adjuvant efficacy is caused by a high proportion of cell clones in micrometastases with innate chemotherapeutic drug resistance. It is striking that in melanoma, as in bronchogenic carcinoma and some other tumors,

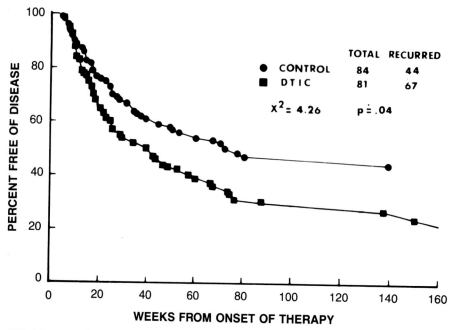

FIG. 11–6 Randomized prospective trial of adjuvant DTIC chemotherapy compared to surgical control that was conducted by the Central Oncology group. Note that the disease-free interval for the treated patients actually was worse than the controls ($P = 0.04$). The overall survival rates were also worse for the treated group, but the difference was not as significant ($P = 0.14$, data not shown). (Hill GJ II, et al: DTIC and combination therapy for melanoma. III. DTIC (NSC 45388) surgical adjuvant study COG protocol 7040. Cancer 47:2557, 1981).

acquisition of drug resistance is a characteristic of the tumor, even before bulky metastases develop, and before hypoxic, poorly vascularized cell populations exist. It is unknown whether drug resistance is a phenotype of all human melanomas (even the primary itself), whether metastases represent select drug-resistant clones of tumor cells, or whether the concentration of DTIC at the tumor bed is subtherapeutic. Regardless of the exact cellular basis for drug resistance, high-risk melanoma patients should be spared the rigors of adjuvant DTIC chemotherapy until more active drugs or combinations of drugs become available. As outlined in Chapter 14, many other drugs have been evaluated in patients with advanced disease, but, unfortunately, there are no new drugs with promising activity at present.

ADJUVANT RADIATION THERAPY

RATIONALE

Melanoma can no longer be considered radioresistant, since higher doses with longer intervals between treatments provide excellent palliation for

metastatic melanoma in the skin, soft tissue, and lymph nodes (see Chap. 15). Radiation therapy can also be effective palliation for metastases in the bone and brain.

CURRENT STUDIES

Only one adjuvant radiation therapy trial has been published, and this had negative results. Creagan and colleagues randomized patients with nodal metastases to treatment with regional radiation therapy to the node-bearing area or no further treatment after lymphadenectomy.[37] The patients received no concomitant immunotherapy or chemotherapy. There was no improvement in survival or regional control of disease in the patients receiving irradiation therapy compared to control patients. In retrospect, this is not surprising, since the risk for recurrence after lymphadenectomy is low after surgical treatment to begin with.

Although there are no published randomized clinical trials, adjuvant radiation therapy is often administered following surgical resection of cerebral metastases.

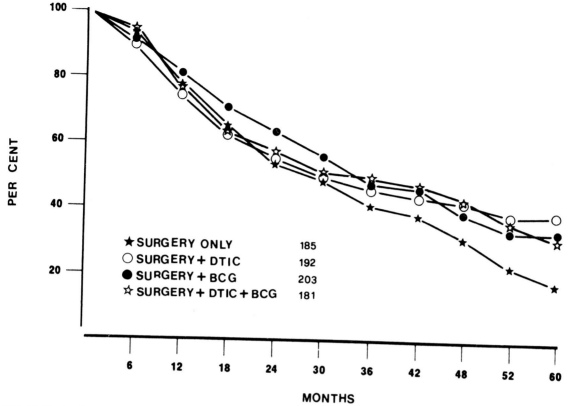

FIG. 11–7 Randomized prospective protocol of adjuvant therapy in 761 stage II melanoma patients conducted by the WHO Melanoma Group. There was no benefit of adjuvant BCG, DTIC, or a combination of the two compared to a surgical control arm. (Veronesi U, et al: A randomized trial of adjuvant chemotherapy and immunotherapy in cutaneous melanoma. N Engl J Med 307:913, 1982).

FIG. 11–8 A randomized prospective trial comparing chemoimmunotherapy (*C. parvum*, DTIC, and cyclophosphamide) with immunotherapy alone (*C. parvum*) in 136 patients with resected metastatic melanoma conducted by SEG. There were no differences between the treatment groups. (From Balch CM, et al: Ineffectiveness of adjuvant chemotherapy using DTIC and cyclophosphamide in patients with resectable metastatic melanoma. Surgery. 95:454, 1984).

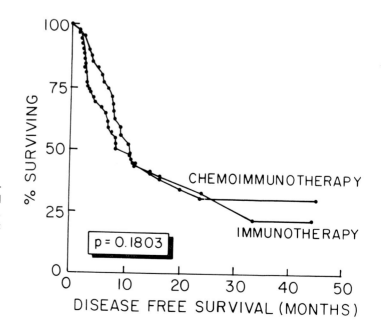

CURRENT AND FUTURE DIRECTIONS

There is considerable potential for clinical trials evaluating the benefit of adjuvant radiation therapy in patients at high risk for local recurrence or after resection of soft-tissue, intransit, or cerebral metastases. Some clinical trials in these areas are now under way. The use of radiosensitizing agents such as quinones, compounds with electron affinity, and glyoxals or pyruvates promises to be a major area of research in treatment of melanoma. This approach may be extended to adjuvant radiation therapy at particular sites, such as metastases in the brain.[61]

SUMMARY

A large number of clinical trials have so far been unable to prove a substantial benefit for any form of adjuvant therapy. In general, the use of adjuvant immunotherapy, chemotherapy, or radiation therapy should be limited to investigational trials to determine their benefit and toxicity. There are some encouraging results with several new forms of immunotherapy. To date, the results with adjuvant chemotherapy have been totally unsuccessful. Further evaluation is needed to determine what benefits there may be for adjuvant radiation therapy in selected patients with skin, subcutaneous, and cerebral metastases.

One important aspect of adjuvant therapy, as with all treatment, is the cost in terms of morbidity to the patient relative to the anticipated benefit. For example, during the WHO trial of adjuvant chemotherapy, the morbidity caused by recurrent treatment with DTIC was so severe that many patients refused to continue it after one or two courses of treatment. The anticipation of treatment with DTIC in 5-day series for a month caused many patients such a severe depression that their work, sex life, marriage, and most pleasures were severely hampered. Most patients are more than prepared to put up with this when they have demonstrable disease but are much more reluctant to do so for a possible slight improvement in prognosis. The potential benefits must, therefore, be considerable before adjuvant therapy becomes standard practice in all but tumors with a very bad prognosis.

REFERENCES

1. Abo T, Balch CM: Characterization of HNK-1$^+$ (Leu-7) human lymphocytes: III. Interferon effects on spontaneous cytotoxicity and phenotypic expression of lymphocyte subpopulations delineated by the monoclonal HNK-1 antibody. Cell Immunol 73:376, 1982

2. Ariyan S, Kirkwood JM, Mitchell MS, Nordlund JJ, Lerner AB, Papac RJ: Intralymphatic and regional surgical adjuvant immunotherapy in high-risk melanoma of the extremities. Surgery 92:459, 1982

3. Asherson GL, Zembala M, Thomas WR, Perera MACC: Suppressor cells and the handling of antigen. Immunol Rev 50:3, 1980

4. Aune TM, Peirce CW: Inhibition of interferon or soluble immune response suppressor (SIRS) mediated suppression by levamisole. Int J Immunopharmacol 5:91, 1983

5. Austin FC, Boone CW: Virus augmentation of the antigenicity of tumor cell extracts. Adv Cancer Res 30:301, 1979

6. Bach JF: The use of regulatory biological products of manipulate immune responses. In Fougereau M, Dausset J (eds): Progress in Immunology, Vol IV, p 1171. London, Academic Press, 1980

7. Balch CM, Durant JR, Bartolucci AA, and the Southeastern Cancer Study Group: The impact of surgical quality control in multi-institutional group trials involving adjuvant cancer treatments. Ann Surg 198:164, 1983

8. Balch CM, Maddox WA: The logic of adjunctive therapy in surgical patients with resectable cancer. South Med J 71:951, 1978

9. Balch CM, Murad TM, Soong S-j, Ingalls AL, Richards PC, Maddox WA: Tumor thickness as a guide to surgical management of clinical stage I melanoma patients. Cancer 43:883, 1979

10. Balch CM, Murray D, Presant C, Bartolucci AA, and the Southeastern Cancer Study Group: Ineffectiveness of adjuvant chemotherapy using DTIC and cyclophosphamide in patients with resectable metastatic melanoma. Surgery 95:454, 1984

11. Balch CM, Smalley RV, Bartolucci AA, Burns D, Presant CA, Durant JR, and the Southeastern Cancer Study Group: A randomized prospective clinical trial of adjuvant C. parvum immunotherapy in 260 patients with clinically localized melanoma (stage I): Prognostic factors analysis and preliminary results of immunotherapy. Cancer 49:1079, 1982

12. Balch CM, Soong S-j, Milton GW, Shaw HM, McGovern VJ, Murad TM, McCarthy WH, Maddox WA: A comparison of prognostic factors and surgical results in 1,786 patients with localized (stage I) melanoma treated in Alabama, USA and New South Wales, Australia. Ann Surg 196:677, 1982

13. Balch CM, Soong S-j, Murad JM, Ingalls AL, Maddox WA: A multifactorial analysis of melanoma. III. Prognostic factors in melanoma patients with lymph node metastases (stage II). Ann Surg 193:377, 1981

14. Balch CM, Tilden AB: Indomethacin, prostaglandin, and immune regulation in melanoma. In Reisfeld RA, Ferrone S (eds): Melanoma Antigens and Antibodies, p 23. New York, Plenum, 1981

15. Banzet P, Jacquillat C, Civatte J, Puissant A, Maral J, Chastang C, Israel L, Belaich S, Jourdain J-C, Weil M, Auclerc G: Adjuvant chemotherapy in the management of primary malignant melanoma. Cancer 41:1240, 1978

16. Bast RC Jr, Reinherz EL, Maver C, Lavin P, Schlossman SF: Contrasting effects of cyclophosphamide and prednisolone on the phenotype of human peripheral blood leukocytes. Clin Immunol Immunopathol 28:101, 1983

17. Bast RC Jr, Zbar B, Borsos T, Rapp HJ: BCG and cancer. N Engl J Med 290:1413, 1974

18. Belardelli F, Gresser I, Maury C, Duvillard P, Prade M, Maunoury MT: Antitumor effects of interferon in mice injected with interferon-sensitive and interferon-resistant friend leukemia cells: III. Inhibition of growth and necrosis of tumors implanted subcutaneously. Int J Cancer 31:649, 1983

19. Bindon C, Czerniecki M, Ruell P, Edwards A, McCarthy WH, Harris R, Hersey P: Clearance rates and systemic effects of intravenously administered interleukin 2 (IL-2) containing preparations in human subjects. Br J Cancer 47:123, 1983

20. Blomgren H: Bestatin, a new immunomodulator augments the release of mitogenic factors from PHA-stimulated human lymphocytes. Biomedicine 34:188, 1981

21. Blume MR, Rosenbaum EH, Cohen RJ, Gershow J, Glassberg AB, Shepley E: Adjuvant immunotherapy of high risk stage I melanoma with transfer factor. Cancer 47:882, 1981

22. Bluming AZ: Current status of clinical immunotherapy. Cancer Chemotherapy Report 59:901, 1975

23. Bodurtha AJ, Chee DO, Laucius JF, Mastrangelo MJ, Prehn RT: Clinical and immunological significance of human melanoma cytotoxic antibody. Cancer Res 35:189, 1975

24. Broder S, Megson M: Interrelationships between immunoregulatory cells, neoplastic diseases and immunodeficiency states. In Saunders JP, Daniels JC, Serrou B, Rosenfeld C, Denney CB (eds): Fundamental Mechanisms in Human Cancer Immunology, p 193. New York, Elsevier/North-Holland, 1981

25. Brown JP, Nishiyama K, Hellstrom I, Hellstrom KE: Structural characterization of human melanoma-associated antigen p97 using monoclonal antibodies. J Immunol 127:539, 1981

26. Bruckner HW, Mokyr MB, Mitchell MS: Effect of imidazole-4-carboxamide, 5-(3,3-dimethyl-1-triazeno) on immunity in patients with malignant melanoma. Cancer Res 34:181, 1974

27. Bukowski RM, Deodhar S, Hewlett JS, Greenstreet R: Randomized controlled trial of transfer factor in stage II malignant melanoma. Cancer 51:269, 1983

28. Burk MW, Saxton RE, Mann BD, Morton DL: Definition of human melanoma-associated cell surface antigens by hybridoma monoclonal antibodies. Surgery 94:84, 1983

29. Camacho ES, Pinsky CM, Braun DW Jr, Golbey RB, Fortner JG, Wanebo HJ, Oettgen HF: DNCB reactivity and prognosis in 419 patients with malignant melanoma. Cancer 47:2446, 1981

30. Carrel S, Mach JP, Accolla RS: Human melanoma-associated antigen(s) detected by monoclonal antibodies. Br J Cancer 43:561, 1981

31. Cassel WA, Murray DR, Phillips HS: A phase II study on the postsurgical management of stage II malignant melanoma with a Newcastle disease virus oncolysate. Cancer 52:856, 1983

32. Cassel WA, Murray DR, Torbin AH, Olkowski ZL, Moore ME: Viral oncolysate in the management of malignant melanoma. I. Preparation of the oncolysate and measurement of immunologic responses. Cancer 40:672, 1977

33. Chouaib S, Fradelizi D: The mechanism of inhibition of human IL 2 production. J Immunol 129:2463, 1982

34. Coates AS, Klopp RG, Zarling JM, Borden EC, Crowley JJ, Carbone PP: Immunologic function during adjuvant BCG immunotherapy for malignant melanoma: Induction of anergy. Cancer Immunol Immunotherapy 7:175, 1979

35. Cochran AJ, Buyse ME, Lejeune FJ, Macher E, Revuz J, Rumke P: Adjuvant reactivity predicts survival in patients with "high risk" primary malignant melanoma treated with systemic BCG. Int J Cancer 28:543, 1981

36. Costanzi JJ: The chemotherapy of human malignant melanoma. In Costanzi JJ (ed): Malignant Melanoma 1, p 259. The Hague, Nijhoff, 1983

37. Creagan ET, Cupps RE, Ivins JC, Pritchard DJ, Sim FH, Soule EH, O'Fallon JR: Adjuvant radiation therapy for regional nodal metastases from malignant melanoma: A randomized, prospective study. Cancer 42:2206, 1978

38. Creasey AA, Bartholomew JC, Merigan JC: Role of G_0-G_1-arrest in the inhibition of tumor cell growth by interferon. Proc Natl Acad Sci USA 77:1471, 1980

39. Cunningham TJ, Schoenfeld D, Nathanson L, Wolter J, Patterson WB, Borden E: A controlled ECOG study of adjuvant therapy in patients with stage I and II malignant melanoma. In Salamon SS, Jones SE (eds): Adjuvant Therapy of Cancer II, p 507. New York, Grune & Stratton, 1979

40. Czarnetzki BM, Macher E, Behrendt H, Lejeune F: Current status of melanoma chemotherapy and immunotherapy. Recent Results Cancer Res 80:264, 1982

41. Dausset J, Contu L: The MHC and immune response in man. In Fougereau M, Dausset J (eds): Progress in immunology IV, p 513. London, Academic Press, 1980

42. deGast GC, The TH, Schraffordt Koops H, Huiges HA, Oldhoff J, Nieweg HO: Humoral and cell-mediated immune response in patients with malignant melanoma. I. In vitro lymphocyte reactivity to

PHA and antigens following immunization. Cancer 36:1289, 1975

43. Dent PB, McCulloch PB, Liao SK, Stone BR, Singal DP: Heterogeneity of melanoma-associated antigens detected by sera from patients receiving adjuvant allogeneic tumor vaccine immunotherapy. Clin Immunol Immunopathol 23:379, 1982

44. Dippold WG, Lloyd KO, Li LTC, Ikeda H, Oettgen HF, Old LJ: Cell surface antigens of human malignant melanoma: Definition of six antigenic systems with mouse monoclonal antibodies. Proc Natl Acad Sci USA 77:6114, 1980

45. Droller MJ, Gomolka D: Inhibition of tumor growth in association with modification of *in vivo* immune response by indomethacin and polyinosinic:polycytidylic acid. Cancer Res 42:5038, 1982

46. Eilber FR, Morton DL, Holmes EC, Sparks FC, Ramming KP: Adjuvant immunotherapy with BCG in treatment of regional lymph node metastases from malignant melanoma. N Engl J Med 294:237, 1976

47. Eilber FR, Nizze JA, Morton DL: Sequential evaluation of general immune competence in cancer patients: Correlation with clinical course. Cancer 35:660, 1975

48. Eilber FR, Townsend CM Jr, Morton DL: Results of BCG adjuvant immunotherapy for melanoma of the head and neck. Am J Surg 132:476, 1976

49. Fisher MS, Kripke ML: Suppressor T lymphocytes control the development of primary skin cancers in ultraviolet-irradiated mice. Science 216:1133, 1982

50. Fisher RI, Terry WD, Hodes RJ, Rosenberg SA, Makuch R, Gordon HG, Fisher SG: Adjuvant immunotherapy or chemotherapy for malignant melanoma. Surg Clin North Am 61:1267, 1981

51. Fleischmann WR, Newton RC, Fleischmann CM, Brysk MM: Discrimination between non-malignant and malignant cells by combined IFN-gamma and IFN-alpha/beta. Third Annual International Congress of Interferon Research, November 1–3, 1982, Miami, Florida

52. Frost P, Prete P, Kerbel R: Abrogation of the in vitro generation of the cytotoxic T-cell responses to a murine tumour: The role of suppressor cells. Int J Cancer 30:211, 1982

53. Garovoy MR, Reddish MA, Rocklin RE: Histamine induced suppressor factor inhibition of helper T cell generation and function. J Immunol 130:357, 1983

54. Garrigues HJ, Tilgen W, Hellstrom I, Franke W, Hellstrom KE: Detection of a human melanoma-associated antigen p97, in histological sections of primary human melanomas. Int J Cancer 29:511, 1982

55. Goeddel DV, Leung DW, Dull TJ, Gross M, Lawn RM, McCandliss R, Seeburg PH, Ullrich A, Yelverlon E, Gray PW: The structure of eight distinct cloned human leukocyte interferon cDNAs. Nature 290:20, 1981

56. Goldstein AL, Chirigos MA: Lymphokines and thymic hormones: Their potential utilization in cancer therapeutics. Prog Cancer Res Therapy, p 201, 1981

57. Golub SH, Dorey F, Hara D, Morton DL, Burk MW: Systemic administration of human leukocyte interferon to melanoma patients. I. Effects on natural killer function and cell populations. J Natl Cancer Inst 68:703, 1982

58. Golub SH, Forsythe AB, Morton DL: Sequential examination of lymphocyte proliferative capacity in patients with malignant melanoma receiving BCG immunotherapy. Int J Cancer 19:18, 1977

59. Golub SH, O'Connell TX, Morton DL: Correlation of in vivo and in vitro assays of immunocompetence in cancer patients. Cancer Res 34:1833, 1974

60. Gonzalez RL, Wong P, Spitler LE: Adjuvant immunotherapy with transfer factor in patients with melanoma metastatic to lung. Cancer 45:57, 1980

61. Gray AJ, Dische S, Adams GE, Flockhart IR, Foster JL: Clinical testing of the radiosensitiser Ro-07-0582. I. Dose tolerance, serum and tumour concentrations. Clin Radiol 27:151, 1976

62. Greene MI, Dorf ME, Peirres M, Beneacerraf B: Reduction of syngeneic tumor growth by an anti I.J. alloantiserum. Proc Natl Acad Sci USA 74:5118, 1977

63. Grimm EA, Mazumder A, Zhang HZ, Rosenberg SA: Lymphokine-activated killer cell phenomenon: Lysis of natural killer resistant fresh solid tumor cells by interleukin 2-activated autologous human peripheral blood lymphocytes. J Exp Med 155:1823, 1982

64. Gutterman JU, Fine S, Quesada J, Horning SJ, Levine JF, Alexanian R, Bernhardt L, Kramer M, Spiegel H, Colburn W, Trown P, Merigan T, Dziewanowski Z: Recombinant leukocyte A interferon: Pharmacokinetics, single-dose tolerance, and biologic effects in cancer patients. Ann Intern Med 96:549, 1982

65. Gutterman JU, McBride C, Freireich EJ, Mavligit G, Frei E III, Hersh EM: Active immunotherapy with BCG for recurrent malignant melanoma. Lancet I, p 1208, 1973

66. Gutterman JU, Richman SP, McBride CM, Burgess MA, Bartold SL, Kennedy A, Gehan EA, Mavligit G, Hersh EM: Immunotherapy for recurrent malignant melanoma: Efficacy of BCG in prolonging the postoperative disease-free interval and survival. Recent Results Cancer Res 68:359, 1979

67. Hedley DW, McElwain TJ, Currie GA: Specific active immunotherapy does not prolong survival in surgically treated patients with stage IIB malignant melanoma and may promote early recurrence. Br J Cancer 37:491, 1978

68. Hefeneider SH, Conlon PJ, Henney CS, Gillis S: In vivo interleukin 2 administration augments the generation of alloreactive cytolytic T lymphocytes and resident natural killer cells. J Immunol 130:222, 1983

69. Hellström I, Hellström KE, Brown JP, Woodbury

RF: Antigens of human tumors particularly melanomas as studied with the monoclonal antibody technique. In Hammerling GJ, Hammerling U, Kearney JF (eds): Research Monographs in Immunology, Vol 3, p 191. New York, Elsevier/North-Holland, Biomedical Press, 1981

70. Hellström KE, Nelson K, Cory J, Forstrom JW, Hellström I: A tumor specific suppressor factor produced by a murine T cell hybridoma. In Mitchell MS, Oettgen HF (eds): Hybridomas in Cancer Diagnosis and Treatment, p 47. New York, Raven Press 1982

71. Herlyn M, Clark WH Jr, Mastrangelo MJ, DuPont G IV, Elder DE, LaRossa D, Hamilton R, Bondi E, Tuthill R, Steplewski Z, Koprowski H: Specific immunoreactivity of hybridoma-secreted monoclonal anti-melanoma antibodies to cultured cells and freshly derived human cells. Cancer Res 40:3602, 1980

72. Hersey P, Bindon C, Czerniecki M, Spurling A, Wass J, McCarthy WH: Inhibition of interleukin 2 production by factors released from tumor cells. J Immunol 131:2837 1983

73. Hersey P, Bindon C, Edwards A, Murray E, Phillips G, McCarthy WH: Induction of cytotoxic activity in human lymphocytes against autologous and allogeneic melanoma cells in vitro by culture with interleukin 2. Int J Cancer 28:695, 1982

74. Hersey P, Bradley M, Hasic E, Haran G, Edwards A, McCarthy WH: Immunological effects of solarium exposure. Lancet 1:545, 1983

75. Hersey P, Edwards AE, Edwards J, Adams E, Nelson DS, Milton GW: Specificity of cell mediated cytotoxicity against human melanoma lines. Evidence for non-specific killing by activated T-cells. Int J Cancer 16:173, 1975

76. Hersey P, Edwards A, McCarthy WH: Tumour-related changes in natural killer cell activity in melanoma patients: Influence of stage of disease, tumour thickness and age of patients. Int J Cancer 25:187, 1980

77. Hersey P, Edwards A, McCarthy WH, Milton GW: Tumor related changes and prognostic significance of natural killer cell activity in melanoma patients. In Herberman RB (ed): NK Cells and Other Natural Effector Cells, p 1167. New York, Academic Press, 1982

78. Hersey P, Edwards AE, Murray E, McCarthy WH, Milton GW: Sequential studies of melanoma leukocyte-dependent antibody activity in melanoma patients. Eur J Cancer 14:629, 1978

79. Hersey P, Edwards A, Murray E, McCarthy WH, Milton GW: Prognostic significance of leukocyte dependent antibody activity in melanoma patients. J Natl Cancer Inst 71:45, 1983

80. Hersey P, Grace J, Murray E, Palmer A, McCarthy WH: Expression of Thy-1 antigen on human melanoma cells. Int J Cancer (in press)

81. Hersey P, Haran G, Hasic E, Edwards A: Alteration of T cell subsets and induction of suppressor T cell activity in normal subjects after exposure to sunlight. J Immunol 131:171, 1983

82. Hersey P, Ho K, Werkmeister J, Abele U: Inhibition of suppressor T cells in pokeweed mitogen-stimulated cultures of T and B cells by levamisole in vitro and in vivo. Clin Exp Immunol 46:340, 1981

83. Hersey P, Honeyman M, Edwards A, Adams E, McCarthy WH: Antigens on melanoma cells detected by leukocyte dependent antibody assays of human melanoma antisera. Int J Cancer 18:564, 1976

84. Hersey P, McCarthy WH: The nature and significance of melanoma antigens recognized by human subjects. In Reisfeld RA, Ferrone S (eds): Melanoma Antigens and Antibodies, p 211. New York, Plenum, 1982

85. Hilal EY, Pinsky CM, Hirshaut Y, Wanebo HJ, Hansen JA, Braun DW Jr, Fortner JG, Oettgen HF: Surgical adjuvant therapy of malignant melanoma with *Corynebacterium parvum*. Cancer 48:245, 1981

86. Hill GJ II, Moss SE, Golomb FM, Grage TB, Fletcher WS, Minton JP, Krementz ET: DTIC and combination therapy for melanoma: III. DTIC (NSC 45388) Surgical Adjuvant Study COG Protocol 7040. Cancer 47:2556, 1981

87. Hollinshead A, Arlen M, Yonemoto R, Cohen M, Tanner K, Kundin WD, Scherrer J: Pilot studies using melanoma tumor-associated antigens (TAA) in specific-active immunochemotherapy of malignant melanoma. Cancer 49:1387, 1982

88. Holtermann OA, Karakousis CP, Berger J, Constantine RI: Adjuvant therapy with DTIC and Estracyt or BCG in malignant melanoma. Proc Am Soc Clin Oncol 21:400, 1980

89. Houghton AN, Eisinger M, Albino AP, Cairncross JG, Old LJ: Surface antigens of melanocytes and melanomas: Markers of melanocyte differentiation and melanoma subsets. J Exp Med 156:1755, 1982

90. Ikeda S, Ishihara K: Randomized controlled study of immunochemotherapy with bestatin, a new small molecular weight immunomodulator and chemotherapy as adjuvant to surgery for stage IB and II malignant melanoma. Presented at 13th International Congress of Chemotherapy, 1983

91. Ikonopisov RL, Lewis MG, Hunter-Craig ID, Bodenham DC, Phillips TM, Cooling CI, Proctor J, Fairley GH, Alexander P: Autoimmunization with irradiated tumour cells in human malignant melanoma. Br Med J 2:752, 1970

92. Imai K, Natali PG, Kay NE, Wilson BS, Ferrone S: Tissue distribution and molecular profile of a differentiation antigen detected by a monoclonal antibody (345-134S) produced against human melanoma cells. Cancer Immunol Immunotherapy 12:159, 1982

93. Irie RF, Giuliano AE, Morton DL: Oncofoetal antigen: A tumor-associated fetal antigen immunogenic in man. J Natl Cancer Inst 63:367, 1979

94. Israel L: Report on 414 cases of human tumors treated with corynebacteria. In Halpern N (ed):

Corynebacterium parvum: Applications in Experimental and Clinical Oncology, p 389. New York, Plenum, 1975

95. Jones PC, Sze LL, Liu PY, Morton DL, Irie RF: Prolonged survival for melanoma patients with elevated IgM antibody to oncofetal antigen. J Natl Cancer Inst 66:249, 1981

96. Kaiser LR, Burk MW, Morton DL: Adjuvant therapy for malignant melanoma. Surg Clin North Am 61:1249, 1981

97. Knost JA, Reynolds V, Greco FA, Oldham RK: Adjuvant chemoimmunotherapy. Stage I/II malignant melanoma. J Surg Oncol 19:165, 1982

98. Lamoureux G, Turcotte R, Portelance V (eds): BCG in Cancer Immunotherapy. New York, Grune & Stratton, 1976

99. Larson SM, Brown JP, Wright PW, Carrasquillo JA, Hellström I, Hellström KE: Imaging of melanoma with I-131-labeled monoclonal antibodies. J Nucl Med 24:123, 1983

100. Larson SM, Carrasquillo JA, Krohn KA, Brown JP, McGuffin RW, Ferens JM, Graham MM, Hill LD, Beaumier PL, Hellström KE, Hellström I: Localization of ^{131}I-labeled p97-specific FAB fragments in human melanoma as a basis for radiotherapy. J Clin Invest 72:2101, 1983

101. Larson SM, Carrasquillo JA, Krohn KA, McGuffin RW, Williams DL, Hellström I, Hellström KE, Lyster D: Diagnostic imaging of malignant melanoma with radiolabeled antitumor antibodies. JAMA 249:811, 1983

102. Lawrence BV, Lipton A, Harvey H, Gottlieb R, Kukrika M, Dixon R, Graham W, Miller S, Heckard R, White D, and the Central Pennsylvania Oncology Group: *Corynebacterium parvum* vs. BCG as adjuvant immunotherapy for stages I and II malignant melanoma. Proceedings 2nd International Conference on the Adjuvant Therapy of Cancer. Tucson, Arizona, 1979

103. Lawrence HS: The transfer in humans of delayed skin sensitivity to streptococcal M substance and to tuberculin with disrupted leukocytes. J Clin Invest 34:219, 1955

104. Levy R, Miller RA: Tumor therapy with monoclonal antibodies. Fed Proc 42:2650, 1983

105. Lewis MG, Ikonopisov RL, Nairn RC, Phillips TM, Fairley GH, Bodenham DC, Alexander P: Tumourspecific antibodies in human malignant melanoma and their relationship to the extent of the disease. Br Med J 3:547, 1969

106. Liao SK, Clarke BJ, Khosravi M, Kwong PC, Brickenden A, Dent PB: Human melanoma-specific oncofetal antigen defined by a mouse monoclonal antibody. Int J Cancer 30:573, 1982

107. Lindemann J: Viruses as immunological adjuvants in cancer. Biochim Biophys Acta 355:49, 1974

108. Lindemann J, Klein PA: Viral oncolysis: Increased immunogenicity of host cell antigen associated with influenza virus. J Exp Med 126:93, 1967

109. Lipton A, Harvey HA, Lawrence B, Gottlieb R, Kukrika M, Dixon R, Graham W, Miller S, Heckard R, Schelzel D, White DS: *Corynebacterium parvum* versus BCG adjuvant immunotherapy in human malignant melanoma. Cancer 51:57, 1983

110. Livingston PO, Takeyama H, Pollack MS, Houghton AN, Albino A, Pinsky CM, Oettgen HF, Old LJ: Serological responses of melanoma patients to vaccines derived from allogeneic cultured melanoma cells. Int J Cancer 31:567, 1983

111. Livingston PO, Watanabe T, Shiku H, Houghton AN, Albino A, Takahashi T, Resnick LA, Michitsch R, Pinsky CM, Oettgen HF, Old LJ: Serological response of melanoma patients receiving melanoma cell vaccines. I. Autologous cultured melanoma cells. Int J Cancer 30:413, 1982

112. Mastrangelo MJH, Berd D: Current status of biological responses modifier therapy of human cancer. Thirteenth International Cancer Congress Proceedings, No. 40, 1982

113. Miller JFAP, Morahan G, Walker ID: T cell antigen receptors: Fact and artefact. Immunology Today 4:141, 1983

114. Milton GW, Shaw HM, McCarthy WH, Pearson L, Balch CM, Soong S-j: Prophylactic lymph node dissection in clinical stage I cutaneous malignant melanoma: Results of surgical treatment in 1,319 patients. Br J Surg 69:108, 1982

115. Misset JL, Delgado M, De Vassal F, Mathe G, Serrou B, Jeanne C, Guerrin J, Plagne R, Schneider M, Le Mevel B, Metz R, Morice V: Immunotherapy or chemoimmunotherapy as adjuvant treatment for malignant melanoma: A G.I.F. trial. In Salmon SE, Jones SE (eds): Adjuvant Therapy of Cancer III, p 225. New York, Grune & Stratton, 1981

116. Murray DR, Cassel WA, Torbin AH, Olkowski ZL, Moore ME: Viral oncolysate in the management of malignant melanoma. II. Clinical Studies. Cancer 40:680, 1977

117. Naor D: Suppressor cells: Permitters and promoters of malignancy. Adv Cancer Res 29:45, 1979

118. Natali PG, Cavaliere R, Bigotti A, Nicotra MR, Russo C, Ng AK, Giacomini P, Ferrone S: Antigenic heterogeneity of surgically removed primary and autologous metastatic human melanoma lesions. J Immunol 130:1462, 1983

119. Nathanson L, Wolter J, Horton J, Colsky J, Shnider BI, Schilling A: Characteristics of prognosis and response to an imidazole carboxamide in malignant melanoma. Clin Pharmacol Ther 12:955, 1971

120. North RJ, Dye ES, Mills CD: T cell-mediated negative regulation of concomitant antitumour immunity as an obstacle to adoptive immunotherapy of established tumors. In Fefer A, Goldstein A (eds): The Potential Role of T Cells in Cancer Therapy, p 65. New York, Raven Press, 1982

121. Oldham RK: Monoclonal antibodies in cancer therapy. J Clin Oncol 1:582, 1983

122. Ortaldo JR, Mantovani A, Hobbs D, Rubinstein M,

Pestka S, Herberman RB: Effects of several species of human leukocyte interferon on cytotoxic activity of NK cells and monocytes. Int J Cancer 31:285, 1983

123. Osband ME, Shen YJ, Shlesinger M, Brown A, Hamilton D, Cohen E, Lavin P, McCaffrey R: Successful tumour immunotherapy with cimetidine in mice. Lancet 1:636, 1981

124. Paterson AHG, Williams D, Jerry LM, McPherson TA: Reduced incidence of loco-regional recurrences in melanoma using BCG immunotherapy after surgery. Proc Am Soc Clin Oncol 1:170, 1982

125. Pinsky CM, Hirshaut Y, Wanebo HJ: Randomized trial of bacillus Calmette-Guerin (percutaneous administration) as surgical adjuvant immunotherapy for patients with stage II melanoma. Ann NY Acad Sci 277:182, 1976

126. Pinsky CM, Oettgen HF: Surgical adjuvant therapy for malignant melanoma. Surg Clin North Am 61:1259, 1981

127. Pross HF, Baines MG: Spontaneous human lymphocyte-mediated cytotoxicity against tumour target cells. I. The effect of malignant disease. Int J Cancer 18:593, 1976

128. Quagliana J, Tranum B, Neidhardt J, Gagliano R: Adjuvant chemotherapy with BCNU, Hydrea and DTIC (BHD) with or without immunotherapy (BCG) in high risk melanoma patients: A SWOG study. Proc Am Assoc Cancer Res 21:399, 1980

129. Quirt IC, and others. Randomized controlled trial of adjuvant chemoimmunotherapy with DTIC and BCG after complete excision of primary melanoma with a poor prognosis or melanoma metastases. Can Med Assoc J 128:929, 1983

130. Reisfeld RA, Ferrone S: Melanoma Antigens and Antibodies. New York, Plenum, 1982

131. Roses DG, Campion JF, Harris MN, Gumport SL: Malignant melanoma: Delayed hypersensitivity skin testing. Arch Surg 114:35, 1979

132. Roth JA, Grimm EA, Gupta RK, Ames R: Immunoregulatory factors derived from human tumors. J Immunol 128:1955, 1982

133. Russell PS, Chase CM, Burton RC: Studies of allogeneic tumor transplants: Induced rejection of advanced tumors by immune alterations of recipients. J Immunol 130:951, 1983

134. Saal JG, Riethmüller G, Rieber EP, Hadam M, Ehinger H, Schneider W: Regional BCG-therapy of malignant melanoma: In vitro monitoring of spontaneous cytolytic activity of circulating lymphocytes. Cancer Immunol Immunotherapy 3:27, 1977

135. Salaman MR: The state of transfer factor. Immunol Today 3:4, 1982

136. Schabel FM Jr: Concepts for systemic treatment of micrometastases. Cancer 35:15, 1975

137. Schabel FM Jr: Rationale for adjuvant chemotherapy. Cancer 39:2875, 1977

138. Seigler HF, Cox E, Mutzner F, Shepherd L, Nicholson E, Shingleton WW: Specific active immu-

notherapy for melanoma. Ann Surg 190:366, 1979

139. Shaw HM, McGovern VJ, Milton GW, Farago GA, McCarthy WH: The female superiority in survival in clinical stage II cutaneous malignant melanoma. Cancer 49:1941, 1982

140. Shiku H, Takahashi T, Oettgen HF, Old LJ: Cell surface antigens of human malignant melanoma. II. Serological typing with immune adherence assays and definition of two new surface antigens. J Exp Med 144:873, 1976

141. Silberberg-Sinakin I, Gigli I, Baer RL, Thorbecke GJ: Langerhans cells: Role in contact hypersensitivity and relationship to lymphoid dendritic cells and to macrophages. Immunol Rev 53:203, 1980

142. Silberman AW, Morton DL: Adjuvant therapy following surgery for primary malignant melanoma. In Costanzi JJ (ed): Malignant Melanoma 1, p 207. The Hague, Nijhoff, 1983

143. Sober AJ, Fitzpatrick TB, Cosimi AB, Wood WC: Adjuvant therapy for melanoma. Surgery 93:726, 1983

144. Spitler LE: BCG, levamisole and transfer factor in the treatment of cancer. Prog Exp Tumor Res 25:178, 1980

145. Spitler LE, Sagebiel R: A randomized trial of levamisole versus placebo as adjuvant therapy in malignant melanoma. N Engl J Med 303:1143, 1980

146. Stuhlmiller GM, Sullivan DC, Vervaert CE, Croker BP, Harris CC, Seigler HF: In vivo tumor localization using tumor-specific monkey xenoantibody, alloantibody and murine monoclonal antibody. Ann Surg 194:592, 1981

147. Sutherland CM, Leong SPL, Cooperband SR, Deckers PJ, Horning MO, Krementz ET: In vivo delayed hypersensitivity reactions to partially purified human melanoma antigens. J Surg Oncol 20:221, 1982

148. Takasugi M, Ramseyer A, Takasugi J: Decline of natural nonselective cell-mediated cytotoxicity in patients with tumor progression. Cancer Res 37:413, 1977

149. Taniguchi T, Matsui H, Fujita T, Takaoka C, Kashima N, Yoshimoto R, Hamuro J: Structure and expression of a cloned cDNA for human interleukin-2. Nature 302:305, 1983

150. Thatcher N, Palmer MK, Gasiunas N, Crowther D: Lymphocyte function and response to chemoimmunotherapy in patients with metastatic melanoma. Br J Cancer 36:751, 1976

151. Thatcher N, Swindell R, Crowther D: Effects of corynebacterium parvum and BCG therapy on immune parameters in patients with disseminated melanoma: A sequential study over 28 days. II. Changes in non-specific (NK, K and T cell) lymphocytoxicity and delayed hypersensitivity skin reactions. Clin Exp Immunol 35:171, 1979

152. Thornes RD, Lynch G, Sheehan MV: Cimetidine and conmarin therapy of melanoma. Lancet 2:328, 1982

153. Tilden AB, Abo T, Balch CM: Suppressor cell function of human granular lymphocytes identified by the HNK-1 (Leu-7) monoclonal antibody. J Immunol 130:1171, 1983

154. Tilden AB, Balch CM: Indomethacin enhancement of immunocompetence in melanoma patients. Surgery 90:77, 1981

155. Tilden AB, Balch CM: A comparison of PGE$_2$ effects on human suppressor cell function and on interleukin 2 function. J Immunol 129:2469, 1982

156. Tilden AB, Balch CM: Immune modulatory effects of indomethacin in melanoma patients are not related to prostaglandin E$_2$-mediated suppression. Surgery 92:528, 1982

157. Trowsdale J, Lee J, McMichael A: HLA-DR bouillabaisse. Immunol Today 4:31, 1983

158. Veronesi U, Adamus J, Aubert C, Bajetta E, Beretta G, Bonadonna G, Bufalino R, Cascinelli N, Cocconi G, Durand J, De Marsillac J, Ikonopisov RL, Kiss B, Lejeune F, MacKie R, Madej G, Mulder H, Mechl Z, Milton GW, Morabito A, Peter H, Priario J, Paul E, Rumke P, Sertoli R, Tomin R: A randomized trial of adjuvant chemotherapy and immunotherapy in cutaneous melanoma. N Engl J Med 307:913, 1982

159. Wagner H, Hardt C, Heeg K, Pfizenmaier K, Solbach W, Bartlett R, Stockinger H, Rollinghoff M: T-T cell interactions during cytotoxic T lymphocyte (CTL) responses: T cell derived helper factor (interleukin 2) as a probe to analyze CTL responsiveness and thymic maturation of CTL progenitors. Immunological Rev 51:215, 1980

160. Wallack MK: Specific immunotherapy with vaccinia oncolysates. Cancer Immunol Immunotherapy 12:1, 1981

161. Wallack MK: Specific tumor immunity produced by the injection of vaccinia viral oncolysates. J Surg Res 33:11, 1982

162. Welk PK, Apperson S, Hamilton E, Stepping N: Biological properties of genetic hybrids of bacteria-derived human leukocyte interferons. J Cell Biochem, Suppl 6, 1982

163. Welte K, Wang CY, Mertelsmann R, Venuta S, Feldmann SP, Moore MAS: Purification of human interleukin 2 to apparent homogeneity and its molecular heterogeneity. J Exp Med 156:454, 1982

164. Werkmeister J, McCarthy WH, Hersey P: Suppressor cell activity in melanoma patients. I. Relation to tumor growth and immunoglobulin levels in vivo. Int J Cancer 28:1, 1981

165. Werkmeister J, Zaunders J, McCarthy WH, Hersey P: Characterization of an inhibitor of cell division released in tumour cell cultures. Clin Exp Immunol 41:487, 1980

166. Winchester RJ, Wang CY, Gibofsky A, Kunkel HG, Lloyd KO, Old LJ: Expression of Ia-like antigens on cultured human malignant melanoma cell lines. Proc Natl Acad Sci USA 75:6235, 1978

167. Wood WC, Cosimi AB, Carey RW, Kaufman SD: Randomized trial of adjuvant therapy for "high risk" primary malignant melanoma. Surgery 83:677, 1978

168. Woodward JG, Fernandez PA, Daynes RA: Cell-mediated immune response to syngeneic UV-induced tumors. III. Requirement for an IA$^+$ macrophage in the *in vitro* differentiation of cytotoxic T lymphocytes. J Immunol 122:1196, 1979

169. Zembala M, Mytar B, Popiela T, Asherson GL: Depressed *in vitro* peripheral blood lymphocyte response to mitogens in cancer patients: The role of suppressor cells. Int J Cancer 19:605, 1977

Part III
Distant Metastases

CHARLES M. BALCH
GERALD W. MILTON

Diagnosis of Metastatic Melanoma at Distant Sites

12

Metastatic melanoma can have a more variable clinical course than almost any other human cancer. Therefore, it is incumbent on the physician who treats melanoma patients to understand the patterns of metastases and methods of evaluation for metastatic disease. This should blend a suitably comprehensive examination of each patient with cost-effectiveness. This chapter concerning diagnosis and Chapter 13 concerning treatment of distant metastases describe the clinical aspects of metastatic melanoma based on our experience at the University of Alabama in Birmingham (UAB) and the Sydney Melanoma Unit (SMU). They also incorporate a review of the literature concerning metastatic melanoma at distant sites (stage III).

CLINICAL EVALUATION OF METASTASES

The clinician must evaluate the patient for the presence and extent of metastases before instituting treatment. In the absence of symptoms or signs of metastases, a minimum number of laboratory and radiologic tests should be ordered, since their costs add further burden to the patient and his family, and the diagnostic yield is often small. Rather than order a battery of expensive tests, an initial screening appraisal should be performed, then the metastatic survey pursued on a more selective basis, depending on the presence of signs or symptoms of disease in a particular area. Such an approach has been described using algorithms.[9,17] Guidelines for metastatic evaluation at specific sites are listed in Table 12-1.

The goals of treatment, cure versus palliation, are important factors in determining the extent of metastatic evaluation to be performed. In general, laboratory tests, except for screening, should not be ordered unless a positive result would lead to a change in the treatment plan. Other factors, such as cost and availability, are involved as well. Finally, knowledge of prognostic factors and the natural history of disease will help decide whether the probability of detecting metastases warrants a more or less comprehensive metastatic evaluation. These same principles are also important postoperatively in deciding how long to follow the patient, how frequent the follow-up visits should be, and what types of screening tests should be used.

HISTORY AND PHYSICAL EXAMINATION

A complete history and physical examination is the most important part of the initial metastatic evaluation. A hallmark of metastatic disease is a symptom complex that progresses either in intensity or frequency. A careful history and physical examination is the most sensitive, specific, and cost-effective means of evaluating possible metastatic disease short

TABLE 12–1
TESTS FOR EVALUATING METASTATIC MELANOMA

Metastatic Site	Symptoms	Initial Studies	Confirmatory Studies (If Necessary)
Lung	Usually none (may have some dyspnea, cough, or hemoptysis)	Chest x-ray film	Tomograms or CT scan
Liver	Weight loss, anorexia, upper abdominal pain	↑ AP ↑ LDH P$_x$: Liver mass or ascites	Liver sonar Abdominal CT scan (or liver scan if CT unavailable)
Skin, SQ	New nodule	P$_x$ examination	Biopsy
GI Tract	Hematemesis, melena, obstruction, abdominal pain	P$_x$ examination Stool guaiac	GI contrast x-ray films Endoscopy
Brain	Headache, numbness, motor weakness	H$_x$ and P$_x$ examination	Brain CT scan (or brain scan if CT unavailable)
Bone	Localized pain	↑ AP	Bone scan Bone x-ray film
Kidneys, Bladder	Hematuria	Urinalysis	Intravenous pyelogram Cystoscopy

SQ, subcutaneous; H$_x$, medical history; P$_x$, physical examination; AP, alkaline phosphatase; LDH, lactic dehydrogenase

of a biopsy. Details of signs and symptoms involving specific metastatic sites are described later in this chapter.

LABORATORY TESTS

In general, liver function tests, including lactic dehydrogenase (LDH), are important screening tests for metastatic disease. An isolated elevation of the serum alkaline phosphatase (AP) or LDH is presumptive evidence of metastatic disease.[1,17,21,40,181]

RADIOLOGIC TESTS

The chest x-ray (CXR) is a radiologic test that should routinely be used for screening purposes. Whole lung tomograms or computed tomography (CT) scans of the chest are useful for evaluating suspected pulmonary, pleural, or mediastinal metastases. For patients who, on the basis of physical examination or abnormal liver chemistries, have suspected intra-abdominal metastases, a CT or ultrasound (US) scan of the abdomen should be obtained if possible.[7,14,56,188,189] Their relative merits are discussed under Liver, Biliary Tract, and Spleen. Contrast studies of the gastrointestinal (GI) tract are indicated if there are signs or symptoms suggesting metastatic disease in this area. However, they should not be used for screening purposes. Similarly, x-rays of the bone should be performed only for symptomatic disease or suspicion of metastases suggested by a radionuclide bone scan. Bone surveys are not indicated for routine metastatic evaluation.

Lymphangiography has been used by some physicians to detect retroperitoneal or nodal metastases. However, it is associated with some morbidity to the patient, is limited in the number of nodes that can be examined, and is not a highly specific test. Lymphangiograms therefore have little, if any, application in the evaluation of metastatic melanoma.

Several excellent reviews of radiologic evaluations for metastases have been published.[6,39]

RADIONUCLIDE SCANS

Bone, brain, and liver radioisotope scans are often used as screening tests for metastatic disease.[3] However, numerous studies have now shown that these scans are not indicated for routine screening of occult metastatic melanoma because their diagnostic yield is less than 1%.[2,18,19,36,40,45,47,54] A typical experience is described by Evans and colleagues,[18] who found no true-positive brain or liver scans in 230 stage I melanoma patients. However, there were two false-positive scans of the liver and two of the brain. One craniotomy, two arteriograms, and numerous follow-up scans were obtained to confirm that these scans were indeed false-positive. The cost of the 322 screening scans was $23,964 (in U.S. dollars in 1980), and the expense of the follow-up tests and unnecessary surgery was considerably greater.

Radionuclide scans may be obtained for specific signs or symptoms of bone, brain, or liver disease. A bone scan is the most sensitive test for skeletal metastatic disease, but a careful history and directed radiographs are necessary to ensure that areas of uptake do not represent old trauma or inflammation.[40,191] Radionuclide brain scans are not as sensitive as CT scans,[9,104] but either test may be indicated in the presence of headache or neurologic abnormalities. Liver scans have a relatively high rate of false-negative and false-positive results but can be diagnostic when the results indicate multiple filling defects.[14,19,40,184,188,189]

Some clinicians have recommended the use of gallium[67] scans for metastatic disease, especially in lymph nodes.[27,37] While this test may detect nodal metastases, it is not sensitive enough or specific enough for screening patients with possible occult nodal metastases.[44,47] Physical examination and CXR are relatively more efficient, more sensitive, and less costly than gallium[67] scanning for assessing the involvement of lymph nodes in most locations. A recent evaluation of tomographic gallium scanning yielded very encouraging results with a high degree of specificity in the identification of clinically occult disease,[30] but these results have not been confirmed.

PATHOLOGIC TESTS

The diagnosis of metastatic disease is definitively made by a biopsy. An excisional or needle biopsy (such as with a Tru-cut needle) is relatively easy to perform when the suspected metastasis is superficially located and has a low complication rate. More deeply situated lesions may also be approached with a thin needle biopsy.[22] In many circumstances, however, the clinical diagnosis is sufficient when made by radiologic studies, especially if the abnormality was absent on previous studies.

Cytologic examination of urine, sputum, or cerebrospinal, peritoneal, or pleural fluid may also yield a diagnosis of metastatic melanoma when there are specific symptoms referable to these areas (Fig. 12-1).[24,58,59,138] Very occasionally, laparotomy and examination of the liver and abdominal organs may be indicated to rule out occult metastatic disease before proceeding with major surgery for locally advanced or metastatic disease elsewhere.

OTHER TESTS

Innovative new tests for detecting metastatic melanoma are currently being evaluated. In general, however, their diagnostic yield is no better and they are more expensive than currently available metastatic tests. In the future, they may be important in monitoring the effects of systemic treatment or for detecting early metastases at distant sites when more effective systemic treatments become available. Some of these tests include elevations of serum γ-glutamyl transpeptidase[39] and urinary chromatography of melanogens.[8] A particularly promising technique is the use of radiolabeled monoclonal antibodies prepared against melanoma-associated antigens, which has been used to detect metastatic melanoma in human patients (Fig 12-2).[31,53]

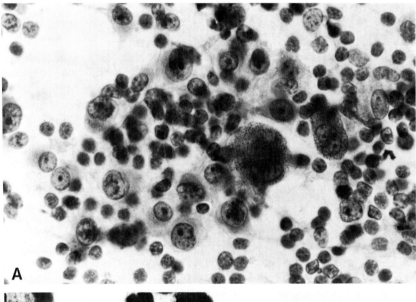

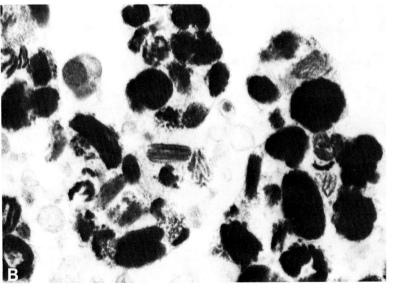

FIG. 12–1 Cytologic examination of a pleural effusion showing metastatic melanoma cells. (A) Light microscopy view. (B) Electron microscopy verifying the diagnosis by the presence of melanosomes in the cytoplasm. (Courtesy of James Wilkerson, M.D., Department of Pathology, UAB).

PATTERNS AND TIMING OF METASTASES

Melanoma can metastasize to virtually any organ or tissue.[5,12,16,36,41] Nevertheless, there are certain patterns of metastases for melanoma that will help the clinician focus on those sites most likely to harbor metastatic disease.

As listed in Table 12-2, the most common first sites of distant metastases are skin, subcutaneous tissues, and lung. The liver, bone, and brain are also commonly diagnosed sites of relapse, but with less frequency. The distribution of metastases is slightly different in autopsied melanoma patients (Table 12-2). Common sites of metastases at autopsy, such as pancreas, thyroid, and adrenal, are clinically silent in most patients prior to death. The two most common causes of death result from metastases involving the lung or brain (Table 12-3).

Patients with stage I disease who relapsed had a median interval of 1.3 years before nodal metastases were diagnosed (Fig. 12-3).[4] Stage I patients who progressed with distant metastases had a median interval of 34 months before distant metastatic dis-

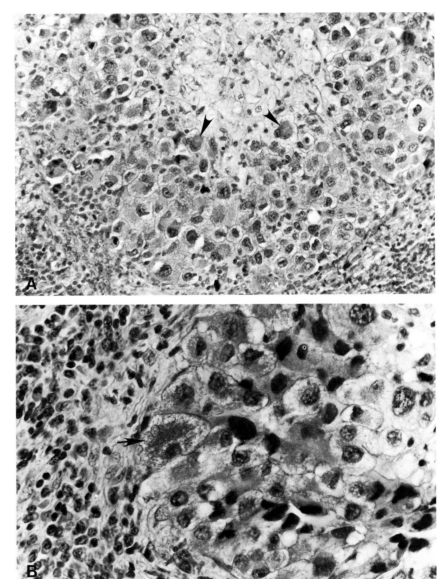

FIG. 12–2 Use of monoclonal antibodies for diagnosing melanoma. This 31-year-old woman has a lymph node metastasis from an unknown primary site in the left axilla. The light microscopic examination was equivocal for melanoma or carcinoma. (A) Immunoperoxidase staining of the specimen with a specific antimelanoma monoclonal antibody (S100) demonstrating the presence of melanoma antigens in the cytoplasm (arrows). (B) Higher-power field, showing the cytoplasmic stain (arrow), which is easily discerned by a brown color within the cytoplasm. (Courtesy of James Wilkerson, M.D., Department of Pathology, UAB).

TABLE 12–2
COMMON DISTANT SITES OF METASTATIC MELANOMA

Site	Clinical Series*	Autopsy Series*
Skin, subcutaneous and lymph node	42%–59%	50%–75%
Lung	18%–36%	70%–87%
Liver	14%–20%	54%–77%
Brain	12%–20%	36%–54%
Bone	11%–17%	23%–49%
Intestine	1%– 7%	26%–58%
Heart	<1%	40%–45%
Pancreas	<1%	38%–53%
Adrenals	<1%	36%–54%
Kidney	<1%	35%–48%
Thyroid	<1%	25%–39%

*See references 1, 5, 10, 12, 13, 16, 20, 21, 36, 41, 45 and 50).

TABLE 12–3
CAUSE OF DEATH IN 216 AUTOPSIED PATIENTS WITH METASTATIC MELANOMA

Cause	Incidence	
	Patel[41] (216 patients)	Budman[10] (139 patients)
Respiratory failure	39%	16%
Brain or cord complication	20%	32%
Cardiac failure	10%	9%
Liver failure	7%	7%
Infection	7%	10%
Renal failure	2%	1%
Bowel obstruction	—	8%
Hemorrhage	—	7%
Miscellaneous	15%	10%

ease was diagnosed, while those with nodal metastases (stage II) that progressed to distant sites did so within 11 months of treatment (Fig. 12-4).[5] The time to relapse is also correlated with tumor thickness.[38] Usually, the thicker the tumor is, the more aggressive its metastatic potential and the earlier its metastases develop. If thinner lesions metastasize, they often do not become manifest for many years after diagnosis (Fig. 12-5). The disease-free period between treatment of the primary melanoma and development of metastases can last as long as 15 to 20 years, but the vast majority of metastases occur within 3 to 5 years. These observations emphasize the importance of long-term follow-up to gain an accurate picture of metastatic disease. Since many recurrences are amenable to treatment, it is important that the follow-up be particularly vigilant during the 3- to 5-year period of greatest risk after the primary treatment. The frequency of examination may vary among patients according to their risk of metastases, but the practice at UAB is to evaluate the patient every 2 to 4 months for the first 2 years, at 6-month intervals to the fifth year, and then at least once a year indefinitely.

The site of first recurrence is also influenced by tumor thickness.[38] If a thin melanoma recurs, first recurrence is a distant metastasis (*e.g.*, lung, liver, or brain) in more than 50% of patients. On the other hand, the first recurrence of a thick melanoma is local or regional in more than 80% of patients (Fig. 12-6).

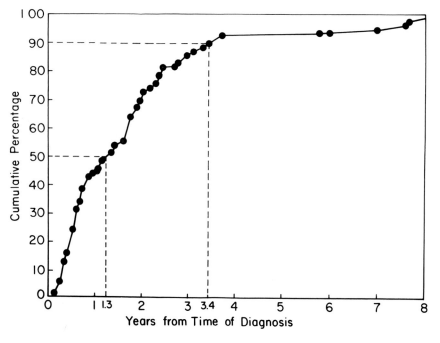

FIG. 12–3 Cumulative incidence of nodal metastases in patients whose initial surgical treatment was wide excision of the primary melanoma alone. The *dotted line* indicates that 50% of these patients developed nodal metastases within 1.3 years after initial diagnosis, while 90% did so within 3.4 years. (Balch CM, et al: A multifactorial analysis of melanoma. III. Prognostic factors in melanoma patients with lymph node metastases (stage II). Ann Surg 193: 377, 1981)

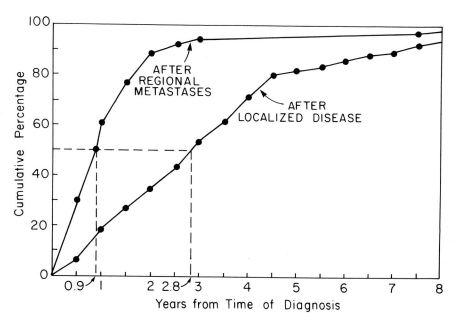

FIG. 12–4 Cumulative incidence curves for distant metastases grouped by initial stage of disease (localized melanoma and regional metastases). The *dotted line* demonstrates that 50% of patients who progressed to distant metastases did so within 10.8 months after regional metastases were diagnosed, and 33.6 months after a localized melanoma was diagnosed. (Balch CM, et al: A multifactorial analysis of melanoma. IV. Prognostic factors in 200 melanoma patients with distant metastases (stage III). J Clin Oncol 1:126, 1983)

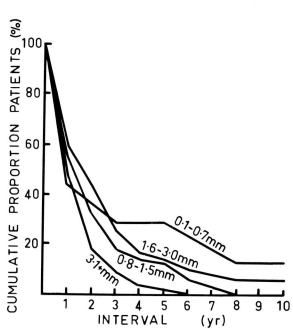

FIG. 12–5 Cumulative proportion of 326 patients treated at SMU whose lesions recurred. Patients with thicker melanomas developed their first recurrence more rapidly than patients with thin tumors. All lesions thicker than 3 mm had recurred within 6 years, while not all the thinnest melanomas had recurred within 10 years (Milton GW, et al: Tumour thickness and the site and time of first recurrence in cutaneous malignant melanoma (stage I). Br J Surg 67:543, 1980)

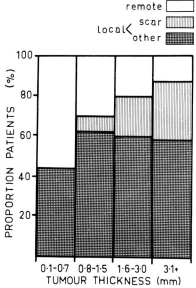

FIG. 12–6 Site of first recurrence in 326 stage I melanoma patients treated at SMU whose lesions recurred, grouped according to tumor thickness. Sites of first recurrence were either remote (*i.e.*, distant sites) or local. The local recurrences were further grouped according to whether the recurrence was at or near the surgical scar or at other sites in the region (intransit or regional node metastases). For melanomas more than 3 mm thick, the site of first recurrence was almost entirely in the scar or at regional sites. None of the thin lesions developed their first metastases locally, but the site of first metastasis for the few lesions in this thickness range developed either at regional sites or at distant sites with approximately equal frequency. (Milton GW, et al: *ibid*, Br J Surg 67:543, 1980)

Finally, melanoma has an unusual growth characteristic in metastatic sites, since it invades as a series of circumscribed deposits with a plane of separation between the tumor border and normal tissues. This information is important to the surgeon, since even large deposits can be enucleated if they are not fixed to surrounding tissues. The exception to this is melanoma that recurs in the scar of previous surgery and may be inextricably bound to adjacent structures.

DISTANT METASTASES

SKIN, SUBCUTANEOUS TISSUES, AND DISTANT LYMPH NODES

The most common sites of distant metastases are skin and subcutaneous tissues, which are often the first sign of hematogenous spread.[5,20,21,50] Skin and subcutaneous metastases are generally 0.5 cm to 2 cm in diameter and are readily detectable by physical examination. Occasionally, it may be clinically difficult to distinguish a cutaneous metastasis from a second primary melanoma. The metastases can be single or multiple and can occur anywhere on the body. Usually they are firm, round, and pigmented, although the pigmentation may not be visible at first

if the nodule is deep in the subcutaneous fat. When the first subcutaneous nodule is felt it may appear to be isolated, but often several more nodules will be detected within a short time. Some patients retain remarkably good health despite large numbers of subcutaneous metastases. Diffuse cutaneous or subcutaneous metastases can be associated with metastases to the heart.[12]

Distant lymph node metastases can occur in any area. The more superficial nodal metastases are easily diagnosed by physical examination. Those within the thorax can usually be detected on CXR, with CT scans or tomograms used as confirmatory tests, while abdominal metastatic nodes are generally detected by CT scans or ultrasonography.[7,14,75] When they involve the retroperitoneum, the pelvis, or the mediastinum, they can become quite large and cause symptoms by invasion or displacement of adjacent tissues (Fig. 12-7).[14,66,72]

LUNG, PLEURA, AND MEDIASTINUM

The second most common initial site of metastases involves the lung and pleura. Nearly all patients with disseminated melanoma will develop metastases in the chest prior to death. These lesions are evaluated by a CXR as the screening test (preoperatively and during follow-up), while suspicious

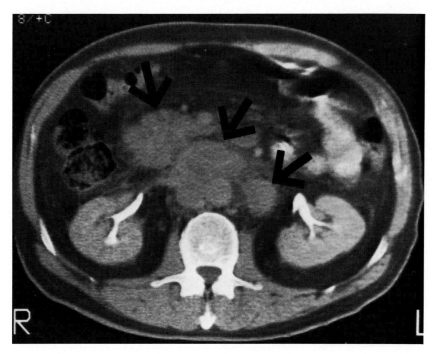

FIG. 12–7 Demonstration of extensive periaortic nodal metastases (*arrows*). This 57-year-old man presented with cervical node metastases from an unknown primary site. He subsequently developed metastases in the liver, periaortic lymph nodes, and the left eye. The metastases were unresponsive to both chemotherapy and radiation therapy, and the patient died 18 months after the initial diagnosis was made.

intrathoracic metastases are further evaluated by tomograms, CT scans, or bronchoscopy.

For screening purposes, a standard CXR (upright PA and lateral views) is sufficiently sensitive and cost-effective to be used in all melanoma patients. The yield of the more expensive pulmonary tomograms or CT scans is too low and the cost too high to justify when the CXR is normal.[36,71,75] Moreover, the false-positive rate of CT scans or tomograms can be as high as 15%. Even in patients with distant metastases (stage III), they are not indicated unless the presence of pulmonary metastases would alter the treatment plan.

Evaluation of suspicious metastases begins when one or more lesions are seen on CXR. This is the usual presentation of pulmonary metastases from melanoma.[5,21,69,74,88,90,94] Webb[94] and Chen[69] have described the frequency and patterns of thoracic metastases seen on CXR (Table 12-4). Most patients had multiple pulmonary nodules; only 22% were solitary. The tumors did not contain calcium deposits, although one melanoma patient at UAB did have documented calcification in a pulmonary metastasis. Hilar and mediastinal adenopathy frequently accompany pulmonary metastases. Patients with hilar nodules or lymphagitic spread have a particularly rapid course, with an average survival of about 1 month.

Whole lung tomograms or CT scans of the chest are of value in evaluating suspicious chest lesions or in determining whether the metastatic disease seen on CXR is also present elsewhere in the chest. Both tomograms and CT scans have advantages and disadvantages for evaluating thoracic metastases from melanoma.[68,75,76,80,83,84,86] Basically, tomograms can detect lesions 6 mm in diameter while CT scans can identify lesions down to 3 mm in diameter, but the increased sensitivity is offset by decreased specificity. Which of these is used by the clinician will often depend on available facilities, the cost of the test, and the skills of the radiologist involved. It also depends on the necessity to detect metastases as small as 3 mm when making an individual patient treatment decision.

Early in their development, pulmonary metastases from melanoma are asymptomatic. Sooner or later, however, they tend to cause one or more of the following symptoms: persistent cough, hemoptysis, shortness of breath, or chest pain. An irritating, dry, and unproductive cough may progress into hemoptysis and to coughing up clots of melanin and tumor.[57] These symptoms are usually caused by small, submucosal bronchial deposits that later enlarge and ulcerate. They may also be caused by (1) a single large extrabronchial deposit, which first compresses and then invades a major bronchus; (2) shortness of breath, which is usually caused by a blood-stained pleural effusion or, less frequently, by a pneumothorax; or (3) chest pain, which is usually caused by pleural or chest wall invasion.[73,97]

Bronchoscopy with biopsy may be considered in an occasional patient when the diagnosis of the pulmonary lesion is in doubt (*e.g.,* metastatic disease, fungal disease, benign tumor, or bronchogenic carcinoma), especially when symptoms suggest bronchial involvement (*e.g.,* a productive cough, a centrally placed lesion or a cavitary lesion). A scalene lymph node biopsy is indicated for palpable nodes. Mediastinoscopy is indicated if mediastinal nodes that are accessible through the instrument are present on CXR, tomograms, or CT scans. Thoracentesis or pleural biopsies may be helpful when evaluating effusions. Thin needle biopsy of a pulmonary lesion may be useful in selected instances under CT scan guidance to establish the histologic diagnosis. If the diagnosis remains in doubt, an exploratory thoracotomy may be necessary.

BRAIN AND SPINAL CORD

Melanoma ranks behind lung and breast carcinoma as the third most common tumor that metastasizes to the brain.[99,136] It is the initial site of metastases in 12% to 20% of patients in different clinical series and is usually associated with more widespread visceral disease.[1,5,12,16,98,110,115,128] At autopsy, cerebral

TABLE 12-4
DISTRIBUTION OF INTRATHORACIC METASTASES SEEN ON CHEST X-RAY FILMS IN MELANOMA PATIENTS

Distribution	Incidence	
	Webb[94] (63 patients)	Chen[69] (130 patients)
Pulmonary metastases	91%	78%
Solitary nodules	22%	26%
Multiple nodules	66%	72%
Miliary nodules	13%	2%
Lymphangitic spread	8%	—
Hilar or mediastinal adenopathy	44%	23%
Pleural effusion	16%	15%
Atelectasis and bronchial obstruction	13%	—
Lytic bone metastases	10%	11%
Cardiomegaly	6%	—

metastases are present in 36% to 54% of patients.[1,10,13,16,41] The hemispheres are generally involved equally, with the cerebrum involved most frequently, usually the frontal lobe, followed by the cerebellum, base of the brain and spinal cord (Fig. 12-8). Hydrocephalus is associated with about 33% of posterior fossa lesions. Cerebral metastases are solitary in only about 25% to 48% of patients.[12,105,115,128,130]

An unusual feature of cerebral metastases is their propensity for hemorrhage, which occurs much more frequently than with other histologic types of metastases. This occurs in 33% to 50% of the melanoma metastases involving the brain.[103,109,114,120] Ginaldi and colleagues found CT evidence of hemorrhage in most of the 93 patients examined, and the hemorrhagic component increased as the tumor nodules became larger.[115]

Brain scans will probably not detect occult metastases in asymptomatic patients in any disease stage. This was demonstrated in five separate series involving 504 stage I and II patients, in which not a single true-positive brain scan was obtained whereas there were 11 (2%) false-positive brain scans.[2,18,19,45,54] In patients with stage III melanomas, cerebral metastases were detected in only 11% to 16% of patients studied, but all patients with positive scans had antecedent symptoms.[40,45,115,123]

Signs and symptoms of brain metastases are listed in Table 12-5. Headache and mental deficits are the most common symptoms in most patients.[12,45,103,107,128,129] Headache resulting from brain metastases characteristically begins as a mild morning headache. As the condition progresses and the intracranial pressure increases, the headache will persist longer into the day and become more severe. It is usually generalized, although it may be slightly worse in the frontal or occipital region and is often associated with visual changes. Seizures are more common in patients with melanoma metastases compared to those with other types of tumors, but they occur in only about 25% of patients, usually later in the course of disease.[103,107,129]

The most common physical sign of brain metastases is a focal neurologic defect.[98,103,107,128] The presence of papilledema is a helpful sign, but its absence is not useful diagnostically. Diabetes insipidus due to meningeal, hypothalamic, or pituitary involvement may be the heralding sign in a few patients. It is also common for patients to present with either subarachnoid or intracerebral hemorrhages.[103,109,115,119,120,126,127,134,140] Massive hemorrhage is a much more frequent complication from brain metastases in melanoma patients compared to brain metastases from other primary tumors.

The radiologic diagnosis of melanoma metastatic to the central nervous system has been reviewed in several published series.[109,115,167] The best single test for the diagnosis of intracerebral metastases is a CT scan with contrast enhancement (Fig 12-9).[101,104,106,109,115,121,129,135] The accuracy and sensitivity of the scan make it unnecessary in most cases to perform either a radionuclide brain scan or an EEG, unless there are some equivocal findings that warrant these complementary studies. A carotid arteriogram may be indicated to rule out possible vas-

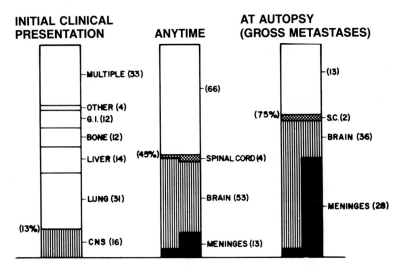

FIG. 12-8 Incidence of CNS metastases in patients with advanced melanoma. The graph represents 122 patients and 53 autopsies. The CNS was the first site of relapse in 13% of patients, occurred later in the clinical course in 45% of patients, and was present in 75% of patients at autopsy. The overlapping proportions indicate patients with more than one site of metastases. (Amer MH, et al: Malignant melanoma and central nervous system metastases. Incidence, diagnosis, treatment and survival. Cancer 42: 660, 1978)

TABLE 12–5
RELATIVE FREQUENCY OF SYMPTOMS AND SIGNS FROM BRAIN METASTASES*

Symptoms		*Signs*	
Headache	+ + + +	Pyramidal signs (paresis, hypertonia Babinski)	+ + +
Higher function loss (memory loss, dementia, personality change)	+ +		
Nausea and vomiting	+ +	Cranial nerve palsy papilledema	+ + + +
Visual changes	+ +		
Paresis	+ +		
Convulsions	+ +	Temporal lobe signs (e.g., grimacing) Seizures	+
Sensory loss	+	Extrapyramidal cerebellar	+

*(Modified from Pennington, reference 128)

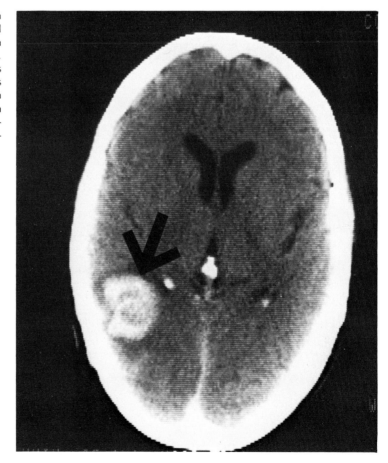

FIG. 12–9   CT scan of a metastatic melanoma in the right cerebral hemisphere (parieto-occipital junction). The scan shows a very large lesion with high attenuation using minimal enhancement. The high-density nature of the lesion suggests hemorrhage into a metastatic melanoma. This was confirmed at the time of craniotomy, when the lesion was removed in this 54-year-old man who presented with severe right-sided headaches. He died 2 months later of widespread metastases.

cular abnormalities. Nuclear magnetic resonance (NMR) scans may be used increasingly in the future. Skull films are unnecessary unless there is a need to identify bone metastases as a possible source of symptoms. A spinal tap to diagnose meningeal involvement is generally not necessary and may involve some risk if there are signs of increased intracranial pressure. On the other hand, cytologic examination of cerebrospinal fluid may be helpful in making a differential diagnosis, especially if the brain scan is equivocal. In some circumstances, a stereotactic-guided biopsy may be performed when the histologic information is essential to patient management.

Meningeal involvement occurs clinically in 3% to 13% of patients but is more frequently observed at autopsy.[13,41,98,105,130] The most common initial symptom in one series was headache (76% of patients) followed by mental confusion (46%) and signs of meningeal irritation such as nuchal rigidity or pain on straight leg raising (45% of patients).[98] The diagnosis can be made by cytologic examination of the cerebrospinal fluid.[138] It is difficult to diagnose this condition by CT scan unless it is associated with parenchymal brain metastases.

Spinal metastases are a devastating but fortunately unusual occurrence. Paraplegia may develop as the tumor grows in one or more areas close to or in the spinal cord or its roots. The most common site is extradural. Less frequently, it may arise in the cord itself or in the meninges associated with nerve roots. Clinically, the development of paraplegia may be preceded by back pain or radicular nerve pain with weakness or numbness of the leg or urinary incontinence.[129] It may progress to complete and irreversible paralysis within 24 hours.

GASTROINTESTINAL TRACT

Melanoma is one of the most frequent types of tumors that metastasize to the GI tract. The distribution of these metastases is shown in Table 12-6. Although metastases here are not often detected clinically, the GI tract is a frequent site of metastasis in autopsy series. This dichotomy exists because the symptoms are generally absent or vague and the GI metastases occur rather late in the course of disease. Most clinical series involving stage III melanoma patients do not mention GI tract as a site of metastasis, although two groups[1,12] diagnosed this condition in 8.5% and 20% (respectively) of their patients. In autopsy series, the small intestine was the most common site of metastases (in 26%–58% of all patients), while they were less frequent in the stomach (7%–26%) and colon (14%–28%) and were unusual in the esophagus (3%–9%) and anus (1%).[10,12,16,35,41,165]

Metastases to the GI tract usually occur in multiple sites simultaneously. The individual lesions are exophytic or polypoid submucosal nodules that can be umbilicated or can undergo central cavitation.[145,149,154,161,162,164,170,173] Less frequent patterns are shallow, ulcerative lesions that usually occur in the stomach and resemble gastric ulcers, or solitary, infiltrative lesions that occur most often in the small bowel and are associated with a more favorable prognosis. In about half of the patients, the metastases are pigmented while the remainder are fleshy and amelanotic.

Metastases in the gastrointestinal tract are difficult to detect by radiologic studies, so their routine use is not indicated for screening purposes. However, the physician should question the patient carefully about symptoms referable to GI metastases and

TABLE 12–6
INCIDENCE OF METASTASES IN THE GASTROINTESTINAL TRACT

Metastatic Site	Clinical Series	Autopsy Series		
	M.D. Anderson Hospital, Goldstein[154] (67 patients)	Memorial Hospital, Das Gupta[149] (100 patients)	M.D. Anderson Hospital, Einhorn[16] (96 patients)	Roswell Park, Patel[41] (216 patients)
Esophagus	7%	4%	3%	9%
Stomach	24%	26%	7%	23%
Duodenum	19%	12%	—	—
Jejunum and ileum	48%	58%	26%	36%
Colon and rectum	5%	27%	14%	28%
Gallbladder or bile ducts	3%	15%	4%	9%
Mesentery and omentum	18%	—	—	—

should consider a stool guaiac in anemic patients or those with a change in bowel habits. Large metastases are sometimes palpable on abdominal examination or can be seen by sigmoidoscopy.

Early involvement of the GI tract usually causes vague and subtle symptoms, so it is necessary to suspect intestinal metastases with persistent, nonspecific complaints such as epigastric distress, nausea, anorexia, or weight loss, which occur in a large number of patients. Only occasionally do some acute and potentially catastrophic symptoms occur. The most common clinical manifestations are the result of (1) chronic bleeding with anemia, anorexia, and weight loss; (2) obstruction of the small bowel with abdominal pain, nausea, and vomiting (Fig. 12-10); or (3) acute bleeding with hematemesis or melena. [16,36,142,147,148,149,151,152,154,155,156,158,159,160,164,169,171] Uncommon clinical presentations are bowel perforation,[145,151,155,158] peptic ulcer symptoms,[145,149,153] malabsorption,[144] and intractable diarrhea.[154] Involvement of the esophagus can cause dysphagia.[154] Occasionally, hemoperitoneum can develop following hemorrhage from subperitoneal deposits.

FIG. 12–10 Metastatic melanoma to the duodenum. This patient first presented with symptoms of anemia and vague epigastric pain. He was subsequently found to have an "ulcer" in the duodenum. This progressed to complete obstruction of the proximal duodenum, which was diagnosed at laparotomy as metastatic melanoma. A palliative gastroenterostomy was performed.

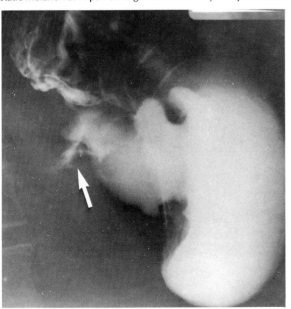

Intussusception is a frequent etiology of obstructive symptoms and other abdominal complaints. Numerous cases have been reported in the literature.[149,154,155,157,158,159,160,163,171] It usually follows a chronic or subacute course, characterized by an insidious onset. The triad of abdominal cramps, nausea without vomiting, and abdominal distention was the most consistent symptom in one series.[157] Frequently, the typical signs of palpable abdominal mass, bloody stools, and abdominal tenderness are lacking in these patients. These symptoms may be obscured if the patient also has symptoms that could be attributable to GI toxicity from chemotherapy. A CT scan can sometimes be helpful in establishing the diagnosis (Fig. 12-11).

The diagnosis of GI metastases is usually made by barium contrast radiographs or, more recently, by endoscopy. Several reviews have been written about the radiologic spectrum of metastatic melanoma involving the GI tract.[143,154,161,162,164,170] All patients undergoing an upper GI series for abdominal complaints should have a small bowel follow-through examination, since metastases are most likely to be present in this area. If the small bowel series is normal but there is a strong clinical suspicion of metastases, a small bowel enteroclysis can be performed.[168]

The largest diversity of radiologic presentations of metastatic melanoma occurs in the small intestine.[154] Usually there are multiple mural nodules, although some patients have large, excavated or ulcerated masses.[154,161,170,173] There is a distinct predilection for these tumors to be on the antimesenteric border of the bowel. In the stomach and duodenum, intramural nodules are the most commonly encountered form of metastases, but almost half of these have central ulceration or umbilication. On barium studies, these lesions can have a "bull's-eye" or "target" appearance when the barium occupies the ulcer cavity (Fig. 12-12).[161,164,166,169] Colonic metastases are generally multiple, submucosal nodules that do not usually cause symptoms.[149,154,167] Esophageal metastases are uncommon, but these patients often present with a bulky, polypoid mass that can cause symptoms of dysphagia.[146,149,154,172]

LIVER, BILIARY TRACT, AND SPLEEN

Hepatic metastases occur in 14% to 20% of patients with metastatic melanoma in different clinical series, but are present in the majority of patients at autopsy.[1,5,12,16,179] As it is unusual for isolated liver

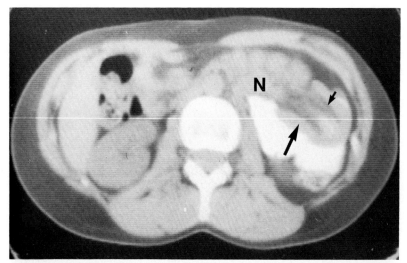

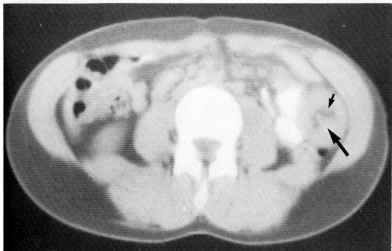

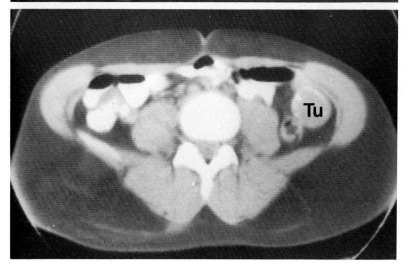

FIG. 12–11 Enteroenteric intussusception due to metastatic melanoma. Longitudinal view of intussusception (*top*). A small amount of contrast material (*small arrowhead*) outlines the lumen of the intussusceptum. *Large arrows* indicate the intussuscipiens. Note the mesentery lymphadenopathy (*N*). At a more caudal level, the intussusception is seen in cross-section (*center*). Note the eccentric lumen of the intussusceptum (*small arrowhead*) and mesentery fat (*large arrowhead*) on one side. Two centimeters caudal to the center scale (*bottom*). The leading tumor mass (*Tu*) is seen within the intussusicipiens. (Mauro MA, Koehler RE: Alimentary tract. In Lee JKT, Sagel SS, Stanley RJ (eds): Computed Body Tomography, p. 307. New York, Raven Press, 1983)

metastases to occur in patients with cutaneous melanoma, the clinical setting is generally widespread melanoma with liver involvement. This is because there are no reliable and accurate tests for detecting liver metastases at an early stage of their evolution. Thus, it is generally not worthwhile to order tests other than liver chemistries for screening purposes unless there are signs or symptoms suggesting metastatic liver disease. Hepatic metastases are usually not detected by radiologic tests until they are large (>3 cm in diameter) and multiple.[188] The prognosis of these patients is poor (*i.e.,* a median survival of 2 to 4 months), and treatment options are so few that there is almost no need to order routine liver scans. However, a radiologic assessment of the liver may be warranted to evaluate the patient's overall status when deciding treatment options for metastases at some other site.

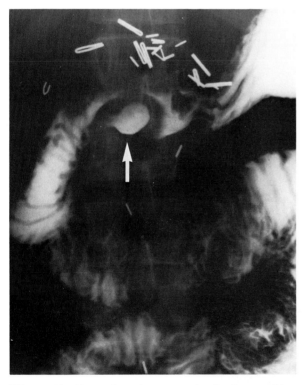

FIG. 12–12 Metastatic melanoma to the duodenum with a "bull's eye" appearance on barium study. This 22-year-old woman previously had multiple small intestinal metastastes and retroperitoneal nodal metastases removed. She later developed upper abdominal pain, and the barium swallow showed a cavitating mass in the inferior portion of the duodenal bulb due to metastatic melanoma (*arrows*).

Screening tests for liver metastases should consist only of a history and physical examination and serum liver chemistries. These are sufficiently accurate and the most cost-effective of all available tests. There are now numerous studies that clearly document the futility of using liver scintiscans, US or CT scans to screen for occult metastases in the liver of melanoma patients.[2,18,19,36,45,47,54] They are therefore neither warranted nor cost-effective as screening tests in any patient with stage I or II melanoma.

The patterns of abnormal liver chemistries that suggest liver metastases are an elevated LDH or AP in the presence of normal or only slightly elevated serum glutamic-oxaloacetic transaminase (SGOT) or bilirubin.[16,21,40,181] An elevated LDH is a clinically useful and specific test for detecting metastatic melanoma. Finck and colleagues[21] found that this was the first abnormality in 74% of melanoma patients, while an additional 18% had a simultaneous elevation of both LDH and AP. Only 8% had an elevation of the AP or SGOT before the LDH became elevated. As an indicator of liver metastases, LDH had a sensitivity and specificity of 95% and 83%, respectively, in stage II patients and 87% and 57% in stage III patients who had autopsy confirmation of hepatic metastases. They emphasized that hemolyzed serum samples can give falsely high LDH values, so radiologic studies are not obtained unless the serum LDH is elevated on at least two consecutive determinations, or the initial elevation is twice the upper limits of normal and the serum sample is not grossly hemolyzed.[21] An elevated serum bilirubin due to liver metastases is uncommon and is usually indicative of an advanced disease state.

Symptoms and physical signs resulting from early liver metastases are uncommon. The patient may experience decreased appetite with loss of weight followed within weeks by general lassitude and debility. The loss of appetite may precede a clinically palpable liver by a month or more. On the other hand, the patient may have an easily palpable liver and feel perfectly well. As the disease in the liver progresses, most distressing nausea and vomiting may develop. The patient may report a vague "dragging" sensation or "fullness" in the upper abdomen. Clinical jaundice with hepatic metastases is not common until the condition is far advanced. Very occasionally, severe sudden pain in the right upper abdomen may develop because of hemorrhage into a necrotic liver tumor. Fever resulting from hepatic necrosis is not uncommon. On physical examination, nodules on the anterior and inferior surfaces of the liver may be felt, or generalized hepatomegaly may be evident. However, more than half of patients with liver metastases do not develop hepatomegaly.[1]

When liver metastases are suspected, the confirmatory radiologic tests to be considered are (1) radionuclide liver scan, (2) ultrasound, (3) CT scan, or (4) hepatic arteriogram.[176] The tests to be used depend on availability and cost at individual hospitals, the interpretive skills of the radiologist, and the generation of equipment used, which is especially important in regard to CT scanners and US units. Most comparative studies have found that the abdominal CT scans are slightly more accurate and reliable than US and radionuclide liver scans for evaluation of liver masses.[14,174,184,188,189] However, the CT scan is more expensive and usually less available than the other two tests. No combination of these three tests increased the accuracy of detection over a single test; lesions 3 cm or greater in diameter were reliably detected by each imaging test, but smaller lesions were usually missed.[188] Ultrasonography has about the same accuracy as CT scans when a technically adequate examination was obtained and is less expensive. However, US examination can be hampered by a study that is technically inadequate because of interfering intestinal gas. Both CT and US have an advantage over radionuclide liver scans in that they can assess the entire abdomen and pelvis during a single examination (whereas the liver scans assess only the liver and spleen), and they can distinguish solid from cystic masses as well as their spatial location within the liver. At both UAB and SMU, suspected liver masses are usually examined first by US (because it is more available and less expensive than CT), while CT scans are reserved for evaluating equivocal masses seen by ultrasound (Fig. 12-13).

Nuclear magnetic resonance (NMR) imaging, a technique that depends on the intrinsic paramagnetic properties of biologic tissue, is beginning to make an impact on the detection and staging of neoplastic disease. This technique produces images that are similar in format to CT images but does not use x-rays.[43] The unique ability of NMR to characterize and display the magnetic relaxation times of various biologic tissues is proving to be a helpful addition to tumor detection, since most neoplastic tissues have considerably longer magnetic relaxation times than benign tissues of the same biologic type.[15,43,49] Even though clinical experience is very limited at this time, NMR images are already of sufficiently good quality to detect tumors that cannot be visualized by CT, and serious studies are in progress comparing the efficacy of NMR to that of CT and ultrasound.

The role of angiography for evaluating suspected metastases in the abdomen and retroperitoneum is generally limited to the few instances

FIG. 12–13   Ultrasound examination of the liver. A parasagittal view demonstrating an echogenic metastatic melanoma in the right liver lobe (*arrow*). Ultrasonography is the preferred method at UAB and SMU for following patients with known liver metastases.

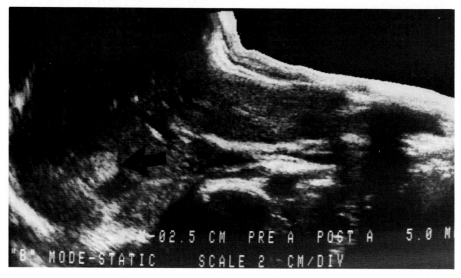

in which the differential diagnosis cannot be resolved by noninvasive techniques and the information gained would be an essential part of the treatment decision. It is also important when hepatic resection is comtemplated.

It is usually not necessary to confirm the diagnosis of liver metastases by biopsy. In the few instances in which the confirmed diagnosis is essential to treatment decisions, a needle biopsy can be performed percutaneously, by laparoscopy or by laparotomy.

Metastatic melanoma involving the gallbladder or bile ducts is present in 4% to 20% of autopsied patients.[12,16,35] It can involve the serosal surfaces or appear as polypoid masses within the gallbladder arising from the mucosa. Rarely, these metastases can cause symptoms of cholecystitis that are diagnosed as fixed filling defects in a cholecystogram.[154,175,177,182,185,186,187,190] Some of these patients presented with jaundice, and the extrahepatic obstruction caused by bile duct metastases was observed by percutaneous transhepatic cholangiogram and confirmed by surgery.[177,178,183] Most of these patients had metastatic melanoma elsewhere as well, particularly in the liver and lungs.

Melanoma is one of the few tumors that metastasizes to the spleen.[1,12,36] It may rarely cause splenomegaly, but is more often diagnosed as an incidental finding on a liver–spleen scan, abdominal CT scan, or laparotomy. Most patients with splenic metastases (up to 88%) have concomitant liver or pancreatic metastases. Rarely, a patient may develop symptoms of massive hemorrhage from a ruptured splenic metastasis.

BONE

Bone metastases occur infrequently in most clinical series (11%–17%) but are more commonly observed in autopsy series (see Table 12-2).[1,12,192,200] They generally occur in patients with widespread metastatic disease but occasionally represent the first evidence of recurrence.[192,200] The life span of these patients is short; however, because effective palliative treatment can be achieved in most cases, it is worthwhile to pursue the diagnosis. In the asymptomatic melanoma patient, particularly one with stage I or II disease, the yield of occult bony metastases on bone scan is too low to justify it as a screening procedure.[2,19,40,45,54,191]

Bony metastases from melanoma are medullary in location and destructive in nature. They are generally osteolytic in appearance on x-ray and pro-

voke little if any bone formation. Some of the roentgenographic patterns of bone metastases have been described previously.[192,197,199,200] The distribution of osseous metastases in two large series is shown in Figure 12-14. Axial metastases account for up to 80% of bony lesions, being most common in the spine.[12,192,200] When they involve the vertebral body, there are often compression fractures that may lead to neurologic symptoms such as radicular back pain, paresthesia or paresis of the legs, or urinary retention. Only about 10% of lytic lesions occur in weight-bearing bones that could result in pathologic fractures.[12,200] Occasionally, a metastasis beneath an articular surface may cause a joint effusion or may occur as a solitary lesion in a toe or a finger (Fig. 12-15).[35,192,193,198]

Bone metastases are most frequently diagnosed

FIG. 12–14 Distribution of 317 skeletal metastases in 166 patients from two patient series (See references 192 and 200). The most common sites involved were the spine (33% of patients) and the ribs (25%).

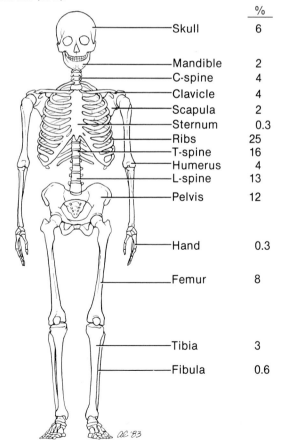

	%
Skull	6
Mandible	2
C-spine	4
Clavicle	4
Scapula	2
Sternum	0.3
Ribs	25
T-spine	16
Humerus	4
L-spine	13
Pelvis	12
Hand	0.3
Femur	8
Tibia	3
Fibula	0.6

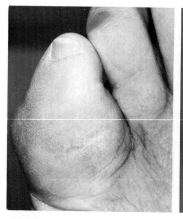
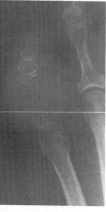
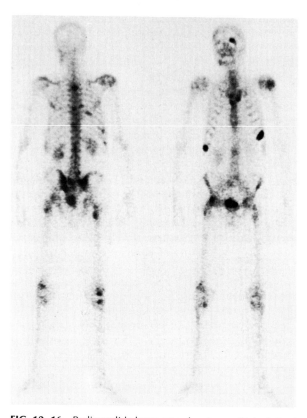

FIG. 12–15   Metastatic melanoma to the fifth toe. This 74-year-old woman presented with a 3-week history of swelling in her left fifth toe after minor trauma that had not improved. Three years previously she had had a 7 mm melanoma excised from the opposite leg. An x-ray film of the toe showed a metastatic melanoma.

in symptomatic patients, although occasionally they are seen incidentally on radiographs (*e.g.*, rib metastases on routine CXR) or a bone scan prompted by an elevated alkaline phosphatase in the absence of liver metastases. The pain from bony metastases is typically nocturnal at first, becoming persistent, progressive, and localized. It is boring in nature and can be quite severe in intensity.

These metastases are imaged radiographically or scintigraphically. The radionuclide bone scan has clearly established itself over radiographic skeletal surveys as the initial test for evaluating suspected bone metastases (Fig. 12-16). Its remarkable sensitivity, which is reported to be 50% to 80% greater than radiographs alone, allows detection of skeletal lesions far earlier than their appearance on skeletal x-rays.[191,192,196] However, scan abnormalities are nonspecific and must be correlated with radiographic study and a patient history (for fractures, trauma, arthritis and so forth) to distinguish between benign and malignant causes. It may be necessary to perform a bone biopsy to establish the diagnosis in some situations before instituting treatment.

Skeletal metastases can involve the bone marrow, sometimes extensively in the vertebrae or sternum.[12,16] Bone marrow aspirates in one series of stage III melanoma patients yielded metastatic disease in 9%,[16] while in another, it was positive in 2 of 14 patients with stage II melanoma.[2]

FIG. 12–16   Radionuclide bone scan showing multiple skeletal metastases. This 37-year-old man had a 4.5-mm melanoma excised from his back. He subsequently developed multiple bony and subcutaneous metastases. This scintigram shows multiple metastatic lesions in the ribs, femur, mandible, sternum, and orbit of the left eye that caused proptosis. The left orbit and a spontaneous rib fracture on the right were treated with radiation therapy.

KIDNEYS AND URINARY TRACT

While metastatic melanoma frequently appears at these sites at autopsy, it rarely causes clinically recognizable symptoms, and these are usually terminal manifestations of disease. Solitary or symptomatic metastases that are amenable to treatment do, however, occur occasionally.

The kidneys contain metastatic melanoma in 35% to 48% of autopsied patients; the bladder, in 13% to 18%; and the ureters and prostate, in only 2% to 5% of patients.[10,12,16,35,41,202]

Renal metastases generally occur as multiple, small (3 mm–10 mm) cortical nodules that are usually asymptomatic but that can cause hematuria or melanuria. It is uncommon that they are large enough for radiographic detection. Lumbar pain can be caused by large deposits in the kidney. Metastases in the renal pelvis and ureters are subepithelial and can cause a confusing roentgenographic appearance resembling one or more filling defects.[209,211,212,213] Some may be large enough to cause obstructive lesions with hydronephrosis or bleeding.[211,213] Although patients with bladder metastases commonly present with multiple subepithelial pedunculated or sessile lesions, solitary lesions can occur.[204,205,207,208,209,214,216,217,218] These metastases are more symptomatic than those at other sites, and patients generally present with hematuria, dysuria, or frequency. Prostate and urethral metastases can also cause hematuria, dysuria, or hesitancy.[202,206,210]

Physical examination and urinalysis are useful screening tests for metastases in these organs, especially in patients with stage III disease. The most common symptom prompting a urinary tract investigation is gross or microscopic hematuria.[1,12,205,217] Abdominal mass, rectal mass, symptoms of urinary tract infection, melanuria, melanospermia, and azotemia can also occur.[202,209,215,217] In the majority of patients, the diagnosis of metastases can be made by intravenous pyelogram, cystogram, cystoscopy, or imaging scans (CT or sonar). Occasionally, cytologic examination of the urine will demonstrate melanoma cells.[205,219]

OTHER SITES

Heart and pericardium

Metastatic melanoma is present in the heart or pericardium in about half of autopsied patients.[12,16,41] Of all malignancies, melanoma has the highest frequency of cardiac metastases.[220,223] Symptoms of cardiac or pericardial metastases may occur in some patients with disseminated disease, but there has not been a reported case of this condition as an isolated finding.[221,223,224,225,226,227] Cardiac metastases generally involve the myocardium and usually do not interfere with its function to an extent that they cause symptoms. Metastases to the pericardium or endocardium, including heart valves, occur less frequently but are more likely to evoke symptomatic changes.[221]

There are six criteria that may suggest the presence of cardiac metastases in a patient previously treated for melanoma who is without previous heart disease. They are (1) acute pericarditis, (2) cardiac tamponade or constriction, (3) rapid increase in the size of the heart on chest x-ray film, (4) onset of an ectopic tachycardia, (5) development of second- or third-degree atrioventricular heart block, and (6) onset of unequivocal cardiac failure.[223] There are no reproducible electrocardiographic patterns that are helpful in diagnosing cardiac metastases.[220] An echocardiogram or cardiac CT with contrast enhancement is probably helpful for detecting pericardial metastases, a condition for which palliative treatment might be considered. Pericardiocentesis is useful in patients with symptomatic pericardial disease demonstrable by echocardiography. Cardiac catheterization may be necessary in some cases to determine the etiology of a cardiac abnormality, especially when there are no signs of metastases elsewhere and another treatable cause of heart disease is suspected.

Pancreas

The pancreas is another common site of metastasis in autopsied patients, being present in 38% to 53% of reported cases.[12,16,36,41] The metastases are generally multiple, discrete lesions throughout the gland that rarely replace it or obstruct its major ducts. Metastases in the pancreas may be diagnosed as an incidental finding by CT scan or ultrasound but rarely cause symptoms (Fig. 12-17). Usually, symptoms occur in the form of an abdominal mass, often with obstruction of the bowel (duodenum) or biliary tract. Large pancreatic deposits can cause very troublesome backache.

Peritoneum and mesentery

Metastases of the peritoneum and mesentery can occur in patients with generalized abdominal metastases, are almost always associated with bowel or hepatic metastases, and are a common finding at autopsy.[16,41,170,251] They may cause symptoms resulting from malignant ascites or from bulky metastases compressing the bowel. Diagnosis of large lesions can be made by CT scan or ultrasonography, or as an incidental finding at laparotomy or an abdominal angiogram.[7,33,154]

Endocrine organs

The adrenal gland in particular is a frequent site of metastases, being found in 36% to 54% of autopsied patients.[12,16,36,41,202,228] Adrenal masses are occasionally seen in patients by CT scan or ultrasonography. The metastases are almost always bilateral. It is unusual for them to cause symptoms, and, should they occur, symptoms are generally vague. One patient had successful palliation for 24 months after adrenalectomy for an isolated metastasis.[12] Adrenal in-

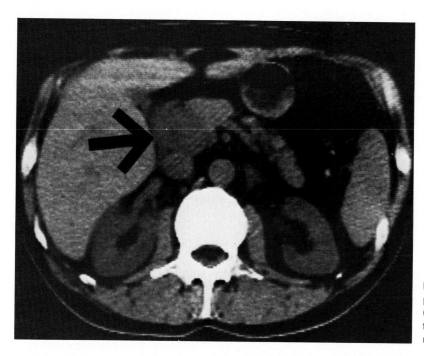

FIG. 12–17 Pancreatic metastasis in a patient with vague upper abdominal pain (arrow). CT-directed needle biopsy confirmed the diagnosis of metastatic melanoma.

sufficiency has been reported as a cause of death in some patients.[10] This probably occurs more often than is suspected clinically, because the symptoms are attributed to the patient's generalized disease.[229]

The thyroid gland is involved with melanoma metastases in 25% to 39% of autopsied patients, but they rarely cause thyroid dysfunction.[12,16,36,41] Both lobes are usually involved in a diffuse manner. Patients may present with an asymptomatic mass in the neck, but this is rarely an isolated finding. Parathyroid involvement is very infrequent, even in autopsied patients in which the incidence is 2% to 4%.

The pituitary gland can also be involved with metastatic melanoma. This is an infrequent occurrence (<5%), however, even in autopsy series. Two cases of diabetes insipidus from metastatic melanoma have been documented clinically.[1,12]

Breast

One of the most common metastatic neoplasms in the breast parenchyma is melanoma.[35,57,230,231,232,233,234,235] The autopsy incidence is 2% to 6% in different series.[12,16,36] It is occasionally diagnosed clinically by palpation. All such patients have abnormal mammograms, but the radiographic appearance more closely resembles benign breast disease.[232] It is not uncommon for these to be associated with skin or subcutaneous metastases elsewhere.

Ovary, uterus, and vagina

Ovarian metastases are rarely detected clinically but may present as a palpable abdominal mass.[12] They are more frequently seen in autopsied cases (7%–16%).[12,16,36,41] Likewise, uterine and vaginal metastases are seen in 2% to 7% of these autopsied cases, but are usually not symptomatic. One reported patient presented with vaginal bleeding from a metastic melanoma extensively involving the uterus.[252]

Testes and penis

Metastases of the testes and penis rarely occur clinically but are detected in about 5% to 7% of autopsied patients.[16,36,236] Melanoma was the most common cause of testicular metastases in one series, in which it occurred in 9 of 22 patients.[237] Patients usually present with a testicular enlargement. A metastatic melanoma involved the corpus cavernosum of the penis in one autopsied patient.[238]

Oral cavity, pharynx, and larynx

Metastases to this area often cause symptoms that may be misinterpreted as an intercurrent illness. Metastases have been documented clinically to the mandible or maxillary bone in patients presenting with a toothache or tooth abscess. It may also involve the tongue, tonsils, or pharynx, simulating an inflammatory process or a sore throat, or the larynx with symptoms of hoarseness.[239,240,241,242,243,244,245,246,247,248,249,250] The physician or dentist evaluating melanoma patients with such symptoms should have a high index of suspicion for metastatic disease.

Other sites

Metastatic melanoma has been reported to occur in the eyes and periorbital tissues, muscle, thymus, bronchus, and parotid gland.[12,16,57,66,194,242,244,253,254,256]

MELANOSIS

Melanosis is a rare complication of advanced melanoma that is characterized by generalized diffuse pigmentary deposits. The entire skin becomes dark gray or slate colored, and melanuria is present as well.[258,259,260,261,262] Only about 20 cases have been reported. All patients had widespread metastatic disease, and the melanosis occurred as a terminal event. The cause of the skin coloration has been debated, but it most likely results from melanin pigment deposition rather than from metastatic tumor cells in the skin. One feature of melanosis frequently noted at the SMU has been that the patient remains in surprisingly good health in spite of a huge liver and dark melanin staining of the skin.

METASTATIC MELANOMA FROM AN UNKNOWN PRIMARY SITE

Occasionally, patients will present with either lymph node metastases or distant metastases, but no detectable primary melanoma can be found. Patients with occult primary melanoma constitute 4% to 12% of patients with metastatic disease.[4,263,264,265,266,267,268] About two thirds of patients with occult primary melanoma will present with a metastatic lymph node (most commonly in the axilla), while one third will present with distant metastases (usually the skin, subcutaneous tissue, lung, or brain).

About 10% to 20% of patients will describe a previous mole on the skin within the lymphatic drainage area of the metastatic node. Typically, this was noticed sometime within the preceding 1 to 3 years when it became raised, itched, bled, or was subjected to minor injury, leaving a pale scar. About one third of patients had had some previous treatment of a mole, such as diathermy or curettage in the draining area; this presumably was the primary melanoma. The majority of patients, however, had no previous history of cutaneous melanoma.

The first step in evaluating such a patient is to search the skin carefully for a possible primary lesion and to biopsy any suspicious-looking skin lesions, especially pigmented ones. A knowledge of the anatomical area drained by the diseased lymph nodes will allow a concentrated search in this area. A Wood's ultraviolet lamp may be useful in revealing areas of depigmentation or a halo nevus. The next step is an examination for clinical evidence of visceral or disseminated disease. This includes a careful physical examination comprising opthalmoscopy, CXR, liver function tests, and other tests depending on the presentation and any signs or symptoms of metastatic disease.

The results in all series in which known and unknown primary melanomas have been examined clearly reveal no difference in outcome when these patients are matched according to prognostic factors (Fig. 12-18). Accordingly, patients with an unknown primary melanoma should be treated in the same manner as a similarly staged patient with a known primary melanoma.

The two usual explanations for metastatic melanoma from an unknown primary origin are the following: (1) it is a melanoma arising *de novo* within a lymph node or a visceral site; or (2) it is caused by spontaneous regression of the primary lesion. There is considerable support for the latter hypothesis. Thus, the disappearance of a primary lesion through the process of spontaneous regression and a later discovery of metastatic melanoma is most consistent with the results obtained to date. It is possible that the tumor immune response to melanoma antigens that caused the destruction of the primary melanoma might be responsible for the long-term survival obtained in some of the reported patients.

When feasible, an aggressive surgical approach is recommended for both cure and palliation of these patients (see Chaps. 7 and 13). In patients with regional metastases, the 5-year survival for those treated by lymphadenectomy who had a metastasis in a single lymph node was significantly better than for those who had involvement of more than one lymph node.[4] Patients with skin and subcutaneous metastases have a better prognosis compared to those with other sites of distant metastases, with a 2-year survival rate of up to 37% reported in one series.[266]

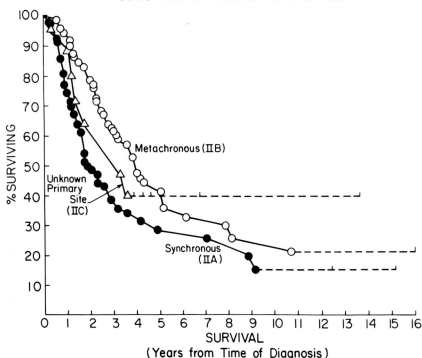

SUBSTAGE OF NODAL METASTASES

FIG. 12–18 Survival curves for substages of patients with nodal metastases, calculated from the time of diagnosis. Those patients with metastatic melanoma in regional lymph nodes arising from an unknown primary site (stage IIC) had the same survival rate as those patients presenting with synchronous nodal metastases (stage IIA) or those with metachronous metastases (stage IIB). (Balch CM, et al: A multifactorial analysis of melanoma. III. Prognostic factors in melanoma patients with lymph node metastases (stage II). Ann Surg 193:377, 1981)

REFERENCES

GENERAL DIAGNOSIS AND TREATMENT

1. Amer MH, Al-Sarraf M, Vaitkevicius VK: Clinical presentation, natural history and prognostic factors in advanced malignant melanoma. Surg Gynecol Obstet 149:687, 1979
2. Aranha GV, Simmons RL, Gunnarsson A, Grage TB, McKhann CF: The value of preoperative screening procedures in stage I and II malignant melanoma. J Surg Oncol 11:1, 1979
3. Balch CM, Karakousis C, Mettlin C, Natarajan N, Donegan WL, Smart CR, Murphy GR: Management of cutaneous melanoma in the United States: Results of the American College of Surgeons' melanoma survey. Surg Gynecol Obstet 158:311, 1984
4. Balch CM, Soong S-j, Murad TM, Ingalls AL, Maddox WA: A multifactorial analysis of melanoma III: Prognostic factors in melanoma patients with lymph node metastases (stage II). Ann Surg 193:377, 1981
5. Balch CM, Soong S-j, Murad TM, Smith JW, Maddox WA, Durant JR: A multifactorial analysis of melanoma IV. Prognostic factors in 200 melanoma patients with distant metastases (stage III). J Clin Oncol 1:126, 1983
6. Bassett LW, Steckel RJ: Imaging techniques in the detection of metastatic disease. Semin Oncol 4:39, 1977
7. Bernardino ME, Goldstein HM: Gray scale ultrasonography in the evaluation of metastatic melanoma. Cancer 42:2529, 1978
8. Blois MS, Banda PW: Detection of occult metastatic melanoma by urine chromatography. Cancer Res 36:3317, 1976
9. Bragg DG: Medical imaging problems in the patient with advanced cancer. JAMA 244:597, 1980
10. Budman DR, Camacho E, Wittes RE: The current causes of death in patients with malignant melanoma. Eur J Cancer 14:327, 1978
11. Cox KR, Hare WSC, Bruce PT: Lymphography in melanoma: Correlation of radiology with pathology. Cancer 19:637, 1966
12. Das Gupta T, Brasfield R: Metastatic melanoma: A clinicopathological study. Cancer 17:1323, 1964
13. de la Monte SM, Moore GW, Hutchins GM: Patterned distribution of metastases from malignant melanoma in humans. Cancer Res 43:3427, 1983
14. Doiron MJ, Bernardino ME: A comparison of noninvasive imaging modalities in the melanoma patient. Cancer 47:2581, 1981
15. Doyle FH, Pennock JM, Banks LM, McDonnell MJ, Bydder GM, Steiner RE, Young IR, Clarke GJ, Pasmore T, Gilderdale DJ: Nuclear magnetic reso-

nance imaging of the liver: Initial experience. Am J Roentgenol 138:193, 1982

16. Einhorn LH, Burgess MA, Vallejos C, Bodey GP Sr, Gutterman J, Mavligit G, Hersh EM, Luce JK, Frei E III, Freireich EJ, Gottlieb JA: Prognostic correlations and response to treatment in advanced metastatic malignant melanoma. Cancer Res 34:1995, 1974

17. Eiseman B, Robinson WA, Steele G Jr: Follow-up of the Cancer Patient. New York, Georg Thieme Verlag, Thieme-Stratton, 1982

18. Evans RA, Bland KI, McMurtrey MJ, Ballantyne AJ: Radionuclide scans not indicated for clinical stage I melanoma. Surg Gynecol Obstet 150:532, 1980

19. Felix EL, Sindelar WF, Bagley DH, Johnston GS, Ketcham AS: The use of bone and brain scans as screening procedures in patients with malignant lesions. Surg Gynecol Obstet 141:867, 1975

20. Feun LG, Gutterman J, Burgess MA, Hersh EM, Mavligit G, McBride CM, Benjamin RS, Richman SP, Murphy WK, Bodey GP, Brown BW, Mountain CF, Leavens ME, Freireich EJ: The natural history of resectable metastatic melanoma (stage IVA melanoma). Cancer 50:1656, 1982

21. Finck SJ, Giuliano AE, Morton DL: LDH and melanoma. Cancer 51:840, 1983

22. Friedman M, Forgione H, Shanbhag V: Needle aspiration of metastatic melanoma. Acta Cytol 24:7, 1980

23. Habermalz HJ, Fisher JJ: Radiation therapy of malignant melanoma: Experience with high individual treatment doses. Cancer 38:2258, 1976

24. Hajdu SI, Savino A: Cytologic diagnosis of malignant melanoma. Acta Cytol 17:320, 1973

25. Hilaris BS, Raben M, Calabrese AS, Phillips RF, Henschke UK: Value of radiation therapy for distant metastases from malignant melanoma. Cancer 16:765, 1963

26. Huffman TA, Sterin WK: Ten-year survival with multiple metastatic malignant melanoma: Primary site unknown. Arch Surg 106:234, 1973

27. Jackson FI, McPherson TA, Lentle BC: Gallium-67 scintigraphy in multisystem malignant melanoma. Radiology 122:163, 1977

28. Karakousis CP: Surgical treatment of recurrent malignant melanoma. Contemp Surg 22:75, 1983

29. Karakousis CP, Temple DF, Moore R, Ambrus JL: Prognostic parameters in recurrent malignant melanoma. Cancer 52:575, 1983

30. Kirkwood JM, Myers JE, Vlock DR, Neumann R, Ariyan S, Gottschalk A, Hoffer P: Tomographic gallium-67 citrate scanning: Useful new surveillance for metastatic melanoma. Ann Surg 198:102, 1983

31. Larson SM, Brown JP, Wright PW, Carrasquillo JA, Hellstrom I, Hellstrom KE: Imaging of melanoma with I-131-labeled monoclonal antibodies. J Nucl Med 24:123, 1983

32. Lawson DH, Nixon DW, Black ML, Tindall GT, Barnes DA, Faraj BA, Ali FM, Camp VM, Richmond A: Evaluation of transsphenoidal hypophysectomy in the management of patients with advanced malignant melanoma. Cancer 51:1541, 1983

33. Levitt RG, Koehler RE, Sagel SS, Lee JKT: Metastatic disease of the mesentery and omentum. Radiol Clin North Am 20:501, 1982

34. Libshitz HI: Symposium on metastatic disease. Radiol Clin North Am 20:417, 1982

35. Meyer JE: Radiographic evaluation of metastatic melanoma. Cancer 42:127, 1978

36. Meyer JE, Stolbach L: Pretreatment radiographic evaluation of patients with malignant melanoma. Cancer 42:125, 1978

37. Milder MS, Frankel RS, Bulkley GB, Ketcham AS, Johnston GS: Gallium-67 scintigraphy in malignant melanoma. Cancer 32:1350, 1973

38. Milton GW, Shaw HM, Farago GA, McCarthy WH: Tumour thickness and the site and time of first recurrence in cutaneous malignant melanoma (stage I): Br J Surg 67:543, 1980

39. Murray JL, Lerner MP, Nordquist RE: Elevated γ-glutamyl transpeptidase levels in malignant melanoma. Cancer 49:1439, 1982

40. Muss HB, Richards F II, Barnes PL, Willard VV, Cowan RJ: Radionuclide scanning in patients with advanced malignant melanoma. Clin Nucl Med 4:516, 1979

41. Patel JK, Didolkar MS, Pickren JW, Moore RH: Metastatic pattern of malignant melanoma: A study of 216 autopsy cases. Am J Surg 135:807, 1978

42. Presant CA, Bartolucci AA, Smalley RV, Vogler WR, the Southeastern Cancer Study Group: Cyclophosphamide plus 5-(3,3-dimethyl-1-triazeno)-imidazole-4-carboxamide (DTIC) with or without corynebacterium parvum in metastatic malignant melanoma. Cancer 44:899, 1979

43. Pykett IL, Newhouse JH, Buonanno FS, Brady TJ, Goldman MR, Kistler JP, Pohost GM: Principles of nuclear magnetic resonance imaging. Radiology 143:157, 1982

44. Romolo JL, Fisher SG: Gallium[67] scanning compared with physical examination in the preoperative staging of malignant melanoma. Cancer 44:468, 1979

45. Roth JA, Eilber FR, Bennett LR, Morton DL: Radionuclide photoscanning: Usefulness in preoperative evaluation of melanoma patients. Arch Surg 110:1211, 1975

46. Sacre R, Lejeune FJ: Pattern of metastases distribution in 173 stage I or II melanoma patients. Anticancer Res 2:47, 1982

47. Seigler HF, Fetter BF: Current management of melanoma. Ann Surg 186:1, 1977

48. Seigler HF, Lucas VS Jr, Pickett NJ, Huang AT: DTIC, CCNU, bleomycin and vincristine (BOLD) in metastatic melanoma. Cancer 46:2346, 1980

49. Smith FW: Two years' clinical experience with NMR imaging. Applied Radiol, 12:29, 1983

50. Stehlin JS Jr, Hills WJ, Rufino C: Disseminated melanoma: Biologic behavior and treatment. Arch Surg 94:495, 1967

51. Storm FK, Kaiser LR, Goodnight JE, Harrison WH, Elliott RS, Gomes AS, Morton DL: Thermo-chemotherapy for melanoma metastases in liver. Cancer 49:1243, 1982

52. Strauss A, Dritschilo A, Nathanson L, Piro AJ: Radiation therapy of malignant melanomas: An evaluation of clinically used fractionation schemes. Cancer 47:1262, 1981

53. Stuhlmiller GM, Sullivan DC, Vervaert CE, Croker BP, Harris CC, Seigler HF: In vivo tumor localization using tumor-specific monkey xenoantibody, alloantibody, and murine monoclonal xenoantibody. Ann Surg 194:592, 1981

54. Thomas JH, Panoussopoulous D, Liesmann GE, Jewell WR, Preston DF: Scintiscans in the evaluation of patients with malignant melanomas. Surg Gynecol Obstet 149:574, 1979

55. Turnbull A, Shah J, Fortner J: Recurrent melanoma of an extremity treated by major amputation. Arch Surg 106:496, 1973

56. Whalen JP: Radiology of the abdomen: Impact of new imaging methods. Am J Roentgenol 133:587, 1979

57. Wheelock MC, Frable WJ, Urnes PD: Bizarre metastases from malignant neoplasms. Am J Clin Pathol 37:475, 1962

58. Yamada T, Itou U, Watanabe Y, Ohashi S: Cytologic diagnosis of malignant melanoma. Acta Cytol 16:70, 1972

59. Zornoza J: Needle biopsy of metastases. Radiol Clin North Am 20:569, 1982

SKIN AND SUBCUTANEOUS METASTASES

60. Cox KR: Regional cutaneous metastases in melanoma of the limb. Surg Gynecol Obstet 139:385, 1974

61. Kim JH, Hahn EW, Ahmed SA: Combination hyperthermia and radiation therapy for malignant melanoma. Cancer 50:478, 1982

62. Luk KH, Francis ME, Perez CA, Johnson RJ: Radiation therapy and hyperthermia in the treatment of superficial lesions: Preliminary analysis: Treatment efficacy and reactions of skin tissues subcutaneous. Am J Clin Oncol 6:399, 1983

63. Overgaard J: Fractionated radiation and hyperthermia: Experimental and clinical studies. Cancer 48:1116, 1981

LUNG, PLEURA, AND MEDIASTINUM

64. Anderson CB, Philpott GW, Ferguson TB: The treatment of malignant pleural effusions. Cancer 33:916, 1974

65. Andrews AH Jr, Caldarelli DD: Carbon dioxide laser treatment of metastatic melanoma of the trachea and bronchi. Ann Otol Rhinol Laryngol 90:310, 1981

66. Braman SS, Whitcomb ME: Endobronchial metastasis. Arch Intern Med 135:543, 1975

67. Cahan WG: Excision of melanoma metastases to lung: Problems in diagnosis and management. Ann Surg 178:703, 1973

68. Chang AE, Schaner EG, Conkle DM, Flye MW, Doppman JL, Rosenberg SA: Evaluation of computed tomography in the detection of pulmonary metastases: A prospective study. Cancer 43:913, 1979

69. Chen JTT, Dahmash NS, Ravin CE, Heaston DK, Putman CE, Seigler HF, Reed JC: Metastatic melanoma to the thorax: Report of 130 patients. Am J Roentgenol 137:293, 1981

70. Cline RE, Young WG Jr: Long term results following surgical treatment of metastatic pulmonary tumors. Am Surg 36:61, 1970

71. Curtis A McB, Ravin CE, Deering TF, Putman CE, McLoud TC, Greenspan RH: The efficacy of full-lung tomography in the detection of early metastatic disease from melanoma. Diagn Radiol 144:27, 1982

72. Feldman L, Kricun ME: Malignant melanoma presenting as a mediastinal mass. JAMA 241:396, 1979

73. Gibbons JA, Devig PM: Massive hemothorax due to metastatic malignant melanoma. Chest 73:123, 1978

74. Gromet MA, Ominsky SH, Epstein WL, Blois MS: The thorax as the initial site for systemic relapse in malignant melanoma: A prospective survey of 324 patients. Cancer 44:776, 1979

75. Heaston DK, Putman CE: Radiographic manifestations of thoracic malignant melanoma. In Seigler HF (ed): Clinical Management of Melanoma, p 62. The Hague, Nijhoff, 1982

76. Libshitz HI, North LB: Pulmonary metastases. Radiol Clin North Am 20:437, 1982

77. McCormack PM, Bains MS, Beattie EJ Jr, Martini N: Pulmonary resection in metastatic carcinoma. Chest 73:163, 1978

78. McCormack PM, Martini N: The changing role of surgery for pulmonary metastases. Ann Thorac Surg 28:139, 1979

79. Mathisen DJ, Flye MW, Peabody J: The role of thoracotomy in the management of pulmonary metastases from malignant melanoma. Ann Thorac Surg 27:295, 1979

80. Mintzer RA, Malave SR, Neiman HL, Michaelis LL, Vanecko RM, Sanders JH: Computed vs. conventional tomography in evaluation of primary and secondary pulmonary neoplasms. Radiology 132:653, 1979

81. Morrow CE, Vassilopoulos PP, Grage TB: Surgical resection for metastatic neoplasms of the lung: Experience at the University of Minnesota Hospitals. Cancer 45:2981, 1980

82. Morton DL, Joseph WL, Ketcham AS, Geelhoed

GW, Adkins PC: Surgical resection and adjunctive immunotherapy for selected patients with multiple pulmonary metastases. Ann Surg 178:360, 1973

83. Muhm JR, Brown LR, Crowe JK: Use of computed tomography in the detection of pulmonary nodules. Mayo Clin Proc 52:345, 1977

84. Neifeld JP, Michaelis LL, Doppman JL: Suspected pulmonary metastases: Correlation of chest x-ray, whole lung tomograms, and operative findings. Cancer 39:383, 1977

85. Reed RJ III, Kent EM: Solitary pulmonary melanomas: Two case reports. J Thorac Cardiovasc Surg 48:226, 1964

86. Schaner EG, Chang AE, Doppman JL, Conkle DM, Flye MW, Rosenberg SA: Comparison of computed and conventional whole lung tomography in detecting pulmonary nodules: A prospective radiologic-pathologic study. Am J Roentgenol 131:51, 1978

87. Sethi SM, Saxton GD: Osteoarthropathy associated with solitary pulmonary metastasis from melanoma. Can J Surg 17:221, 1974

88. Simeone JF, Putman CE, Greenspan RH: Detection of metastatic malignant melanoma by chest roentgenography. Cancer 39:1993, 1977

89. Sonoda T, Krauss S: Hypertrophic osteoarthropathy associated with pulmonary metastasis of malignant melanoma. J Tenn Med Assoc 68:716, 1975

90. Sutton FD Jr, Vestal RE, Creagh CE: Varied presentations of metastatic pulmonary melanoma. Chest 65:415, 1974

91. Turney S, Haight C: Pulmonary resection for metastatic neoplasms. J Thorac Cardiovasc Surg 61:784, 1971

92. Vidne BA, Richter S, Levy MJ: Surgical treatment of solitary pulmonary metastasis. Cancer 38:2561, 1976

93. Webb WR: Hilar and mediastinal lymph node metastases in malignant melanoma. Am J Roentgenol 133:805, 1979

94. Webb WR, Gamsu G: Thoracic metastasis in malignant melanoma: A radiographic survey of 65 patients. Chest 71:176, 1977

95. Wilkins EW Jr, Head JM, Burke JF: Pulmonary resection for metastatic neoplasms in the lung: Experience at the Massachusetts General Hospital. Am J Surg 135:480, 1978

96. Wilson KS, Naidoo A: Hypertrophic osteoarthropathy. Mayo Clin Proc 54:208, 1979

97. Yeung KY, Bonnet JD: Spontaneous pneumothorax with metastatic malignant melanoma. Chest 71:435, 1977

BRAIN AND SPINAL CORD

98. Amer MH, Al-Sarraf M, Baker LH, Vaitkevicius VK: Malignant melanoma and central nervous system metastases: Incidence, diagnosis, treatment and survival. Cancer 42:660, 1978

99. Aronson SM, Garcia JH, Aronson BE: Metastatic neoplasms of the brain: Their frequency in relation to age. Cancer 17:558, 1964

100. Atkinson L: Melanoma of the central nervous system. Aust NZ J Surg 48:14, 1978

101. Bardfeld PA, Passalaqua AM, Braunstein P, Raghavendra BN, Leeds NE, Kricheff II: A comparison of radionuclide scanning and computed tomography in metastatic lesions of the brain. J Comput Assist Tomogr 1:315, 1977

102. Bauman ML, Price TR: Intracranial metastatic malignant melanoma: Long-term survival following subtotal resection. South Med J 65:344, 1972

103. Bremer AM, West CR, Didolkar MS: An evaluation of the surgical management of melanoma of the brain. J Surg Oncol 10:211, 1978

104. Buell U, Niendorf HP, Kazner E, Lanksch W, Wilske J, Steinhoff H, Gahr H: Computerized transaxial tomography and cerebral serial scintigraphy in intracranial tumors—rates of detection and tumor-type identification: Concise communication. J Nucl Med 19:476, 1978

105. Bullard DE, Cox EB, Seigler HF: Central nervous system metastases in malignant melanoma. Neurosurgery 8:26, 1981

106. Butler AR, Kricheff II: Non-contrast CT scanning: Limited value in suspected brain tumor. Radiology 126:689, 1978

107. Carella RJ, Gelber R, Hendrickson F, Berry HC, Cooper JS: Value of radiation therapy in the management of patients with cerebral metastases from malignant melanoma: Radiation Therapy Oncology Group brain metastases study I and II. Cancer 45:679, 1980

108. Cooper JS, Carella R: Radiotherapy of intracerebral metastatic malignant melanoma. Radiology 134:735, 1980

109. Enzmann DR, Kramer R, Norman D, Pollock J: Malignant melanoma metastatic to the central nervous system. Radiology 127:177, 1978

110. Fell DA, Leavens ME, McBride CM: Surgical versus nonsurgical management of metastatic melanoma of the brain. Neurosurgery 7:238, 1980

111. Fletcher JW, George EA, Henry RE, Donati RM: Brain scans, dexamethasone therapy, and brain tumors. JAMA 232:1261, 1975

112. Galicich JH, Sundaresan N, Arbit E, Passe S: Surgical treatment of single brain metastasis: Factors associated with survival. Cancer 45:381, 1980

113. Gelber RD, Larson M, Borgelt BB, Kramer S: Equivalence of radiation schedules for the palliative treatment of brain metastases in patients with favorable prognosis. Cancer 48:1749, 1981

114. Gildersleeve N Jr, Koo AH, McDonald CJ: Metastatic tumor presenting as intracerebral hemorrhage: Report of 6 cases examined by computed tomography. Radiology 124:109, 1977

115. Ginaldi S, Wallace S, Shalen P, Luna M, Handel S: Cranial computed tomography of malignant melanoma. Am J Roentgenol 136:145, 1981

116. Gottlieb JA, Frei E III, Luce JK: An evaluation of the management of patients with cerebral metastases from malignant melanoma. Cancer 29:701, 1972

117. Greenberg HS, Kim J, Posner JB: Epidural spinal cord compression from metastatic tumor: Results with a new treatment protocol. Ann Neurol 8:361, 1980

118. Hafström L, Jönsson P-E, Strömblad L-G: Intracranial metastases of malignant melanoma treated by surgery. Cancer 46:2088, 1980

119. Hayward RD: Malignant melanoma and the central nervous system: A guide for classification based on the clinical findings. J Neurol Neurosurg Psychiatry 39:526, 1976

120. Hayward RD: Secondary malignant melanoma of the brain. Clin Oncol 2:227, 1976

121. Holtås S, Cronqvist S: Cranial computed tomography of patients with malignant melanoma. Neuroradiology 22:123, 1981

122. Lang EF, Slater J: Metastatic brain tumors: Results of surgical and nonsurgical treatment. Surg Clin North Am 44:865, 1964

123. Lewi HJ, Roberts MM, Donaldson AA, Forrest APM: The use of cerebral computer assisted tomography as a staging investigation of patients with carcinoma of the breast and malignant melanoma. Surg Gynecol Obstet 151:385, 1980

124. McCann WP, Weir BKA, Elvidge AR: Long-term survival after removal of metastatic malignant melanoma of the brain: Report of two cases. J Neurosurg 28:483, 1968

125. McNeel DP, Leavens ME: Long-term survival with recurrent metastatic intracranial melanoma: Case report. J Neurosurg 29:91, 1968

126. Madonick MJ, Savitsky N: Subarachnoid hemorrhage in melanoma of the brain. Arch Neurol Psych 65:628, 1951

127. Mandybur TI: Intracranial hemorrhage caused by metastatic tumors. Neurology 27:650, 1977

128. Pennington DG, Milton GW: Cerebral metastasis from melanoma. Aust NZ J Surg 45:405, 1975

129. Posner JB: Management of central nervous system metastases. Semin Oncol 4:81, 1977

130. Posner JB, Chernik NL: Intracranial metastases from systemic cancer. Adv Neurol 19:579, 1978

131. Ransohoff J: Surgical management of metastatic tumors. Semin Oncol 2:21, 1975

132. Reyes V, Horrax G: Metastatic melanoma of the brain: Report of a case with unusually long survival period following surgical removal. Ann Surg 131:237, 1950

133. Ruderman NB, Hall, TC: Use of glucocorticoids in the palliative treatment of metastatic brain tumors. Cancer 18:298, 1965

134. Scott M: Spontaneous intracerebral hematoma caused by cerebral neoplasms: Report of eight verified cases. J Neurosurg 42:338, 1975

135. Solis OJ, Davis KR, Adair LB, Roberson GR, Kleinman G: Intracerebral metastatic melanoma: CT evaluation. Comput Tomogr 1:135, 1977

136. Vieth RG, Odom GL: Intracranial metastases and their neurosurgical treatment. J Neurosurg 23:375, 1965

137. Vlock DR, Kirkwood JM, Leutzinger C, Kapp DS, Fischer JJ: High-dose fraction radiation therapy for intracranial metastases of malignant melanoma: A comparison with low-dose fraction therapy. Cancer 49:2289, 1982

138. Wasserstrom WR, Glass JP, Posner JB: Diagnosis and treatment of leptomeningeal metastases from solid tumors: Experience with 90 patients. Cancer 49:759, 1982

139. Winston KR, Walsh JW, Fischer EG: Results of operative treatment of intracranial metastatic tumors. Cancer 45:2639, 1980

140. Wolpert SM, Zimmer A, Schechter MM, Zingesser LH: The neuroradiology of melanomas of the central nervous system. Am J Roentgenol 101:178, 1967

141. Young RF, Post EM, King GA: Treatment of spinal epidural metastases: Randomized prospective comparison of laminectomy and radiotherapy. J Neurosurg 53:741, 1980

GASTROINTESTINAL TRACT

142. Backman H: Metastases of malignant melanoma in the gastrointestinal tract. Geriatrics 24:112, 1969

143. Beckly DE: Alimentary tract metastases from malignant melanoma. Clin Radiol 25:385, 1974

144. Benisch BM, Abramson S, Present DH: Malabsorption and metastatic melanoma. Mt Sinai J Med 39:474, 1972

145. Booth JB: Malignant melanoma of the stomach: Report of a case presenting as an acute perforation and review of the literature. Br J Surg 52:262, 1965

146. Butler ML, Van Heertum RL, Teplick SK: Metastatic malignant melanoma of the esophagus: A case report. Gastroenterology 69:1334, 1975

147. Byrd BF Jr, Morton CE III: Malignant melanoma metastatic to the gastrointestinal tract from an occult primary tumor. South Med J 71:1306, 1978

148. Calderon R, Ceballos J, McGraw JP: Metastatic melanoma of the stomach. Am J Roentgenol 74:242, 1955

149. Das Gupta TK, Brasfield RD: Metastatic melanoma of the gastrointestinal tract. Arch Surg 88:969, 1964

150. Davis GH, Zollinger RW: Metastatic melanoma of the stomach. Am J Surg 99:94, 1960

151. Fraser-Moodie A, Hughes RG, Jones SM, Shorey BA, Snape L: Malignant melanoma metastases to the alimentary tract. Gut 17:206, 1976

152. Giler S, Kott I, Urca I: Malignant melanoma metastatic to the gastrointestinal tract. World J Surg 3:375, 1979

153. Goldman SL, Pollak EW, Wolfman EF Jr: Gastric

ulcer: An unusual presentation of malignant melanoma. JAMA 237:52, 1977

154. Goldstein HM, Beydoun MT, Dodd GD: Radiologic spectrum of melanoma metastatic to the gastrointestinal tract. Am J Roentgenol 129:605, 1977

155. Goodman PL, Karakousis CP: Symptomatic gastrointestinal metastases from malignant melanoma. Cancer 48:1058, 1981

156. Harris MN: Massive gastrointestinal hemorrhage due to metastatic malignant melanoma of small intestine. Arch Surg 88:1049, 1964

157. Karakousis C, Holyoke ED, Douglass HO Jr: Intussusception as a complication of malignant neoplasm. Arch Surg 109:515, 1974

158. Klausner JM, Skornick Y, Lelcuk S, Baratz M, Merhav A: Acute complications of metastatic melanoma to the gastrointestinal tract. Br J Surg 69:195, 1982

159. Macbeth WAAG, Gwynne JF, Jamieson MG: Metastatic melanoma in the small bowel. Aust NZ J Surg 38:309, 1969

160. May ARL, Edwards JM: Surgical excision of visceral metastases from malignant melanoma. Clin Oncol 2:233, 1976

161. Meyers MA, McSweeney J: Secondary neoplasms of the bowel. Radiology 105:1, 1972

162. Oddson TA, Rice RP, Seigler HF, Thompson WM, Kelvin FM, Clark WM. The spectrum of small bowel melanoma. Gastrointest Radiol 3:419, 1978

163. Paglia MA, Exelby PE: Recurrent intussusception from metastatic melanoma. NY State J Med, December 1, 1968

164. Pomerantz H, Margolin HN: Metastases to the gastrointestinal tract from malignant melanoma. Am J Roentgenol 88:712, 1962

165. Potchen EJ, Khung CL, Yatsuhashi M: X-ray diagnosis of gastric melanoma. N Engl J Med 271:133, 1964

166. Reeder MM, Cavanagh RC: "Bull's-eye" lesions: Solitary or multiple nodules in the gastrointestinal tract with larger central ulceration. JAMA 229:825, 1974

167. Sacks BA, Joffe N, Antonioli DA: Metastatic melanoma presenting clinically as multiple colonic polyps. Am J Roentgenol 129:511, 1977

168. Sanders DE, Ho CS: The small bowel enema: Experience with 150 examinations. Am J Roentgenol 127:743, 1976

169. Shah SM, Smart DF, Texter EC Jr, Morris WD: Metastatic melanoma of the stomach: The endoscopic and roentgenographic findings and review of the literature. South Med J 70:379, 1977

170. Thompson WH: Radiographic manifestations of metastatic melanoma to the gastrointestinal tract, hepatobiliary system, pancreas, spleen and mesentery. In Seigler HF (ed): Clinical Management of Melanoma, p 133. The Hague, Nijhoff, 1982

171. Willbanks OL, Fogelman MJ: Gastrointestinal melanosarcoma. Am J Surg 120:602, 1970

172. Wood CB, Wood RAB: Metastatic malignant melanoma of the esophagus. Dig Dis Sci 20:786, 1975

173. Zornoza J, Goldstein HM: Cavitating metastases of the small intestine. Am J Roentgenol 129:613, 1977

LIVER, BILIARY TRACT AND SPLEEN

174. Alderson PO, Adams DF, McNeil BJ, Sanders R, Siegelman SS, Finberg H, Hessel SJ, Abrams HL: A prospective comparison of computed tomography, ultrasound and scintigraphy of the liver in patients with colon or breast carcinoma. Radiology 146: 439, 1983.

175. Balthazar EJ, Javors B: Malignant melanoma of the gallbladder. Am J Gastroenterol 64:332, 1975

176. Bernardino ME, Thomas JL, Barnes PA, Lewis E: Diagnostic approaches to liver and spleen metastases. Radiol Clin North Am 20:469, 1982

177. Bowdler DA, Leach RD: Metastatic intrabiliary melanoma. Clin Oncol 8:251, 1982

178. Daunt N, King DM: Metastatic melanoma in the biliary tree. Br J Radiol 55:873, 1982

179. Felix EL, Bagley DH, Sindelar WF, Johnston GS, Ketcham AS: The value of the liver scan in preoperative screening of patients with malignancies. Cancer 38:1137, 1976

180. Fortner JG, Kallum BO, Kim DK: Surgical management of hepatic vein occlusion by tumor: Budd-Chiari syndrome. Arch Surg 112:727, 1977

181. Garg R, McPherson TA, Lentle B, Jackson F: Usefulness of an elevated serum lactate dehydrogenase value as a marker of hepatic metastases in malignant melanoma. Can Med Assoc J 120:1114, 1979

182. Herrington JL Jr: Metastatic malignant melanoma of the gallbladder masquerading as cholelithiasis. Am J Surg 109:676, 1965

183. MacCarty RL, Stephens DH, Hattery RR, Sheedy PF II: Hepatic imaging by computed tomography: A comparison with ^{99m}Tc-sulfur colloid, ultrasonography, and angiography. Radiol Clin North Am 17:137, 1979

184. McArthur MS, Teergarden DK: Metastatic melanoma presenting as obstructive jaundice with hemobilia. Am J Surg 145:830, 1983

185. McFadden PM, Krementz ET, McKinnon WMP, Pararo LL, Ryan RF: Metastatic melanoma of the gallbladder. Cancer 44:1802, 1979

186. Ostick DG, Haqqani MT: Obstructive cholecystitis due to metastatic melanoma. Postgrad Med J 52:710, 1976

187. Shimkin PM, Soloway MS, Jaffe E: Metastatic melanoma of the gallbladder. Am J Roentgenol 116:393, 1972

188. Smith TJ, Kemeny MM, Sugarbaker PH, Jones AE, Vermess M, Shawker TH, Edwards BK: A prospective study of hepatic imaging in the detection of metastatic disease. Ann Surg 195:486, 1982

189. Snow JH Jr, Goldstein HM, Wallace S: Comparison

of scintigraphy, sonography, and computed tomography in the evaluation of hepatic neoplasms. Am J Roentgenol 132:915, 1979

190. Zemlyn S: Metastatic melanoma of the gallbladder. Radiology 87:744, 1966

BONE

191. Devereux D, Johnston G, Blei L, Head G, Makuch R, Burt M: The role of bone scans in assessing malignant melanoma in patients with stage III disease. Surg Gynecol Obstet 151:45, 1980
192. Fon GT, Wong WS, Gold RH, Kaiser LR: Skeletal metastases of melanoma: Radiographic, scintigraphic, and clinical review. Am J Roentgenol 137:103, 1981
193. Gelberman RH, Stewart WR, Harrelson JM: Hand metastasis from melanoma: A case study. Clin Orthop 136:264, 1978
194. Harrelson JM: Orthopaedic considerations in the treatment of malignant melanoma. In Seigler HF (ed): Clinical Management of Melanoma, p 435, The Hague, Nijhoff, 1982
195. Nussbaum H, Allen B, Kagan AR, Gilbert HA, Rao A, Chan P: Management of bone metastasis—multidisciplinary approach. Semin Oncol 4:93, 1977
196. Pagani JJ, Libshitz HI: Imaging bone metastases. Radiol Clin North Am 20:545, 1982
197. Selby HM, Sherman RS, Pack GT: A roentgen study of bone metastases from melanoma. Radiology 67:224, 1956
198. Shenberger KN, Morgan GJ Jr: Recurrent malignant melanoma presenting as monoarthritis. J Rheumatol 9:328, 1982
199. Steiner GM, MacDonald JS: Metastases to bone from malignant melanoma. Clin Radiol 23:52, 1972
200. Stewart WR, Gelberman RH, Harrelson JM, Seigler HF: Skeletal metastases of melanoma. J Bone Joint Surg 60A:645, 1978
201. Tong D, Gillick L, Hendrickson FR: The palliation of symptomatic osseous metastases: Final results of the study by the Radiation Therapy Oncology Group. Cancer 50:893, 1982

KIDNEYS, URETER, AND BLADDER

202. Abeshouse BS: Primary and secondary melanoma of the genitourinary tract. South Med J 51:994, 1958
203. Agnew CH: Metastatic malignant melanoma of the kidney simulating a primary neoplasm: A case report. Am J Roentgenol 80:813, 1958
204. Amar AD: Metastatic melanoma of the bladder. J Urol 92:198, 1964
205. Bartone FF: Metastatic melanoma of the bladder. J Urol 91:151, 1964
206. Berry NE, Reese L: Malignant melanoma which had its first clinical manifestations in the prostate gland. J Urol 69:286, 1953
207. Das Gupta T, Grabstald H: Melanoma of the genitourinary tract. J Urol 93:607, 1965

208. deKernion JB, Golub SH, Gupta RK, Silverstein M, Morton DL: Successful transurethral intralesional BCG therapy of a bladder melanoma. Cancer 36:1662, 1975
209. Goldstein HM, Kaminsky S, Wallace S, Johnson DE: Urographic manifestations of metastatic melanoma. Radiology 121:801, 1974
210. Lowsley OS: Melanoma of the urinary tract and prostate gland. South Med J 44:487, 1951
211. McKenzie DJ, Bell R: Melanoma with solitary metastasis to ureter. J Urol 99:399, 1968
212. Nakazono M, Iwata S, Kuribayashi N: Disseminated metastatic ureteral melanoma: A case report. J Urol 114:624, 1975
213. Samellas W, Marks AR: Metastatic melanoma of the urinary tract. J Urol 85:21, 1961
214. Sheehan EE, Greenberg SD, Scott R Jr: Metastatic neoplasms of the bladder. J Urol 90:281, 1963
215. Smith GW, Griffith DP, Pranke DW: Melanospermia: An unusual presentation of malignant melanoma. J Urol 110:314, 1973
216. Su C-T, Prince CL: Melanoma of the bladder. J Urol 87:365, 1962
217. Walsh EJ, Ockuly EA, Ockuly EF, Ockuly JJ: Treatment of metastatic melanoma of the bladder. J Urol 96:472, 1966
218. Weston PAM, Smith BJ: Metastatic melanoma in the bladder and urethra. Br J Surg 51:78, 1964
219. Woodard BH, Ideker RE, Johnston WW: Cytologic detection of malignant melanoma in urine. Acta Cytol 22:350, 1978

OTHER SITES
Heart

220. Berge T, Sievers J: Myocardial metastases: A pathological and electrocardiographic study. Br Heart J 30:383, 1968
221. Bryant J, Vuckovic G: Metastatic tumors of the endocardium: Report of three cases. Arch Pathol Lab Med 102:206, 1978
222. Cham WC, Freiman AH, Carstens PHB, Chu FCH: Radiation therapy of cardiac and pericardial metastases. Radiology 114:701, 1975
223. Glancy DL, Roberts WC: The heart in malignant melanoma: A study of 70 autopsy cases. Am J Cardiol 21:555, 1968
224. Hanfling SM: Metastatic cancer to the heart: Review of the literature and report of 127 cases. Circulation 22:474, 1960
225. Moragues V: Cardiac metastasis from malignant melanoma: Report of 4 cases. Am Heart J 18:579, 1939
226. Smith LH: Secondary tumors of the heart. Review of Surgery 33:223, 1976
227. Thomas JH, Panoussopoulos DG, Jewell WR, Pierce GE: Tricuspid stenosis secondary to metastatic melanoma. Cancer 39:1732, 1977

Endocrine organs

228. Twersky J, Levin DC: Metastatic melanoma of the adrenal: An unusual cause of adrenal calcification. Radiology 116:627, 1975
229. Seidenwurm D, Elmer EB, Kaplan LM, Williams EK, Morris DG, Hoffman AR: Metastases to the adrenal glands and the development of Addison's disease. Cancer (in press)

Breast

230. Charache H: Metastatic tumors in the breast with a report of ten cases. Surgery 33:385, 1953
231. Jochimsen PR, Brown RC: Metastatic melanoma in the breast masquerading as fibroadenoma. JAMA 236:2779, 1976
232. Paulus DD, Libshitz HI: Metastasis to the breast. Radiol Clin North Am 20:561, 1982
233. Pressman PI: Malignant melanoma and the breast. Cancer 31:784, 1973
234. Sandison AT: Metastatic tumours in the breast. Br J Surg 47:54, 1959
235. Silverman EM, Oberman HA: Metastatic neoplasms in the breast. Surg Gynecol Obstet 138:26, 1974

Testes and penis

236. Hanash KA, Carney JA, Kelalis PP: Metastatic tumors to testicles: Routes of metastasis. J Urol 102:465, 1969
237. Johnson DE, Jackson L, Ayala AG: Secondary carcinoma of the testis. South Med J 64:1128, 1971
238. Paquin AJ Jr, Roland SI: Secondary carcinoma of the penis: A review of the literature and a report of nine new cases. Cancer 9:629, 1956

Oral cavity and larynx

239. Aisenberg MS, Inman CL Sr: Tumors that have metastasized to the jaws. Oral Surg 9:1210, 1956
240. Ashur H, Mizrahi S, Ben-Hur N, Dolberg L: Metastatic malignant melanoma to the palatine tonsils: Report of case. J Oral Surg 37:110, 1979
241. Bluestone LI: Malignant melanoma metastatic to the mandible: Report of a case. Oral Surg 6:237, 1953
242. Chamberlain D: Malignant melanoma, metastatic to the larynx. Arch Otolaryngol 83:231, 1966
243. Craig RM, Glass BJ, Rhyne RR: Malignant melanoma: Metastasis to the tonsil. J Am Dent Assoc 104:893, 1982
244. Fisher GE, Odess JS: Metastatic malignant melanoma of the larynx. AMA Arch Otolaryngol 54:639, 1951
245. Meyer I, Shklar G: Malignant tumors metastatic to mouth and jaws. Oral Surg 20:350, 1965
246. Miller AS, Pullon PA: Metastatic malignant melanoma of the tongue. Arch Dermatol 103:201, 1971
247. Mosby EL, Sugg WE Jr, Hiatt WR: Gingival and pharyngeal metastasis from a malignant melanoma: Report of a case. Oral Surg 36:6, 1973
248. Pliskin ME, Mastrangelo MJ, Brown AM, Custer RP: Metastatic melanoma of the maxilla presenting as a gingival swelling. Oral Surg 41:101, 1976
249. Samit AM, Falk HJ, Ohanian M, Leban SG, Mashberg A: Malignant melanoma metastatic to the mandible. J Oral Surg 36:816, 1975
250. Trodahl JN, Sprague WG: Benign and malignant melanocytic lesions of the oral mucosa: An analysis of 135 cases. Cancer 25:812, 1970

Peritoneum and mesentery

251. Zboralske FF, Bessolo RJ: Metastatic carcinoma to the mesentery and gut. Radiology 88:302, 1967

Uterus

252. Casey JH, Shapiro RF: Metastatic melanoma presenting as primary uterine neoplasm: A case report. Cancer 33:729, 1974

Eye

253. Fishman ML, Tomaszewski MM, Kuwabara T: Malignant melanoma of the skin metastatic to the eye: Frequency in autopsy series. Arch Ophthalmol 94:1309, 1976
254. Font RL, Naumann G, Zimmerman LE: Primary malignant melanoma of the skin metastatic to the eye and orbit: Report of ten cases and review of the literature. Am J Ophthalmol 63:738, 1967
255. Liddicoat DA, Wolter JR, Wilkinson WC: Retinal metastasis of malignant melanoblastoma: A case report. Am J Ophthalmol 48:172, 1959
256. Riffenburgh RS: Metastatic malignant melanoma to the retina. Arch Ophthalmol 66:487, 1961
257. Sobol S, Druck NS, Wolf M: Palliative orbital decompression for metastatic melanoma to the orbit. Laryngoscope 90:329, 1980

MELANOSIS

258. Gebhart W, Kokoschka EM: Generalized diffuse melanosis secondary to malignant melanoma. In Ackerman AB (ed): Pathology of Malignant Melanoma, p 243. New York, Masson, 1981
259. Goodall P, Spriggs AI, Wells FR: Malignant melanoma with melanosis and melanuria, and with pigmented monocytes and tumour cells in the blood: Autoradiographic demonstration of tyrosinase in malignant cells from peritoneal fluid. Br J Surg 48:549, 1960
260. Konrad K, Wolff K: Pathogenesis of diffuse melanosis secondary to malignant melanoma. Br J Dermatol 91:635, 1974
261. Silberberg I, Kopf AW, Gumport SL: Diffuse melanosis in malignant melanoma: Report of a case and

of studies by light and electron microscopy. Arch Dermatol 97:671, 1968

262. Sohn N, Gang H, Gumport SL, Goldstein M, Deppisch LM: Generalized melanosis secondary to malignant melanoma: Report of a case with serum and tissue tyrosinase studies. Cancer 24:897, 1969

METASTASES FROM UNKNOWN PRIMARY MELANOMA

263. Baab GH, McBride CM: Malignant melanoma: The patient with an unknown site of primary origin. Arch Surg 110:896, 1975

264. Chang P, Knapper WH: Metastatic melanoma of unknown primary. Cancer 49:1106, 1982

265. Das Gupta T, Bowden L, Berg JW: Malignant melanoma of unknown primary origin. Surg Gynecol Obstet 117:341, 1963

266. Giuliano AE, Moseley HS, Morton DL: Clinical aspects of unknown primary melanoma. Ann Surg 191:98, 1980

267. Milton GW, Shaw HM, McCarthy WH: Occult primary malignant melanoma: Factors influencing survival. Br J Surg 64:805, 1977

268. Reintgen DS, McCarty KS, Woodard B, Cox E, Seigler HF: Metastatic malignant melanoma with an unknown primary. Surg Gynecol Obstet 156:335, 1983

CHARLES M. BALCH
GERALD W. MILTON

Treatment for Advanced Metastatic Melanoma

13

The average patient with systemic metastatic melanoma has only 6 months to live.[5] Cure is not a realistic aim, so the treatment must therefore reflect a carefully considered judgment that will endeavor to preserve the quality of life while attempting to prolong it. Even though advanced melanoma cannot be cured, effective measures can often be used to relieve or prevent debilitating symptoms. The purpose of this chapter is to describe an overall treatment philosophy for such patients. More specific details concerning systemic chemotherapy, radiation therapy, and care of the dying patient are described in Chapters 14 to 16. A detailed description of prognostic factors that predict the clinical course of a patient with advanced metastatic melanoma is described in Chapter 19.

INITIAL ASSESSMENT AND PATIENT COUNSELING

GENERAL APPROACH

The treatment of a patient with advanced melanoma depends on several factors, including the site(s) and number of metastases, their rate of growth, any previous treatment, and the age, overall condition, and desires of the patient. For example, a more vigorous treatment might be recommended for a slowly growing solitary metastasis. On the other hand, only symptomatic treatment or none at all might be considered in a debilitated patient with multiple metastases who has failed prior treatment.

The number of organs or tissues containing metastases is the most significant factor predicting survival in patients with distant metastases.[5] The median survival is 7 months for one metastatic site, 4 months for two sites, and only 2 months for three or more metastatic sites. The location of the metastasis is also important. The relatively favorable sites include (in approximately descending order) skin, subcutaneous tissue, distant lymph nodes, lung, and bone. Unfavorable sites are the liver and brain.[5]

The estimated rate of tumor growth can also be an important part of the initial assessment. The relative rapidity of the metastatic process can be estimated only in general terms. Nevertheless, the patient may be able to give an accurate history about the duration of superficially located metastases. The duration of symptoms, previous laboratory tests, scans, or x-rays may also be useful in making this estimation. If the patient has received previous treatment for a systemic metastasis (such as chemo-

therapy or surgery), the survival is likely to be shorter (in the range of 2 to 4 months). Older patients and those in a debilitated state are less likely to withstand vigorous treatments than younger patients and those who have not suffered the constitutional ravages of metastatic disease. Finally, the patient's desires regarding his or her treatment after counseling about benefits and risks should be strongly considered when choosing alternative forms of palliative treatment.

DEFINING GOALS, RISKS, AND BENEFITS OF TREATMENT

Defining goals of treatment is an especially important consideration that should be incorporated into the overall assessment of the patient and the treatment plan. The goals of treatment are (1) relief of symptoms if present, (2) prolongation of life, and (3) staging to determine subsequent treatment. Treatment directed at relieving symptons is generally worthwhile, especially when the anticipated benefit of relieving symptoms exceeds the toxicity and risk of the treatment itself. In addition, the effectiveness of the treatment can be monitored by both subjective and objective assessment of the symptoms caused by the metastases. The benefit: risk ratio must be even higher in the asymptomatic patient with metastases. The goal of treatment here is to prolong life, and it is important that the treatment itself does not severely limit the patient's quality of life. This is especially true for melanoma patients, since systemic control of disease usually cannot be achieved with currently available chemotherapy. Each treatment has its own set of risks, and the physician employing these treatments must thoroughly understand these potential risks as they apply to each individual patient setting.

PATIENT COUNSELING

In general, the patient should know about his situation and participate in decisions concerning treatment alternatives (see Chap. 16). One of the greatest causes of anxiety is uncertainty. Therefore, if the patient is made aware of his situation, he may be able to cope with it more appropriately and suitably arrange his personal life. It is recognized that there are some patients who are unable to cope if a completely honest approach is adopted. However, some discussion is important, as it is difficult to initiate treatment without explaining the reasons for it. Otherwise, the patient may lose his trust in the physician and may not accept subsequent treatment recommendations.

When counseling patients and their families, it is important for the physician to be sympathetic and realistic but hopeful about the results of treatment. It is important for a patient to have hope, and even in grim situations there can be realistic goals of treatment, if only to relieve symptoms. In other words, the physician should continue treating the patient even when it is no longer possible to treat the cancer. The approach taken for each patient depends on his prognosis, physical condition, and emotional stability. Each approach must therefore be individualized.

TREATMENT MODALITIES AVAILABLE

Multiple treatment modalities are available for patients with metastatic disease. These are listed in Table 13-1 with their indications and risks.

NO TREATMENT

Providing no treatment is an important consideration, especially in asymptomatic patients, those who are terminally ill, or those of advanced age.

There are two situations to consider. First is the asymptomatic patient with a tumor in a favorable site, such as lung or bone (but not brain). The physician may elect to observe these lesions if they are growing slowly and are not causing symptoms. Quality of life is maintained in this instance, and treatment can be deferred until the lesions begin to progress, either by size or multiplicity, or until the patient develops symptoms. The second situation is the patient who is terminally ill or at an extreme age, when the benefit:risk ratio is small. The decision to forgo treatment can be difficult but is often best made by the patient himself, assisted by close relatives or medical or nursing advisers. Naturally, a patient should not be denied treatment in an individual circumstance when there is a reasonable expectation that the treatment will be successful and the risk or toxicity is low.

SURGERY

Surgery is a very effective palliative treatment for isolated metastases, especially since melanoma often metastasizes sequentially and effective chemotherapy is not presently available. Surgical excision of metastatic melanoma probably gives the patient the best, quickest, and longest-lasting palliation. On

TABLE 13–1
TREATMENT OPTIONS FOR SYSTEMIC METASTATIC MELANOMA

Treatment Option	General Indications	Possible Risks	Comment
Surgery	Superficial lesions Brain Symptomatic visceral Occasional lung	Anesthesia Infection Hemorrhage	Best for isolated lesions, especially symptomatic, low risk patients
Radiation therapy	Superficial lesions Brain Bone	Normal tissue injury	Dose fraction important; often very effective
Chemotherapy	Widespread disease Symptomatic lesions	Severe vomiting, marrow depression	Low activity for most drugs; widespread effect
Hyperthermia	Liver lesions Large superficial lesions	Normal tissue injury	An experimental treatment
Limb perfusion	Local recurrences Intransit metastases Satellites	Muscle necrosis Skin burns Vascular thrombosis	Usually effective; restricted to extremity lesions; requires major surgery
Cryotherapy or diathermy	Skin and subcutaneous lesions	Poor wound healing	
Intralesional chemotherapy or immunotherapy	Skin and subcutaneous lesions	Tissue necrosis, fever, allergic reactions, generalized infectious disease	Can be locally effective in some lesions
Systemic immunotherapy	Nonvisceral lesions	Fever, allergic reactions	Little benefit so far; experimental treatment

some occasions, the palliative effect can last for 5 to 10 years (Fig. 13-1).[26] Surgery can therefore prevent symptoms from occurring, can relieve symptoms, and can prolong life. The favorable experience with surgical resection of distant metastases in selected patients treated at the M. D. Anderson Hospital is shown in Table 13-2.

The obvious limitation of surgery is that it is a local form of treatment, and the patient will eventually succumb from metastatic disease in other sites. Careful patient selection is therefore important. Sometimes a period of observation for several weeks may provide relevant information about the rate of tumor growth and the possibility of multiple other metastases present that would emerge during an observation period. Surgery should be confined to situations involving accessible lesions that are limited in amount and to patients in whom the operation can be safely performed. Some examples include isolated visceral metastases, especially brain and occasionally lung metastases. Gastrointestinal metastates that are obstructing and most superficially located lesions in the skin, subcutaneous tissues, or distant lymph nodes are also amenable to this approach. Liver metastases are associated with such a short survival (*i.e.*, 2 to 4 months) that excision is generally not indicated.

The choice of surgical excision as a means of palliation depends on the site of the disease and the duration of anticipated survival. If the patient's life is likely to be measured in weeks, the surgical ablation of a large growth is not justified, whereas longer anticipated survival renders excision of gross disease worth considering. Eash case has to be considered on its own merit.

RADIATION THERAPY

Irradiation has an important role in the treatment of patients with advanced melanoma when the lesions are located in particular sites. This treatment modality is described further in Chapter 15, and the indications will only be summarized here.

Radiation can be effective palliative treatment for patients with bone or brain metastases and for those lesions located on the skin, subcutaneous tissues, or lymph nodes. Radiation with high-energy beams will relieve the pain from bony metastases, usually within 1 week. Indeed, if the pain has not been substantially improved by that time, it is wise to seek an alternative explanation for the symptoms. Cranial (whole brain) and spinal cord irradiation can be extremely effective for central nervous sys-

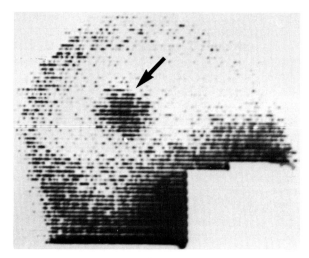

FIG. 13–1 Remarkable case of a patient living 10 years with multiple metastatic melanomas that were surgically excised. The figure shows a brain scan (taken in 1970) of a 57-year-old man who had a melanoma previously excised from the forearm in 1963. A solitary cerebral metastasis was surgically removed in 1970, and the patient received postoperative radiation therapy. In 1972, he presented with symptoms of small bowel obstruction and had a large solitary intestinal metastasis excised. Later in 1972, a left thoracotomy was performed to remove a solitary pulmonary metastasis. The patient did well until 1977, when he had a right thoracotomy for another pulmonary metastasis. In 1977, he also developed chronic lymphocytic leukemia. The patient had no evidence of metastatic melanoma and did not require any treatment for his leukemia until 1979. He died in December 1980 with pleural and pulmonary metastases. The patient had excellent palliative results from surgical excision of the sequential solitary metastases and was symptom free during 10 of the 10.5 years he lived with metastatic melanoma.

tem metastases, especially when used with dexamethasone (up to 16 mg to 24 mg per day).

Irradiation can be extremely effective treatment for superficially located metastatic disease in the skin or soft tissues where they can be treated with high-energy photon beams using a linear accelerator. The dose fraction schedule is important, however. A suggested dose fraction schedule is 600 rads given twice a week for 3 weeks. In most cases, high-dose, low-fraction irradiation will completely sterilize metastases located on the skin, subcutaneous tissues, or lymph nodes.[23,52]

CHEMOTHERAPY

There is a paucity of drugs available for treating systemic melanoma (see Chap. 14). Imidazole carboximide (DTIC) is the only drug with significant

TABLE 13–2
MEDIAN SURVIVAL IN 103 MELANOMA PATIENTS AFTER SURGICAL RESECTION OF DISTANT METASTASES AT THE M. D. ANDERSON HOSPITAL*

Site	Number of Patients[†]	Survival from Onset of Metastases (Months)	
		Median	Range
Subcutaneous or lymph nodes	64	23	3–180
Lung	26	16	1–132
Brain	16	15	1–84
Gastrointestinal	9	18	4–192
Bone	2		1–61
Throat	1		9

* About two thirds of patients received adjuvant chemotherapy, immunotherapy, or both.

† Some patients had multiple sites excised.

(Feun LG, Gutterman J, Burgess MA, Hersh EM, Mavligit G, McBride CM, Benjamin RS, Richman SP, Murphy WK, Bodey GP, Brown BW, Mountain CF, Leavens ME, Freireich EJ: The natural history of resectable metastatic melanoma (stage IV A melanoma). Cancer 50:1656, 1982)

activity in melanoma. The response rates are only 15% to 20% in most series, and the toxicity is high (especially with protracted vomiting). Nevertheless, in individual cases with measurable lesions chemotherapy may be considered, especially in symptomatic patients. If there is not a dramatic response after two courses of chemotherapy, it can be discontinued or another drug combination evaluated. In general, nonvisceral metastases respond better to DTIC chemotherapy combinations than do visceral metastases. Often, chemotherapy is used only in patients whose lesions are not amenable to surgery or irradiation therapy, and only sparingly in asymptomatic patients.

HYPERTHERMIA

Hyperthermia is an investigational treatment for large tumors, especially those that are either superficially located or are in the liver. It is probably not a very effective treatment by itself. It may, however, increase the effectiveness of other treatments, such as radiation therapy for superficial lesions[61,62,63] or regional chemotherapy for liver metastases.[51] Toxicity to surrounding normal tissues is generally minimal.

SYSTEMIC IMMUNOTHERAPY

Nonspecific immunotherapy using such agents as BCG or *Corynebacterium parvum* is not effective in palliative management of patients with metastatic melanoma.[42] Newer agents such as interferon and active-specific immunotherapy with melanoma

vaccines are currently under investigation (see Chap. 11).

HORMONAL MANIPULATIONS

Attempts to use hormone therapy, either ablative or supplemental, involving estrogen or progesterone hormones have been unsuccessful. This includes pituitary and hypophysis ablation (see Chap. 14).[32]

SELECTING TREATMENT OPTIONS

There is no standard approach to treating systemic metastases that would apply to all circumstances. The general guidelines and sequence of treatment options that are used at UAB and the SMU are listed in Table 13–3.

SITES OF TREATMENT

SKIN, SUBCUTANEOUS TISSUES, AND LYMPH NODES

When lesions in the skin, subcutaneous tissues, and lymph nodes are isolated (one or a few), surgical excision is the treatment of choice, for they can be treated safely, quickly, and effectively by surgery. They should be excised before they become bulky and symptomatic, when they would require an even more extensive operation. These lesions should be excised with a rim of normal-appearing tissue (0.5 cm–1 cm) to minimize the risk of recurrence. Sequential metastases in these areas can be excised sur-

TABLE 13–3
GENERAL GUIDELINES FOR TREATMENT SEQUENCES

Metastatic Site	First Option	Second Option	Third Option
Skin, Subcutaneous (Trunk, head, neck)			
Isolated	Surgery	Radiation	Drugs
Multiple	Radiation	Drugs	Drugs
Skin, Subcutaneous (Extremity)			
Isolated	Surgery	Limb perfusion	Radiation or drugs
Multiple	Limb perfusion (± surgery)	Radiation	Drugs
Lung			
Isolated	Surgery	Drugs	Drugs
Multiple	Drugs	Drugs	Drugs
Liver	Drugs	Drugs	Drugs
Bone	Radiation (± surgery)	Drugs	Drugs
Brain			
Isolated	Surgery (± irradiation)	Radiation	
Multiple	Radiation	Radiation	
Gastrointestinal Tract			
Isolated	Surgery	Drugs	Drugs
Multiple	Drugs	Drugs	Drugs

gically unless they multiply or appear in short succession. In the latter situation (multiple or recurrent lesions), irradiation therapy may be considered as a second option.[23,52] Symptomatic nodal or soft-tissue metastases in surgically inaccessible sites (*e.g.*, mediastinum, retroperitoneum, pelvis) might also be considered for radiotherapy (Fig. 13-2). Patients who have widespread lesions or symptomatic deep lymph nodes not accessible to radiotherapy might be considered for chemotherapy.

Excellent results are obtained with surgical excision of subcutaneous or distant lymph node metastases. Many patients require repeated excisions, but the median survival from the onset of these metastases can be up to 23 months (range 3 months–18 months).[20]

One very distressing aspect of disseminated melanoma is the presence of large fungating tumors involving the skin, which rapidly acquire secondary infection and, as a consequence, produce a foul-smelling, bloody discharge. Such tumors should be excised if at all possible, or treated by irradiation or chemotherapy. As a temporary measure, the tumor mass can sometimes be reduced by applying a powder made of equal parts of ground copper sulfate and sugar. This also reduces surface hemorrhage. A commercially available wound-cleaning paste (Debrisan)* is also useful in this situation. Odor from the discharge can often be controlled by washing the surface of the mass with soft soap and water and then applying a thick layer of yoghurt twice daily.

LUNG, PLEURA, AND MEDIASTINUM

The lung is one of the most frequent sites of visceral metastases. Relative to other visceral sites, however, pulmonary metastases are associated with a longer survival, with a median survival of 10 to 11 months from their onset.[5,16,29]

Pulmonary metastases are usually multiple and bilateral; often they are associated with hilar or mediastinal nodal metastases.[12,67,69,75,93] The treatment approach should be determined by the site and number of thoracic metastases.

For solitary pulmonary metastases in asymptomatic patients, surgical excision may be indicated if an observation period of 3 to 4 weeks demonstrates no new lesions and the tumor has a relatively slow growth rate (Fig. 13-3). Morton and colleagues have recommended excision of solitary metastases

*Johnson & Johnson, Inc.

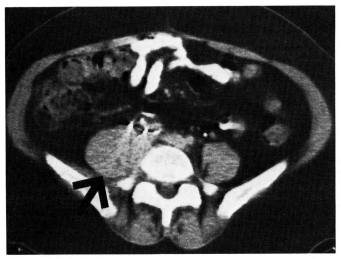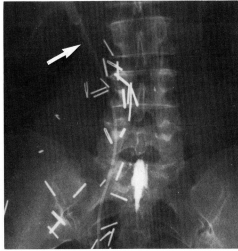

FIG. 13–2 Soft-tissue metastases treated by radiation therapy. (*Left*) CT scan showing a soft-tissue metastasis involving the right psoas muscle (*arrow*). This lesion entrapped the right ureter, causing obstruction and pyuria. (*Right*) A ureteral stent (*arrow*) was temporarily placed while the metastases were treated with irradiation therapy.

FIG. 13–3 Successful palliative surgery for pulmonary metastases. This 53-year-old man presented with a subcutaneous metastasis on the back from an unknown primary site. Three years later, he developed three pulmonary metastases (two in the right lung, one in the left lung). They were unchanged in size over a 6-week period of observation. He underwent a median sternotomy for removal of five pulmonary metastases located in both lungs. The patient is still disease-free 2½ years after surgical excision. (*Left*) Preoperative x-ray film of two pulmonary metastases in the right lung (*arrow*). (*Right*) Postoperative x-ray film demonstrating no recurrence in either lung field 2½ years later.

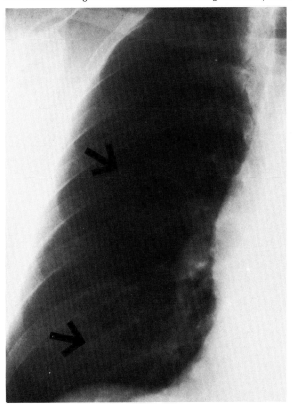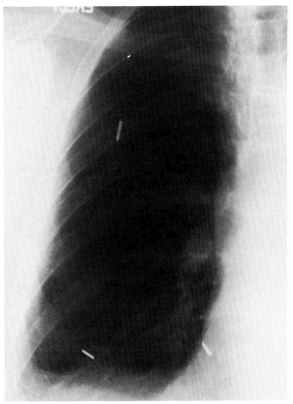

for tumors with a doubling time exceeding 40 days.[82] Whole lung tomograms or CT scans are essential, for often a patient with a solitary lesion on chest x-ray film actually has other pulmonary or intrathoracic lesions as well.[67,84,94] The operation is safe (1% mortality), but careful patient selection is important, as only a minority of patients will benefit. Surgical excision of solitary pulmonary metastases is justified in selected patients, for truly long-term survival can be achieved.[12,20,67,70,74,77,78,85,91,92] The median survival ranges from 16 to 24 months, with 5-year survival rates of 12% to 21% in some large series (Fig. 13-4).[20,77,78,79,81] Not all institutions, however, have had such favorable results.[79,95]

The extent of resection is determined by the location and number of metastases and the pulmonary function status. In most cases, a wedge or segmental resection will suffice, but a lobectomy is sometimes necessary when the lesions are larger or more central, or when a diagnosis of primary lung carcinoma is possible. A pneumonectomy is rarely indicated. An interesting clinical setting for which palliative surgery might be considered is the combination of pulmonary metastases and osteoarthro-pathy. Several patients with this condition have been reported whose symptoms were relieved by pulmonary resection of the metastases.[87,89,96]

Another justification for excising solitary pulmonary lesions is to confirm that they do not represent a second primary malignancy or a benign process. This situation can occur in up to one third of patients whose workup culminates in a thoracotomy.[67,79]

Patients who are not considered for surgery, such as those with multiple, slow-growing tumors, might be followed with no treatment at all while they are asymptomatic. If the pulmonary metastases progress rapidly, especially if multiple visceral sites of metastases are also involved or if the patient is symptomatic, an initial course of chemotherapy might be given. The response rate for DTIC chemotherapy is particularly poor for pulmonary metastases, and there is no evidence that life is prolonged with this drug.[16,42] Seigler[48] has recently described a four-drug combination of chemotherapy (BOLD) with a 40% response rate, and this has been beneficial to some patients with pulmonary metastases treated at UAB. A disappointing consequence to a

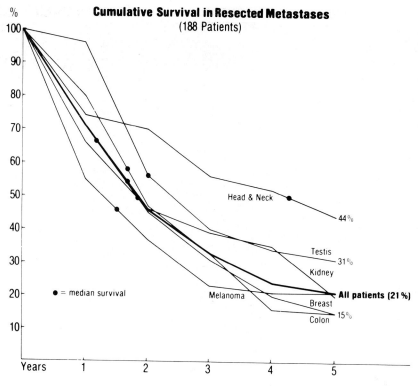

Cumulative Survival in Resected Metastases
(188 Patients)

FIG. 13-4 Actuarial survival curves calculated from treatment of pulmonary metastases in 188 patients treated at the Memorial Sloan-Kettering Cancer Center, New York City. The median survival for the 29 melanoma patients was 29 months (range, 4 months to 28 years). The 5-year survival rate for the melanoma patients was 21%, the same as for all patients with resected metastases of other histological types. (McCormack PM, et al: Pulmonary resection in metastatic carcinoma. Chest 73:163, 1978)

good chemotherapy response for pulmonary metastases is that the disease recurs within 3 to 12 months either in the brain or in the lungs (Fig. 13-5). In either event, the recurrent tumor is not likely to respond to a second course of treatment.

Metastases involving a bronchus, the trachea, or larynx are unusual. Such patients may present with hemoptysis, persistent cough, or atelectasis on chest x-ray film. The diagnosis is confirmed by endoscopy and biopsy. Depending on the size and location of the lesion, the degree of symptoms, and the patient's overall state of health, such lesions might be treated (1) endoscopically by fulgeration or laser excision when the upper trachea is involved,[65] (2) by radiation therapy, (3) by chemotherapy, or (4) surgically by segmental resection or pneumonectomy. Pleural effusions are generally associated with a short survival. If symptomatic, they can be treated by thoracentesis or by tube thoracostomy and chemical pleurodesis.[64] Hemothorax is rare but may be treated by tube thoracostomy or by thoracotomy and cauterization if bleeding persists and the patient is a suitable candidate.[73]

LIVER, BILIARY TRACT, AND SPLEEN

Patients with liver metastases have a particularly poor prognosis, with an average life expectancy of only 2 to 4 months.[1,5,16,29] Rarely, a patient may have an isolated liver metastasis that can be surgically resected,[180] but the duration of palliation is generally short. In most patients, either systemic or regional chemotherapy using a combination of DTIC could be considered. This would be continued if the patient had an objective tumor response. Otherwise, no further treatment would be offered. Hyperthermia has been used in a few patients on an experimental basis.[51]

Patients with symptoms from gallbladder metastases should be considered for cholecystectomy if the metastasis is confined to the gallbladder. Such patients should be medically fit and should have a

FIG. 13–5 Palliative response to combination chemotherapy using DTIC, bleomycin, vincristine, and CCNU.[48] (*Left*) Pretreatment chest x-ray film showing multiple pulmonary metastases (*arrows*). (*Right*) Five months later, the patient still had a complete response in the lungs but developed brain metastases that were unresponsive to radiation therapy. She died 1 month later in a coma. In the UAB experience, over 40% of patients who respond to this combination chemotherapy regimen develop brain metastases later in the course of their disease.

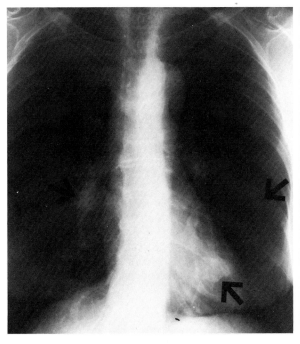
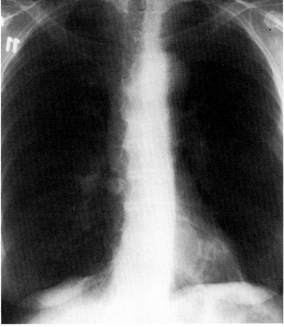

life expectancy exceeding several months. Short-term relief of symptoms is usually successful, but all reported patients died within a year.[177,182,185,186,187,190] Hematobilia and jaundice from metastatic melanoma in the distal common bile duct (the first site of metastases) have been treated by pancreatoduodenectomy.[184] Finally, patients with symptomatic, isolated splenic metastases might be considered for splenectomy. One case of satisfactory long-term palliation after splenectomy has been reported.[12]

BONE

The life expectancy of melanoma patients with bony metastases is 4 to 6 months on the average, and even shorter when other sites are involved as well.[5,192,200] The treatment depends on (1) the degree of symptoms, (2) the location and magnitude of bony lesions, and (3) the life expectancy. The goals should be to relieve pain, to maximize ambulation, and to minimize nursing care. In general, patients without symptoms should be followed to assess the progression of their lesions without any major treatment intervention unless they become symptomatic.

Symptomatic metastases generally involve non-weight-bearing bones, particularly the spine or ribs. In these cases, radiotherapy to the lesions will usually give relief for up to 6 months; however, the fields should generally be restricted to the area of symptomatic involvement (Fig. 13-6). A high-dose, short-course dose schedule will minimize patient travel time or hospitalization (see Chap. 15).[52,201] If pain relief is not obtained with the first course of radiation therapy, a second course usually does not succeed. If the first response was excellent and the recurrence interval exceeded 6 months, bony lesions might be reirradiated if symptoms later recur. Currently available chemotherapy is not effective for palliation of skeletal metastases.[194]

Symptomatic metastases in weight-bearing bones (*e.g.*, femur) require special consideration. If the lesion is large, and especially if there is evidence of cortical destruction, the patient might be considered for prophylactic stabilization and irradiation if his life expectancy is at least 2 months. Stabilization includes operative metallic fixation (*e.g.*, intramedullary rods), joint replacement, repair with methyl methacrylate, or external braces or casts.[194,195] Radiation therapy is generally given postoperatively. Alternatively, the lesion could be treated with irradiation alone. The patient should then be followed closely for evidence of pathologic fracture. In the presence of pathologic fracture of a weight-bearing

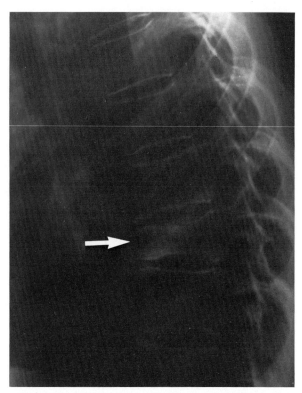

FIG. 13–6 Palliative radiation therapy for symptomatic bony metastases. This 47-year-old woman had a 3.2-mm ulcerated melanoma on her back. She subsequently developed symptomatic bone metastases with a compression fracture of the ninth thoracic vertebrae. This lesion and an asymptomatic metastasis of the femoral head were treated with palliative irradiation therapy. The patient's back pain completely subsided. She subsequently developed multiple subcutaneous metastases that responded to chemotherapy, and later died of brain metastases.

bone, stabilization is the best alternative, as it maximizes quality of life and decreases hospital or nursing home costs, unless the risk of surgery is high or the life expectancy is short.

Patients with compression fractures of the vertebrae that result in cord compression require prompt recognition and treatment if paralysis is to be avoided. This may require decompressive laminectomy with postoperative radiation therapy, or irradiation alone, depending on the extent of the disease and the patient's overall medical condition.

An occasional patient will have an isolated but symptomatic bony metastasis. This might be treated by surgical excision or minor amputation, such as that of a digit, especially if it is not responsive to an initial course of irradiation.[20,193]

BRAIN AND SPINAL CORD

Cerebral metastases are among the most common causes of death from melanoma, ranging from 20% to 54% of patients among different series. The life expectancy is relatively short, ranging from 2 to 7 months depending on the extent of metastatic disease and its response to treatment.[5,10,16,41,98,100,115]

The mainstay of initial treatment is corticosteroids, the most effective being dexamethasone (up to 16 mg–24 mg per day). This will reduce the edema around the tumor and relieve symptoms in most patients, at least temporarily.[111,116,133] The steroid dose should be tapered over 2 to 4 weeks and then stopped after definitive treatment unless symptoms exacerbate with steroid withdrawal. Lack of improvement after a trial of steroids in patients with rapid neurologic deterioration is usually caused by intratumor hemorrhage with intracerebral hematoma. Radiation therapy is the treatment of choice for multiple tumors. Surgical excision with cranial irradiation is the most definitive treatment option in the case of a solitary metastasis. Chemotherapy is not effective for brain metastasis from melanoma.[16,98,107,116]

Surgical excision is preferred for solitary and surgically accessible lesions. A craniotomy is a relatively safe procedure (operative mortality of about 5%) that alleviates symptoms in most patients and prevents further neurologic damage in patients with demonstrable metastases. It should also be considered in some patients with disease at other sites plus symptomatic brain metastases, since their estimated life expectancy can exceed 2 to 3 months and their neurologic status usually improves.

One reason surgical excision is preferred to irradiation in most patients is the hemorrhagic nature of the metastatic tumor.[103,109,115,125] Bleeding in and around the tumor can occur both before and during the surgery. For this reason, the use of laser beam excision in combination with the tulip biopsy technique is often safer and quicker and is accompanied by less blood loss than suction and coagulation. Tumor spillage must be minimized, since metastases in the scalp incision can occur in up to 10% of patients.[110] Whole brain irradiation is generally given postoperatively. While this combined approach appears to improve survival rates compared to surgery alone, there is a paucity of data concerning the use of adjunctive irradiation (Fig. 13-7).

Survival in different series averages about 6 months for surgically treated patients (Table 13-4) and ranges from 2 to 20 months.[20,28,98,100,103,105,108,118,122,128,131,136,139] Satisfactory improvement in the neurologic condition occurred in the majority of patients. Survival results were influenced by the remission duration and the neurologic status at the time of surgery and presence of metastases at other sites.[112] Although long-term successes are uncommon, a few patients will live 3 to 5 years or longer after surgery.[12,102,103,105,118,124,125,132] Examples of two long-term survivors at UAB are shown in Figures 13-1 and 13-8. No studies have directly proved whether surgery, radiation, or both provide more effective palliation for solitary metastases. Long-term survival is not seen in patients treated by irradiation ther-

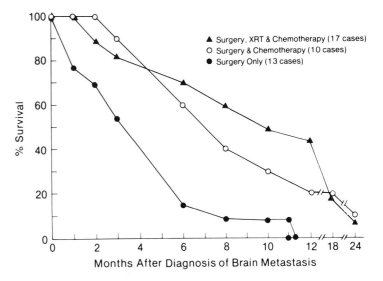

FIG. 13–7 Palliative surgery for cerebral metastases. Actuarial survival curves for 40 patients who underwent surgical excision of cerebral metastases at the M. D. Anderson Hospital and Tumor Institute, Houston. Those patients who received adjuvant radiation therapy or chemotherapy did better than those patients treated by surgery alone. (Fell DA, Leavens ME, McBride CM: Surgical versus nonsurgical management of metastatic melanoma of the brain. Neurosurgery 7:238, 1980)

▲ Surgery, XRT & Chemotherapy (17 cases)
O Surgery & Chemotherapy (10 cases)
● Surgery Only (13 cases)

% Survival

Months After Diagnosis of Brain Metastasis

TABLE 13-4
MEDIAN SURVIVAL AFTER SURGICAL OR IRRADIATION TREATMENT FOR
METASTATIC MELANOMA OF THE BRAIN*

Series	Number of Patients	Median Survival (Months)	
		Surgery (±Radiation Therapy)	Radiation Alone
Amer[98]	20	20 (4 patients)	4.6
Bremer[103]	19	5.5	
Atkinson[100]	21	5.6	
Hafström[118]	25	6	
Winston[139]	8	2	
Ransohoff[131]	14	12	
Feun[20]	16	15	
Vlock[137]	46	5	3
Gottlieb[116]	41		3
Carella[107]	60		3
Cooper[108]	29		3
Fell[110]	80	5	1.5

*This table exemplifies the insufficient comparative data for surgical excision (± adjuvant brain irradiation) versus irradiation alone for limited extent brain metastases. A randomized clinical trial addressing this problem is needed.

apy, however. Although overall results and quality of life are probably similar with the two treatment options, surgery occasionally offers greater prolongation of life.

Radiation therapy should be considered if the lesions are multiple or are located in an area that would preclude a safe operation. A rapid fraction course is probably as effective as higher doses over longer time periods (see Chap. 15).[52,113,137] There is some risk of hemorrhage into a necrotic brain metastasis, especially if it is large (*i.e.,* >2 cm in diameter). Objective response rates in most series average only about 30% to 40%, but a higher proportion of patients (up to 76%) experience improvement or complete relief of symptoms.[16,25,98,107,108,116]

Surgical decompression of obstructing spinal cord lesions is indicated in selected patients, although there is some evidence that radiation therapy might be an effective alternative in some patients.[117,129,141] High doses of corticosteroids should be given as well. Early treatment intervention is essential, since the best results for both surgery and irradiation treatments occurred in patients with mild neurologic symptoms; there have been very few treatment responses in totally paraplegic patients. Patients with symptomatic but nonobstructive disease might be considered for irradiation therapy to the local area.[52] Usually, this is caused by extension of bony metastases to the surrounding spinal cord. Treatment results for meningeal metastases by either radiotherapy or intrathecal chemotherapy are dismal, although there have been a few transient successes.[98,138]

GASTROINTESTINAL TRACT

Although solitary metastases occasionally occur in the gastrointestinal tract, multiple lesions in each affected organ are most common. Moreover, these metastases usually occur in disseminated disease, with an average survival of only 2 to 4 months. Despite these facts, there are situations in which successful and effective palliative treatments can be offered to the patient.

One of the most common symptomatic consequences of gastrointestinal metastases is chronic bleeding. In anemic patients, this can be treated with repeated blood transfusions. Chemotherapy can be considered for patients with multiple gastrointestinal lesions, and surgical excision for solitary metastases, if the patient's condition permits and there are no other visceral metastases (Fig. 13-9).

Surgery is recommended for most patients with the acute complications of obstruction, massive bleeding, or perforation. These cannot be treated by other modalities, and the only other alternative is to allow the patient to die. The final decision depends on the patient's overall clinical condition, but symptoms can be successfully alleviated in most cases, and survival after surgical excision of the offending metastases averaged 4 to 8 months.[1,35,147,149,151,152,155,156,157,158,159,160,171] In the case of multiple gastrointestinal metastases, only lesions causing immediate symptoms should be removed unless those remaining are relatively few in number and can be safely removed. Even major operative procedures such as esophagogastrectomy or sub-

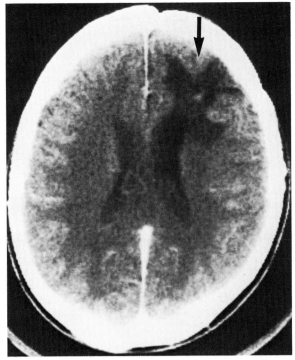

FIG. 13–8 Long-term palliative surgery for brain metastases. This 25-year-old white man had a melanoma excised from his leg along with nodal metastases in 1975. In 1976, he presented with expressive aphasia. A CT scan showed a large hematoma in the left frontal lobe surrounding a metastatic melanoma. This was excised surgically, and the patient underwent postoperative irradiation therapy. He also participated in a clinical protocol, receiving 6 months of DTIC and cyclophosphamide chemotherapy plus 2 years of *Corynebacterium parvum* immunotherapy. The figure shows the last CT scan, demonstrating a residual surgical defect in the right frontal lobe but no evidence of metastatic melanoma. The patient has remained disease free and is entirely asymptomatic 7½ years after surgical excision of his cerebral metastases.

total gastrectomy have been successfully performed, but these should be reserved for the rare patients in whom long-term results are expected. Survival of 2 to 5 years after excision of gastrointestinal metastases has been reported in a few patients, most of whom had palliative excision for symptomatic solitary gastric or intestinal metastases.[1,35,151,152,155,158,159,160,171]

Obstruction is usually caused by large polypoid lesions that mechanically obstruct the bowel or act as a leading point for intussusception (Fig. 13-10).[149,155,157,159,163,171] These submucosal lesions are generally removed with a bowel resection or, occasionally, through enterotomies, depending on the site and number of lesions. An intestinal bypass pro-

cedure may be sufficient for some patients with extensive disease that would otherwise require an extensive or risky resection. Bowel obstruction was the immediate cause of death in 8% of patients in one autopsy series.[10]

Massive or repeated episodes of bleeding requiring transfusions are uncommon and are likely to result from gastric metastases. Surgical treatment generally consists of segmental bowel resection or partial gastrectomy, although sometimes more extended operations are required.[12,147,148,151,152,155,158] Repeated transfusions required by continual bleeding tax both patient and physician with the difficult question of when to suspend treatment.

KIDNEY AND URINARY TRACT

Only solitary or symptomatic metastatic tumors in the kidney and urinary tract should be considered for treatment by surgical excision or chemotherapy. Radiation therapy is generally not helpful, but immunotherapy may be beneficial in occasional patients.[208] Kidney and urinary tract metastases are generally asymptomatic until the terminal stages of disease, and death usually occurs in 1 to 4 months after the clinical diagnosis is made. Metastatic melanoma can occasionally mimic primary renal or bladder carcinomas, both endoscopically and radiographically.[203,209]

Bladder metastases can be treated by transurethral resection or partial cystectomy, depending on their number, size, and location.[202,204,205,207,213,217] Symptoms are usually relieved, but survival after treatment averages only 3 to 6 months for most patients. Rarely do patients survive more than 1 year.

Kidney and ureteral metastases presenting with bleeding or obstruction can be treated by ureteronephrectomy in selected patients,[211,212] or by a ureteral stent if the patient is not an operative candidate. In most cases, survival averages only 4 months.

Symptomatic prostate metastases occur rarely but can be treated by transurethral resection or open prostatectomy.[210,211] Obstructive urethral disease could also be decompressed by a suprapubic cystostomy in poor-risk patients.

OTHER SITES

Heart and pericardium

In almost all patients with metastases to the heart and pericardium, the disease is untreatable and survival ranges from a few weeks to a few months after diagnosis. Pericardial metastases with symptomatic

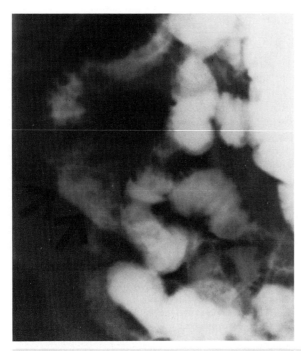

FIG. 13–9 This 50-year-old white man presented with a 3.5-mm ulcerated melanoma of the back. He underwent an elective lymph node dissection and postoperatively received 2 years of *C. parvum* immunotherapy as part of a randomized clinical trial. Six years later, he developed anemia. (*Top*) An upper gastrointestinal series with small bowel follow through demonstrated a possible metastatic lesion in the ileum (*arrows*). Effacement of the mucosa in this area was seen consistently on spot x-ray films. (*Bottom*) The pathology specimen showing one of two large intestinal metastases that were completely resected. The patient has had no further evidence of relapse 12 months after this surgery.

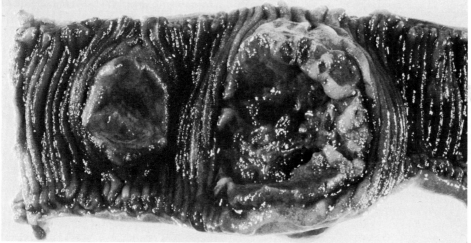

effusions might be treated by either open pericardiectomy or radiation therapy.[222] A few patients respond temporarily to chemotherapy.

Pancreas

Occasionally, patients with metastases to the pancreas may have biliary or duodenal obstructive symptoms. Surgical bypass procedures or radiation therapy might be considered as first choice in selected patients, with a trial course of chemotherapy as a second choice. All such treatments would usually be deferred while patients are asymptomatic.

Peritoneum and mesentery

In patients with metastases to the peritoneum and mesentery, survival is short. However, chemotherapy would be considered for treatment of symptomatic patients (*e.g.,* ascites), while asymptomatic patients would not be treated.

Endocrine organs

Solitary metastases in endocrine organs should be surgically excised, especially if the patient is symptomatic. Occasionally, surgical palliation can be successful for adrenal or pituitary metastases.[12,207,228]

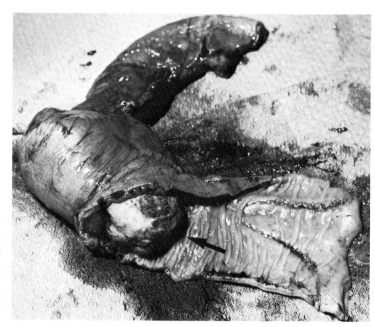

FIG. 13–10 Operative specimen excised from a 24-year-old woman who had recurrent periumbilical cramping pains and was treated at SMU. She then developed abdominal distention and vomiting over a 2-week period. There is a large tumor deposit at the apex of an intussusception. This is one of the two commonest complications seen in patients presenting with a small intestinal metastasis, the other being hemorrhage and consequent anemia.

One patient had successful palliation for 24 months after adrenalectomy for an isolated metastasis.[12] Radiation therapy or chemotherapy might also be considered in symptomatic patients, especially those with multiple metastases.

Breast

Lesions in the breast should be surgically excised as a first choice or treated with irradiation or chemotherapy as a second choice. Most patients survive less than 6 months, although some live more than a year.[230,233,234] Since these tumors can simulate primary breast carcinoma by physical examination, mammography, and frozen section biopsy, it is important to distinguish between these two entities before embarking on radical breast surgery.[231,235]

Ovary, uterus, and vagina

Lesions in the ovary, uterus, and vagina could be treated by surgical excision or irradiation if the patient is symptomatic but has a reasonable life expectancy. There are a few reports of successful, although temporary, palliation.[12,231]

Testis and penis

Surgical excision may be considered if the lesions in the testis or penis are symptomatic or isolated.[236]

Oral cavity and larynx

Surgical excision or irradiation may be considered in those few patients with clinically isolated disease of the oral cavity or larynx, especially if it is symptomatic.[243,244,246,249] In one report, a melanoma patient

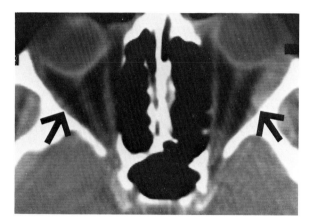

FIG. 13–11 Symptomatic metastases of the eye. This 39-year-old white man had a 4.5-mm ulcerated melanoma of his trunk with axillary and inguinal nodal metastases. Three years later he developed pulmonary, subcutaneous, bone, and orbital metastases. He had pain, proptosis, and decreased vision in his left eye that was treated with irradiation therapy (600 rad twice a week for 2 weeks). This relieved his symptoms during the remaining 4 months of his life. The figure shows a sagittal CT view of the orbits. The *right arrow* points to a metastatic lesion involving the lateral rectus muscle and the globe of the right eye. The *left arrow* points to the normal anatomy in the left orbit.

was alive 6 years after irradiation of laryngeal metastasis from a primary tumor on the chest.[242]

Eye

Symptomatic metastases in or behind the eye should be treated with irradiation after considering vision in that eye to be impaired or lost (Fig. 13-11). Enucleation should be reserved for failures after treatment with irradiation or chemotherapy. Orbital decompression may be required with evacuation of the tumor mass if the globe is grossly displaced and the patient has a reasonable life expectancy.[257]

REFERENCES

GENERAL DIAGNOSIS AND TREATMENT

1. Amer MH, Al-Sarraf M, Vaitkevicius VK: Clinical presentation, natural history and prognostic factors in advanced malignant melanoma. Surg Gynecol Obstet 149:687, 1979
2. Aranha GV, Simmons RL, Gunnarsson A, Grage TB, McKhann CF: The value of preoperative screening procedures in stage I and II malignant melanoma. J Surg Oncol 11:1, 1979
3. Balch CM, Karakousis C, Mettlin C, Natarajan N, Donegan WL, Smart CR, Murphy GR: Management of cutaneous melanoma in the United States: Results of the American College of Surgeons' melanoma survey. Surg Gynecol Obstet 158:311, 1984
4. Balch CM, Soong S-j, Murad TM, Ingalls AL, Maddox WA: A multifactorial analysis of melanoma III: Prognostic factors in melanoma patients with lymph node metastases (stage II). Ann Surg 193:377, 1981
5. Balch CM, Soong S-j, Murad TM, Smith JW, Maddox WA, Durant JR: A multifactorial analysis of melanoma IV. Prognostic factors in 200 melanoma patients with distant metastases (stage III). J Clin Oncol 1:126, 1983
6. Bassett LW, Steckel RJ: Imaging techniques in the detection of metastatic disease. Semin Oncol 4:39, 1977
7. Bernardino ME, Goldstein HM: Gray scale ultrasonography in the evaluation of metastatic melanoma. Cancer 42:2529, 1978
8. Blois MS, Banda PW: Detection of occult metastatic melanoma by urine chromatography. Cancer Res 36:3317, 1976
9. Bragg DG: Medical imaging problems in the patient with advanced cancer. JAMA 244:597, 1980
10. Budman DR, Camacho E, Wittes RE: The current causes of death in patients with malignant melanoma. Eur J Cancer 14:327, 1978
11. Cox KR, Hare WSC, Bruce PT: Lymphography in melanoma: Correlation of radiology with pathology. Cancer 19:637, 1966
12. Das Gupta T, Brasfield R: Metastatic melanoma: A clinicopathological study. Cancer 17:1323, 1964
13. de la Monte SM, Moore GW, Hutchins GM: Patterned distribution of metastases from malignant melanoma in humans. Cancer Res 43:3427, 1983
14. Doiron MJ, Bernardino ME: A comparison of noninvasive imaging modalities in the melanoma patient. Cancer 47:2581, 1981
15. Doyle FH, Pennock JM, Banks LM, McDonnell MJ, Bydder GM, Steiner RE, Young IR, Clarke GJ, Pasmore T, Gilderdale DJ: Nuclear magnetic resonance imaging of the liver: Initial experience. Am J Roentgenol 138:193, 1982
16. Einhorn LH, Burgess MA, Vallejos C, Bodey GP Sr, Gutterman J, Mavligit G, Hersh EM, Luce JK, Frei E III, Freireich EJ, Gottlieb JA: Prognostic correlations and response to treatment in advanced metastatic malignant melanoma. Cancer Res 34:1995, 1974
17. Eiseman B, Robinson WA, Steele G Jr: Follow-up of the Cancer Patient. New York, Georg Thieme Verlag, Thieme-Stratton, 1982
18. Evans RA, Bland KI, McMurtrey MJ, Ballantyne AJ: Radionuclide scans not indicated for clinical stage I melanoma. Surg Gynecol Obstet 150:532, 1980
19. Felix EL, Sindelar WF, Bagley DH, Johnston GS, Ketcham AS: The use of bone and brain scans as screening procedures in patients with malignant lesions. Surg Gynecol Obstet 141:867, 1975
20. Feun LG, Gutterman J, Burgess MA, Hersh EM, Mavligit G, McBride CM, Benjamin RS, Richman SP, Murphy WK, Bodey GP, Brown BW, Mountain CF, Leavens ME, Freireich EJ: The natural history of resectable metastatic melanoma (stage IVA melanoma). Cancer 50:1656, 1982
21. Finck SJ, Giuliano AE, Morton DL: LDH and melanoma. Cancer 51:840, 1983
22. Friedman M, Forgione H, Shanbhag V: Needle aspiration of metastatic melanoma. Acta Cytol 24:7, 1980
23. Habermalz HJ, Fisher JJ: Radiation therapy of malignant melanoma: Experience with high individual treatment doses. Cancer 38:2258, 1976
24. Hajdu SI, Savino A: Cytologic diagnosis of malignant melanoma. Acta Cytol 17:320, 1973
25. Hilaris BS, Raben M, Calabrese AS, Phillips RF, Henschke UK: Value of radiation therapy for distant metastases from malignant melanoma. Cancer 16:765, 1963
26. Huffman TA, Sterin WK: Ten-year survival with multiple metastatic malignant melanoma: Primary site unknown. Arch Surg 106:234, 1973
27. Jackson FI, McPherson TA, Lentle BC: Gallium-67 scintigraphy in multisystem malignant melanoma. Radiology 122:163, 1977
28. Karakousis CP: Surgical treatment of recurrent malignant melanoma. Contemp Surg 22:75, 1983
29. Karakousis CP, Temple DF, Moore R, Ambrus JL: Prognostic parameters in recurrent malignant melanoma. Cancer 52:575, 1983
30. Kirkwood JM, Myers JE, Vlock DR, Neumann R, Ariyan S, Gottschalk A, Hoffer P: Tomographic

gallium-67 citrate scanning: Useful new surveillance for metastatic melanoma. Ann Surg 198:102, 1983

31. Larson SM, Brown JP, Wright PW, Carrasquillo JA, Hellstrom I, Hellstrom KE: Imaging of melanoma with I-131-labeled monoclonal antibodies. J Nucl Med 24:123, 1983

32. Lawson DH, Nixon DW, Black ML, Tindall GT, Barnes DA, Faraj BA, Ali FM, Camp VM, Richmond A: Evaluation of transsphenoidal hypophysectomy in the management of patients with advanced malignant melanoma. Cancer 51:1541, 1983

33. Levitt RG, Koehler RE, Sagel SS, Lee JKT: Metastatic disease of the mesentery and omentum. Radiol Clin North Am 20:501, 1982

34. Libshitz HI: Symposium on metastatic disease. Radiol Clin North Am 20:417, 1982

35. Meyer JE: Radiographic evaluation of metastatic melanoma. Cancer 42:127, 1978

36. Meyer JE, Stolbach L: Pretreatment radiographic evaluation of patients with malignant melanoma. Cancer 42:125, 1978

37. Milder MS, Frankel RS, Bulkley GB, Ketcham AS, Johnston GS: Gallium-67 scintigraphy in malignant melanoma. Cancer 32:1350, 1973

38. Milton GW, Shaw HM, Farago GA, McCarthy WH: Tumour thickness and the site and time of first recurrence in cutaneous malignant melanoma (stage I): Br J Surg 67:543, 1980

39. Murray JL, Lerner MP, Nordquist RE: Elevated γ-glutamyl transpeptidase levels in malignant melanoma. Cancer 49:1439, 1982

40. Muss HB, Richards F II, Barnes PL, Willard VV, Cowan RJ: Radionuclide scanning in patients with advanced malignant melanoma. Clin Nucl Med 4:516, 1979

41. Patel JK, Didolkar MS, Pickren JW, Moore RH: Metastatic pattern of malignant melanoma: A study of 216 autopsy cases. Am J Surg 135:807, 1978

42. Presant CA, Bartolucci AA, Smalley RV, Vogler WR, the Southeastern Cancer Study Group: Cyyclophosphamide plus 5-(3,3-dimethyl-1-triazeno)-imidazole-4-carboxamide (DTIC) with or without *Corynebacterium parvum* in metastatic malignant melanoma. Cancer 44:899, 1979

43. Pykett IL, Newhouse JH, Buonanno FS, Brady TJ, Goldman MR, Kistler JP, Pohost GM: Principles of nuclear magnetic resonance imaging. Radiology 143:157, 1982

44. Romolo JL, Fisher SG: Gallium[67] scanning compared with physical examination in the preoperative staging of malignant melanoma. Cancer 44:468, 1979

45. Roth JA, Eilber FR, Bennett LR, Morton DL: Radionuclide photoscanning: Usefulness in preoperative evaluation of melanoma patients. Arch Surg 110:1211, 1975

46. Sacre R, Lejeune FJ: Pattern of metastases distribu-

tion in 173 stage I or II melanoma patients. Anticancer Res 2:47, 1982

47. Seigler HF, Fetter BF: Current management of melanoma. Ann Surg 186:1, 1977

48. Seigler HF, Lucas VS Jr, Pickett NJ, Huang AT: DTIC, CCNU, bleomycin and vincristine (BOLD) in metastatic melanoma. Cancer 46:2346, 1980

49. Smith FW: Two years' clinical experience with NMR imaging. Applied Radiol, 12:29, 1983

50. Stehlin JS Jr, Hills WJ, Rufino C: Disseminated melanoma: Biologic behavior and treatment. Arch Surg 94:495, 1967

51. Storm FK, Kaiser LR, Goodnight JE, Harrison WH, Elliott RS, Gomes AS, Morton DL: Thermochemotherapy for melanoma metastases in liver. Cancer 49:1243, 1982

52. Strauss A, Dritschilo A, Nathanson L, Piro AJ: Radiation therapy of malignant melanomas: An evaluation of clinically used fractionation schemes. Cancer 47:1262, 1981

53. Stuhlmiller GM, Sullivan DC, Vervaert CE, Croker BP, Harris CC, Seigler HF: In vivo tumor localization using tumor-specific monkey xenoantibody, alloantibody, and murine monoclonal xenoantibody. Ann Surg 194:592, 1981

54. Thomas JH, Panoussopoulous D, Liesmann GE, Jewell WR, Preston DF: Scintiscans in the evaluation of patients with malignant melanomas. Surg Gynecol Obstet 149:574, 1979

55. Turnbull A, Shah J, Fortner J: Recurrent melanoma of an extremity treated by major amputation. Arch Surg 106:496, 1973

56. Whalen JP: Radiology of the abdomen: Impact of new imaging methods. Am J Roentgenol 133:587, 1979

57. Wheelock MC, Frable WJ, Urnes PD: Bizarre metastases from malignant neoplasms. Am J Clin Pathol 37:475, 1962

58. Yamada T, Itou U, Watanabe Y, Ohashi S: Cytologic diagnosis of malignant melanoma. Acta Cytol 16:70, 1972

59. Zornoza J: Needle biopsy of metastases. Radiol Clin North Am 20:569, 1982

SKIN AND SUBCUTANEOUS METASTASES

60. Cox KR: Regional cutaneous metastases in melanoma of the limb. Surg Gynecol Obstet 139:385, 1974

61. Kim JH, Hahn EW, Ahmed SA: Combination hyperthermia and radiation therapy for malignant melanoma. Cancer 50:478, 1982

62. Luk KH, Francis ME, Perez CA, Johnson RJ: Radiation therapy and hyperthermia in the treatment of superficial lesions: Preliminary analysis: Treatment efficacy and reactions of skin tissues subcutaneous. Am J Clin Oncol 6:399, 1983

63. Overgaard J: Fractionated radiation and hyperthermia: Experimental and clinical studies. Cancer 48:1116, 1981

LUNG, PLEURA, AND MEDIASTINUM

64. Anderson CB, Philpott GW, Ferguson TB: The treatment of malignant pleural effusions. Cancer 33:916, 1974

65. Andrews AH Jr, Caldarelli DD: Carbon dioxide laser treatment of metastatic melanoma of the trachea and bronchi. Ann Otol Rhinol Laryngol 90:310, 1981

66. Braman SS, Whitcomb ME: Endobronchial metastasis. Arch Intern Med 135:543, 1975

67. Cahan WG: Excision of melanoma metastases to lung: Problems in diagnosis and management. Ann Surg 178:703, 1973

68. Chang AE, Schaner EG, Conkle DM, Flye MW, Doppman JL, Rosenberg SA: Evaluation of computed tomography in the detection of pulmonary metastases: A prospective study. Cancer 43:913, 1979

69. Chen JTT, Dahmash NS, Ravin CE, Heaston DK, Putman CE, Seigler HF, Reed JC: Metastatic melanoma to the thorax: Report of 130 patients. Am J Roentgenol 137:293, 1981

70. Cline RE, Young WG Jr: Long term results following surgical treatment of metastatic pulmonary tumors. Am Surg 36:61, 1970

71. Curtis A McB, Ravin CE, Deering TF, Putman CE, McLoud TC, Greenspan RH: The efficacy of full-lung tomography in the detection of early metastatic disease from melanoma. Diagn Radiol 144:27, 1982

72. Feldman L, Kricun ME: Malignant melanoma presenting as a mediastinal mass. JAMA 241:396, 1979

73. Gibbons JA, Devig PM: Massive hemothorax due to metastatic malignant melanoma. Chest 73:123, 1978

74. Gromet MA, Ominsky SH, Epstein WL, Blois MS: The thorax as the initial site for systemic relapse in malignant melanoma: A prospective survey of 324 patients. Cancer 44:776, 1979

75. Heaston DK, Putman CE: Radiographic manifestations of thoracic malignant melanoma. In Seigler HF (ed): Clinical Management of Melanoma, p 62. The Hague, Nijhoff, 1982

76. Libshitz HI, North LB: Pulmonary metastases. Radiol Clin North Am 20:437, 1982

77. McCormack PM, Bains MS, Beattie EJ Jr, Martini N: Pulmonary resection in metastatic carcinoma. Chest 73:163, 1978

78. McCormack PM, Martini N: The changing role of surgery for pulmonary metastases. Ann Thorac Surg 28:139, 1979

79. Mathisen DJ, Flye MW, Peabody J: The role of thoracotomy in the management of pulmonary metastases from malignant melanoma. Ann Thorac Surg 27:295, 1979

80. Mintzer RA, Malave SR, Neiman HL, Michaelis LL, Vanecko RM, Sanders JH: Computed vs. conventional tomography in evaluation of primary and secondary pulmonary neoplasms. Radiology 132:653, 1979

81. Morrow CE, Vassilopoulos PP, Grage TB: Surgical resection for metastatic neoplasms of the lung: Experience at the University of Minnesota Hospitals. Cancer 45:2981, 1980

82. Morton DL, Joseph WL, Ketcham AS, Geelhoed GW, Adkins PC: Surgical resection and adjunctive immunotherapy for selected patients with multiple pulmonary metastases. Ann Surg 178:360, 1973

83. Muhm JR, Brown LR, Crowe JK: Use of computed tomography in the detection of pulmonary nodules. Mayo Clin Proc 52:345, 1977

84. Neifeld JP, Michaelis LL, Doppman JL: Suspected pulmonary metastases: Correlation of chest x-ray, whole lung tomograms, and operative findings. Cancer 39:383, 1977

85. Reed RJ III, Kent EM: Solitary pulmonary melanomas: Two case reports. J Thorac Cardiovasc Surg 48:226, 1964

86. Schaner EG, Chang AE, Doppman JL, Conkle DM, Flye MW, Rosenberg SA: Comparison of computed and conventional whole lung tomography in detecting pulmonary nodules: A prospective radiologic-pathologic study. Am J Roentgenol 131:51, 1978

87. Sethi SM, Saxton GD: Osteoarthropathy associated with solitary pulmonary metastasis from melanoma. Can J Surg 17:221, 1974

88. Simeone JF, Putman CE, Greenspan RH: Detection of metastatic malignant melanoma by chest roentgenography. Cancer 39:1993, 1977

89. Sonoda T, Krauss S: Hypertrophic osteoarthropathy associated with pulmonary metastasis of malignant melanoma. J Tenn Med Assoc 68:716, 1975

90. Sutton FD Jr, Vestal RE, Creagh CE: Varied presentations of metastatic pulmonary melanoma. Chest 65:415, 1974

91. Turney S, Haight C: Pulmonary resection for metastatic neoplasms. J Thorac Cardiovasc Surg 61:784, 1971

92. Vidne BA, Richter S, Levy MJ: Surgical treatment of solitary pulmonary metastasis. Cancer 38:2561, 1976

93. Webb WR: Hilar and mediastinal lymph node metastases in malignant melanoma. Am J Roentgenol 133:805, 1979

94. Webb WR, Gamsu G: Thoracic metastasis in malignant melanoma: A radiographic survey of 65 patients. Chest 71:176, 1977

95. Wilkins EW Jr, Head JM, Burke JF: Pulmonary resection for metastatic neoplasms in the lung: Experience at the Massachusetts General Hospital. Am J Surg 135:480, 1978

96. Wilson KS, Naidoo A: Hypertrophic osteoarthropathy. Mayo Clin Proc 54:208, 1979

97. Yeung KY, Bonnet JD: Spontaneous pneumothorax

with metastatic malignant melanoma. Chest 71:435, 1977

BRAIN AND SPINAL CORD

98. Amer MH, Al-Sarraf M, Baker LH, Vaitkevicius VK: Malignant melanoma and central nervous system metastases: Incidence, diagnosis, treatment and survival. Cancer 42:660, 1978
99. Aronson SM, Garcia JH, Aronson BE: Metastatic neoplasms of the brain: Their frequency in relation to age. Cancer 17:558, 1964
100. Atkinson L: Melanoma of the central nervous system. Aust NZ J Surg 48:14, 1978
101. Bardfeld PA, Passalaqua AM, Braunstein P, Raghavendra BN, Leeds NE, Kricheff II: A comparison of radionuclide scanning and computed tomography in metastatic lesions of the brain. J Comput Assist Tomogr 1:315, 1977
102. Bauman ML, Price TR: Intracranial metastatic malignant melanoma: Long-term survival following subtotal resection. South Med J 65:344, 1972
103. Bremer AM, West CR, Didolkar MS: An evaluation of the surgical management of melanoma of the brain. J Surg Oncol 10:211, 1978
104. Buell U, Niendorf HP, Kazner E, Lanksch W, Wilske J, Steinhoff H, Gahr H: Computerized transaxial tomography and cerebral serial scintigraphy in intracranial tumors—rates of detection and tumor-type identification: Concise communication. J Nucl Med 19:476, 1978
105. Bullard DE, Cox EB, Seigler HF: Central nervous system metastases in malignant melanoma. Neurosurgery 8:26, 1981
106. Butler AR, Kricheff II: Non-contrast CT scanning: Limited value in suspected brain tumor. Radiology 126:689, 1978
107. Carella RJ, Gelber R, Hendrickson F, Berry HC, Cooper JS: Value of radiation therapy in the management of patients with cerebral metastases from malignant melanoma: Radiation Therapy Oncology Group brain metastases study I and II. Cancer 45:679, 1980
108. Cooper JS, Carella R: Radiotherapy of intracerebral metastatic malignant melanoma. Radiology 134:735, 1980
109. Enzmann DR, Kramer R, Norman D, Pollock J: Malignant melanoma metastatic to the central nervous system. Radiology 127:177, 1978
110. Fell DA, Leavens ME, McBride CM: Surgical versus nonsurgical management of metastatic melanoma of the brain. Neurosurgery 7:238, 1980
111. Fletcher JW, George EA, Henry RE, Donati RM: Brain scans, dexamethasone therapy, and brain tumors. JAMA 232:1261, 1975
112. Galicich JH, Sundaresan N, Arbit E, Passe S: Surgical treatment of single brain metastasis: Factors associated with survival. Cancer 45:381, 1980
113. Gelber RD, Larson M, Borgelt BB, Kramer S: Equivalence of radiation schedules for the palliative treatment of brain metastases in patients with favorable prognosis. Cancer 48:1749, 1981
114. Gildersleeve N Jr, Koo AH, McDonald CJ: Metastatic tumor presenting as intracerebral hemorrhage: Report of 6 cases examined by computed tomography. Radiology 124:109, 1977
115. Ginaldi S, Wallace S, Shalen P, Luna M, Handel S: Cranial computed tomography of malignant melanoma. Am J Roentgenol 136:145, 1981
116. Gottlieb JA, Frei E III, Luce JK: An evaluation of the management of patients with cerebral metastases from malignant melanoma. Cancer 29:701, 1972
117. Greenberg HS, Kim J, Posner JB: Epidural spinal cord compression from metastatic tumor: Results with a new treatment protocol. Ann Neurol 8:361, 1980
118. Hafström L, Jönsson P-E, Strömblad L-G: Intracranial metastases of malignant melanoma treated by surgery. Cancer 46:2088, 1980
119. Hayward RD: Malignant melanoma and the central nervous system: A guide for classification based on the clinical findings. J Neurol Neurosurg Psychiatry 39:526, 1976
120. Hayward RD: Secondary malignant melanoma of the brain. Clin Oncol 2:227, 1976
121. Holtås S, Cronqvist S: Cranial computed tomography of patients with malignant melanoma. Neuroradiology 22:123, 1981
122. Lang EF, Slater J: Metastatic brain tumors: Results of surgical and nonsurgical treatment. Surg Clin North Am 44:865, 1964
123. Lewi HJ, Roberts MM, Donaldson AA, Forrest APM: The use of cerebral computer assisted tomography as a staging investigation of patients with carcinoma of the breast and malignant melanoma. Surg Gynecol Obstet 151:385, 1980
124. McCann WP, Weir BKA, Elvidge AR: Long-term survival after removal of metastatic malignant melanoma of the brain: Report of two cases. J Neurosurg 28:483, 1968
125. McNeel DP, Leavens ME: Long-term survival with recurrent metastatic intracranial melanoma: Case report. J Neurosurg 29:91, 1968
126. Madonick MJ, Savitsky N: Subarachnoid hemorrhage in melanoma of the brain. Arch Neurol Psych 65:628, 1951
127. Mandybur TI: Intracranial hemorrhage caused by metastatic tumors. Neurology 27:650, 1977
128. Pennington DG, Milton GW: Cerebral metastasis from melanoma. Aust NZ J Surg 45:405, 1975
129. Posner JB: Management of central nervous system metastases. Semin Oncol 4:81, 1977
130. Posner JB, Chernik NL: Intracranial metastases from systemic cancer. Adv Neurol 19:579, 1978
131. Ransohoff J: Surgical management of metastatic tumors. Semin Oncol 2:21, 1975
132. Reyes V, Horrax G: Metastatic melanoma of the

brain: Report of a case with unusually long survival period following surgical removal. Ann Surg 131:237, 1950

133. Ruderman NB, Hall, TC: Use of glucocorticoids in the palliative treatment of metastatic brain tumors. Cancer 18:298, 1965

134. Scott M: Spontaneous intracerebral hematoma caused by cerebral neoplasms: Report of eight verified cases. J Neurosurg 42:338, 1975

135. Solis OJ, Davis KR, Adair LB, Roberson GR, Kleinman G: Intracerebral metastatic melanoma: CT evaluation. Comput Tomogr 1:135, 1977

136. Vieth RG, Odom GL: Intracranial metastases and their neurosurgical treatment. J Neurosurg 23:375, 1965

137. Vlock DR, Kirkwood JM, Leutzinger C, Kapp DS, Fischer JJ: High-dose fraction radiation therapy for intracranial metastases of malignant melanoma: A comparison with low-dose fraction therapy. Cancer 49:2289, 1982

138. Wasserstrom WR, Glass JP, Posner JB: Diagnosis and treatment of leptomeningeal metastases from solid tumors: Experience with 90 patients. Cancer 49:759, 1982

139. Winston KR, Walsh JW, Fischer EG: Results of operative treatment of intracranial metastatic tumors. Cancer 45:2639, 1980

140. Wolpert SM, Zimmer A, Schechter MM, Zingesser LH: The neuroradiology of melanomas of the central nervous system. Am J Roentgenol 101:178, 1967

141. Young RF, Post EM, King GA: Treatment of spinal epidural metastases: Randomized prospective comparison of laminectomy and radiotherapy. J Neurosurg 53:741, 1980

GASTROINTESTINAL TRACT

142. Backman H: Metastases of malignant melanoma in the gastrointestinal tract. Geriatrics 24:112, 1969

143. Beckly DE: Alimentary tract metastases from malignant melanoma. Clin Radiol 25:385, 1974

144. Benisch BM, Abramson S, Present DH: Malabsorption and metastatic melanoma. Mt Sinai J Med 39:474, 1972

145. Booth JB: Malignant melanoma of the stomach: Report of a case presenting as an acute perforation and review of the literature. Br J Surg 52:262, 1965

146. Butler ML, Van Heertum RL, Teplick SK: Metastatic malignant melanoma of the esophagus: A case report. Gastroenterology 69:1334, 1975

147. Byrd BF Jr, Morton CE III: Malignant melanoma metastatic to the gastrointestinal tract from an occult primary tumor. South Med J 71:1306, 1978

148. Calderon R, Ceballos J, McGraw JP: Metastatic melanoma of the stomach. Am J Roentgenol 74:242, 1955

149. Das Gupta TK, Brasfield RD: Metastatic melanoma of the gastrointestinal tract. Arch Surg 88:969, 1964

150. Davis GH, Zollinger RW: Metastatic melanoma of the stomach. Am J Surg 99:94, 1960

151. Fraser-Moodie A, Hughes RG, Jones SM, Shorey BA, Snape L: Malignant melanoma metastases to the alimentary tract. Gut 17:206, 1976

152. Giler S, Kott I, Urca I: Malignant melanoma metastatic to the gastrointestinal tract. World J Surg 3:375, 1979

153. Goldman SL, Pollak EW, Wolfman EF Jr: Gastric ulcer: An unusual presentation of malignant melanoma. JAMA 237:52, 1977

154. Goldstein HM, Beydoun MT, Dodd GD: Radiologic spectrum of melanoma metastatic to the gastrointestinal tract. Am J Roentgenol 129:605, 1977

155. Goodman PL, Karakousis CP: Symptomatic gastrointestinal metastases from malignant melanoma. Cancer 48:1058, 1981

156. Harris MN: Massive gastrointestinal hemorrhage due to metastatic malignant melanoma of small intestine. Arch Surg 88:1049, 1964

157. Karakousis C, Holyoke ED, Douglass HO Jr: Intussusception as a complication of malignant neoplasm. Arch Surg 109:515, 1974

158. Klausner JM, Skornick Y, Lelcuk S, Baratz M, Merhav A: Acute complications of metastatic melanoma to the gastrointestinal tract. Br J Surg 69:195, 1982

159. Macbeth WAAG, Gwynne JF, Jamieson MG: Metastatic melanoma in the small bowel. Aust NZ J Surg 38:309, 1969

160. May ARL, Edwards JM: Surgical excision of visceral metastases from malignant melanoma. Clin Oncol 2:233, 1976

161. Meyers MA, McSweeney J: Secondary neoplasms of the bowel. Radiology 105:1, 1972

162. Oddson TA, Rice RP, Seigler HF, Thompson WM, Kelvin FM, Clark WM. The spectrum of small bowel melanoma. Gastrointest Radiol 3:419, 1978

163. Paglia MA, Exelby PE: Recurrent intussusception from metastatic melanoma. NY State J Med, December 1, 1968

164. Pomerantz H, Margolin HN: Metastases to the gastrointestinal tract from malignant melanoma. Am J Roentgenol 88:712, 1962

165. Potchen EJ, Khung CL, Yatsuhashi M: X-ray diagnosis of gastric melanoma. N Engl J Med 271:133, 1964

166. Reeder MM, Cavanagh RC: "Bull's-eye" lesions: Solitary or multiple nodules in the gastrointestinal tract with larger central ulceration. JAMA 229:825, 1974

167. Sacks BA, Joffee N, Antonioli DA: Metastatic melanoma presenting clinically as multiple colonic polyps. Am J Roentgenol 129:511, 1977

168. Sanders DE, Ho CS: The small bowel enema: Experience with 150 examinations. Am J Roentgenol 127:743, 1976

169. Shah SM, Smart DF, Texter EC Jr, Morris WD: Metastatic melanoma of the stomach: The endo-

scopic and roentgenographic findings and review of the literature. South Med J 70:379, 1977

170. Thompson WH: Radiographic manifestations of metastatic melanoma to the gastrointestinal tract, hepatobiliary system, pancreas, spleen and mesentery. In Seigler HF (ed): Clinical Management of Melanoma, p 133. The Hague, Nijhoff, 1982

171. Willbanks OL, Fogelman MJ: Gastrointestinal melanosarcoma. Am J Surg 120:602, 1970

172. Wood CB, Wood RAB: Metastatic malignant melanoma of the esophagus. Dig Dis Sci 20:786, 1975

173. Zornoza J, Goldstein HM: Cavitating metastases of the small intestine. Am J Roentgenol 129:613, 1977

LIVER, BILIARY TRACT AND SPLEEN

174. Alderson PO, Adams DF, McNeil BJ, Sanders R, Siegelman SS, Finberg H, Hessel SJ, Abrams HL: A prospective comparison of computed tomography, ultrasound and scintigraphy of the liver in patients with colon or breast carcinoma. Radiology 146: 439, 1983.

175. Balthazar EJ, Javors B: Malignant melanoma of the gallbladder. Am J Gastroenterol 64:332, 1975

176. Bernardino ME, Thomas JL, Barnes PA, Lewis E: Diagnostic approaches to liver and spleen metastases. Radiol Clin North Am 20:469, 1982

177. Bowdler DA, Leach RD: Metastatic intrabiliary melanoma. Clin Oncol 8:251, 1982

178. Daunt N, King DM: Metastatic melanoma in the biliary tree. Br J Radiol 55:873, 1982

179. Felix EL, Bagley DH, Sindelar WF, Johnston GS, Ketcham AS: The value of the liver scan in preoperative screening of patients with malignancies. Cancer 38:1137, 1976

180. Fortner JG, Kallum BO, Kim DK: Surgical management of hepatic vein occlusion by tumor: Budd-Chiari syndrome. Arch Surg 112:727, 1977

181. Garg R, McPherson TA, Lentle B, Jackson F: Usefulness of an elevated serum lactate dehydrogenase value as a marker of hepatic metastases in malignant melanoma. Can Med Assoc J 120:1114, 1979

182. Herrington JL Jr: Metastatic malignant melanoma of the gallbladder masquerading as cholelithiasis. Am J Surg 109:676, 1965

183. MacCarty RL, Stephens DH, Hattery RR, Sheedy PF II: Hepatic imaging by computed tomography: A comparison with ^{99m}Tc-sulfur colloid, ultrasonography, and angiography. Radiol Clin North Am 17:137, 1979

184. McArthur MS, Teergarden DK: Metastatic melanoma presenting as obstructive jaundice with hemobilia. Am J Surg 145:830, 1983

185. McFadden PM, Krementz ET, McKinnon WMP, Pararo LL, Ryan RF: Metastatic melanoma of the gallbladder. Cancer 44:1802, 1979

186. Ostick DG, Haqqani MT: Obstructive cholecystitis due to metastatic melanoma. Postgrad Med J 52:710, 1976

187. Shimkin PM, Soloway MS, Jaffe E: Metastatic melanoma of the gallbladder. Am J Roentgenol 116:393, 1972

188. Smith TJ, Kemeny MM, Sugarbaker PH, Jones AE, Vermess M, Shawker TH, Edwards BK: A prospective study of hepatic imaging in the detection of metastatic disease. Ann Surg 195:486, 1982

189. Snow JH Jr, Goldstein HM, Wallace S: Comparison of scintigraphy, sonography, and computed tomography in the evaluation of hepatic neoplasms. Am J Roentgenol 132:915, 1979

190. Zemlyn S: Metastatic melanoma of the gallbladder. Radiology 87:744, 1966

BONE

191. Devereux D, Johnston G, Blei L, Head G, Makuch R, Burt M: The role of bone scans in assessing malignant melanoma in patients with stage III disease. Surg Gynecol Obstet 151:45, 1980

192. Fon GT, Wong WS, Gold RH, Kaiser LR: Skeletal metastases of melanoma: Radiographic, scintigraphic, and clinical review. Am J Roentgenol 137:103, 1981

193. Gelberman RH, Stewart WR, Harrelson JM: Hand metastasis from melanoma: A case study. Clin Orthop 136:264, 1978

194. Harrelson JM: Orthopaedic considerations in the treatment of malignant melanoma. In Seigler HF (ed): Clinical Management of Melanoma, p 435, The Hague, Nijhoff, 1982

195. Nussbaum H, Allen B, Kagan AR, Gilbert HA, Rao A, Chan P: Management of bone metastasis—multidisciplinary approach. Semin Oncol 4:93, 1977

196. Pagani JJ, Libshitz HI: Imaging bone metastases. Radiol Clin North Am 20:545, 1982

197. Selby HM, Sherman RS, Pack GT: A roentgen study of bone metastases from melanoma. Radiology 67:224, 1956

198. Shenberger KN, Morgan GJ Jr: Recurrent malignant melanoma presenting as monoarthritis. J Rheumatol 9:328, 1982

199. Steiner GM, MacDonald JS: Metastases to bone from malignant melanoma. Clin Radiol 23:52, 1972

200. Stewart WR, Gelberman RH, Harrelson JM, Seigler HF: Skeletal metastases of melanoma. J Bone Joint Surg 60A:645, 1978

201. Tong D, Gillick L, Hendrickson FR: The palliation of symptomatic osseous metastases: Final results of the study by the Radiation Therapy Oncology Group. Cancer 50:893, 1982

KIDNEYS, URETER, AND BLADDER

202. Abeshouse BS: Primary and secondary melanoma of the genitourinary tract. South Med J 51:994, 1958

203. Agnew CH: Metastatic malignant melanoma of the kidney simulating a primary neoplasm: A case report. Am J Roentgenol 80:813, 1958

204. Amar AD: Metastatic melanoma of the bladder. J Urol 92:198, 1964

205. Bartone FF: Metastatic melanoma of the bladder. J Urol 91:151, 1964

206. Berry NE, Reese L: Malignant melanoma which had its first clinical manifestations in the prostate gland. J Urol 69:286, 1953

207. Das Gupta T, Grabstald H: Melanoma of the genitourinary tract. J Urol 93:607, 1965

208. deKernion JB, Golub SH, Gupta RK, Silverstein M, Morton DL: Successful transurethral intralesional BCG therapy of a bladder melanoma. Cancer 36:1662, 1975

209. Goldstein HM, Kaminsky S, Wallace S, Johnson DE: Urographic manifestations of metastatic melanoma. Radiology 121:801, 1974

210. Lowsley OS: Melanoma of the urinary tract and prostate gland. South Med J 44:487, 1951

211. McKenzie DJ, Bell R: Melanoma with solitary metastasis to ureter. J Urol 99:399, 1968

212. Nakazono M, Iwata S, Kuribayashi N: Disseminated metastatic ureteral melanoma: A case report. J Urol 114:624, 1975

213. Samellas W, Marks AR: Metastatic melanoma of the urinary tract. J Urol 85:21, 1961

214. Sheehan EE, Greenberg SD, Scott R Jr: Metastatic neoplasms of the bladder. J Urol 90:281, 1963

215. Smith GW, Griffith DP, Pranke DW: Melanospermia: An unusual presentation of malignant melanoma. J Urol 110:314, 1973

216. Su C-T, Prince CL: Melanoma of the bladder. J Urol 87:365, 1962

217. Walsh EJ, Ockuly EA, Ockuly EF, Ockuly JJ: Treatment of metastatic melanoma of the bladder. J Urol 96:472, 1966

218. Weston PAM, Smith BJ: Metastatic melanoma in the bladder and urethra. Br J Surg 51:78, 1964

219. Woodard BH, Ideker RE, Johnston WW: Cytologic detection of malignant melanoma in urine. Acta Cytol 22:350, 1978

OTHER SITES

Heart

220. Berge T, Sievers J: Myocardial metastases: A pathological and electrocardiographic study. Br Heart J 30:383, 1968

221. Bryant J, Vuckovic G: Metastatic tumors of the endocardium: Report of three cases. Arch Pathol Lab Med 102:206, 1978

222. Cham WC, Freiman AH, Carstens PHB, Chu FCH: Radiation therapy of cardiac and pericardial metastases. Radiology 114:701, 1975

223. Glancy DL, Roberts WC: The heart in malignant melanoma: A study of 70 autopsy cases. Am J Cardiol 21:555, 1968

224. Hanfling SM: Metastatic cancer to the heart: Review of the literature and report of 127 cases. Circulation 22:474, 1960

225. Moragues V: Cardiac metastasis from malignant melanoma: Report of 4 cases. Am Heart J 18:579, 1939

226. Smith LH: Secondary tumors of the heart. Review of Surgery 33:223, 1976

227. Thomas JH, Panoussopoulos DG, Jewell WR, Pierce GE: Tricuspid stenosis secondary to metastatic melanoma. Cancer 39:1732, 1977

Endocrine organs

228. Twersky J, Levin DC: Metastatic melanoma of the adrenal: An unusual cause of adrenal calcification. Radiology 116:627, 1975

229. Seidenwurm D, Elmer EB, Kaplan LM, Williams EK, Morris DG, Hoffman AR: Metastases to the adrenal glands and the development of Addison's disease. Cancer (in press)

Breast

230. Charache H: Metastatic tumors in the breast with a report of ten cases. Surgery 33:385, 1953

231. Jochimsen PR, Brown RC: Metastatic melanoma in the breast masquerading as fibroadenoma. JAMA 236:2779, 1976

232. Paulus DD, Libshitz HI: Metastasis to the breast. Radiol Clin North Am 20:561, 1982

233. Pressman PI: Malignant melanoma and the breast. Cancer 31:784, 1973

234. Sandison AT: Metastatic tumours in the breast. Br J Surg 47:54, 1959

235. Silverman EM, Oberman HA: Metastatic neoplasms in the breast. Surg Gynecol Obstet 138:26, 1974

Testes and penis

236. Hanash KA, Carney JA, Kelalis PP: Metastatic tumors to testicles: Routes of metastasis. J Urol 102:465, 1969

237. Johnson DE, Jackson L, Ayala AG: Secondary carcinoma of the testis. South Med J 64:1128, 1971

238. Paquin AJ Jr, Roland SI: Secondary carcinoma of the penis: A review of the literature and a report of nine new cases. Cancer 9:629, 1956

Oral cavity and larynx

239. Aisenberg MS, Inman CL Sr: Tumors that have metastasized to the jaws. Oral Surg 9:1210, 1956

240. Ashur H, Mizrahi S, Ben-Hur N, Dolberg L: Metastatic malignant melanoma to the palatine tonsils: Report of case. J Oral Surg 37:110, 1979

241. Bluestone LI: Malignant melanoma metastatic to the mandible: Report of a case. Oral Surg 6:237, 1953

242. Chamberlain D: Malignant melanoma, metastatic to the larynx. Arch Otolaryngol 83:231, 1966

243. Craig RM, Glass BJ, Rhyne RR: Malignant melanoma: Metastasis to the tonsil. J Am Dent Assoc 104:893, 1982

244. Fisher GE, Odess JS: Metastatic malignant melanoma of the larynx. AMA Arch Otolaryngol 54:639, 1951

245. Meyer I, Shklar G: Malignant tumors metastatic to mouth and jaws. Oral Surg 20:350, 1965

246. Miller AS, Pullon PA: Metastatic malignant melanoma of the tongue. Arch Dermatol 103:201, 1971

247. Mosby EL, Sugg WE Jr, Hiatt WR: Gingival and pharyngeal metastasis from a malignant melanoma: Report of a case. Oral Surg 36:6, 1973

248. Pliskin ME, Mastrangelo MJ, Brown AM, Custer RP: Metastatic melanoma of the maxilla presenting as a gingival swelling. Oral Surg 41:101, 1976

249. Samit AM, Falk HJ, Ohanian M, Leban SG, Mashberg A: Malignant melanoma metastatic to the mandible. J Oral Surg 36:816, 1975

250. Trodahl JN, Sprague WG: Benign and malignant melanocytic lesions of the oral mucosa: An analysis of 135 cases. Cancer 25:812, 1970

Peritoneum and mesentery

251. Zboralske FF, Bessolo RJ: Metastatic carcinoma to the mesentery and gut. Radiology 88:302, 1967

Uterus

252. Casey JH, Shapiro RF: Metastatic melanoma presenting as primary uterine neoplasm: A case report. Cancer 33:729, 1974

Eye

253. Fishman ML, Tomaszewski MM, Kuwabara T: Malignant melanoma of the skin metastatic to the eye: Frequency in autopsy series. Arch Ophthalmol 94:1309, 1976

254. Font RL, Naumann G, Zimmerman LE: Primary malignant melanoma of the skin metastatic to the eye and orbit: Report of ten cases and review of the literature. Am J Ophthalmol 63:738, 1967

255. Liddicoat DA, Wolter JR, Wilkinson WC: Retinal metastasis of malignant melanoblastoma: A case report. Am J Ophthalmol 48:172, 1959

256. Riffenburgh RS: Metastatic malignant melanoma to the retina. Arch Ophthalmol 66:487, 1961

257. Sobol S, Druck NS, Wolf M: Palliative orbital decompression for metastatic melanoma to the orbit. Laryngoscope 90:329, 1980

ALAN S. COATES
JOHN R. DURANT

Chemotherapy for Metastatic Melanoma
14

The overall contribution of chemotherapy to the treatment of metastatic melanoma remains marginal. There is little evidence that it alters survival duration; objective responses are rare and usually brief. The strategy that has been used with considerable success in the development of effective chemotherapy for other tumor types has been to identify active single agents, then to apply them in combination. In melanoma, the same strategy has been followed but has largely failed at both levels. Few active single agents have been discovered, and evidence that any combination is superior to single-agent treatment remains unsatisfactory. Clinical trials to identify new active agents must therefore continue.

In the opinion of many clinicians, including the authors, the poor results obtained with standard agents make it ethical to consider trial of investigational agents in previously untreated patients. Outside clinical trials, the place of chemotherapy in routine management of metastatic melanoma is limited. Any decision to use chemotherapy must be made after balancing the potential benefits against the side-effects. In general, asymptomatic patients should not receive chemotherapy. In patients with symptoms, a trial of treatment may be given. Should there be a failure of one chemotherapy regimen, it is doubtful that a second trial would be of value.

The purpose of this chapter is to discuss available evidence for the activity of conventional and newer agents in metastatic melanoma, to propose reasonable guidelines for chemotherapy outside clinical trials, and to consider research strategies that might lead to the discovery of better treatment for this disease. The principles governing design and evaluation of clinical trials to detect the efficacy of a drug or drug combination have been well reviewed,[50,51] but not all reports adhere to them. In assessing the reported response rate for any study, it is important to bear in mind the influence of prognostic factors and trial size.[8,50] Apparent superiority of any regimen should be treated with caution if it has not been confirmed in a prospective randomized trial comparing the new regimen to a standard agent or combination. Moreover, response rates must not be taken as the only measure of the result of a trial. The effect of therapy on duration of survival should also be considered, and the side-effects, inconvenience, and cost weighed against the benefit.[15,16] Since survival is influenced by the inherent prognosis of patients admitted to a study,[65] comparison of survival in uncontrolled phase-II trials is of little value;

the impact, if any, of a particular chemotherapeutic regimen on survival can best be determined in prospective controlled trials.

STANDARD SINGLE AGENTS

DACARBAZINE

The nearest approach to standard chemotherapy for metastatic melanoma is undoubtedly dacarbazine (5-[3,3-dimethyltriazeno]-imidazole-4-carboxamide; DTIC; NSC-45388). Various schedules and dosages have been employed, ranging from 2 mg/kg daily for 10 days every 4 weeks[9] to 850 mg/m^2 or 1450 mg/m^2 as a single infusion every 4 to 6 weeks.[26,67] Most studies use criteria of response similar to those of the World Health Organization working party,[57] although some exclude patients who did not receive two cycles of therapy when calculating response rates, thus inflating the proportion of responses. The most popular dosage has been 250 mg/m^2 (150 mg/m^2–400mg/m^2) daily for 5 days every 4 weeks.[19,23,39] Overall (complete plus partial) response rates of 14% to 25% have been compiled by several reviewers,[20,34,54] while cooperative group results have tended toward the lower figure.[13,23] Very few of the responses are complete.[20,34]

The major side-effects of dacarbazine are nausea and vomiting, which are the most severe on the first day of each course. Local pain at the injection site is common and may be worse if the drug has undergone photodegradation. Dacarbazine should therefore be protected from light during preparation and administration. Hematologic side-effects are dose limiting, with nadir neutrophil and platelet counts on the 10th to 14th day, but recovery is usually rapid, and the effects are not cumulative. This is a major advantage over the nitrosoureas, which may cause progressive irreversible marrow failure. As with many anticancer drugs, dacarbazine is a potent carcinogen.

A derivative of dacarbazine, TIC mustard, although more active in animal models, was significantly less effective than dacarbazine in a prospective trial in human malignant melanoma.[21]

Several factors have been shown to influence the probability of response and the duration of survival.[65] Women respond more frequently than men do. Metastases in subcutaneous tissue and lymph nodes are more likely to respond than those in brain, liver, or bone, with pulmonary metastases intermediate between these two extremes.[19,23,34,65] Performance status is an important prognostic factor for response[19,23] and survival.[65] Prior exposure to chemotherapy reduces the probability of response to less than 10%, a level difficult to distinguish from random measurement error.[48,58] These factors must be borne in mind when comparing regimens that have not been evaluated in the same prospective randomized trial. They can account for differences in response rate at least as great as those claimed for different regimens.

The impact of objective response on survival remains uncertain. While it is true that patients responding to chemotherapy survive longer than those who do not respond,[13,23] this may merely reflect an inherently better prognosis rather than an effect of treatment.

As noted above, it is the authors' policy to enter patients into clinical trials of investigational agents whenever possible; but when standard chemotherapy is required, as for example in a symptomatic patient who is unsuitable for investigational therapy for medical, psychological, or geographical reasons or who refuses such therapy, dacarbazine may be used as a single agent either as a 30-minute infusion of 750 mg/m^2 every 3 weeks, escalating as tolerated, or in an intravenous push dose of 250 mg/m^2 five times daily every 4 weeks. The choice between these approaches is not important and depends on convenience.

NITROSOUREAS

Carmustine (1, 3-bis-[2-chloroethyl]-1-nitrosourea; BCNU; NSC-409962), semustine (1-[2-chloroethyl]-3-[4-methylcyclohexyl]-1-nitrosourea; methyl-CCNU; NSC-9544), and lomustine (1-[2-chloroethyl]-3-cyclohexyl-1-nitrosourea; CCNU; NSC-79037) are the best-studied members of this class. Although the reported response rates for carmustine and semustine are slightly higher than for lomustine,[11,31,53,68,86] the commercial availability of lomustine and its ease of oral administration combine to make it the most popular of the three. It may be preferred to dacarbazine in patients for whom intravenous therapy is inconvenient, but its use requires close surveillance. A common dose is 100 mg/m^2 orally every 6 to 8 weeks. Side-effects are usually mild; nausea and vomiting are controllable with oral antinauseants. Myelosuppression may be severe, prolonged, and cumulative. It is not safe to give further therapy at the same dosage level to a patient who has recovered from severe myelosuppression caused by nitrosourea, since stem cell damage may lead to more dangerous toxicity on the next cycle. Indeed, it may not be safe to use any myelosuppressive agent in such patients. Occasional side-effects include pulmonary fibrosis and renal failure.

A newer nitrosourea studied for the treatment of melanoma is chlorozotocin,[73,81] but there is no evidence that it offers any significant advantage over other nitrosoureas.

There seems to be little difference between semustine and dacarbazine as single agents for previously untreated patients,[23] but the response rate to either drug after failure of the other is very low.

OTHER STANDARD AGENTS

Conventional doses of alkylating agents produce only modest response rates,[72] but McElwain and associates[55] reported a response rate of 70% using high doses of melphalan. Such treatment requires intensive support, with or without autologous bone marrow rescue. Since the responses were not durable, it remains a research rather than a routine procedure.

The *Vinca* alkaloids vincristine, vinblastine, and vindesine all produce responses,[71,72,78] but as with other drugs, these responses occur more often in subcutaneous and lymph node metastases than in visceral metastatic disease. Antimetabolites have not produced useful response rates, even when methotrexate was used in high dosage.[36,44] Mitolactol (dibromodulcitol; DBD) produced responses in 5 of 25 patients reported by Bellet and associates[7] and in 4 of 47 patients in an Australian trial,[18] but other reports have been negative.[42,56] However, since all reported patients responding to mitolactol had received prior chemotherapy, and few side-effects were observed, it remains an option for second-line treatment. The related drug dianhydrogalactitol appears inactive.[2,80]

CHEMOTHERAPY COMBINATIONS

Most combinations of the above drugs as well as other standard agents have been tried. Before reviewing the results claimed, it is important to emphasize that there is no prospective controlled trial conclusively showing superiority for any combination of drugs over the same drugs used singly.

Important trials that fail to show such superiority include the Eastern Cooperative Oncology Group (ECOG) study of semustine versus dacarbazine versus a combination of semustine and dacarbazine.[23] The response rate for semustine was 15%, for dacarbazine 14%, and for the combination 14%. Duration of response was the same in all groups. Toxicity was more severe in the group receiving the combination, and all three drug-related deaths were in this group.[23] An earlier study by the same group failed to demonstrate any advantage for the combination of carmustine and dacarbazine over dacarbazine alone.[22]

Perhaps the best suggestion of possible benefit from a combination drug therapy is the trial reported by Costanzi and associates for the Southwest Oncology Group.[25] They had previously shown a response rate of 30% for the combination of carmustine, hydroxyurea, and dacarbazine (BHD). In a prospective trial, they compared BHD against BHD plus immunotherapy with bacillus Calmette Guérin (BCG), and against a combination of dacarbazine plus BCG. The response rate for BHD was 31%, for BHD plus BCG 27%, and for dacarbazine plus BCG 18%. Survival rates were not significantly different between the two treatment arms.[25] If one assumed that the BCG had no adverse effect, the study would support a benefit for BHD over dacarbazine. However, this is not altogether a safe assumption.[14,17,47] It is unfortunate that there was no treatment arm with dacarbazine alone in this study.

A study conducted by the Central Oncology Group failed to show any difference in response rate between BHD and dacarbazine alone, or two other combinations.[13] This conflict in results may reflect dosage differences, but a later study by the Central Oncology Group found no improvement in response rates for similar combinations when the doses were escalated to produce toxicity.[41] Nonetheless, BHD remains one of the more popular combinations used for the treatment of metastatic melanoma.

It must be remembered that these trials might not have detected a difference in favor of combination chemotherapy even if such a difference were in fact present. The most powerful of them[23] would have only a 90% accuracy of detecting a difference in a response rate as great as between 20% and 37%, certainly still within the range of differences claimed by the proponents of combination chemotherapy. A study comparing standard BHD to the same drugs given sequentially in an attempt to exploit cell kinetics showed no benefit for the sequential approach.[24]

Another combination of growing popularity is bleomycin, vincristine, lomustine, and dacarbazine (BOLD), for which response rates of 39% to 48% have been reported.[3,75] Other combinations reported to have favorable response rates in trials of reasonable size include cyclophosphamide plus vincristine with or without procarbazine,[12] and various other combinations of dacarbazine, bleomycin, nitrosoureas, and vincristine,[1,13,32,35,41] although one group has reported that further experience did not confirm an early high response rate.[7] The latter report is to be commended, as the literature too often becomes unbalanced by the preferential publication of early "promising" results of regimens that do not prove in the long run to be therapeutic advances.

NEWER AGENTS

CISPLATIN

Cisplatin has been reported to be active as a single agent.[4,40] This has led to studies of combinations including cisplatin, particularly the combination of vinblastine, bleomycin, and cisplatin (VBD), which has been effective in other tumors. Nathanson and associates[60] reported 16 responses among 34 evaluable patients, a response rate of 47%, including complete responses in visceral metastatic deposits, but Bajetta and associates[5] observed only eight responses among 29 evaluable patients, a rate of 28%, without responses in visceral sites. Although the latter authors correctly interpret their study as not confirming that VBD is superior to other combinations, the difference between their overall response rate and that reported by Nathanson and associates is only marginally significant (p = 0.09; Fisher's exact test). The combination of cisplatin with dacarbazine with or without other agents seems to offer little advantage over single-agent therapy,[38,45] and the combination of cisplatin with the alkylating agent ifosfamide, which was regarded favorably after a report of eight responses in 15 cases,[74] failed to produce responses in 14 later cases.[6,10]

AGENTS EXPLOITING THE MELANIN SYNTHETIC PATHWAY

The melanin synthetic pathway offers several theoretical targets for rationally designed chemotherapy,[63,84] since most other melanin-synthesizing cells serve a nonessential role. Albinism would be a small price for the cure of metastatic melanoma, provided that no unforeseen complications occur in the central nervous system. Melanin is a heteropolymer synthesized from tyrosine through intermediates including dihydroxyphenylalanine (dopa) and various toxic quinones. The process is controlled at several steps by the enzyme tyrosinase[63] and is stimulated by the hormone melanotropin (MSH). Stimulation of melanin synthesis by a combination of MSH and tyrosine is mildly cytotoxic, and levodopa and dopamine, which are accumulated preferentially in melanoma tissues, also inhibit the growth of melanoma cells in the B-16 model. Clinical application of this approach is at an early stage, but Wick[85] has reported inhibition of DNA synthesis in biopsies of human malignant melanoma after dopamine infusion. Substituted phenols such as 4-hydroxyanisole have been used as false precursors that are converted by tyrosinase to toxic metabolites.[59] Thiouracil can also be incorporated into the melanin synthetic pathway, and could thus act as a carrier for radioactive or other cytotoxic agents.[30]

OTHER DRUGS

All other new agents have proved disappointing, including diglycoaldehyde,[82] amsacrine,[27,43] piperazinedione,[64,66] etoposide,[2] teniposide,[19] and maytansine.[19]

HORMONAL THERAPY

Several lines of evidence suggest that melanoma is responsive hormonally. Human pigmentation is increased at puberty and during pregnancy; women with melanoma have a better prognosis than men do[33,69,76,77] and anecdotes describe the remission or exacerbation of melanoma metastases during pregnancy. Various persons have described receptors for estrogen in melanoma cells,[61] although it is possible that this finding is an artifact owing to the enzymatic liberation of isotope from labeled ligand by tyrosinase.

Diethylstilbestrol was reported to produce response in 2 of 35 patients with metastatic malignant melanoma.[37] The nonsteroidal antiestrogen tamoxifen has also been reported to be active, producing responses in 4 of 26 patients in one study, and 3 of 17 in another.[46,62] This raised considerable interest, especially because of the low morbidity associated with tamoxifen therapy, but the majority of later reports suggest a very low response rate,[29,49,52,70,79,83] even when doses as high as 100 mg/m^2 were used.[28] The cumulative response rate in these negative studies was 2:146. Hormonal therapy may be useful as a

placebo, but its contribution to therapeutic advancement is minimal.

CONCLUSIONS

The chemotherapeutic treatment of metastatic melanoma remains a challenge both to the investigator attempting to develop improved regimens and to the clinician. Future progress will demand the identification of new active agents. While these may emerge from the empirical investigation of new compounds, the past results of this approach are unimpressive. The rational exploitation of the biochemical differences between melanoma and normal nonpigmented cells may offer more hope.

REFERENCES

1. Abele R, Bernheim J, Cumps E, Buyse M, Kenis Y: Re-evaluation of the combination of CCNU, vincristine and bleomycin in the treatment of malignant disseminated melanoma. Cancer Treat Rep 65:505, 1981
2. Ahmann DL, Bisel HF, Edmonson JH, Hahn RG, O'Connell MJ, Frytak S: Phase II study of VP-16-213 versus dianhydrogalactitol in patients with metastatic malignant melanoma. Cancer Treat Rep 60:1681, 1976
3. Ahn SS, Morton DL: Preliminary results of BOLD for disseminated melanoma. Proc Am Soc Clin Oncol 1:179, 1982
4. Al-Sarraf M, Fletcher W, Oishi N, Pugh R, Hewlett JS, Balducci L, McCracken J, Padilla F: Cisplatin hydration with and without mannitol diuresis in refractory disseminated malignant melanoma: A Southwest Oncology Group study. Cancer Treat Rep 66:31, 1982
5. Bajetta E, Rovej R, Buzzoni R, Vaglini M, Bonadonna G: Treatment of advanced malignant melanoma with vinblastine, bleomycin and cisplatin. Cancer Treat Rep 66:1299, 1982
6. Balda BR, Jehn U, Klövekorn W, Wohlrab A: Kombinationschemotherapie malinger melanome mit cis-diamino-dichloro-platin (II) und Ifosfamid. Klin Wochenschr 59:781, 1981
7. Bellet RE, Catalano RB, Mastrangelo MJ, Berd D: Positive phase II trial of dibromodulcitol in patients with metastatic melanoma refractory to DTIC and a nitrosourea. Cancer Treat Rep 62:2095, 1978
8. Bellet RE, Mastrangelo MJ, Berd D, Lustbader E: Chemotherapy of metastatic malignant melanoma. In Clark WH Jr, Goldman LI, Mastrangelo MJ (eds): Human Malignant Melanoma, p 325. New York, Grune & Stratton, 1979

9. Bellet RE, Mastrangelo MJ, Laucius JF, Bodurtha AJ: Randomized prospective trial of DTIC (NSC-45388) alone versus BCNU (NSC-409962) plus vincristine (NSC-67574) in the treatment of metastatic malignant melanoma. Cancer Treat Rep 60:595, 1976

10. Berdel WE, Fink U, Emmerich B, Maubach PA, Busch U, Remy W, Rastetter J: Chemotherapie malinger melanoma mit cis-diaminodichloroplatinum und Ifosfamid. Dtsch Med Wochenschr 107:26, 1982

11. Broder LE, Hansen HH: 1-(2-chloroethyl)-3-cyclohexyl-1-nitrosourea (CCNU, NSC-79037): A comparison of drug administration at four-week and six-week intervals. Eur J Cancer 9:147, 1973

12. Bryne MJ: Cyclophosphamide, vincristine and procarbazine in the treatment of malignant melanoma. Cancer 38:1922, 1976

13. Carter RD, Krementz ET, Hill GJ II, Metter GE, Fletcher WS, Golomb FM, Grage TB, Minton JP, Sparks FC: DTIC (NSC-45388) and combination therapy for melanoma. I. Studies with DTIC, BCNU (NSC-409962), CCNU (NSC-79037), vincristine (NSC-67574), and hydroxyurea (NSC-32065). Cancer Treat Rep 60:601, 1976

14. Coates AS: BCG immunotherapy. Med J Aust 2:143, 1977

15. Coates AS, Abraham S, Kaye SB: On the receiving end: Patient perception of the side effects of cancer chemotherapy. Eur J Cancer Clin Oncol 19:202, 1983

16. Coates AS, Fisher DC, McNeil DR: On the receiving end. II. Linear analogue self assessment (LASA) in the evaluation of quality of life in cancer patients receiving therapy. Eur J Cancer Clin Oncol 19:1633, 1983

17. Coates AS, Klopp RG, Zarling JM, Borden EC, Crowley JJ, Carbone PP: Immunologic function during adjuvant BCG immunotherapy for malignant melanoma: Induction of anergy. Cancer Immunology and Immunotherapy 7:175, 1979

18. Coates AS, McCarthy WH, Milton GW: Dibromodulcitol (DBD) chemotherapy of malignant melanoma—a phase II study. Proceedings of the Clinical Oncologic Society of Australia, 1981

19. Comis RL: Systemic therapy of malignant melanoma. Current Concepts in Oncology 4:18, 1982

20. Comis RL, Carter SK: Integration of chemotherapy into combined modality therapy of solid tumors. IV. Malignant melanoma. Cancer Treat Rep 1:285, 1974

21. Costanza ME, Nathanson L, Costello WG, Wolter J, Brunk F, Colsky J, Hall T, Oberfield RA, Regelson W: Results of a randomized study comparing DTIC with TIC mustard in malignant melanoma. Cancer 37:1654, 1976

22. Costanza ME, Nathanson L, Lenhard R, Wolter J, Colsky J, Oberfield RA, Schilling A: Therapy of malignant melanoma with an imidazole carboxamide and Bis-Chloroethyl Nitrosourea. Cancer 30:1457, 1972

23. Costanza ME, Nathanson L, Schoenfeld D, Wolter J, Colsky J, Regelson W, Cunningham T, Sedransk N: Results with methyl-CCNU and DTIC in metastatic melanoma. Cancer 40:1010, 1977

24. Costanzi J, Fabian C, Wilson H, Dixon D: Sequential combination chemotherapy for disseminated melanoma: A Southwest Oncology Group study. Cancer Treat Rep 65:732, 1981

25. Costanzi JJ, Vaitkevicius VK, Quagliana JM, Hoogstraten B, Coltman CA Jr, Delaney FC: Combination chemotherapy for disseminated malignant melanoma. Cancer 35:342, 1975

26. Cowan DH, Bergsagel DE: Intermittent treatment of metastatic malignant melanoma with high-dose 5-(3,3-dimethyl-1-triazeno)imidazole-4-carboxamide (NSC-45388). Cancer Chemother Rep 55:175, 1971

27. Creagan ET, Ahmann DL, Ingle JN, Purvis JD, Green SJ: Phase II evaluation of PALA and AMSA for patients with disseminated malignant melanoma. Cancer Treat Rep 65:169, 1981

28. Creagan ET, Ingle JN, Ahmann DL, Green SJ: Phase II study of high-dose tamoxifen (NSC-180973) in patients with disseminated malignant melanoma. Cancer 49:1353, 1982

29. Creagan ET, Ingle JN, Green SJ, Ahmann DL, Jiang NS: Phase II study of tamoxifen in patients with disseminated malignant melanoma. Cancer Treat Rep 64:199, 1980

30. Dencker L, Larsson B, Olander K, Ullberg S: A new melanoma seeker for possible clinical use: Selective accumulation of radiolabelled thiouracil. Br J Cancer 45:95, 1982

31. DeVita VT, Carbone PP, Owens AH Jr, Gold GL, Krant MJ, Edmonson J: Clinical trials with 1,3-bis (2-chloro-ethyl)-1-nitrosourea, NSC-409962. Cancer Res 25:1876, 1965

32. DeWasch G, Bernheim J, Michel J, Lejeune F, Kenis Y: Combination chemotherapy with three marginally effective agents, CCNU, vincristine and bleomycin, in the treatment of stage III melanoma. Cancer Treat Rep 60:1273, 1976

33. Drzewiecki KT, Andersen PK: Survival with malignant melanoma. A regression analysis of prognostic factors. Cancer 49:2414, 1982

34. Einhorn LH, Burgess MA, Vallejos C, Bodey GP Sr, Gutterman J, Mavligit G, Hersh EM, Luce JK, Frei E III, Freireich EJ, Gottlieb JA: Prognostic correlations and response to treatment in advanced metastatic malignant melanoma. Cancer Res 34:1995, 1974

35. Everall JD, Dowd PM: Use of combination chemotherapy with CCNU, bleomycin and vincristine in the treatment of metastatic melanoma in patients resistant to DTIC therapy. Cancer Treat Rep 63:151, 1979

36. Fisher RI, Chabner BA, Myers CE: Phase II study of high dose methotrexate in patients with advanced malignant melanoma. Cancer Treat Rep 63:147, 1979

37. Fisher RI, Young RC, Lippmann ME: Diethylstilbestrol therapy of surgically non-resected malignant melanoma. Proc Am Assoc Cancer Res 19:339, 1978

38. Friedman MA, Kaufman DA, Williams JE, Resser KJ, Rosenbaum EH, Cohen RJ, Glassberg AB, Blume MR, Gershow J, Chan EYC: Combined DTIC and cis-dichloro-diammineplatinum(II) therapy for patients with disseminated melanoma: A Northern California Oncology Group study. Cancer Treat Rep 63:493, 1979

39. Golomb FM: Chemotherapy of Melanoma. In McCarthy WH (ed): Melanoma and Skin Cancer, p 497. Sydney, Blight, 1972

40. Goodnight JE Jr, Moseley HS, Eilber FR, Sarna G, Morton DL: Cis-dichloro-diammineplatinum II alone and combined with DTIC for treatment of disseminated malignant melanoma. Cancer Treat Rep 63:2005, 1979

41. Hill GJ II, Metter GE, Krementz ET, Fletcher WS, Golomb FM, Ramirez G, Grage TB, Moss SE: DTIC and combination therapy for melanoma. II. Escalating schedules of DTIC with BCNU, CCNU and vincristine. Cancer Treat Rep 63:1989, 1979

42. Hopkins J, Richards F II, Case D, Pope E, Spurr C, White D, Jackson D, Stuart J, Muss H, Cooper MR: A phase II study of dibromodulcitol (DBD) in stage IV melanoma. Proc Am Soc Clin Oncol 1:179, 1982

43. Houghton AN, Camacho F, Wittes R, Young CW: Phase II study of AMSA in patients with metastatic malignant melanoma. Cancer Treat Rep 65:170, 1981

44. Karakousis CP, Carlson M: High-dose methotrexate in malignant melanoma. Cancer Treat Rep 63:1405, 1979

45. Karakousis CP, Getaz EP, Bjornsson S, Henderson ES, Irequi M, Martinez L, Ospina J, Cavins J, Preisler H, Holyoke E, Holtermann O: Cis-dichlorodiammineplatinum(II) and DTIC in malignant melanoma. Cancer Treat Rep 63:2009, 1979

46. Karakousis CP, Lopez RE, Bhakoo HS, Rosen F, Moore R, Carlson M: Estrogen and progesterone receptors and tamoxifen in malignant melanoma. Cancer Treat Rep 64:819, 1980

47. Lamoureux G, Poisson R, Desrosiers M: An antagonistic side-effect of BCG immunotherapy: Induction of immunological anergy. In Lamoureux G, Turcotte R, Portelance V (eds): BCG in Cancer Immunotherapy, p 167. New York, Grune & Stratton, 1976

48. Lavin PT, Flowerdew G: Studies in variation associated with the measurement of solid tumors. Cancer 46:1286, 1980

49. Leake RE, Laing L, Calman KC, Macbeth FR: Estrogen receptors and anti-estrogen therapy in selected human solid tumors. Cancer Treat Rep 64:797, 1980

50. Lee YJ, Catane R, Rozencweig M, Bono VH Jr, Muggia FM, Simon R, Staquet MJ: Analysis and interpretation of response rates for anticancer drugs. Cancer Treat Rep 63:1713, 1979

51. Lee YJ, Staquet MJ, Simon R, Catane R, Muggia F: Two-stage plans for patient accrual in phase II cancer clinical trials. Cancer Treat Rep 63:1732, 1979

52. Leichman CG, Samson MK, Baker LH: Phase II trial of tamoxifen in malignant melanoma. Cancer Treat Rep 66:1447, 1982

53. Lessner HE: BCNU (1,3,bis[B-chloroethyl]-1-nitrosourea): Effects on advanced Hodgkin's disease and other neoplasia. Cancer 22:451, 1968

54. Luce JK: Chemotherapy of melanoma. Semin Oncol 2:179, 1975

55. McElwain TJ, Hedley DW, Burton G, Clink HM, Gordon MY, Jarman M, Juttnen CA, Millar JL, Milsted RA, Prentice G, Smith IE, Spence D, Woods M: Marrow autotransplantation accelerates haematological recovery in patients with malignant melanoma treated with high-dose Melphalan. Br J Cancer 40:72, 1979

56. Medina W, Kirkwood JM: Phase II trial of mitolactol in patients with metastatic melanoma. Cancer Treat Rep 66:195, 1982

57. Miller AB, Hoogstraten B, Staquet M, Winkler A: Reporting results of cancer treatment. Cancer 47:207, 1981

58. Moertel CG, Hanley JA: The effects of measuring error on the results of therapeutic trials in advanced cancer. Cancer 38:388, 1976

59. Morgan BDG, O'Neill T, Dewey DL, Galpine AR, Riley PA: Treatment of malignant melanoma by intravascular 4-hydroxyanisole. Clin Oncol 7:227, 1981

60. Nathanson L, Kaufman SD, Carey RW: Vinblastine, infusion, bleomycin, and cis-dichlorodiammineplatinum chemotherapy in metastatic melanoma. Cancer 48:1290, 1981

61. Neifeld JP, Lippman ME: Steroid hormone receptors and melanoma. J Invest Dermatol 74:379, 1980

62. Nesbit RA, Woods RL, Tattersall MHN, Fox RM, Forbes JF, MacKay IR, Goodyear M: Tamoxifen in malignant melanoma. N Engl J Med 301:1241, 1979

63. Pawelek J, Korner A, Bergstrom A, Bologna J: New regulators of melanin biosynthesis and the autodestruction of melanoma cells. Nature 286:617, 1980

64. Presant CA, Bartolucci AA, Balch CM, Troner M, the Southeastern Cancer Study Group: A randomized comparison of cyclophosphamide, DTIC with or without piperazinedione in metastatic malignant melanoma. Cancer 49:1355, 1982

65. Presant CA, Bartolucci AA, the Southeastern Cancer Study Group: Prognostic factors in metastatic malignant melanoma: The Southeastern Cancer Study Group experience. Cancer 49:2192, 1982

66. Presant CA, Bartolucci AA, Ungaro P, Oldham R: Phase II trial of piperazinedione in malignant melanoma: A report by the Southeastern Cancer Study Group. Cancer Treat Rep 63:1367, 1979

67. Pritchard KI, Quirt IC, Cowan DH, Osoba D, Kutas GJ: DTIC therapy in metastatic malignant melanoma:

A simplified dose schedule. Cancer Treat Rep 64: 1123, 1980

68. Ramirez G, Wilson W, Grage T, Hill G: Phase II evaluation of 1,3-bis(2-chloro-ethyl)-1-nitrosourea (BCNU: NSC-409962) in patients with solid tumors. Cancer Chemother Rep 56:787, 1972

69. Rampen F: Malignant melanoma: Sex differences in survival after evidence of distant metastasis. Br J Cancer 42:52, 1980

70. Reimer RR, Costanzi J, Fabian C: Southwest Oncology Group experience with tamoxifen in metastatic melanoma. Cancer Treat Rep 66:1680, 1982

71. Retsas S, Peat I, Ashford R, Coe M, Maher J, Drury A, Hanham IWF, Phillips RH, Newton KA, Westbury G: Updated results of vindesine as a single agent in the therapy of advanced malignant melanoma. Cancer Treat Rev (Suppl)7:87, 1980

72. Rumke P: Malignant melanoma. In Pinedo HM (ed): Cancer Chemotherapy 1979, p 412. Amsterdam–Oxford, Excerpta Medica, 1979

73. Samson MK, Baker LH, Cummings G, Talley RW, McDonald B, Bhathena DB: Clinical trial of chlorozotocin, DTIC, and dactinomycin in metastatic malignant melanoma. Cancer Treat Rep 66:371, 1982

74. Schmidt CG, Becher R: Kombinierte chemotherapie des metastasierenden Melanoblastoms mit Ifosfamid und cis-diamino-dichloro-platin(II). Dtsch Med Wochenschr 104:872, 1979

75. Seigler HF, Lucas VS Jr, Pickett NJ, Huang AT: DTIC, CCNU, bleomycin and vincristine (BOLD) in metastatic melanoma. Cancer 46:2346, 1980

76. Shaw HM, McGovern VJ, Milton GW, Farago GA, McCarthy WH: Malignant melanoma: Influence of site of lesion and age of patient in the female superiority in survival. Cancer 46:2731, 1980

77. Shaw HM, McGovern VJ, Milton GW, Farago GA, McCarthy WH: The female superiority in survival in clinical stage II cutaneous malignant melanoma. Cancer 49:1941, 1982

78. Smith IE, Hedley DW, Powles TJ, McElwain TJ: Vindesine: A phase II study in the treatment of breast carcinoma, malignant melanoma, and other tumors. Cancer Treat Rep 62:1427, 1978

79. Telhaug R, Klepp O, Bormer O: Phase II study of tamoxifen in patients with metastatic malignant melanoma. Cancer Treat Rep 66:1437, 1982

80. Thigpen JT, Al–Sarraf M, Hewlett JS: Phase II trial of dianhydrogalactitol in metastatic malignant melanoma. A Southwest Oncology Group study. Cancer Treat Rep 63:525, 1979

81. Van Amburg AL III, Presant CA, Burns D: Phase II study of chlorozotocin in malignant melanoma: A Southeastern Cancer Study Group report. Cancer Treat Rep 66:1431, 1982

82. Vosika GJ, Briscoe K, Carey RW, O'Donnell JF, Perry MC, Budman D, Richards F III, Coleman M: Phase II study of diglycoaldehyde in malignant melanomas and soft tissue sarcomas. Cancer Treat Rep 65:823, 1981

83. Wagstaff J, Thatcher N, Rankin E, Crowther D: Tamoxifen in the treatment of metastatic malignant melanoma. Cancer Treat Rep 66:1771, 1982

84. Wick MM: An experimental approach to the chemotherapy of melanoma. J Invest Dermatol 74:63, 1980

85. Wick MM: Inhibitory effect of dopamine on human malignant melanoma. Proc Am Soc Clin Oncol 21:328, 1980

86. Young RC, Canellos GP, Chabner BA, Schein PS, Brereton HD, DeVita VT: Treatment of malignant melanoma with methyl CCNU. Clin Pharmacol Ther 15:617, 1974

DONN J. BRASCHO

Radiotherapy for Metastatic Melanoma
15

Radiation Biology and Melanoma
Dose Schedules and Energy Sources
Combination Therapy
Radiation Treatment of Specific Metastatic
        Sites
    Skin, Subcutaneous, and Lymph Nodes
    Central Nervous System (CNS)
    Bone
    Abdomen and Pelvis
    Lung and Mediastinum
Radiation Treatment of Primary Cutaneous
        Melanoma
Experience of the University of Alabama
        Radiation Therapy Department
Summary

Melanomas have a long-standing reputation of being radioresistant tumors. A frequently quoted reference supporting this view is an article about 400 cases of melanoma treated at the Memorial Sloan-Kettering Hospital in New York between 1917 and 1935.[1] In that series, radiation was used only when the disease was far advanced or when a surgical operation would have been very mutilating. No details were given as to the type of irradiation or the dosages that were used. It was noted that in only 2.5% of cases was there evidence of radiation response, and the treatment nearly always failed to provide palliation. The author concluded that melanoma was much more radioresistant than most other tumors and, therefore, that radiation was not considered as proper treatment for this disease.

During the next decade, several investigators, largely from the European radiation therapy centers, advocated irradiation for treating melanoma.[15,33,35] Dickson was one of the first to question the prevailing 1950s concept that all melanomas were radioresistant.[13] In a combined series of patients treated at the Johns Hopkins Hospital and Toronto General Hospital, he reported the treatment results of wide surgical excision of the primary tumor and the regional lymph nodes, plus postoperative radiation therapy to areas containing metastases on histologic examination. High doses of radiation were generally used. This was not a controlled randomized study, but the survival results suggested some value for postoperative radiation therapy. This article stimulated more interest in the adjunctive use of radiation therapy in melanoma patients.

Hilaris and associates reported in 1963 that radiation therapy offered effective palliation for selected patients with distant metastases.[21] In their series, measurable responses were obtained in 57% of patients with osseous, cerebral, and visceral metastases. One case of particular interest was treated with interstitial irradiation for an ulcerated soft-tissue lesion of the lower leg. Using this high-dose technique, they noted a complete response with no evidence of disease 6 years after implant and 10 years after diagnosis. This example demonstrated that excellent regression of soft-tissue masses could be obtained with high doses of radiation.

In retrospect, one reason melanoma was so often considered radioresistant was that the unique biologic properties of the tumor were not recognized at first, and optimal dose schedules for this type of cancer were not consistently used.

RADIATION BIOLOGY AND MELANOMA

Hellriegel treated both primary and metastatic melanoma with large doses of irradiation and concluded in 1963 that, while melanoma could be successfully treated by radiation therapy, "high" doses were necessary for successful treatment.[20] This was perhaps the first clinical reference to support the current concept of high individual dose irradiation for treating metastatic melanoma.

It was not until the early 1970s that *in vitro*[3,12] and *in vivo*[22] studies suggested that the observed "radioresistance" of melanoma was the result of an unusually "large shoulder" in the radiation cell survival curve (Fig. 15-1). Such observations supported the view that optimal radiation treatment should use a dose schedule of relatively few fractions, but high doses. Habermalz and Fischer, in 1976, first used individual doses of 600 rad, or greater, given once or twice weekly for skin metastases; partial or complete regression occurred in 29 of 33 treated lesions.[17] Hornsey, in 1978, showed that dose fractions of 400 rad to 800 rad were significantly more effective than 200 rad to 300 rad.[23] He suggested that the high individual dose needed for response in melanomas reflected the cell's large capacity to re-

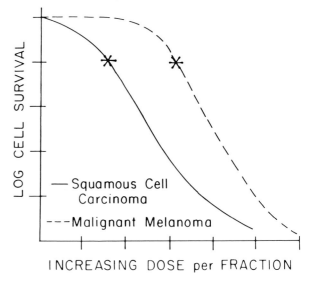

FIG. 15–1 Comparison of the relative log cell survival as determined by the capacity to undergo sublethal damage repair for a hypothetical squamous cell carcinoma and a melanoma. The *asterisks* indicate the radiation dose per fraction required to eventuate an observable response (*i.e.*, isoeffect).

pair sublethal damage and, further, that this effect might result from hypoxia.

DOSE SCHEDULES AND ENERGY SOURCES

Overgaard compared different doses per fraction and different total doses in patients with cutaneous and lymph node metastases from melanoma.[28] He found that an increased dose per treatment resulted in an increased response, but the response did not correlate with the total dose of irradiation. The response was significantly better with fraction sizes greater than 800 rad when compared to doses less than 400 rad per fraction. He also referred to the presence of a large shoulder of the radiation survival curve of melanoma cells *in vitro* and recommended a dose of 900 rad administered three times over 8 days.[28] Such a treatment schedule was sufficient to control tumors up to 9 cm × 10 cm in size completely, even though the cumulative dose was rather small.

Another study supporting higher radiation dose-fraction size was reported by Strauss and associates.[32] This was a retrospective review over an 8-year period in which the dose-fractionation schemes evolved from standard fraction size to large-dose techniques. They observed that the radiation fraction size was a major factor in determining the treatment response. The sites of metastatic lesions evaluated were brain, spinal cord, soft tissue, and bone. The large dose per fraction of 400 rad to 700 rad appeared to be more effective than the other fractionation programs in providing good overall palliation for specific symptoms. Individual treatments of 600 rad to 800 rad resulted in the best overall response rate (80%).

Doss and co-workers also reviewed radiation response rates for metastatic melanoma with particular attention to the time/dose fractionation schedules.[14] Osseous and cerebral metastases were the most common recurrences treated. The overall complete response rate was 37%. For regimens using more than 400 rad per fraction, a 67% response rate was noted. When primary soft-tissue recurrences were treated, the patients with small-volume lesions did best. In spite of high dose per fraction, the toxicity was not significantly different from that of standard radiation courses.

Harwood and Cummings[18] reported treatment results in 54 patients divided into three clinical categories of disease: (1) microscopic residual melanoma following surgery, (2) gross residual melanoma after surgery, and (3) recurrent melanoma. Selected high-risk patients with resected regional lymph node metastases were also treated. A high-dose fractionated radiation treatment was given on days 0, 7, and 21 with a daily dose fraction of 800 rad. This regimen was found to be suitable for treating large volumes of tissues such as the axillae, supraclavicular fossae, inguinal-iliac regions, and neck. However, they warned that it is not applicable to visceral metastases in the brain, lung, or liver, where such a radiation dose is above the limits of normal tissue tolerance. While the local control rates were improved by radiation, there was a high rate of systemic failure at other sites in such patients, emphasizing the need for more effective systemic therapy for melanoma. In their experience, the response rate using this high-dose fractionation regimen was substantially greater than had been previously observed with conventional fractionated radiotherapy.

COMBINATION THERAPY

The unique properties of melanoma radiosensitivity to large-dose fractions of irradiation have stimulated interest in combined treatment to maximize the cell's susceptibility to irreversible radiation damage. It has been postulated that the high individual dose treatments overwhelm the mechanisms by which sublethal radiation damage is repaired by the melanoma cell.[23,28] For example, there is radiobiologic evidence that superoxide dismutase, which occurs at high levels in melanin granules, effectively scavenges and neutralizes the free radicals produced by ionizing radiation.[26,27] With such an enzyme present in melanoma cells, massive single doses are necessary to counteract the loss of free radicals caused by the enzyme's reparative actions. Furthermore, large lesions, whether primary or secondary, may not be responsive to high total dose or high individual dose therapy because of hypoxic and resistant cell compartments within the tumor.

Because of these biologic properties, there has been an intensified interest in either adjunctive methods or new treatment modalities to overcome these influences on the radiation effect. New approaches that minimize the repair mechanisms for irradiation damage include high-energy transfer radiation such as neutrons, hyperbaric oxygen,[31] chemical radiosensitizers,[30] BCG (bacille Calmette-

Guérin) treatment, or hyperthermia in combination with conventional radiation.

One of the earliest studies was by Thomson and colleagues,[34] who evaluated the relative biologic effectiveness of fast-neutron beams relative to cobalt 60 radiation for a human melanoma cell system *in vitro*. This study did not confirm that fast-neutron radiotherapy *per se* would have a significant treatment effect on melanoma. The differential response of the melanoma cell line to fast-neutron radiation compared to standard x-irradiation was similar to that reported for a variety of normal and tumor-cell systems assayed *in vitro* or *in vivo*. However, their *in vitro* data supported the findings by others that melanoma does not exhibit the radioresistance previously attributed to it from *in vivo* studies.

Another *in vitro* study by Damsker and associates[10] evaluated the radiosensitizing effects of the 7-hydroxy metabolite of chlorpromazine (7-OHCPZ). Previous *in vitro* studies indicated that there was selective localization of chlorpromazine (CPZ) in melanin-rich tissues and that CPZ was an effective radiosensitizing agent against certain melanoma lines. The mechanism of this radiosensitizing effect is unknown. The authors chose to evaluate this particular CPZ metabolite, since it had a greater melanin affinity than its parent compound. Their study showed that 7-OHCPZ was more effective than CPZ as a radiosensitizer for treating transplanted melanoma in animals. Further structural modification of CPZ is under way in an effort to arrive at a molecular substitution pattern that could provide optimal sensitizing capacity. Work within the Radiation Therapy Department of the University of Alabama in Birmingham (UAB) indicates that an alternative mechanism of CPZ action may be modulated by its calmodulin binding activity within cells.* Structural analogues are currently being analyzed to characterize this phenomenon further. This may provide the groundwork for future clinical studies to evaluate the sensitizing effect of these compounds *in vivo*.

A new treatment combination with considerable clinical success is the use of hyperthermia plus radiation therapy for metastatic melanoma in the soft tissues. Kim and associates initiated a clinical trial in 1975 to evaluate the effects of hyperthermia used either alone or in combination with radiation therapy.[24,25] Eligible patients had multiple recurrent melanomas, with the majority of metastases being subcutaneous and in regional lymph nodes. Radio-

frequency heating of lesions for 30 minutes at 42°C to 43.5°C was used immediately prior to radiation therapy. Most patients were irradiated with electron beams in a variety of radiation time/dose fractionation schedules. The radiation schedule for the majority of the lesions was once or twice a week.

There was a 70% overall complete tumor response rate following the combination hyperthermia and radiation therapy. This was significantly greater than that achieved with radiation therapy alone (46%). For tumor volumes less than 10 cc, high dose per fraction radiotherapy alone yielded an 80% control rate. However, for lesions greater than 10 cc, the control rate declined to only 30% when treated with radiation therapy alone. For all tumor volumes, the combination of heat with radiation yielded 80% local tumor control. The best tumor-control rate was obtained when hyperthermia was combined with radiation fractions of 550 rad to 660 rad. The initial rate of tumor regression was characteristically more prompt for tumors treated with combination therapy than with radiation alone. An important observation was that skin or subcutaneous toxicities were not disproportionately enhanced after the combined treatment compared with radiation alone. This was attributed in part to the focal differential temperature induced within the tumor bed by the radiofrequency heating. These studies again supported the concept that large doses per fraction are essential in obtaining adequate responses in melanoma. Additionally, this report documented the importance of tumor volume in disease control. While further experience is necessary in the technical application of hyperthermia to lesions in various parts of the body, this study demonstrates that the addition of hyperthermia can augment the therapeutic effect of radiation in melanoma treatment for metastases.

The combination of radiation with BCG for the treatment of skin metastases was studied by Plesnicar and Rudolf.[29] Both agents were applied in reduced dosages predicted to cause minimal side-effects. This was done to enhance the BCG-mediated skin reaction by percutaneous irradiation. Their clinical experiments were based on laboratory data indicating a more consistent inhibition of tumor growth resulting from BCG treatment combined with irradiation. This preliminary investigation was the first to report the efficacy of intralesional BCG injections into metastatic skin nodules combined with irradiation; however, survival results are not yet available.

At this time, there is no convincing evidence

---

*Lawson A: Personal communication

that standard chemotherapeutic agents significantly enhance the radiation effect on melanoma; however, such adjunctive chemotherapy trials have been meager.[6] Theoretically, there may be some potential advantage in combining irradiation with cytotoxic drugs such as Adriamycin or cisplatinum. It is likely that the use of such combination treatment will be limited by the combined effects on normal tissues.

RADIATION TREATMENT OF SPECIFIC METASTATIC SITES

In this section, specific recommendations for radiation therapy are made for various metastatic sites. The reader is also referred to Chapters 12 and 13 for a general discussion of diagnosis and treatment of melanoma metastases. A summary of dose schedules for radiation therapy at these metastatic sites is listed in Table 15-1.

SKIN, SUBCUTANEOUS, AND LYMPH NODES

Radiation therapy can be quite effective for palliative control of metastases in these areas. Generally, it is used in the setting of multiple or confluent skin or subcutaneous lesions that cannot be surgically ex-

cised, or for nodal metastases that are not surgically accessible (see Chap. 13). Radiation therapy might also be considered in selected patients after multiple or recurring metastases have been excised, but the risk of further recurrence is great (*e.g.,* recurrent intransit metastases on the trunk).

High-dose fractionated irradiation treatment is generally indicated. A dose of 600 rad twice weekly to a total dose of 3600 rad to 4200 rad is well tolerated (Fig. 15-2). Another scheme is to give 800 rad on days 0, 7, and 21. This is tolerable even in large treatment volumes of tissue and does provide long-term palliation. More rapid palliation can be obtained by delivering 800 rad on day 0 and 400 rad on the next 2 consecutive days. The choice of radiation energy will depend on the depth and thickness of the tumor. The majority of these lesions are within 4 cm of the skin surface and can be adequately treated with electron-beam irradiation. Deeper tumors will require a more penetrating beam, such as photons from a cobalt or linear accelerator machine. For tumors that have a large volume (*i.e.,* greater than 10 cc), the addition of hyperthermia to irradiation should be considered. The tumor can be heated and irradiated in succession daily on the 2-day weekly scheme.

Radiation therapy might also be considered empirically as adjuvant postoperative treatment in

TABLE 15–1
RECOMMENDATIONS FOR RADIATION THERAPY OF MELANOMA

Situation	Time/Dose Technique	Total Dose
Cutaneous and Soft Tissue Metastases		
Postoperative, high risk	600 rad twice weekly	3600 rad–4200 rad in 21–28 days
Recurrent or metastatic	Same	Same
Alternate plans		
Rapid palliation	800 rad–400 rad–400 rad on 3 consecutive days	1600 rad in 3 days
Long-term palliation	800 rad on days 0, 7, 21	2400 rad in 21 days
Cerebral Metastases		
(Use adjunctive steroids prior to and during treatment)		
Long-term palliation	300 rad daily for 10 fractions, followed by a boost of 1800 rad–2400 rad in 600-rad fractions given twice weekly	4800 rad–5400 rad in 23–28 days
Short-term palliation	400 rad daily for 5 fractions	2000 rad in 5–7 days
Osseous Metastases	Same as for cutaneous and soft tissue	Same as for cutaneous and soft tissue
Intra-abdominal and Pelvic Nodal and Visceral Metastases		
Small volume	500 rad–600 rad twice weekly	2000 rad–4000 rad in 14–28 days
Large volume	200 rad–400 rad daily	3000 rad–4000 rad in 21–28 days
Head and Neck Melanoma	450 rad daily for 10 fractions	4500 rad in 14 days
(Postoperative or recurrence)		
Cord Compression, Airway Obstruction	500-rad–600-rad fractions twice weekly	2400 rad–3600 rad in 14–21 days

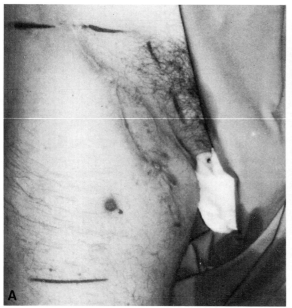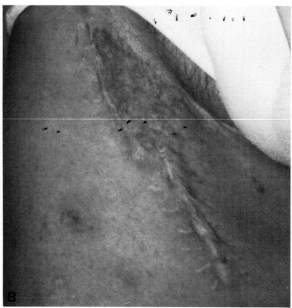

FIG. 15–2 Metastatic cutaneous melanoma after right inguinal dissection. (A) Radiation field marked and treated with electrons at a dose of 600 rad per fraction, twice weekly to 3600 rad in 19 days. (B) Six months later. The lesions are flat and have decreased pigmentation and size. No new areas of disease have developed.

selected patients who have resected lymph node metastases that are massive in size or number, or who have considerable soft-tissue extension of tumor into adjacent structures with close or incomplete margins of excision. Another possible indication for postoperative radiation at the primary cutaneous site would be microscopic or gross residual tumor after surgery.

A randomized prospective study involving adjuvant radiation therapy after surgical excision of regional nodal metastases was conducted by Creagan and colleagues at the Mayo Clinic.[8] They compared adjuvant radiation therapy to the regional lymph node area following lymphadenectomy with lymphadenectomy alone. Patients were treated with supervoltage radiation therapy using 5000 rad in 28 treatment days. The results indicated that adjuvant irradiation did not significantly affect either overall survival or disease-free survival.[8] However, the high-individual-dose technique now recommended for soft-tissue metastases was not used then.

CENTRAL NERVOUS SYSTEM (CNS)

The need for effective treatment of CNS metastases is amply evident, since they are a common cause of death from melanoma.[4] The therapeutic objectives are palliation of distressing symptoms and prolongation of life. In the recent literature, a variety of time/dose schemes have been evaluated to determine the efficacy of conventional radiation or more intensive radiation schedules in patients with metastatic melanoma in the CNS.[2,7,16] The response rates ranged from 37% to 100%, with an average of 68%. The mean duration of response varied from 2 to 5 months, with a mean of 3.5 months. The mean survival following radiation varied from 2 to 7.6 months, with an average of 3.8 months.

Carella and associates (1980) reported the results of 60 patients with CNS metastases treated according to two protocols from the Radiation Therapy Oncology Group.[5] Various radiation schemes were evaluated, but the small number of patients in each group precluded any definite conclusions about the optimal total dose and fractionation schedules that should be employed. However, their results did indicate a significant benefit from radiation therapy both in terms of symptom relief and improved neurologic function. Symptomatic improvement was observed in 76%, with 31% obtaining complete relief of symptoms. Of the four most frequent symptoms, complete or partial improvement was observed in 73% of patients with headache, 61% with motor dysfunction, 62% with impaired mentation, and 83% with convulsions. An improvement in neurologic function class occurred in 41% of the patients. The median survival was only 10 to 14 weeks, and 57% of the patients died from CNS metastases. The authors concluded that radiation therapy can improve neurologic symptoms and function in the majority (70%–90%) of patients. These results are comparable to those obtained for other histologic types of CNS metastases treated by irradiation, thus indicating that melanoma is not inherently a more radioresistant type of CNS metastases.

Vlock and colleagues (1982) also evaluated large-dose fraction schedules of radiation therapy for CNS metastases.[36] Based on two similar cohorts of patients with metastatic melanoma treated with megavoltage radiation to whole-brain fields and concomitant steroids, they concluded that large-dose fractions of radiation therapy achieved palliation similar to that achieved with low-dose fraction radiotherapy. There was no significant difference in the rate of improvement, maximum degree of response, or survival curves of patients treated with high-dose fractions as compared with low-dose fraction radiotherapy. Median survival was 3 months in the high-dose fraction group and 2.5 months in the low-dose fraction group. Patients treated with a high-dose technique had more significant side-effects, especially headache. However, in no instance did side-effects require discontinuation of therapy. These authors considered that the ease of treatment by the high-dose fraction method makes it suitable for application, even in the absence of a significant difference in the ultimate results.

The dose schedule most commonly used at UAB for long-term palliation of cerebral metastases is 300 rad daily for 10 fractions, followed by a boost of 1800 rad to 2400 rad in 600-rad fractions given twice weekly (see Table 15-1). Short-term palliation can be achieved by giving 2000 rad in 5 to 7 days. High-dose steroids are given prior to and during all radiation treatment in an attempt to prevent increased brain edema by the tumor. Usually dexamethasone (Decadron) in dosages of 16 mg/day to 24 mg/day is used.

In patients with solitary brain metastases, the relative efficacy and risk of radiation, surgical excision, or combined treatment is still not defined. Generally, however, surgical excision followed by whole brain irradiation is recommended in this situation (see Chap. 13).

There has been some interest in elective (prophylactic) cranial metastases in patients responding to systemic chemotherapy for metastases at other sites. Pilot studies have indicated that up to 45% of patients responding to intensive polychemotherapy will relapse in the brain. Prospective clinical trials to evaluate this concept are now in progress in the Southeastern Cancer Study Group.

Not infrequently, melanoma will metastasize to the spinal cord, resulting in neurologic deficits. Functional loss is usually preceded by pain. Early diagnosis is essential because loss of cord or nerve function is not usually reversible. Stabilization of tumor growth can be achieved with doses of 500 rad to 600 rad twice weekly to a total of 2400 rad to 3600 rad. A myelogram is usually necessary to localize the site of compression, and the radiation fields should be limited to the area of disease with 3-cm margins. A dose of 4200 rad to the spinal cord should not be exceeded, as cord damage may result.

BONE

Metastatic lesions in extremities can be easily treated using opposing radiation fields and high individual doses of supravoltage irradiation. Six hundred rad twice weekly to a total dose of 3600 rad to 4200 rad is well within normal-tissue tolerance. At least 80% of patients treated with this technique will have palliation of their pain. This response rate is similar to that of other types of metastatic bone lesions.

For osseous metastases to the vertebral column, a slower treatment scheme is usually necessary unless the intra-abdominal organs can be avoided. If large opposing fields are used, large amounts of small bowel will be included in the treatment volume, and high daily-dose fractions are not well tolerated. Usually, conventional palliative fractions of 200 rad to 400 rad daily to total doses within normal tissue tolerance are delivered. One should avoid doses to the intestine exceeding 4000 rad. If the kidneys are in the radiation field, the maximum tolerable dose is in the range of 2000 rad.

ABDOMEN AND PELVIS

Metastatic melanoma can occur anywhere in the abdominal and pelvic region in the form of retroperitoneal, intestinal, liver, spleen, or pancreatic metastases. Usually, radiation is not given unless symptoms are present. If the metastatic lesion requires only small-volume fields, a dose of 500 rad to 600 rad twice weekly to a total dose of 2000 rad to 4000 rad can be given without undue side-effects. However, if larger treatment volumes are necessary, conventional palliative fractions of 200 rad to 400 rad per day to a dose of 3500 rad to 4000 rad is generally all that can be tolerated. There has been no significant experience with adjunctive hyperthermia for lesions of this type. Melanoma metastatic to the liver is not suitable for palliative radiation, as the maximum tolerable dose to liver parenchyma is in the range of 3000 rad using conventional fractionation. High daily doses are not well tolerated, and adequate doses of radiation would result in loss of liver function owing to radiation effect. The volume of functioning tissue lost is usually greater than the loss caused by the tumor itself.

LUNG AND MEDIASTINUM

Melanoma metastatic to the lung cannot be treated by radiation, because the dose required to control disease will cause radiation fibrosis and loss of function. However, mediastinal metastases causing pain or airway obstruction can be treated for palliation with 500-rad to 600-rad fractions twice weekly to a total dose of 2400 rad to 3600 rad in 14 to 21 days.

RADIATION TREATMENT OF PRIMARY CUTANEOUS MELANOMA

The mainstay of treating primary cutaneous melanomas is surgical excision. However, there are selected patients in whom the anatomical site, the extensiveness of the lesion, or the risk of the operation prohibits a complete or safe resection. In such instances, radiation therapy might be considered as an alternative treatment either for residual disease after a narrow excision or as primary treatment of an unresectable melanoma. This approach particularly applies to melanomas arising in the head and neck area.

Creagan and associates[9] reported a retrospective study of 31 patients with head and neck melanomas treated with radiation at the Mayo Clinic. The radiation was directed to the primary tumor or recurrent disease and contiguous lymph nodes, using a total dose of 5000 rad to 6000 rad. Their technique called for a conventional daily dose of 200 rad, but the overall treatment program was given in two courses with a brief rest period. They had a 5-year survival rate of 28%, but it is not possible to compare these results with surgery alone. They were unable to demonstrate any benefit from irradiating minimal residual melanoma, and, furthermore, there was no survival difference in patients with gross tumors versus patients with no clinical evidence of disease at the start of radiation therapy. The lack of benefit may have been caused by the low daily-dose fractions used.

In a nonrandomized radiation study by Harwood and co-workers, a large dose per fraction schedule was used following local excision of recurrent tumors or primary melanomas of the head and neck.[19] Both the local control rate and cosmetic results were good using this combined approach of surgery and irradiation. In patients irradiated for local or regionally recurrent disease following incomplete surgical excision, local control was 70% when a dose per fraction of greater than 400 rad was used, compared to only 25% when a dose per fraction of less than 400 rad was used. For patients referred within 3 months of incomplete surgery with either gross residual tumor left behind or potential microscopic residual tumor, 15 of 17 (88%) had local control when treated by large dose per fraction radiotherapy. These authors recommended that local excision followed by large dose per fraction radiotherapy be considered in patients with head and neck melanomas for whom wide excision would be hazardous or grossly mutilating.

In some European centers, radiotherapy is regarded as the treatment of choice for lentigo maligna (LM) and lentigo maligna melanomas (LMM). Dancuart and associates[11] reported the experience at the Princess Margaret Hospital using conventional orthovoltage irradiation for primary treatment of LM and LMM. Total doses ranged between 3500 rad in 5 fractions to 4500 rad to 5000 rad in 10 to 15 fractions. Only one of the eight cases of LM recurred following irradiation, and this recurrence was controlled with additional radiotherapy. Of 15 cases of LMM, 14 were controlled for periods ranging from 2 months to 6 years after radiotherapy, and one recurrence was salvaged with local excision. They recommended conventional orthovoltage irradiation using 4500 rad to 5000 rad in 10 to 15 fractions and noted that these lesions may take up to 24 months to regress completely following irradiation. Since they are frequently large and occur in older persons, irradiation might be considered as an alternative to surgery, as it produces minimal morbidity, gives excellent cosmetic results, and can be given on an outpatient basis. It is anticipated that similar results could be achieved using electron-beam irradiation for these lesions.

TABLE 15–2
EXPERIENCE IN RADIATION OF MALIGNANT MELANOMA AT THE UNIVERSITY OF ALABAMA IN BIRMINGHAM, 1975–1983
(25 Cases and 27 Treatment Sites)

	Number of Rx Sites	Evaluable	CR	PR	NR
Soft Tissue	9	9	—	7*	2
Brain	10	9	2	6**	1
Bone	5	3	1	2***	—
Prophylactic (soft tissue)	3	2	2	—	—
Totals	27	23	5	15	3

CR, complete response; *, greater than 50% reduction of soft-tissue mass; **, partial neurologic improvement; ***, partial or temporary (greater than 3 months) relief of pain; NR, no response.

EXPERIENCE OF THE UNIVERSITY OF ALABAMA RADIATION THERAPY DEPARTMENT

Twenty-five patients with metastatic melanoma have been treated by the UAB Department of Radiation Therapy during the last eight years (Table 15-2). Twenty-seven sites of disease were treated, the most common being soft-tissue metastases. Nine patients had palliative treatment for unresectable soft-tissue tumors, and three had prophylactic irradition to prevent further recurrences after surgery. Ten patients were referred for palliation of CNS metastases, but no prophylactic brain irradiation was given. Five patients were referred for treatment of osseous metastases.

The majority of patients received a partial or temporary response to their treatment program. In some cases, it was difficult to evaluate response within the treated area because of the rapid clinical progression of generalized disease.

Of the ten patients treated for CNS metastases, six had a partial response. There was one nonresponder and one patient who was not evaluable because he was lost to follow-up. One patient had a large brain metastasis resected, followed by whole-brain irradiation. The patient later developed chronic lymphocytic leukemia and died from this 10 years later without evidence of metastatic melanoma.

Of the five patients treated for bone metastases, there were two partial responders, while one patient with femur metastases is alive without evidence of disease clinically or radiographically at 5 months after irradiation. No follow-up information was available on the other two patients. For soft-tissue metastatic disease, seven of nine patients had partial response and two had no response. No consistent time/dose pattern was used in the treatment of these patients, so it was impossible to compare techniques. The majority of the soft-tissue lesions were treated with electron-beam therapy.

Overall, there were 23 evaluable sites of treatment, with 20 responders and 2 nonresponders. Granted, some of the responses were temporary, but results indicate that radiation therapy can play an important role in the palliation of metastatic melanoma. There were insufficient cases in this series to evaluate the use of prophylactic irradiation in the management of melanoma.

SUMMARY

The following conclusions can be made:

1. There is both *in vitro* and *in vivo* evidence that melanoma responds best to large individual radiation dose fractions and that the response is influenced by the tumor volume, not by the total dose.
2. Large dose per fraction radiotherapy does produce a high response rate and significant long-term control of melanoma that is unresectable or recurrent after surgery.
3. Radiotherapy can provide palliative benefit in patients with symptomatic metastatic melanoma.
4. In cutaneous melanomas of the head and neck, local excision followed by large dose per fraction radiation treatment should be considered when wide excision would be either hazardous or grossly mutilating.
5. Further investigative studies of combination effects of radiation with radiation modifiers or hyperthermia are indicated in an attempt to increase the response rates for metastatic melanoma.

REFERENCES

1. Adair FE: Treatment of melanoma: Report of four hundred cases. Surg Gynecol Obstet 62:406, 1936
2. Amer MH, Al-Sarraf M, Baker LH, Vaitkevicius VK: Malignant melanoma and central nervous system metastases: Incidence, diagnosis, treatment and survival. Cancer 42:660, 1978
3. Barranco SC, Romsdahl MM, Humphrey RM: The radiation response of human malignant melanoma cells grown in vitro. Cancer Res 31:830, 1971
4. Bullard DE, Cox EB, Seigler HF: Central nervous system metastases in malignant melanoma. Neurosurgery 8:26, 1981
5. Carella RJ, Gelber R, Hendrickson F, Berry HC, Cooper JS: Value of radiation therapy in the management of patients with cerebral metastases from malignant melanoma. Radiation Therapy Oncology Group brain metastasis study I and II. Cancer 45:679, 1980
6. Cohen SM, Greenspan EM, Ratner LH, Weiner MJ: Combination chemotherapy of malignant melanoma with imidazole carboxamide, BCNU and vincristine. Cancer 39:41, 1977
7. Cooper JS, Carella R: Radiotherapy of intracerebral metastatic malignant melanoma. Radiology 134:735, 1980
8. Creagan ET, Cupps RE, Ivins JC, Pritchard DJ, Sim FH, Soule EH, O'Fallon JR: Adjuvant radiation therapy for regional nodal metastases from malignant melanoma: A randomized, prospective study. Cancer 42:2206, 1978
9. Creagan ET, Woods JE, Cupps RE, O'Fallon JR: Radiation therapy for malignant melanoma of the head and neck. Am J Surg 138:604, 1979
10. Damsker JI, Macklis R, Brady LW: Radiosensitization of malignant melanoma. I. The effect of 7-hydroxy-chlorpromazine on the in vivo radiation response of Fortner's melanoma. Int J Radiat Oncol Biol Phys 4:821, 1978
11. Dancuart F, Harwood AR, Fitzpatrick PJ: The radiotherapy of lentigo maligna and lentigo maligna melanoma of the head and neck. Cancer 45:2279, 1980
12. Dewey DL: Letter: The radiosensitivity of melanoma cells in culture. Br J Radiol 44:816, 1971
13. Dickson RJ: Malignant melanoma: A combined surgical and radiotherapeutic approach. Am J Roentgenol 79:1063, 1958
14. Doss LL, Memula N: The radioresponsiveness of melanoma. Int J Radiat Oncol Biol Phys 8:1131, 1982
15. Ellis F: The radiosensitivity of malignant melanomata. Br J Radiol 12:327, 1939
16. Gottlieb JA, Frei E III, Luce JK: An evaluation of the management of patients with cerebral metastases from malignant melanoma. Cancer 29:701, 1972
17. Habermalz HJ, Fischer JJ: Radiation therapy of malignant melanoma: Experience with high individual treatment doses. Cancer 38:2258, 1976
18. Harwood AR, Cummings BJ: Radiotherapy for malignant melanoma: A re-appraisal. Cancer Treat Rev 8:271, 1981
19. Harwood AR, Dancuart F, Fitzpatrick PJ, Brown T: Radiotherapy in nonlentiginous melanoma of the head and neck. Cancer 48:2599, 1981
20. Hellriegel W: Radiation therapy of primary and metastatic melanoma. Ann NY Acad Sci 100:131, 1963
21. Hilaris BS, Raben M, Calabrese AS, Phillips RF, Henschke UK: Value of radiation therapy for distant metastases from malignant melanoma. Cancer 16:765, 1963
22. Hornsey S: The radiation response of human malignant melanoma cells in vitro and in vivo. Cancer Res 32:650, 1972
23. Hornsey S: The relationship between total dose, number of fractions and fraction size in the response of malignant melanoma in patients. Br J Radiol 51:905, 1978
24. Kim JH, Hahn EW, Ahmed SA: Combination hyperthermia and radiation therapy for malignant melanoma. Cancer 50:478, 1982
25. Kim JH, Hahn EW, Tokita N: Combination hyperthermia and radiation therapy for cutaneous malignant melanoma. Cancer 41:2143, 1978
26. McCord JM, Fridovich I: The biology and pathology of oxygen radicals. Ann Intern Med 89:122, 1978
27. Oberley LW, Buettner GR: Role of superoxide dismutase in cancer: A review. Cancer Res 39:1141, 1979
28. Overgaard J: Radiation treatment of malignant melanoma. Int J Radiat Oncol Biol Phys 6:41, 1980
29. Plesnicar S, Rudolf Z: Combined BCG and irradiation treatment of skin metastases originating from malignant melanoma. Cancer 50:1100, 1982
30. Rofstad EK, Brustad T: The radiosensitizing effect of metronidazole and misonidazole (Ro-07-0582) on a human malignant melanoma grown in the athymic mutant nude mouse. Br J Radiol 51:381, 1978
31. Sealy R, Hockley J, Shepstone B: The treatment of malignant melanoma with cobalt and hyperbaric oxygen. Clin Radiol 25:211, 1974
32. Strauss A, Dritschilo A, Nathanson L, Piro AJ: Radiation therapy of malignant melanomas: An evaluation of clinically used fractionation schemes. Cancer 47:1262, 1981
33. Sylven B: Malignant melanoma of the skin: Report of 341 cases treated during the years 1929–1943. Acta Radiol (Diagn) (Stockh) 32:33, 1949
34. Thomson LF, Smith AR, Humphrey RM: The response of a human malignant melanoma cell line to high LET radiation. Radiology 117:155, 1975
35. Tod MC: Radiological treatment of malignant melanoma. Br J Radiol 19:223, 1946
36. Vlock DR, Kirkwood JM, Leutzinger C, Kapp DS, Fischer JJ: High-dose fraction radiation therapy for intracranial metastases of malignant melanoma: A comparison with low-dose fraction therapy. Cancer 49:2289, 1982

GERALD W. MILTON

Care of the Dying Patient
16

The management of a dying melanoma patient and the emotional support required by the patient and his family are much the same as for any dying person. However, some features of melanoma cause special problems that may protract the dying process and make it more distressing for the patient and his family.

THE STIGMA OF MELANOMA

In many communities, the word *melanoma* has a deadly connotation, a sort of fatal black spot. Indeed, the black color of the primary tumor and of some metastases gives it a particularly fearsome appearance. Both the primary disease and many of its metastases are mainly at the surface so that they can be observed or felt by the patient. Before a melanoma kills, the patient may live for months, sometimes longer, with good health and the hope of cure, only to have his expectations dashed by the appearance of another metastasis. The patient and the family fluctuate from hope to despair. Most melanoma patients dying of their disease are in the prime of life, with an average age of about 45 years. They have the feeling that much of their life and responsibilities are still before them. Finally, the process of dying can be very protracted because the disease is not usually associated with serious secondary infection or gross interference with vital functions. Metastases in the brain, and, to a lesser extent, those in the lungs and liver often kill reasonably quickly (*i.e.,* in a period of months), but the patient and family frequently realize that their situation is hopeless long before central deposits cause symptoms.

ATTITUDES AND ADJUSTMENTS TOWARD DEATH

The attitude toward death of people living in Western societies is, generally, to ignore it except when it is presented on television as entertainment. A hundred years ago, death in its real form confronted everyone with some frequency, but not so today. Furthermore, many people have difficulty communicating with one another about death and the dying process.

A person realizes that he is the victim of incurable disease either quite suddenly or over a period of time. If the realization occurs slowly, the person is able to become acclimatized to his misfortune by events that may evolve over months. He had a melanoma removed, was reassured that his doctor "got it all out," and was well for months before an enlarged lymph node is resected. Once again he is reassured. Subsequently, the patient may start to develop more lumps and begins to realize that his condition is very serious. Alternatively, the patient may be in perfect health and visits his doctor, who unexpectedly finds evidence of incurable melanoma. Such a patient requires time to adjust mentally to the reality of his situation.

From the early stages of melanoma to the time the disease kills, the patient goes through many mental stages, either one after the other or several simultaneously. These stages have been described elsewhere in detail by Kübler-Ross and Cecily Saunders and, to a lesser extent, by myself. A full appreciation of these stages in the mind of the melanoma patient is, nevertheless, important to his management, so a brief recapitulation seems warranted.

Disbelief that such a terrible misfortune could befall a person leads to expressions such as "I can't believe this is happening to me" or "I'll wake up and find it's all a dream." But after the diagnosis of the primary tumor is established, and especially after the first definitive treatment, the patient is no longer able to disbelieve or to deny that he has cancer, even though at this stage it appears to have been cured. However, the knowledge that he has cancer and has had an operation for it often causes a patient to be moderately to severely depressed in the first weeks after major surgery, which usually resolves without active treatment. If the disease recurs, the patient's hopes are shattered, and sometime during this period, if not before, he will ask "Why me?" or "What have I done to deserve this?" As recurrence follows recurrence, many of which are first observed by the patient, his hopes dwindle; and anger, resentment, bitterness, jealousy, and fear occupy, in differing degrees, part of the patient's mind. These emotions, apart from fear, develop because of the patient's perception of the unfairness of it all and the feeling of being unfavorably selected by unknown and dangerous forces against which he may be helpless. Jealousy has a particular relevance. It is usually directed not against those in the outer circles, but against the next of kin because they will go on living no matter what happens to the patient and no matter how distressed they will be by his death. Memories of friends or acquaintances who have made happy and successful marriages after the death of one member do little to reassure the patient. Jealousy can result in vicious and deliberately hurtful remarks to an already tired and distraught spouse, who may, in turn, have feelings of guilt.

Some of the anxieties endured by patients with

melanoma are aggravated by the superficial nature of the disease. Each palpable lump is another obvious manifestation of a malignant process involving inexorable bodily decay or destruction. Fear may be experienced by some patients, especially by strong men—both strong willed and physically developed. Such men may cover their fear with lighthearted flippancy that may be sustained for months. When the "cover" breaks down, the patient bitterly turns his face to the wall. His expressions and responses become those of total indifference, and he soon dies.

The process of dying with cancer is often an undignified, distressing, and protracted event. The fear and the uncertainties of death are almost universal. Some people hold to their religion with such certainty that their confidence sustains them completely.

Fear of pain often lurks in the back of the patient's mind. Cancer, after all, is widely thought to cause a painful death. Also, there is the fear of showing fear: of appearing to be a coward at one's final hour. This may be reinforced by relatives' praising the patient's stoic attitude to such an extent that he may not verbalize his fears rather than cause their disappointment. Finally, both fear and sadness visit all who know that they are about to leave friends, family, and a pleasant life. This is a far cry from death in elderly persons, when the weakness and the memory of departed old friends may make the dying less traumatic.

Self-pity and loneliness are emotional responses that also arise as the dying patient approaches his grave more alone than at any other time of his life. This loneliness, often accompanied by self-pity, may be at its worst if the patient lies awake for long hours at night with a silent house or hospital ward as the only company to his thoughts. It is worth stressing this loneliness, which has been very well described in literature, because many of the other feelings stem from it. Although good management cannot obliterate the patient's sense of isolation, it can help the patient a great deal, whereas bad management will make his and his family's misfortune much harder to bear.

THE CONCEPT OF TEAM MANAGEMENT

The management of a patient dying from melanoma commences on the first day the disease is diagnosed, even though at that time there is every indication that the melanoma will not prove fatal. The reason for this approach is that, should the disease recur and become lethal, the understanding and trust between the patient and his family on one side and the doctor as part of the management team on the other are already established. It is not so easy for medical or nursing personnel to establish close rapport with the patient and his relatives once the crisis of impending death is real.

The management of the patient with melanoma, fatal or not, is carried out by a team, and it is necessary to mention briefly the attributes of a good team. First, the members of the team know, understand, and trust one another, each member being roughly aware of what each other member is likely to say to the patient and his family and the words they will use. This is important because the cancer patient analyzes the words, phrases, and even expressions of the professionals to try to extract meaning. If the patient, in particular, and, to a lesser extent, his family misunderstand or are confused by what has been said to them by different members of the team, their sense of isolation is increased.

The decisions regarding patient management are ultimately made by the patient himself after hearing recommendations from the medical team and consulting with family and friends. In almost all situations, the doctor (specialist or family physician) provides the leadership in the decision-making process. In some cases, the leader is a nurse, a priest or pastor, the spouse, or the patient himself. The leadership role is not relinquished because of confrontation between members of a good team but by mutual understanding and consent. An open, honest, and compassionate tone of conversation is essential, or the confidence the patient has in the team could be weakened and his isolation and frustration increased. It is acknowledged that all the members of the team are human and come from a diversity of backgrounds, education, and personal experience. As a consequence, they will often have differing emotional responses as well as legitimate differences in philosophy, outlook, and attitudes concerning dying and available treatment options. Some team members may have, to be sure, more specialized knowledge of technicalities than others, but even the most experienced physician can be wrong.

A patient who has apparently incurable melanoma does not invariably die of the disease if he goes against medical opinion. So the patient who refuses to submit to a treatment such as amputation is perfectly within his rights, and events may justify his taking the leadership role for that decision. The doctor does not lose face by acquiescing to the patient's rejection of his advice, and if the patient is proved wrong he may be more prepared to accept the doctor's leadership. The doctor can only advise what he thinks is right for his patient. On the other hand, his knowledge will be suspect if his opinions vacillate through apparent indecision. The patient needs support from all the team and especially from the doctor.

The team should also include the patient himself. He should believe that he is an active participant in his care. Family members, including children, are important members of the team. The healthy spouse may have feelings of guilt and, as a result, may desperately want to help the patient in a doting or overbearing manner. Considerable strain is placed on the spouse, because the patient may rest during the day while the partner must handle the daily responsibilities of the home as well as coping with anxieties. Lack of sleep, constant activities, defense against jealously, and caring for the children may lead to breakdown unless other members see that the spouse has some rest. This applies especially to death from melanoma, because the prehospital terminal illness can be lengthy.

The most common mistake made with children is to underestimate their resilience and capabilities. Even very young children appreciate being considered as team members. They can support the dying patient because they represent his continuity and give him something other than himself to think about. Children are unlikely to say the wrong thing; and even if they do, the patient rarely takes offense. Children should be allowed to speak as they think and generally should not be forbidden to interact with the patient. It is common to meet adults who regretted the fact that, as children, they were not allowed to speak frankly to a dying parent of whom they were very fond. They express this by such phrases as "I wish I had had a really good talk with my father before he died." It is recognized, however, that there are situations when the child's exposure to gross disfigurement or physical changes of a dying family member may have an adverse psychological impact on the child.

The number of professionals in the team varies at different stages of the illness. The medical personnel are the ones who offer the most hope but are also the biggest threat to the patient, because many of the decisions appear to be theirs alone. The family doctor may be an old friend who has known the patient for years, and his advice may be sought even when his knowledge of the technical problems is limited. It is therefore important that he be well informed by the specialists, particularly by verbal communication. A telephone conversation will permit the family physician to make his suggestions about the patient or his family. The specialist, often considered the patient's last hope, has a difficult role, especially when he knows that there is little chance for prolonged survival. He has to engender the trust of other members of the team, and he can do this by being frank. His explanations must be clear, and if other team members wish to comment or question his remarks the specialist must not resent it. He should be the first to seek other help if he is not getting through to the patient, and he may rely heavily on the nurses to keep him informed of the patient's attitudes and fears. The nurses have an important part in the team's activities because of their special position. Many are women and, as such, offer a sympathetic supporting image. The nurses are not a threat in the same way that the physicians can be, and they often have more time to spend with the patient. Frequently, a specialist may explain something as clearly as possible to a patient, only to be told the next day by the nurse that he did not understand it. There are at least two reasons for this. The explanation may have been badly given because of the unconscious use of technical language. Alternatively, the patient may have been simply unable to understand what was said to him because of his emotional state, or was coping by self-denial about his plight.

Several kinds of professional support staff may be very helpful in the care of the dying. Psychiatric advice may be valuable in selected instances. There are some circumstances, for example, in which psychotropic medication is helpful, but it should not be used as a substitute for support, discussion, and problem-solving. There are other occasions, however, when a patient or a relative is so anxious that a period of treatment with a tranquilizing drug such as benzodiazepine may be required to reduce anxiety to a level compatible with coping. The question of using antidepressants is more complex. These drugs should not be used to treat the appropriate sadness and sense of loss experienced by patients or relatives facing death or bereavement. Antidepressant drugs should be reserved for treating depression that is accompanied by the biologic changes seen in endogenous depression, particularly delayed insomnia; diurnal mood variation; loss of energy, appetite, and libido; and slowness of thinking and movement. This type of depressive illness is not uncommon, can be precipitated by stress in predisposed people, and will, therefore, inevitably be present in the response pattern of some patients and relatives. In particular, people with a past history or a family history of depressive illness should be assessed carefully in this area. Untreated depressive illness creates great difficulty in day-to-day coping and is a gross handicap for anyone trying to cope with terminal illness or bereavement.

Members of the church, as nonmedical professionals, help by giving reassurance, moral support, kindness, and concern. A priest or a pastor may have known the patient and his family for years, during good times and bad, and this experience will help him in his supportive role for the family. It is important that the priest or pastor should feel a member of the team and not an outsider, if this can be arranged.

COUNSELING THE PATIENT

OVERALL APPROACH

It is a wise policy always to see the patient with the next of kin or a close friend at all major interviews so that the patient does not have the feeling that he is being told one thing while the family is being told something else. The only conclusion the patient can draw from a separate interview is that the real news is so bad that he must be shielded from it. Hence, a wedge is driven between the patient and those he most needs for support, thus increasing his isolation. If there is reason to believe that the patient and family are totally ignorant of the gravity of the situation, they should be allowed at least a week to suspect the truth. It is not difficult to imply at the first interview that the condition is very serious and that one or two tests are needed. Then at the second interview, this time with the spouse present, the truth can be discussed.

Ian Aird once wrote, "The truth is a tall order," and so it is. The esteem, trust, and perceived authority of the doctor, particularly if he is the specialist, has to be used delicately and the truth given to the patient up to a point. For example, if the patient has liver metastases and is beginning to lose appetite, there is little to be gained by discussing the suffering this will ultimately cause.

GENERAL PRINCIPLES

1. It is important to listen carefully and with interest to what the patient has to say and to avoid interruptions. This is a very important moment in the patient's life, and he deserves full attention.

Care must also be taken not to sound patronizing or condescending.

2. It is prudent to avoid precise statistics, unless pressed by the patient to give them. If a person has a 30% chance of surviving 5 years, it must be explained to him that statistics are estimates relating to populations of patients, not to individual patients. Thus, it is not possible to know whether the patient will be in the 30% group who will live or the 70% who will not.

3. The patient should be told that physicians work with a team and that he can ask questions of the staff.

4. It is useful to have a printed handout to give the patient after the first interview so that he may read it at leisure, discuss it with his family, and possibly come up with further questions.

5. The patient and his family should understand that at all stages of disease he will be looked after by the team as long as he wishes it. This can be implied rather than stated. The continuity of personal relationships developed by the patient to the team members facilitates his care as the disease progresses. With this progression, especially when it has definitely become incurable, all professional members of the team must retain their interest in the symptoms or signs mentioned by the patient. Nothing is so disheartening to a fatally ill person as to believe that he has lost the interest of those caring for him solely because of his perception that "nothing can be done." Even when the physician is unable to treat the cancer, there are many meaningful and important treatments he can offer the patient for relief of symptoms, especially pain.

6. Sleep, necessary at all times, becomes imperative to both patient and spouse and must be achieved no matter what doses of drugs are necessary.

7. Care must be taken by members of the team to avoid appearing to pity the patient. The patient is always on the verge of self-pity. It makes him feel worse if all around him express, "I'm so sorry for you."

8. The quality of life of a patient undergoing cancer chemotherapy is difficult to measure, because it will depend on the patient as well as on the drugs used. However, in general, cancer chemotherapeutic drugs are extremely depressing, and many patients have refused to continue adjuvant therapy because of the side-effects. Sometimes the patient will be reluctant to admit to the severity of the depression, but family members will often point out the poor quality of his life. Hence,

overenergetic treatment is usually unjustified. The patient should always know that he has the right to refuse chemotherapy at any stage.

9. Fatigue and lassitude tend to be very prominent features of advancing malignancy, and the family must not try to force activities on the patient that he is incapable of carrying out. Failure from exhaustion is very depressing.

QUESTIONS AND STATEMENTS BY THE PATIENT OR NEXT OF KIN AND HOW TO ANSWER THEM

Q: "How long do I have?"

A: It is unwise to answer this question directly with a definite time because the patient regards this as an execution date that he watches coming closer, destroying his peace of mind. Second, estimates are often inaccurate. In any case, the patient may be in good health almost to the end or may have a month or more of life that is literally intolerable. If the patient insists on an estimate, it is wise to err on the hopeful side.

S: "Please don't tell my wife I cannot be cured" or "Don't tell Dad the truth about his illness."

A: 1. It is not possible to deceive the patient for long because the reactions of all relations and friends will reveal the truth to him. The patient is very watchful of all that is going on around him, and the same applies to the relatives. In both situations, deception aggravates the distress of all parties because once the patient or family feel they are being deliberately deceived, they lose trust in other team members.

   2. Unless the patient has some understanding of his illness, much of the advised treatment will appear to him as unnecessary or absurd, and his cooperation would be harder to obtain.

Q: "How will I die?"

A: It is difficult to predict how any patient will die, because the disease may spread in a number of ways. Many people worry about pain, but melanoma as a rule is not particularly painful, and there are many methods of pain control. Any symptoms that arise should certainly be treated, and the patient should be cared for as long as he desires.

Q: "Will I have much pain?"

A: An answer similar to the above is usually given.

Q: "Is it catching?" or "Will my children get it?"

A: Melanoma is not contagious, but the risk of a blood relative's developing the disease, albeit very small, is certainly greater than for the general public. However, the patient's family can be taught what to look for so that, if they ever do develop melanoma, it can be treated early while treatment is very effective.

Q: "Where does it spread, and how does it do it?"

A: This is a difficult question, since the mechanism of spread is only partly understood. The site of recurrence cannot really be predicted in any one person, and there is little point in going into all the possibilities, as it will only cause needless anxiety. The answer "If you want to know more about this later, please ask either me or one of the nurses" is vague but usually satisfies the patient, provided one has good rapport with him and supplements the answer if he asks more questions later.

Q: "It seemed to spread after the first operation. What would have happened if I had not had it treated?"

A: The patient must be assured that it is unlikely that the treatment encouraged the spread. Indeed, he came for advice because the disease had already become active and had started to spread before he had treatment.

"QUACKS," FAITH HEALERS, DIETICIANS, AND SPECIAL CLINICS

The patient with remorseless cancer often turns to unlikely sources for help with such remarks as, "Well, if it doesn't do me any good, at least it can do no harm." This remark is partly right and partly wrong, because "quack" remedies can do harm in a variety of ways. First, they can deprive the patient of time better spent with his family. Second, in a vain pursuit of prolonged life, the patient may be stripped of much of his savings, which in calmer moments he would want spent on his family. But the "quack" does provide a service by bolstering the patient's hopes, and this may give him a feeling of well-being that sometimes lasts a surprisingly long time. This demonstrates that much of the decline in health of some patients is caused by attitudes of mind rather than by progress of the disease. The boost in morale after attending a special clinic can make the patient feel better for a while. This means that the assessment of treatment of the special clinics has to be very carefully checked by the physician to be sure he understands the mechanisms of improvement.

It is unwise to be too dogmatic in condemnation of "quacks." When orthodox medicine has failed, it is equally unwise to advise patients to try any of the current fads such as holistic medicine simply because these methods grab the center stage when modern medicine has failed. Any doctor in practice for 20 years or longer will have seen many so-called cures, each in time put on the scrap heap of curiosities as some other treatment approach becomes fashionable. Hence, if a patient with an incurable melanoma asks advice about some supposed remedy, it appears reasonable to reply as follows:

You have observed, Mr. Smith, that we have tried to cure your disease and have used all the methods that have been scientifically tested and others that are still being tested. All I can offer you are help, support, ways of relieving symptoms, and if any new method becomes available, offer that to you as soon as possible. It is reasonable that you should want to try everything. If you do try any of these new methods, I will be most interested to know how you progress. If it is of benefit to you, it could be of benefit to others. But—and this is a big *but*—there is no good evidence that these unorthodox methods are really valuable. The faithful who believe in such methods almost always avoid acknowledging failure. So I do not think this will benefit you, but I have no claim to infallibility, and I could be wrong. This advice I would give you: observe carefully what is done and beware if it appears that money passing from you to them is more important than the treatment. Be careful not to throw away your life's savings so that your family will be destitute. Keep your wits about you; they may be able to offer you help. I think it unlikely they can cure you, because if they could, they have merely to show they can cure cancer and all the honors of the scientific, medical, and political world would be theirs, as well as wealth beyond most people's dreams. The fact that they have none of these suggests that their claims are fraudulent. But you may get peace of mind and a feeling that something is being done, and this could be valuable to you.

CONCLUSIONS

The management of patients with advancing or fatal melanoma is a team effort. The members of the team understand one another and have frank discussions with the patient and his family. The choice of words used in these discussions is always important, and it is essential to use words the patient understands. Certainly, many patients put up a defense when they cannot accept their situation, but it is both unnecessary and inhumane to try to break down this defense deliberately. The patient will accept his situation in his own time.

Part IV
Epidemiology and Prognostic Features

JOHN A. H. LEE

The Causation of Melanoma
17

Although much is known about the causes of melanoma, many of the epidemiologic features of the disease are difficult to reconcile into a consistent, coherent pattern of causation. This chapter describes some factors related to the etiology of melanoma, but it should be emphasized at the outset that this is a complex, multifaceted problem, and many concepts are still evolving.*

ENVIRONMENTAL FACTORS

LATITUDE OF RESIDENCE

The importance of intense and continued sunlight as a potential cause of skin cancer, particularly among fair-skinned persons, was recognized in the 19th century. Among the various types of melanoma, those associated with lentigo maligna satisfactorily fit this causative model. However, the more common superficial spreading and nodular growth patterns of melanoma have different epidemiologic features compared with other forms of skin cancers (*e.g.,* squamous and basal-cell carcinoma). They occur at an earlier age; they are typically not located on the head and neck; they do not occur more frequently among outdoor workers; and they are not associated with solar damage to the skin around the lesions. However, like nonmelanoma skin cancers, the incidence among white-skinned populations directly increases as their residence approaches the equator.[14,33,34] The white population in the more tropical zones of Northern Australia has no higher incidence rates for melanoma[29] or nonmelanoma skin cancer[3,10] than do their neighbors in the subtropics. This apparent exception to the general trend may be an expression of living conditions rather than environment (see Chap. 22 for more details). One Australian epidemiologist has commented, "When the distribution of erythemal ultraviolet doses in Queensland is examined, taking into account the effects of cloud cover, surface reflectance, and human behavior, the observed regional differences in incidence may yet be explained by variations in actual ultraviolet exposure received by the population."[25] Direct measurements of the intensity and duration of the ultraviolet light flux have been related to melanoma incidence and mortality in a few places, with results comparable to the latitude relationship.[48]

*The reader is also referred to the epidemiology sections from each of the 14 Melanoma Centers reporting from 9 countries in Chapters 21 to 35.

MIGRATION PATTERNS

People who have lived some part of their lives in a country in which the melanoma rate is lower have a reduced risk of the disease compared with people who have lived all their lives in the sunshine, as in Israel[32] or Australia.[16] Furthermore, risk among migrants is related to duration of residence in the sun.[3,32] Data from Israel (Table 17-1) illustrate this effect. Within each age group, the advantage of migrating later in life is apparent.

WHO IS AT RISK?

SKIN PIGMENTATION

It has long been clear that skin pigmentation is important in the etiology of melanoma. In 1896, Matas wrote about the low rate of melanoma among American blacks,[40] and this observation was probably not new then. People of African or Asian descent are known to have a lower incidence of melanoma.[13,22] People of Mediterranean descent have lower rates than do those of northern European extraction even though they live closer to the equator, and regardless of whether they live in their countries of origin or elsewhere, such as North America.[34] Cutaneous melanomas may thus be a burden that white persons in a sunny environment have to endure owing to their skin's inability to shield a high proportion of incident UV photons that penetrate into its active layers.[42] Pale pigmentation increases the skin's capacity to synthesize vitamin D and to prevent rickets,[11] but it can also lead to problems such as wrinkling of skin and skin cancers.

As far as American blacks are concerned, the incidence of cutaneous melanoma is quite low and the advantage of pigmented skin seems to extend to the mucosal sites and uveal tract as well.[49] Whether the influence of pigmentation is a primary or secondary phenomenon will become clear only when studies have been done that control for socioeconomic differences and other factors, including genetic ones. Because of these and other confounding differences such as anatomical site, pathologic type, and tumor thickness, the answer is not simple. This question is addressed further in Chapters 24 and 25 by the Alabama and Duke investigators. After the elimination of numerous factors through an appropriate statistical model, the lower survival of the black patient appeared to continue in the Duke study. An alternative explanation is that blacks have a greater predisposition for developing acral lentigi-

TABLE 17–1
INCIDENCE OF MELANOMA IN ISRAEL FOR JEWS BORN IN EUROPE OR AMERICA BY AGE, PERIOD OF IMMIGRATION, AND DIAGNOSIS*

Year of Diagnosis	Age (In Years)				
	15–29	30–44	45–64	65 +	All Ages
Immigration Before 1948					
1960–1964	4.99	5.81	6.54	6.18	6.24
1965–1974	12.36	10.28	10.52	12.26	10.90
Immigration After 1948					
1960–1964	1.09	4.05	4.05	3.95	3.19
1965–1974	2.34	4.86	6.72	8.86	5.40
Ratio of Rates in Post-1948 Migrants to Pre-1948 Migrants					
1960–1964	0.22	0.70	0.62	0.64	0.51
1965–1974	0.19	0.47	0.64	0.72	0.50

* Rates per 100,000 per year.

(Adapted from Katz L, Ben-Tuvla S, Steinitz R: Malignant melanoma of the skin in Israel: Effect of migration. In Magnus K (ed): Trends in Cancer Incidence, p 419. Washington, Hemisphere, 1982)

nous melanomas that occur on the palms, soles, and fingernails,[14,45] while more densely pigmented areas of the skin are less susceptible. The same relationships appear to hold true for Japanese and Chinese (see Chaps. 34 and 35).

This problem occurs both in simple communities in Africa and among American blacks and is not, as was once thought, related to barefoot walking. Acral lentiginous melanomas have been described as a separate entity for less than a decade,[46] and the trends of their incidence, age and sex distribution, and other influences are quite obscure. Apparent precursor lesions have been described on some African feet, and the whole problem awaits a more systematic collection of clinical experience.

FAMILY HISTORY OF MELANOMA

One of the earliest patients with a recognized melanoma reported to Norris in 1832 that his father suffered from a similar condition (see Chap. 1).[44] More recent data also quite clearly suggest that melanoma can have a familial pattern.[17] However, this association appears to work in two distinct ways. Either the familial link may operate through the aggregation of dysplastic nevi (see below), or it may work independently of visible precursor lesions. Whether this suggested distinction is a viable hypothesis or should be discarded because of the recent recognition of dysplastic nevi is as yet uncertain. An increased prevalence of one of the HLA phenotypes (DR-4) and Bf complement allotypes has been reported among Alabama melanoma patients (see Chap. 24). This association was strongest among patients with low-risk disease (thin, nonulcerated stage I melanoma).

Familial patients typically have a somewhat better prognosis than those patients whose melanoma occurs sporadically, and some new genetic relationship may emerge from studying these patients.

ANATOMICAL SITE AND GENDER

Melanomas are generally distributed across the whole skin surface but are concentrated to some degree on the skin of the head and neck.[20] They occur less frequently on those areas of skin that are covered by several layers of clothing, especially the bathing-trunk area and the female breast.[12,15,50] Differences in clothing among men and women have led to a higher incidence of melanomas on the lower legs of women, while the chest, abdomen, and back are relatively spared compared with those of men. Also, men tend to have more melanomas on the external ear than do women, possibly owing in part to differences in hairstyle.

Elwood and Gallagher[19] related the unit area of skin, the patient's age, and a statement about the skin exposure with the incidence of melanoma (Table 17-2). The lowest incidence occurred in unexposed anatomical sites. However, it appears that intermittent skin exposure was as important as permanent exposure. Other similar studies to corroborate these results would be of great interest.

OCCUPATION AND SOCIAL STATUS

In general, there are few relationships that could be demonstrated between melanoma incidence and occupation in studies from Scandinavia,[54] Britain,[36] or

TABLE 17–2
ESTIMATED ANNUAL INCIDENCE RATES PER 100,000 POPULATION FROM MELANOMA OF SKIN IN BRITISH COLUMBIA (1976–1979), PER UNIT AREA OF SKIN, BY AGE, AND BY SITE GROUPING*

Site Group	Age (in years)[†]			
	15–34	35–49	50 +	All Ages
Exposed	1.8 (10)	6.3 (11)	20.6 (20)	8.8
Intermittently exposed	2.8 (69)	9.2 (73)	16.1 (70)	8.5
Unexposed	0.9 (8)	3.1 (9)	6.9 (11)	3.3
All sites	2.2 (87)	7.4 (93)	14.6 (101)	7.3

* Exposed sites are face, neck, scalp, and hand in both sexes; intermittently exposed are the upper arm, back, thigh, leg, and forearm in both sexes and the male chest; unexposed are the abdomen, foot, and female chest.

† Figures in parentheses indicate numbers of patients.

(Adapted from Elwood JM, Gallagher RP: Site distribution of malignant melanoma. Can Med Assoc J 128:1400, 1983)

Australia.[30] There are two exceptions: (1) an excess risk of dying from melanoma among veterinarians,[9] and (2) an increased incidence of head and neck melanomas among outdoor workers.[8] What emerges from these studies is a link between risk and increased social status, whether measured by job, income, or education. Further, this gradient is present when married women are classified by their husband's occupation. This is not a matter of overdiagnosis, since the social gradient is similar for death rates and incidence.

SPECIFIC OCCUPATIONAL FACTORS

Specific occupational risks are represented by a scatter of isolated reports of the increased risk of ocular melanoma at a single chemical plant.[2] The problem at the Lawrence Livermore National Laboratory[4] was not found at the comparable Los Alamos National Laboratory[1] and was unrelated to ionizing radiation of any sort. There are hints about exposure of workers to PCBs[5] or to fluorescent lights.[7] Any of these may represent a genuine specific cause of the disease, but it is clear that the etiology of these tumors is generally unrelated to the workplace.

PRECURSOR LESIONS

XERODERMA PIGMENTOSUM

The relationship of xeroderma to an increased risk of all types of skin malignancy, including melanoma, is classical. Its intensity has been much mitigated by the protection of such patients from the sun. It is of interest that melanomas occur only on the exposed areas of skin. The defective repair mechanism does not lead to malignant change in melanocytes not exposed to solar radiation.

NEVI

It was recognized early that melanomas were frequently associated with preexisting nevi. There was a historical period when the majority of melanomas were thought to arise from nevi showing proliferative activity at the dermoepidermal junction.[50] This view has not stood the test of time. The precise relationship has never been clearly established because of the destruction of the original nevus by the growth of the tumor and the unreliability of patients' histories. Above-average numbers of nevi have been reported to be as strong a risk factor as having red hair. In a modern series of very small melanomas, a preexisting nevus was recognizable in about half of the patients.[47] However, in the course of studies on patients with strong family histories of melanoma, it was found that these patients had enlarged, peculiar-looking nevi.[37,46] Further, such dysplastic nevi have been found in a proportion of patients treated for melanoma but having no family history of the disease.[18] It is as yet unclear whether their recognition and removal can make a major contribution to the control of sporadic melanoma. McGovern and associates[38] found that about 40% of superficial spreading melanomas originated from dysplastic nevi and that these were thicker and had a higher mitotic rate than those arising from melanoma *in situ*.

Immunosuppressed patients seem to have a high risk for developing melanoma, and this appears to involve dysplastic nevi.[26]

CHANGING EPIDEMIOLOGIC FEATURES OF MELANOMA

INCREASED INCIDENCE AND MORTALITY RATES

Both the incidence and mortality from cutaneous melanoma are rising steadily among white populations throughout the world.[31] This appears to have been going on since the early years of the century[24] and is driven by successively higher lifetime risks in those born later in the century.[29] In other words, the lifetime risk of getting a melanoma or dying from it is established sometime before adulthood. This is not surprising if precursor nevi are as important as they seem. It perhaps accounts for the lack of obvious etiologic relationships in the patient's living habits nearer the time of diagnosis. The magnitude of the increase in melanoma mortality risk between successive birth cohorts seems broadly similar among prosperous white countries. The increase

appears to be getting smaller, however, as if a series of plateaus is being reached.[55] This may represent a function of the disease incidence, or it may indicate that earlier diagnosis is improving control to a substantial extent.

The increased incidence of melanoma is not the same for different anatomical sites. Most recent studies indicate that the rates for the head and neck are changing much more slowly than those for the trunk and limbs.[39,41] The changes with age of three groups of birth cohorts in Norway are shown in Figure 17-1. As in Table 17-2, anatomical sites are compared per unit area. The site-specific differences in time trends rule out any general or systemic basis for the current rise in incidence and suggest the importance of changing habits of dress and leisure activities. Differences in cohort effects necessarily lead to differences in the age distribution of patients. It has been shown that the differences in age distribution of patients with head and neck melanomas

FIG. 17–1 Age-specific incidence rates per unit skin area by birth cohort in Norway between 1955 and 1977 for melanoma of the face and trunk in men and the lower limb in women. (Magnus K: Habits of sun exposure and risk of malignant melanoma: An analysis of incidence rates in Norway, 1955–57, by color, sex, age, and primary tumor site. In Magnus K (ed): Trends in Cancer Incidence, p 387. Washington, Hemisphere, 1982)

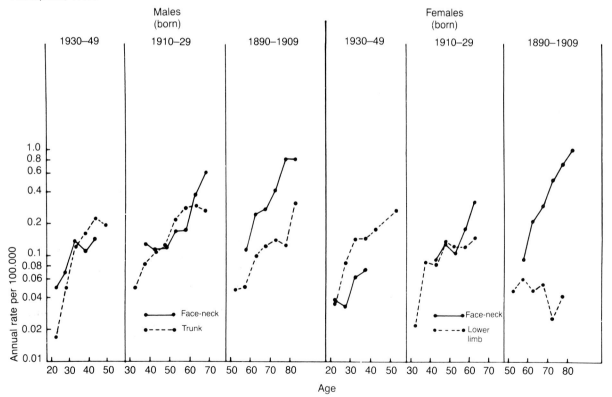

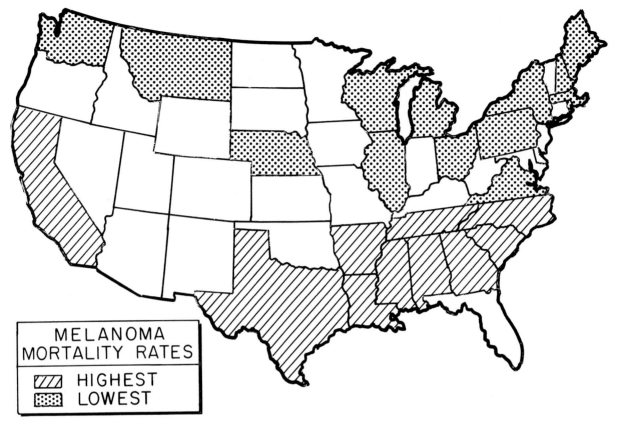

FIG. 17–2 States with the highest and lowest mortality from melanoma in the United States (1950 to 1969). The predominance of melanoma in the south is consistent with increased exposure to solar ultraviolet radiation, but other factors probably play a role as well. (Adapted from Fraumeni JF: The face of cancer in the United States. Hosp Pract, p. 81, December 1983)

compared with those with trunk and limb melanomas can indeed be explained by their different time trends. No special anatomical or pathologic phenomena need be postulated.[51]

Because the nonmelanoma skin cancers seldom cause death and their treatment is rarely a major procedure, registry data about them tend to be less satisfactory than those for melanomas. However, it is now clear that the incidence of these tumors is also rising.[21] Increasing exposure to sunlight could account for this trend in all the common types of skin malignancies.

In contrast to melanomas of the skin, ocular melanomas (which almost all occur in the uveal tract and are thus protected from ultraviolet light by the cornea) do not show the same latitude gradient,[49] nor is mortality from them increasing.[52] Also, the incidence rates for ocular melanomas are either stationary,[52] rising,[53] or flat (Chap. 31). The reported rising trend of melanoma in Japan (mainly unexposed acral lentiginous melanomas) is an interesting finding that does not fit the above hypothesis (see Chap. 35).

CHANGES IN PROGNOSTIC FEATURES

There is a clear trend for melanomas of the skin to be diagnosed when they are less invasive than in the past as gauged by their thickness and level of invasion (see Chap. 18). Part of this trend is the result of increased public awareness to changing lesions of the skin. This has been brought about by notable efforts at public education in some parts of the world. However, suspicion remains that there is an underlying biologic relationship—that, as incidence increases, the extra tumors are less aggressive.[34]

This is evidenced by the shift to a higher proportion of superficial spreading melanoma.

INTERACTIONS

The combination of a susceptible population and an adequate level of sunshine produces a higher incidence of mortality from cutaneous melanoma (Fig. 17-2). For example, the Irish are at an increased risk of melanoma when they migrate to Australia or Boston compared with persons emigrating from other parts of the British Isles. The melanoma rate in Ireland itself is relatively low but is rising. It is possible that the dose–response curves of ultraviolet irradiation for the different populations (*e.g.,* Irish versus Scandinavians) are sufficiently different to account for differences in incidence rates.

These complexities are also illustrated by data from Israel (Table 17-3). The non-Jews, who are mostly indigenous Arabs, are well pigmented and tend to have reduced economic circumstances. This is also true of the Jews who arrive from Africa or Asia. Jews arriving from Europe or America are poorly pigmented and are generally better situated economically, but their state of pigmentation has the advantage of being adapted to a milder climate. Hence, those at highest risk for melanoma are the Jews born in Israel, who are mostly of European stock, fair-skinned, and generally prosperous, and who have passed their whole lives under more intense sunlight.

THE PROSPECTS

As knowledge increases, the paradoxes of the distribution of melanoma seems to be slowly resolving. Outdoor workers *do* have more melanomas of the head and neck than indoor workers have; the skins of those who develop melanomas *do* differ from those who do not; the rates for nonmelanomas *are* increasing along with those of skin melanomas, while melanomas of the protected uveal tract or the protected germinal layer in pigmented persons are not.[27] However, much of the current epidemiologic evidence is still tentative. For example, knowledge of age relationships and cutaneous nevi is based on a single study,[43] as is the information about the relationship of skin tanning to melanoma.[6] Some things do not seem to have been investigated at all. For example, does the habit of taking winter holidays in the sun make an important contribution to the high risk of melanoma among the prosperous? The relationship of social status to ocular melanomas is quite unknown. The interaction between duration of residence in the sun and the age at which migration occurred needs to be clarified for the migrant studies to make their full contribution. Finally, effort directed toward the clinical description and characterization of those patients with melanoma whose disease behaves in an unexpected way (*e.g.,* the occasional patient who recovers after treatment with vaccinia, or who has vitiligo associated with melanoma, or who has a melanoma that runs an indolent course through several pregnancies) could lead to useful insights into this most variable of tumors.

TABLE 17–3
INCIDENCE OF MELANOMA IN ISRAEL BY COUNTRY OF ORIGIN, SEX, AND PERIOD OF DIAGNOSIS*

	Calendar Period		
	1960–1966	*1967–1971*	*1972–1976*
Men			
Non-Jews	0.3	0.7	0.8
Jews born in Africa or Asia	0.7	0.9	1.5
Jews born in Europe or America	1.5	3.4	4.7
Jews born in Israel	2.5	4.7	6.0
Women			
Non-Jews	0.2	0.1	0.5
Jews born in Africa or Asia	0.2	0.6	1.3
Jews born in Europe or America	2.1	4.8	5.6
Jews born in Israel	3.1	7.0	6.8

* Per 100,000 at all ages adjusted to the UICC "World Population."

Our predecessors regarded melanoma as capricious in its behavior. The unpredictability of prognosis has been reduced; but the long silent intervals, the more biologically favorable tumors that occur in women,[28,35] and the occasional reversal of advancing disease remind us that melanoma is potentially vulnerable to defense mechanisms that have not yet been exploited.

REFERENCES

1. Acquavella JF, Tietjen GL, Wilkinson GS, Key CR, Voelz GL: Malignant melanoma incidence at the Los Alamos National Laboratory. Lancet 1:883, 1982

2. Albert DM, Puliafito CA, Fulton AB, Robinson NL, Zakov ZN, Dryja TP: Increased incidence of choroidal malignant melanoma occurring in a single population of chemical workers. Am J Ophthalmol 89:323, 1980

3. Armstrong BK, Holman CDJ, Ford J, Woodings TL: Trends in melanoma incidence and mortality in Australia. In Magnus K (ed): Trends in Cancer Incidence, p 399. Washington, Hemisphere, 1982

4. Austin DJ, Reynolds PJ, Snyder MA, Biggs MW, Stubbs HA: Malignant melanoma among employees of Lawrence Livermore National Laboratory. Lancet 2:712, 1981

5. Bahn AK, Rosenwaike I, Herrmann N, Grover P, Stellman J, O'Leary K: Melanoma after exposure to PCB's. N Engl J Med 295:450, 1976

6. Beitner H, Ringborg U, Wennersten G, Lagerlöf B: Further evidence for increased light sensitivity in patients with malignant melanoma. Br J Dermatol 104:289, 1981

7. Beral V, Evans S, Shaw H, Milton G: Malignant melanoma and exposure to fluorescent lighting at work. Lancet 2:290, 1982

8. Beral V, Robinson N: The relationship of malignant melanoma, basal and squamous skin cancers to indoor and outdoor work. Br J Cancer 44:886, 1981

9. Blair A, Hayes HM Jr: Mortality patterns among US veterinarians, 1974–1977: An expanded study. Int J Epidemiol 11:391, 1982

10. Carmichael GG, Silverstone H: The epidemiology of skin cancer in Queensland: The incidence. Br J Cancer 15:409, 1961

11. Clemens TL, Adams JS, Henderson SL, Holick MF: Increased skin pigment reduces the capacity of skin to synthesize vitamin D. Lancet 1:74, 1982

12. Committee on Impacts of Stratospheric Change: Protection against depletion of stratospheric ozone chlorofluorocarbons, p 339. Washington, National Academy of Sciences, 1979

13. Crombie IK: Racial differences in melanoma incidence. Br J Cancer 40:185, 1979

14. Crombie IK: Variation of melanoma incidence with latitude in North America and Europe. Br J Cancer 40:774, 1979

15. Crombie IK: Distribution of malignant melanoma on the body surface. Br J Cancer 43:842, 1981

16. Dobson AJ, Leeder SR: Mortality from malignant melanoma in Australia: Effects due to country of birth. Int J Epidemiol 11:207, 1982

17. Duggleby WF, Stoll H, Priore RL, Greenwald P, Graham S: A genetic analysis of melanoma—polygenic inheritance as a threshold trait. Am J Epidemiol 114:63, 1981

18. Elder DE, Goldman LI, Goldman SC, Greene MH, Clark WH Jr: Dysplastic nevus syndrome: A phenotypic association of sporadic cutaneous melanoma. Cancer 46:1787, 1980

19. Elwood JM, Gallagher RP: Site distribution of malignant melanoma. Can Med Assoc J 128:1400, 1983

20. Elwood JM, Lee JAH: Recent data on the epidemiology of malignant melanoma. Semin Oncol 2:149, 1975

21. Fears TR, Scotto J: Changes in skin cancer morbidity between 1971–72 and 1977–78. J Natl Cancer Inst 69:365, 1982

22. Feibleman CE, Maize JC: Racial differences in cutaneous melanoma incidence and distribution. In Ackerman AB (ed): Pathology of Malignant Melanoma, p 47. New York, Masson, 1981

23. Fraumeni JF Jr: The face of cancer in the United States. Hosp Pract, p 81, Dec 1983

24. Gordon T, Critenden M, Haenszel W: End results and mortality trends in cancer. II. Cancer mortality trends in the United States. Washington, USDHEW; National Cancer Institute Monograph no 6, p 265, 1961

25. Green A, Siskind V: Geographical distribution of cutaneous melanoma in Queensland. Med J Aust 1:407, 1983

26. Greene MH, Young TI, Clark WH Jr: Malignant melanoma in renal-transplant recipients. Lancet 1:1196, 1981

27. Hinds MW, Kolonel LN: Cutaneous malignant melanoma in Hawaii: An update. West J Med 138:50, 1983

28. Holly EA, Weiss NS, Liff JM: Cutaneous melanoma in relation to exogenous hormones and reproductive factors. J Natl Cancer Inst 70:827, 1983

29. Holman CDJ, James IR, Gattey PH, Armstrong BK: An analysis of trends in mortality from malignant melanoma of the skin in Australia. Int J Cancer 26:703, 1980

30. Holman CDJ, Mulroney CD, Armstrong BK: Epidemiology of pre-invasive and invasive malignant melanoma in Western Australia. Int J Cancer 25:317, 1980

31. Jensen OM, Bolander AM: Trends in malignant melanoma of the skin. World Health Stat 33:2, 1980

32. Katz L, Ben-Tuvla S, Steinitz R: Malignant melanoma of the skin in Israel: Effect of migration. In

Magnus K (ed): Trends in Cancer Incidence, p 419. Washington, Hemisphere, 1982

33. Lee JAH: Melanoma in cancer epidemiology and prevention. In Schottenfeld D, Fraumeni, JF Jr (eds): Cancer, Epidemiology and Prevention, p 984. Philadelphia, WB Saunders, 1982

34. Lee JAH: Melanoma and exposure to sunlight. Epidemiol Rev 4:110, 1982

35. Lee JAH, Storer BE: Further studies of skin melanomas apparently dependent on female sex hormones. Int J Epidemiol 11:127, 1982

36. Lee JAH, Strickland D: Malignant melanoma: Social status and outdoor work. Br J Cancer 41:757, 1980

37. Lynch HT, Fusaro RM, Pester J, Lynch JF: Familial atypical multiple mole melanoma (FAMMM) syndrome: Genetic heterogeneity and malignant melanoma. Br J Cancer 42:58, 1980

38. McGovern VJ, Shaw HM, Milton GW: Histogenesis of malignant melanoma with an adjacent component of the superficial spreading type. Pathology (in press)

39. Magnus K: Habits of sun exposure and risk of malignant melanoma: An analysis of incidence rates in Norway, 1955–57, by color, sex, age, and primary tumor site. In Magnus K (ed): Trends in Cancer Incidence, p 387. Washington, Hemisphere, 1982

40. Matas R: The surgical peculiarities of the Negro. In De Forest W, Dornan WJ (eds): Trans Am Surg Assoc 14:493, 501, 567, 581, 1896

41. Muir CS, Nectoux J: Time trends: Malignant melanoma of skin. In Magnus K (ed): Trends in Cancer Incidence, p 365. Washington, Hemisphere, 1982

42. Murray FG: Pigmentation, sunlight and nutritional disease. Am Anthropol 36:438, 1934

43. Nicholls EM: Development and elimination of pigmented moles, and the anatomical distribution of primary malignant melanoma. Cancer 32:191, 1973

44. Norris W: Case of fungoid disease. Edin Med Surg J 16:562, 1820

45. Reed RJ: New Concepts in Surgical Pathology of the Skin, p 73. New York, Wiley, 1976

46. Reimer RR, Clark WH Jr, Greene MH, Ainsworth AM, Fraumeni JF Jr: Precursor lesions in familial melanoma: A new genetic preneoplastic syndrome. JAMA 239:744, 1978

47. Sagebiel RW: Histopathology of borderline and early malignant melanomas. Am J Surg Pathol 3:543, 1979

48. Scotto J, Fraumeni JF Jr: Skin (other than melanoma). In Schottenfeld D, Fraumeni JF Jr (eds): Cancer Epidemiology and Prevention, p 996. Philadelphia, WB Saunders, 1982

49. Scotto J, Fraumeni JF Jr, Lee JAH: Melanomas of the eye and other noncutaneous sites: Epidemiologic aspects. J Natl Cancer Inst 56:489, 1976

50. Sober AJ, Fitzpatrick TB, Mihm MC Jr: Primary melanoma of the skin: Recognition and management. J Am Acad Dermatol 2:179, 1980.

51. Stevens RG, Moolgavkar SH: Trends by anatomic site of melanoma incidence. Am J Epidemiol (in press)

52. Strickland D, Lee JAH: Melanomas of eye: Stability of rates. Am J Epidemiol 113:700, 1981

53. Swerdlow AJ: Epidemiology of eye cancer in adults in England and Wales 1962–67. Am J Epidemiol 118:294, 1983

54. Teppo L, Pukkala E, Hakama M, Hukulinen T, Herva A, Faxen E: Way of life and cancer incidence in Finland. Scand J Soc Med 19:50, 1980

55. Venzon DJ, Moolgavkar SH: Cohort analysis of malignant melanoma in five countries. Am J Epidemiol 119:62, 1984

CHARLES M. BALCH
HELEN M. SHAW
SENG-JAW SOONG
GERALD W. MILTON

Changing Trends in the Clinical and Pathologic Features of Melanoma

18

The incidence of melanoma has been increasing rapidly, especially during the past two decades (see Chap. 17). At the same time, there have also been major changes in both the clinical and the pathologic features of the disease. There have been few attempts to document changing trends in the various facets of melanoma systematically, probably because of insufficient long-term follow-up information in most series. The primary objective of this chapter is to review changes in prognostic factors of greatest importance examined from the perspective of date of diagnosis. This analysis made from data bases involving 1648 stage I melanoma patients treated over 27 years by the authors at the University of Alabama in Birmingham (UAB) and at the Sydney Melanoma Unit (SMU) in New South Wales, with updated material from a previous report.[2] This is a largely prospective accumulation of data from two referral institutions. There were insufficient numbers of patients presenting with nodal metastases (stage II) to analyze trends over time.

CHANGES IN CLINICAL PRESENTATION

STAGE

The overall incidence of patients presenting with localized (stage I) melanoma increased in the SMU data from 73% of all patients before 1960 to 81% in the 1976 to 1980 period. Although there was a sim-ilar tendency for the proportion of stage I patients to increase in UAB data, the upward trend was not so consistent. Thus, the incidence of stage I patients rose from 83% to 91% from 1955 until 1975 but decreased slightly to 86% for the last 5-year period. The Queensland Melanoma Project (QMP), which reflects a population-based study, has also noted a marked increase in the proportion of melanoma patients with localized disease treated between 1966 and 1977.[4]

SEX RATIO

The male to female ratio at the SMU from 1961 to 1970 was 0.83:1. The proportion of men with melanoma increased between 1971 and 1980, when the male to female ratio was 1.11:1. In the UAB series, the corresponding ratios were 0.78:1 and 1.04:1 (Table 18-1). Studies in Queensland, Australia, Alberta, Canada, and New Haven, Connecticut, have also observed an increase in the male to female ratio between 1966 and 1977.[3,4,5]

ANATOMICAL SITE

In both the SMU series and the UAB series, there was a consistent increase in the proportion of melanomas located on the trunk and a decrease in the proportion on the head and neck (Table 18-1). There were no significant changes in the proportions of melanomas located on the upper or lower extremity. The data were then further subdivided by site

TABLE 18–1
CHANGES IN CLINICAL PRESENTATION OF LOCALIZED MELANOMA NOTED AT THE UNIVERSITY OF ALABAMA IN BIRMINGHAM AND AT THE SYDNEY MELANOMA UNIT, 1960–1980

	<1960		1961–1965		1966–1970		1971–1975		1976–1980		Total	
	UAB*	SMU*	UAB	SMU	UAB	SMU	UAB	SMU	UAB	SMU	UAB	SMU
Number of Patients	32	76	65	89	92	155	114	298	234	492	537	1110
Male	56%	32%	42%	46%	46%	45%	43%	54%	51%	52%	47%	50%
Female	44%	68%	58%	54%	54%	55%	57%	46%	49%	48%	53%	50%
Median Age (Years)	50	48	46	38	47	43	49	45	46	45	48	44
< 30	9%	17%	9%	21%	13%	21%	14%	23%	17%	20%	14%	21%
30–60	60%	57%	62%	45%	64%	69%	58%	63%	55%	61%	58%	61%
> 60	31%	26%	29%	34%	23%	10%	28%	14%	28%	19%	28%	18%
Lesion Location												
Lower extremity	9%	32%	20%	41%	32%	30%	26%	37%	21%	31%	23%	33%
Upper extremity	9%	13%	20%	13%	13%	21%	18%	11%	22%	14%	19%	14%
Head and neck	41%	29%	38%	15%	32%	14%	25%	16%	22%	11%	27%	14%
Trunk	38%	21%	22%	31%	21%	33%	26%	34%	32%	42%	28%	37%
Other	3%	4%	0%	0%	3%	2%	5%	2%	3%	2%	3%	2%

* UAB = University of Alabama in Birmingham; SMU = Sydney Melanoma Unit.

and sex. There was a significant increase in melanomas located on the trunk in men, where the proportion increased from 40% to 56% (p = 0.0004). There was a corresponding significant decrease in head and neck melanomas in men from 36% to 17% (p = 0.001). No significant changes in the site distribution of melanomas were observed for extremity melanomas in men or for any anatomical site in women.

In a study of 5108 melanoma patients diagnosed in Norway between 1955 and 1977, Magnus found a greater increase in the incidence of trunk and lower extremity melanomas compared with face and neck melanomas, but these relationships in site distribution were similar for both men and women.[6] McGregor, in a Canadian study of 519 patients, also found an increase in trunk melanomas for both men and women and an increase in upper extremity melanomas in men only.[5] In contrast again, whatever was responsible for the doubled incidence of melanoma in Queensland affected anatomical sites uniformly. However, there was a reduction in the proportion of leg melanomas in women living in the tropical parts of Queensland.[4]

AGE

There were no consistent changes over time in the ages of melanoma patients (Table 18-1). The median ages were 44 years for SMU patients and 48 years for UAB patients. Throughout the entire period, women tended to present at an earlier age than men at first diagnosis. The age distribution in Queensland also remained steady over time,[4] whereas the median age in Alberta, Canada, increased for men.[5]

CHANGES IN THE PATHOLOGIC FEATURES

TUMOR THICKNESS

Tumor thickness has changed markedly over the past 27 years (Table 18-2). The median thickness (Fig. 18-1) has decreased from a predominance of thick lesions (>3 mm thick) prior to 1960 to an average of 1-mm-thick lesions after 1980 (p < 0.0001). Conversely, the proportion of thin (<0.76 mm) melanomas has steadily increased from 11% before 1960 to 39% during the 1981 to 1982 period (Fig. 18-2). Similarly, Bagley and colleagues also noted a twofold increase in incidence of thin melanomas (from 23% to 53%) over approximately the same time span in their Massachusetts series.[1] An even more dramatic fivefold increase in the proportion of thin melanomas (from 11% to 58%) between 1970 and 1979 was reported from Israel.[7]

TABLE 18–2
CHANGES IN THE PATHOLOGIC CHARACTERISTICS OF LOCALIZED MELANOMA NOTED AT THE UNIVERSITY OF ALABAMA IN BIRMINGHAM AND AT THE SYDNEY MELANOMA UNIT, 1960–1980

	<1960		1961–1965		1966–1970		1971–1975		1976–1980		Total	
	UAB*	SMU*	UAB	SMU	UAB	SMU	UAB	SMU	UAB	SMU	UAB	SMU
Number of Patients	11	76	27	89	54	155	66	298	203	492	361	1110
Median Tumor Thickness (mm)	3.3	2.5	2.0	1.7	1.4	1.4	1.6	1.3	1.4	1.5	1.5	1.3
<0.76	9%	12%	26%	20%	22%	24%	24%	23%	26%	31%	24%	26%
0.76–3.99	45%	63%	48%	65%	70%	65%	56%	65%	63%	59%	62%	62%
≥4.0	45%	25%	26%	15%	8%	11%	20%	12%	11%	10%	14%	12%
Level of Invasion												
II	9%	8%	19%	11%	21%	16%	17%	15%	26%	25%	23%	19%
III	36%	35%	31%	20%	34%	23%	35%	29%	27%	29%	30%	28%
IV	36%	44%	31%	61%	38%	53%	42%	50%	41%	42%	40%	47%
V	18%	12%	19%	8%	8%	7%	6%	5%	6%	4%	7%	6%
Ulceration												
Present	55%	45%	48%	34%	35%	17%	36%	23%	35%	19%	37%	22%
Absent	45%	55%	52%	66%	65%	83%	64%	77%	65%	81%	63%	78%
Growth Pattern												
Superficial spreading	45%	35%	11%	45%	22%	58%	32%	69%	57%	77%	43%	67%
Others	55%	65%	89%	55%	78%	42%	68%	31%	43%	23%	57%	33%

* UAB = University of Alabama in Birmingham; SMU = Sydney Melanoma Unit.

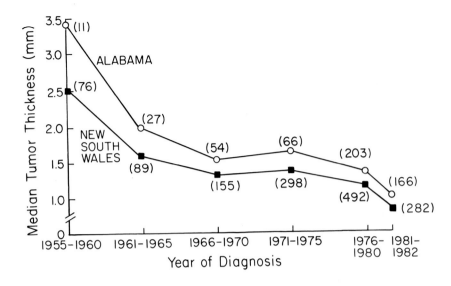

FIG. 18–1 Changes in the median tumor thickness of melanomas treated from 1955 to 1982 (number of patients in *parentheses*).

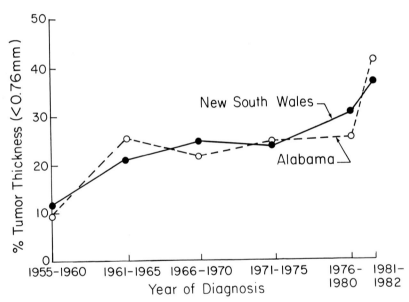

FIG. 18–2 The proportion of "thin" melanomas (<0.76 mm thick) has increased steadily. Such lesions have a very favorable prognosis, with a 5 year survival rate exceeding 97%.

ULCERATION

The presence of ulceration (either macroscopic or microscopic) is generally associated with a poor prognosis. The incidence of ulceration has decreased both in the UAB series from 54% to 32% and in the SMU series from 47% to 15% (p > 0.001, Fig. 18-3).

LEVEL OF INVASION

The levels of invasion have also changed (Table 18-2). Thus, the incidence of melanomas that involved only the papillary dermis (level II) increased

from 9% to 34% (Fig. 18-4), while those deeper lesions with invasion to the reticular dermis (level IV) have decreased from 54% to 32% (p > 0.0001). Although no data exist from either the SMU or UAB regarding changes in level I (*in situ*) melanoma, the QMP has reported a threefold increase in these tumors between 1966 and 1977 (from 8% to 24%).

GROWTH PATTERN

The incidence of nodular melanomas (with a predominant vertical growth phase) has also decreased, while the incidence of superficial spreading melano-

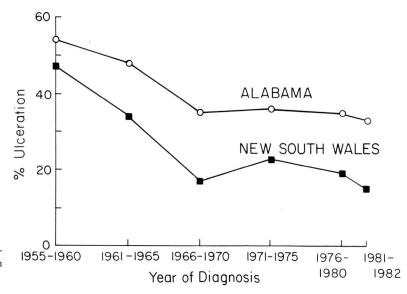

FIG. 18–3 Decreasing incidence of ulcerated melanomas, which are associated with a poor prognosis.

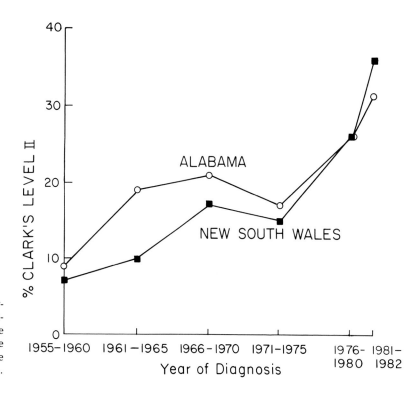

FIG. 18–4 Increasing incidence of favorable melanomas invading only into the papillary (upper) dermis (Clark's level II). There has been a corresponding decrease in the incidence of melanomas invading into the reticular dermis (level IV), from 54% to 32%.

mas (with a predominant radial growth phase) has increased significantly (p > 0.0001, Fig. 18-5) in both Alabama and New South Wales. In contrast, the proportion of superficial spreading melanomas remained uniformly high in Queensland, while the proportion of nodular melanomas also fell between 1966 and 1977, from 28% to 14%. In addition, they recorded a concomitant doubling in the proportion of melanomas arising in lentigo maligna (from 7% to 15%). It is possible, however, that some of these

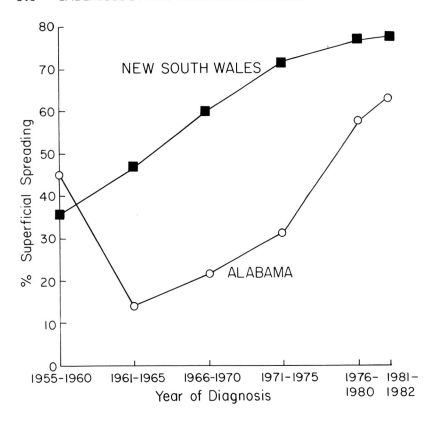

FIG. 18–5 Increasing incidence of superficial spreading melanomas with a predominantly radial growth phase.

discrepancies may reflect differences in pathologic interpretation, especially since histologic reports for the QMP were made by numerous pathologists.

CHANGES IN SURVIVAL RATES (1955–1982)

Despite the marked increase in the number of melanoma patients treated each year, the 8-year survival rate for stage I patients actually increased by 5% over two decades. This was true for both the SMU series and the UAB series (Table 18-3).

EARLIER DIAGNOSIS VERSUS BIOLOGIC CHANGES IN THE DISEASE

During the past several decades, there have been changing trends in the histopathologic characteristics and site distribution of melanoma. These changes are likely caused by earlier diagnosis as well as by changes in the biologic nature of the disease.

It seems certain that in Australia at least, melanoma is now diagnosed and treated at an earlier biologic stage of the disease than in previous years.[4] This is attributable to the active melanoma educational program for both the public and medical profession that has been launched in Australia. At the Sydney Melanoma Unit, the proportion of patients presenting for melanoma treatment with asymptomatic lesions has increased from 6% prior to 1960 to 38% in 1980. The main reasons given by patients for seeking specialist medical attention for asymptomatic lesions were that they had either read or heard about the existence of melanoma or that their local medical officer had noticed a suspicious mole.[*] Greater public and medical awareness of the dangers of cutaneous lesions also probably caused a higher frequency of favorable melanomas in Israel.[7] The results from the SMU series probably represent about the maximum effect that can be achieved by public education, since patients who present with large tumors today rarely do so because they are ignorant but rather because they are frightened. The likelihood

* Shaw HM: Unpublished data

TABLE 18–3
EIGHT-YEAR SURVIVAL RATE OF STAGE I MELANOMA PATIENTS

Patient Series	Diagnosis	
	Before 1970	After 1970
University of Alabama in Birmingham	68% ± 6% (n = 92)	73% ± 5% (n = 269)
Sydney Melanoma Unit	70% ± 3% (n = 320)	75% ± 3% (n = 790)

that the biologic nature of the disease has changed is suggested by the increasing proportion of superficial spreading melanomas. Both events have undoubtedly contributed to the more favorable features of melanoma that are encountered at present.

SUMMARY

Clinical and pathologic characteristics of melanoma were studied between 1955 and 1980 to determine what changes had occurred over a quarter of a century. Over this period, the number of patients treated annually has increased substantially. There was a steady increase in the proportion of patients presenting with localized disease (clinical stage I). Melanomas became thinner, less invasive, less ulcerative, and thus more curable. Also, more of them exhibited a radial growth phase. The median thickness of melanomas in the SMU patients decreased from 2.5 mm prior to 1960 to 0.8 mm during the period 1981–1982, while in the UAB patients, it has decreased from 3.3 mm to 1 mm. In men, there was a significant increase in melanomas located on the trunk and a corresponding decrease in head and neck melanomas. No significant change in the site distribution was observed for any major anatomical area on women. For the most part, similar reports came from both referral practices and a population-based study of melanoma. Long-term survival rates in patients with localized disease were found to increase slightly during the 27-year time frame of this analysis. The changes that have occurred probably result from earlier diagnosis and changes in the biologic nature of the disease.

REFERENCES

1. Bagley FH, Cady B, Lee A, Legg MA: Changes in clinical presentation and management of malignant melanoma. Cancer 47:2126, 1981
2. Balch CM, Soong S-j, Milton GW, Shaw HM, McGovern VJ, McCarthy WH, Murad TM, Maddox WA: Changing trends in cutaneous melanoma over a quarter century in Alabama, USA, and New South Wales, Australia. Cancer 52:1748, 1983
3. Houghton A, Flannery J, Viola MV: Malignant melanoma in Connecticut and Denmark. Int J Cancer 25:95, 1980
4. Little JH, Holt J, Davis N: Changing epidemiology of malignant melanoma in Queensland. Med J Aust 1:66, 1980
5. McGregor SE, Birdsell JM, Grace MA, Jerry LM, Hill GB, Paterson AHG, McPherson TA: Cutaneous malignant melanoma in Alberta: 1967–1976. Cancer 52:755, 1983
6. Magnus K: Habits of sun exposure and risk of malignant melanoma: An analysis of incidence rates in Norway 1955–1977 by cohort, sex, age, and primary tumor site. Cancer 48:2329, 1981
7. Shafir R, Hiss J, Tsur H, Bubis JJ: The thin malignant melanoma: Changing patterns of epidemiology and treatment. Cancer 50:817, 1982

CHARLES M. BALCH
SENG-JAW SOONG
HELEN M. SHAW
GERALD W. MILTON

An Analysis of Prognostic Factors in 4000 Patients with Cutaneous Melanoma

19

A hallmark of melanoma is the multiplicity of prognostic factors that are known to predict the risk of metastatic disease. In fact, the myriad of clinical and pathologic features that appear to affect melanoma survival rates has given the disease a reputation for being very capricious. A prognostic factors analysis of melanoma is therefore essential to identify the dominant variables that can be used for evaluating results of clinical research trials involving adjunctive systemic therapy and for making certain surgical decisions. Also, when these treatments are evaluated, it is important to account for those prognostic variables that can accurately categorize patients into different risk groups for metastatic disease. Otherwise, differences (or lack of differences) between treatment regimens being compared may not result from the treatments themselves but rather may only reflect imbalances of prognostic factors.

This chapter reviews in detail a prognostic factors analysis involving over 4000 patients with cutaneous melanoma treated at the University of Alabama in Birmingham (UAB) and the University of Sydney Melanoma Unit (SMU) over a 25-year period of time (1955–1980). The median follow-up of all patients is 8 years. The results are subdivided into 14 or more clinical and pathologic factors specific for each stage of melanoma (I, II, and III).

DESCRIPTION OF DATA BASE

The SMU melanoma data have been collected prospectively since 1969, while the UAB melanoma data base began in 1975 as a prospective study. Additional data from melanoma patients treated at these units were collected retrospectively to 1950 (see Chaps. 21 and 24). There are now over 4000 melanoma patients with clinical, pathologic, and genetic data recorded in a computerized format. Follow-up information is available for over 95% of patients.

The surgical procedures were performed by one of five surgical oncologists (C. M. Balch, W. A. Maddox, and M. M. Urist at UAB; G. W. Milton and W. H. McCarthy at SMU) for over 95% of the patients. Virtually all the melanomas were examined by two pathologists (T. M. Murad and V. J. McGovern) who did not have knowledge of the clinical course in any of these patients. A small minority of these patients has received adjunctive immunotherapy or chemotherapy during the past few years. This additional treatment modality had little or no influence on survival or prognostic factors reported in this study.

A description of the statistical methods used in this study has been published.[1,4] Survival curves were calculated according to the method of Kaplan and Meier.[25] A generalized Wilcoxon test and the log-rank test were used to determine if significant differences existed between curves. Chi-square tests were employed in statistical assessments where appropriate. The multiple regression procedure proposed by Cox was used in a multifactorial (multivariate) analysis of prognostic factors. The analysis in this study used the more recent of the two regression models proposed by Cox.[12] Wherever appropriate, subgroups of patients were analyzed as both linear and as dichotomous variables.

In this analysis, a three-stage system was used that categorizes patients into clinically localized disease (stage I), regional metastases (stage II), and distant metastases (stage III). The majority of melanoma patients (87%) initially had stage I disease, and their 10-year survival rate was 71%.

PROGNOSTIC FACTORS IN PATIENTS WITH LOCALIZED (STAGE I) MELANOMA

Characteristics of the 3505 stage I patients and their primary melanomas are listed in Table 19-1. When analyzing prognostic factors of stage I melanoma, it is essential to use actuarial methods and survival data with a minimum of 8 to 10 years. A number of investigators have published data about prognostic variables with as little as a 2-year follow-up. Such studies may yield a distorted weighting of prognostic factors, since only the higher-risk patients will have relapsed. Recurrences from less aggressive melanomas usually take place more than 5 years after treatment.

As described in Chapter 18, the prognosis in melanoma changed considerably between 1955 and 1980. Lesions are now thinner, less invasive, less likely to be ulcerated, and exhibit more of a radial growth phase (*i.e.,* a superficial spreading growth pattern). This information is useful in understanding the changing proportions of high- and low-risk melanoma patients, but the year of diagnosis itself is not an important prognostic factor, as long as the dominant variables are accounted for.

TABLE 19–1
DATA BASE FOR PATIENTS WITH LOCALIZED MELANOMA (STAGE I)

	Male	Female	All Patients	Number of Patients with Available Data
Primary Lesion Site				3505
Lower extremity	8%	23%	31%	
Upper extremity	5%	10%	15%	
Head and neck	10%	7%	17%	
Trunk	24%	11%	35%	
Other	1%	1%	2%	
Median Age (Yr)			45	3553
Sex				3554
Male			47%	
Female			53%	
Tumor Thickness				2635
<0.76 mm			27%	
0.76 mm–1.50 mm			30%	
1.51 mm–2.50 mm			20%	
2.51 mm–3.99 mm			12%	
≥4.0 mm			11%	
Median			1.3 mm	
Level of Invasion				2765
II			24%	
III			25%	
IV			45%	
V			6%	
Ulceration				2270
Present			24%	
Absent			76%	
Growth Pattern				2633
Nodular			32%	
Superficial spreading			64%	
Lentigo maligna			4%	
Lymphocyte Infiltration				2687
Absent/mild			35%	
Moderate/heavy			65%	
Pigmentation				2486
Present			93%	
Minimal			7%	

CLINICAL FACTORS

Sex

Overall, melanomas were divided almost equally between men and women (47% versus 53%). When the data were further categorized by the anatomical site of the primary melanoma, some important sex differences in site distribution were seen, as shown in Table 19-1. For example, 73% of all lower extremity lesions occurred in women, while 68% of all chest and back lesions occurred in men. Numerous studies have shown that female patients have a better survival than do men with melanoma.[1,10,21,34,35,36] In this analysis, there was an overall survival advantage in women with melanomas over that for men that was statistically significant (Fig. 19-1A; $p < 0.00001$). However, a primary reason for better survival rates in women is that their melanomas occurred more commonly on the extremities (a more favorable prognostic site) and were less frequently ulcerated.

(*Text continued on page 326*)

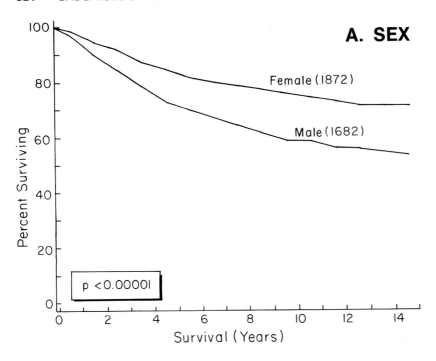

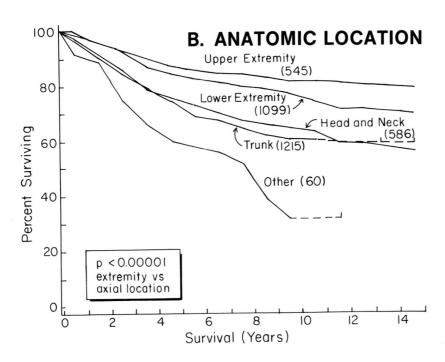

FIG. 19–1 Survival for stage I melanoma patients according to four clinical factors. In this and succeeding figures, the number of patients is indicated in *parentheses*. The *P* value is calculated for the correlation with survival. All survival rates are calculated by the actuarial method and are drawn as *solid lines* to the point of longest survival before death from melanoma; continued *broken lines* indicate the survival duration of patients remaining alive.

C. AGE

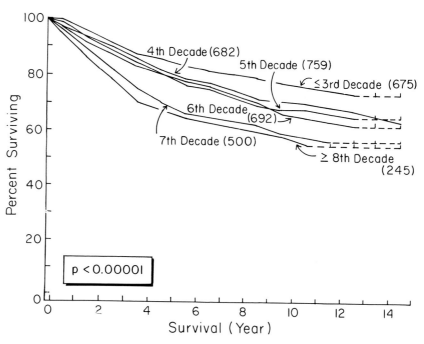

D. INITIAL SURGICAL TREATMENT

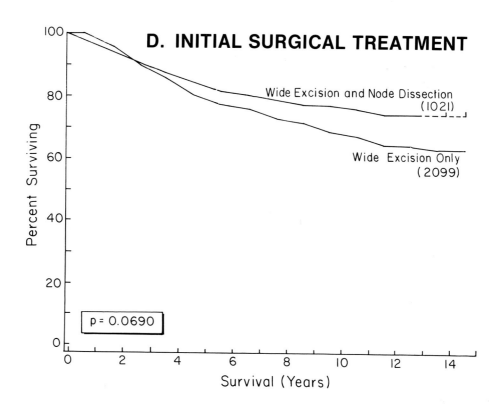

Anatomical location of primary lesion

Melanomas were divided evenly among the four major anatomical locations: 46% of all melanomas were on the upper and lower extremities, while 52% occurred on the trunk or head and neck (Table 19-1).

Patients with extremity melanomas had a better survival rate than those with trunk or head and neck melanomas (Fig. 19-1B; $p < 0.00001$), and those with upper extremity melanomas had a slightly better survival than those with melanomas on the lower extremity ($p = 0.08$).

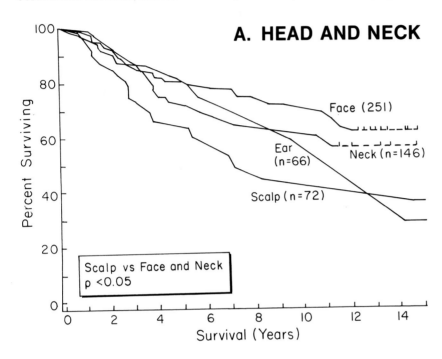

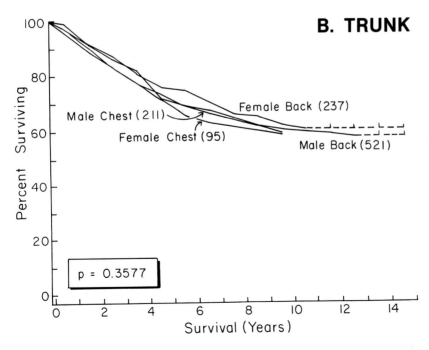

FIG. 19–2 Survival for stage I melanoma patients according to anatomical subsite and sex.

Analysis of anatomical subsites revealed some further differences in prognosis. In the head and neck region, patients with melanomas located on the scalp had a worse prognosis than those with lesions on the face or neck (Fig. 19-2A). These dif-ferences remained even after accounting for sex and tumor thickness.[39] There was no sex difference in prognosis for patients with lesions on these head and neck subsites. There was no survival difference for patients with back and chest lesions, even when sub-

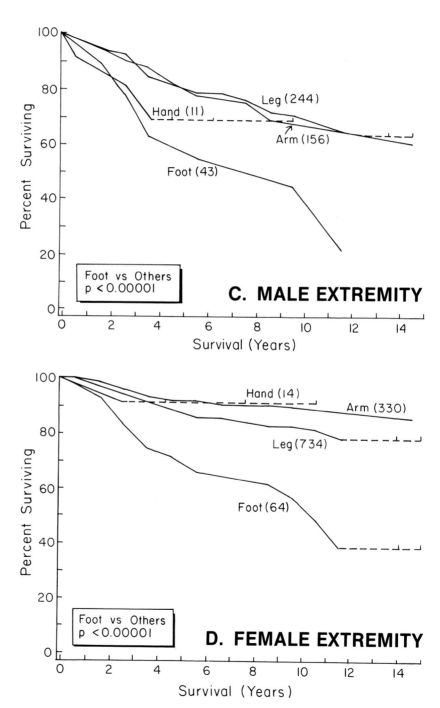

FIG. 19–2 (continued)

grouped by sex (Fig. 19-2B). Patients with melanomas located on the hands and feet had a significantly worse prognosis than those with lesions on the arm or leg.[17,19] In all these anatomical subsites, women had a better prognosis than men did (Figs. 19-2C and D; p < 0.00001). Part of this sex difference in prognosis could be accounted for by the higher proportion of men with ulcerated melanomas (29% versus 19%). Overall, there was no sex difference in prognosis in patients with ulcerated lesions. However, women had a better prognosis for each extremity subsite.

Finally, the four specific subsites reported by Day and colleagues[16] to have a poor prognosis were analyzed in this patient series. These were upper back, upper outer arm, neck, or scalp (BANS). Except for the scalp,[39] these subsites did not have a worse prognosis than other anatomical subsites.

Age

The median age of stage I melanoma patients was 45 years. Advancing age correlated significantly with a shortened length of survival (Fig. 19-1C; p < 0.00001). Patient age also correlated with melanoma thickness (p < 0.00001), with older patients presenting with thicker lesions. Thus, the median thickness for melanoma patients in their third decade was 1.1 mm, whereas it was 1.5 mm for those in the fifth decade and 2.8 mm for those in the seventh decade.

Surgical treatment

In this patient series, there were subgroups of melanoma patients that had statistically improved survival rates with elective regional lymph node dissection (ELND) compared with patients whose initial management was only a wide local excision (WLE) of the primary melanoma (Fig. 19-1D). These results are described in detail in Chapter 8. It is therefore important to include the type of initial surgical treatment (WLE alone or WLE plus ELND) as a prognostic factor in patients with stage I melanoma.

PATHOLOGIC FACTORS

Tumor thickness

The total vertical height of a melanoma is the single most important prognostic factor in stage I melanoma.[1,3,4,8] It is a quantitative parameter that can narrowly define subsets of patients with different survival (Fig. 19-3A; p < 0.00001). In fact, most other prognostic variables derive their predictive ability by a secondary correlation with tumor thickness (as described below). Numerous groups of thickness subsets have been measured for their prognostic value (e.g., <1 mm, 1 mm–4 mm, >4 mm), and only one was found to have more discriminating value than those originally advocated by Breslow.[8] As demonstrated by actuarial survival curves, a more significant survival difference was found using 4 mm rather than 3 mm.[1] It appears, however, that there are no "natural breakpoints,"[14] but rather statistically defined subgroups that will vary from one data set to another depending on the number of patients, the duration of follow-up, and the distribution of other factors (e.g., ulceration, anatomical site of primary lesion, and sex). The large number of patients in the present series has permitted the derivation of a simple nonlinear mathematical model that describes the relationship between tumor thickness and 10-year mortality rate as a continuous event (Fig. 19-4; $R^2 = 0.988$).

There are several important advantages of thickness microstaging that bear directly on the treatment approach. First, the risk of local recurrence, satellites, and intransit metastases correlated proportionately to increased thickness, so that decisions regarding surgical excision margins for the primary melanoma and the selection of patients for isolated limb perfusion can be made based on this parameter (see Chaps. 6 and 10). Second, tumor thickness can accurately predict the risk of metastases and may even be able to distinguish patient groups with isolated regional node metastases from those with a high risk for distant metastases. Patients can therefore be better selected who might benefit from ELND (see Chap. 8) and, in the future, adjuvant immunotherapy or chemotherapy (see Chap. 11).

Level of invasion

There was an inverse correlation between increasing level of melanoma invasion and survival (Fig. 19-3B). The level of invasion is a significant prognostic factor by single factor analysis (p < 0.00001), and it will discriminate patients at various risks for metastases. However, when each of the levels of invasion was further subdivided by tumor thickness, there was still heterogeneity within each level of invasion, both with respect to tumor thickness measurements (Fig. 19-5A) and survival (Fig. 19-6A). For example, level IV melanomas have a wide range of tumor thicknesses (0.6 mm–12.6 mm; median 2.7 mm) and survival. Almost one fourth of the level IV lesions had thickness measurements

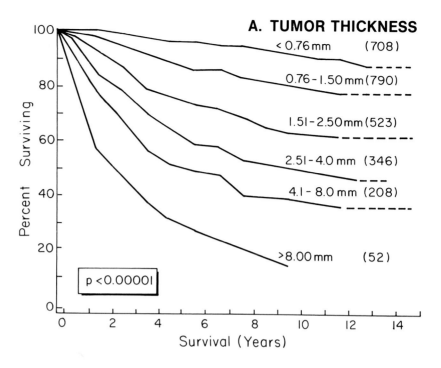

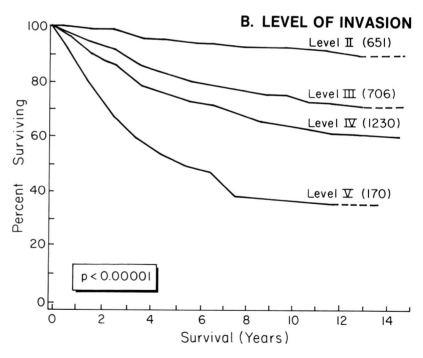

FIG. 19–3 Survival for stage I melanoma patients according to (A) tumor thickness and (B) level of invasion.

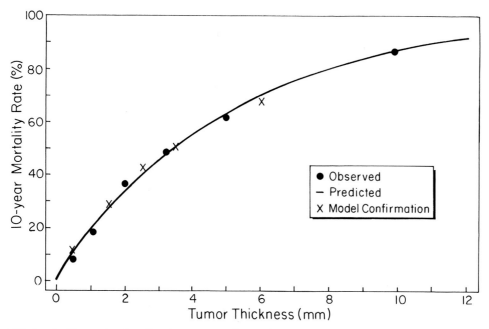

FIG. 19–4 Observed and predicted 10-year mortality rate based on a mathematical model derived from tumor thickness. The mathematical model is $9(T) = 1 - 0.966 \cdot e^{-0.2016T}$ and is described in more detail in Chapter 20. The *solid line* represents that predicted by the model, while the *closed circles* demonstrate the actual observed survival for 2627 patients in the combined Alabama and Sydney data. The accuracy of the model was confirmed by applying it to 747 stage I melanoma patients from the World Health Organization Melanoma Group (data that were not used in the derivation of the model). The linear nature of the curve demonstrates that there are no natural breakpoints but, rather, a continuous correlation of survival with tumor thickness.

< 1.5 mm, and these patients fared much better than did the majority of patients with thicker level IV melanomas (Fig. 19-5*B*).

Comparison of level versus thickness as prognostic indicators

A direct comparison of the two microstaging methods, level of invasion and tumor thickness, was made comparing each level of invasion subdivided by thickness. Within levels III, IV, and V, there were gradations of thickness that influenced survival (Fig. 19-6*A*). Converse relationships were not observed when analyzing sets of melanoma thickness subdivided by levels of invasion (Fig. 19-6*B*). For example, the 10-year survival rate for patients with lesions measuring 1.5 mm to 4 mm was not significantly different for level III, IV, and V lesions. These observations demonstrate that the tumor thickness measurement is a relatively more accurate prognostic factor.[1,2,3,4,10,17,18,19,21,22,31,33,34,40] It is more quantitative, easier to measure, and predicts the risk of metastatic disease better than the level of invasion does. These results were confirmed in a multifactorial analysis (see below).

Ulceration

About one fourth of stage I melanomas were ulcerated (see Table 19-1). Men had a higher proportion of ulcerated lesions that did women (29% versus 19%). The presence of ulceration in the microscopic sections of melanoma is a significant adverse determinant of survival (Fig. 19-7*A*; $p < 0.00001$). Stage I melanoma patients with ulceration had a 10-year survival rate of 50%, while those without ulceration had a 78% 10-year survival rate ($p < 0.0001$). There was a positive correlation of ulceration with thickness ($p < 0.0001$). The median thickness for patients with ulcerated lesions was 3 mm, while those without ulcerated lesions had a median thickness of 1.3 mm. Lesions > 1.5 mm thick were associated with

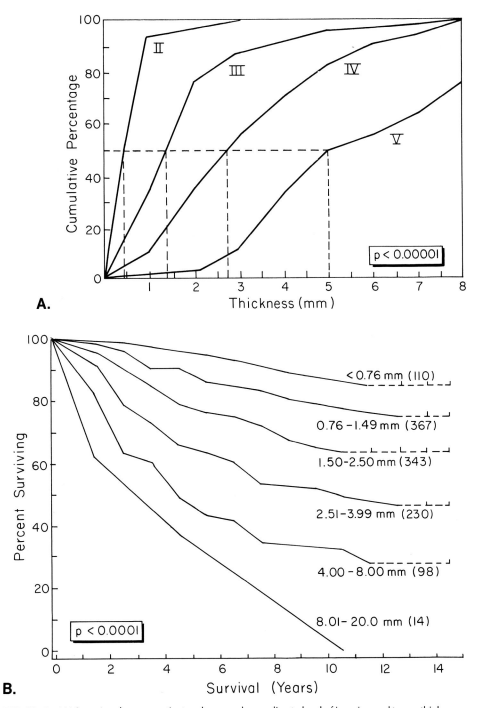

FIG. 19–5 (A) Stage I melanoma patients subgrouped according to level of invasion and tumor thickness. Median thickness for each level is shown by the *dotted lines*. There was a particularly wide range of tumor thickness for level III and IV melanomas. (B) Survival for stage I melanoma patients with level IV lesions according to tumor thickness. The minority of patients with thin level IV melanomas had a relatively favorable prognosis.

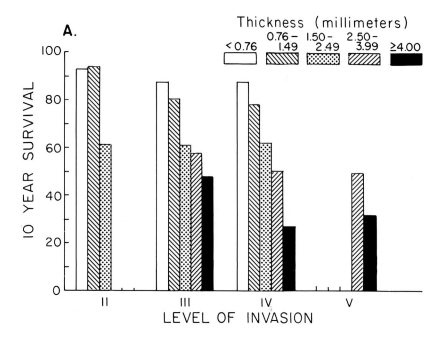

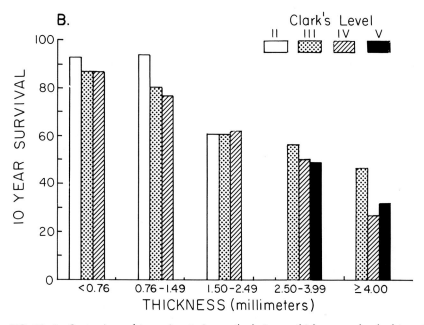

FIG. 19–6 Comparison of two microstaging methods (tumor thickness vs. level of invasion). (*Top*) Ten-year survival rates for stage I melanoma patients according to levels of invasion subgrouped by tumor thickness. There were statistically significant differences in survival rates for patients with lesions of various thicknesses within levels III, IV, and V. (*Bottom*) Ten-year survival rates for stage I melanoma patients according to tumor thickness subgrouped by levels of invasion. There were no statistically significant differences in survival rates for patients with lesions of various levels of invasion within each thickness subgroup.

a 44% incidence of ulceration. The width of the ulceration delineated two prognostic subgroups when analyzed in the UAB data.[7] Melanomas with ulcerated areas < 6 mm wide were thinner overall and had a more shallow ulcer crater than melanomas with ulcers ≥ 6 mm wide; 5-year survival rates for these patients were higher as well (44% versus 5%; p < 0.001).

There is a complex interaction of three important prognostic variables: ulceration, anatomical location of the primary lesion, and sex of the patient. As mentioned before, there is a female superiority in survival, but most of this can be accounted for by the fact that men have a high proportion of lesions that are ulcerative and are located on less favorable anatomical sites (*i.e.,* trunk, head, and neck). When these differences were minimized by grouping patients according to these two variables, there was still a female superiority in 10-year survival for p' tients with extremity lesions (Table 19-2). Women with nonulcerative, extremity lesions had an excellent 10-year survival rate of 89% (Table 19-2). Whether there is or is not an inherently better prognosis for women is still controversial, since women have thinner melanomas than men have.

Growth pattern

Survival rates for patients with three growth patterns of melanoma are shown in Figure 19-7*B*. While acral lentiginous melanomas are also known to represent a distinct growth pattern, this has only been recently appreciated; thus, long-term follow-up results are not available. Patients with superficial spreading (SSM) and lentigo maligna (LMM) lesions had the best survival, whereas those with nodular lesions (NM) had the worst prognosis. The

most statistically significant difference among these groups was between SSM and NM (p < 0.0001).

When patients with SSM and NM were matched for thickness and their 10-year survival rates calculated, no difference was found in these two growth patterns as prognostic factors (Fig. 19-8). Patients with SSM appear to have a better prognosis than those with NM only because SMM are thinner lesions.

Lentigo maligna melanomas constituted only a small number of patients (4%). These lesions were all located on the face or neck and were generally thinner lesions. When matched thickness for thickness, patients with LMM lesions had a better prognosis than the other growth patterns (Fig. 19-8) as described previously.[29] Even LMM lesions ≥ 3 mm thick had an 80% 10-year survival rate.

Lymphocyte infiltration

Lymphocyte infiltration is a prognostic parameter that was categorized in three grades as described.[1] Those patients with the most intense degree of lymphocyte infiltrate had the best survival (Fig. 19-7*C*). There was an inverse correlation with thickness and the amount of lymphocyte infiltrate beneath the primary melanoma lesion.[4,28] Patients with absent-to-minimal lymphocyte infiltration had lesions with a median thickness of 2.3 mm compared with 1.1-mm lesions in those with a heavy lymphocyte infiltration. After adjustment for tumor thickness, the prognostic significance of lymphocyte infiltration disappeared.[3,4,27]

Pigmentation

Pigmentation was present if melanoma cells or macrophages contained melanin pigment in their cytoplasm. Lesions were classified as amelanotic if virtually all cells lacked cytoplasmic melanin. Only 7% of melanomas were amelanotic, and this feature was a significant adverse determinant of survival (Fig. 19-7*D*). Ten-year survival rates of patients with lesions lacking pigmentation was 54%, whereas those patients with pigmentation had a 73% 10-year survival rate. Amelanotic tumors tended to be considerably thicker than highly pigmented tumors, thus accounting for their poor prognosis.[26]

Regression

Regression of the primary melanoma is an interpretive pathologic entity. Signs of regression include increased vascularity with scattered melanin-laden

TABLE 19–2
ULCERATION AND PROGNOSIS IN STAGE I MELANOMA

	10-Year Survival Rate	
	Ulcerated	Nonulcerated
Axial Melanoma*		
Male	26%	61%
Female	25%	70%
Extremity Melanoma		
Male	23%	70%[†]
Female	41%	89%[†]

* Trunk and head and neck regions.

[†] Survival differences in nonulcerated extremity melanomas: male versus female, p = 0.01.

(*Text continued on page 336*)

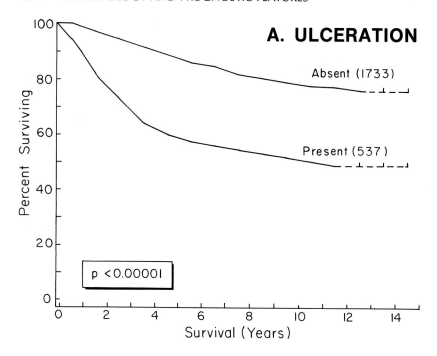

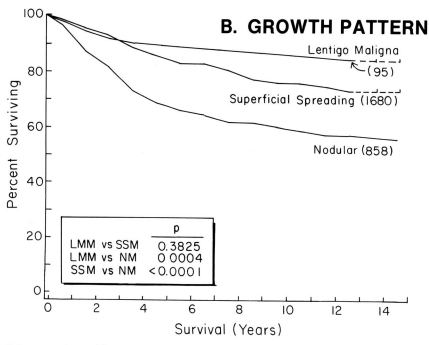

FIG. 19–7 Survival for stage I melanoma patients according to four histopathologic factors.

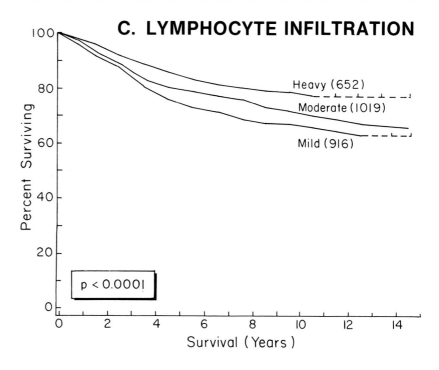

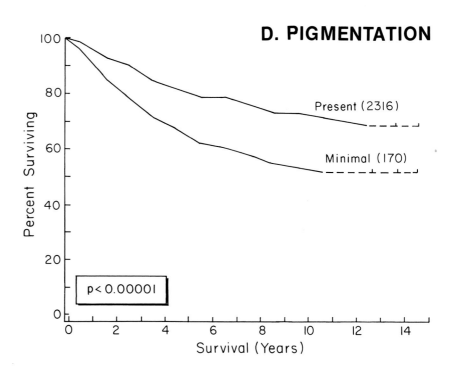

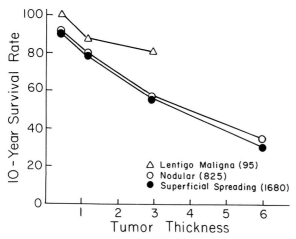

FIG. 19–8 Ten-year survival rates for stage I melanoma patients according to growth pattern and tumor thickness. In patients with melanomas of equivalent tumor thickness, those with nodular and superficial spreading melanomas had similar survival rates, while those with lentigo maligna melanomas had a much more favorable prognosis.

macrophages in the dermis and signs of fibrosis.[37] Typically, the overlying epidermis in the area of regression lacks melanin pigment, whereas pigment is recognized in normal epidermis. There has been considerable controversy regarding the metastatic potential of thin regressing melanomas, with some investigators concluding that there is increased risk[23,30] and others concluding that there is no increased risk.[28,38] An important reason for these different findings is the interpretive nature of defining regression and the variable length of follow-up in different series.

In both the UAB and the SMU data, regression was not an adverse prognostic factor.[1,28] For thin melanomas (0.1 mm–0.75 mm), there was no difference in survival of patients with and without regression. Patients with thin regressing melanomas did have a slightly lower survival rate at 5 years than those with thin unregressed melanomas, but the survival curves merged after 10 years of follow-up (Fig. 19-9), again emphasizing the importance of long-term follow-up. Those patients with regressing melanomas that measured 0.76 mm to 1.49 mm in thickness actually had a significantly better survival than those without regression (Fig. 19-9).

Pathologic stage

There were 22 clinical stage I patients who had occult nodal metastases (clinical stage I, pathologic stage II) identified after ELND. These patients had

a 58% 10-year survival rate compared to 80% for those patients without nodal metastases and 16% for those patients with clinically evident nodal metastases (p = 0.0032; Fig. 19-10). Several investigators have found that tumor thickness can delineate different risk groups among those patients with occult nodal metastases.[20] However, no correlation with thickness was found in this subgroup of patients in the present series.[3] This may be a result of the relatively small sample size, since thickness was predictive in some patients with clinically detectable nodal metastases (see below).

MULTIFACTORIAL ANALYSIS

The above clinical and pathologic parameters were simultaneously compared for their prognostic strength using both single-factor and multifactorial analyses. For the purposes of these analyses, only the 2151 patients for whom *all* clinical and pathologic information was available were included. While almost all data were available for the other patients, their data were excluded from the multifactorial analysis because information for one or more factors was not available. Table 19-3 presents the relative importance of each single factor unadjusted for other factors. A multifactorial analysis

TABLE 19–3
PROGNOSTIC FACTORS ANALYSIS OF CLINICAL STAGE I MELANOMA

Analysis	*Probability*
Single Factor Analysis	
Tumor thickness	< 0.00001
Ulceration	< 0.00001
Level of invasion	< 0.00001
Primary melanoma site	< 0.00001
Sex	< 0.00001
Age	< 0.00001
Pathologic stage	< 0.00001
Pigmentation	< 0.00001
Regression	< 0.00001
Surgical treatment	0.0006
Lymphocyte infiltration	0.0066
Growth pattern	0.0451
Multifactorial Analysis	
Tumor thickness	< 0.00001
Surgical treatment	< 0.00001
Primary melanoma site	< 0.00001
Ulceration	< 0.00001
Pathologic stage	< 0.00001
Level of invasion	0.0026
Sex	0.0029
Regression	0.0327

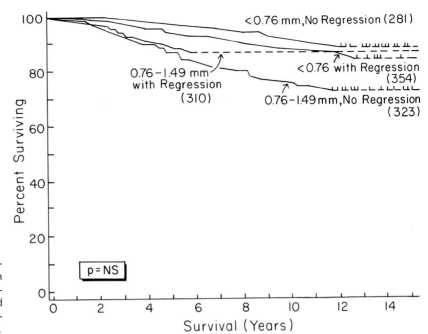

FIG. 19–9 Survival for stage I melanoma patients according to regression and tumor thickness <1.5 mm. Patients with regressing melanomas had essentially the same prognosis as patients with nonregressing melanomas.

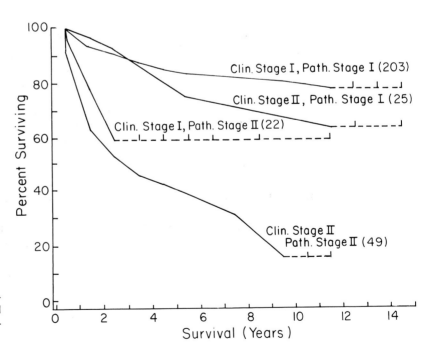

FIG. 19–10 Survival for UAB melanoma patients based on both clinical and pathologic staging (± nodal metastases).

was then performed to examine the primary predictive factors that independently correlated with survival, while simultaneously accounting for the contribution of the other factors listed above (Table 19-3). Each variable was analyzed in sequence for the additive prognostic value after the preceding factor had been accounted for. In the UAB data, for example, when the level of invasion was ranked in the first position followed by tumor thickness, the p values for each variable were 0.003 and 0.001, respectively. This indicated that the parameter of tumor thickness contributed additional prognostic information *after* level of invasion had been accounted for. On the other hand, when these variables were arranged in reverse order, thickness was a highly predictive factor (p < 0.001), but the level of invasion had no additional predictive influence after the thickness was accounted for (p = 0.255).

The influence of these factors on survival was examined using a cohort of 2151 stage I patients for whom information was available for all prognostic factors being analyzed. There were five dominant factors predicting survival in stage I melanoma patients: (1) *thickness* of the melanoma, (2) the type of *initial surgical management* (WLE ± ELND), (3) *pathologic stage* (I versus II), (4) melanoma *ulceration* (present or absent), and (5) *anatomical location* (upper extremity versus lower extremity versus trunk versus head and neck) (Table 19-3). Three other variables also correlated to a lesser extent with survival in certain subgroups of patients: (1) *level of invasion,* (2) *sex,* and (3) *tumor regression* (present or absent) (Table 19-3).

The multifactorial analysis was then repeated within eight separate subgroups to verify these findings (Table 19-4). Melanoma thickness and ulceration had the greatest correlation with survival rates (p < 10^6) for the entire stage I patient population and for all subgroups examined. Most of the other prognostic factors examined derived their prognostic strength through a secondary correlation with tumor thickness. While these and other factors may be important biologically in determining outcome, they were not useful as prognostic factors as long as some of the other features described above were accounted for.

Most other major studies using multifactorial analyses have established *tumor thickness* to be the most important prognostic factor in their series of stage I melanoma patients.[10,13,17,18,19,22,24,31,33,34,40] Similarly, *ulceration* was found to be another strong predictor of survival in eight other patient series.[13,15,19,21,22,31,34,40] Three of these series confirmed

that anatomical location of the primary lesion was another major predictor of survival.[17,19,22]

Other factors analyzed by multivariate analysis that emerged as important variables overall or within selected subgroups in other series included *sex*[10,21,24] and *age* of the patient,[22] as well as tumor features such as lymphocytic infiltrate,[18,21] *tumor diameter,*[22,33,34] *cell type,*[21,40] *microscopic satellites,*[15] *mitotic activity,*[17,18,22,24,31,33,34,40] and *level of invasion.*[22] The timing of the biopsy prior to first definitive treatment was also found to have a significant influence on survival in one series.[21]

Schmoeckel and associates[33,34] considered that the combination of different parameters should improve the degree of prognostic information. They performed multivariate and discriminant analyses in efforts to determine those patients at low or high risk for developing metastases. The product of mitotic activity and tumor thickness, which they termed "prognostic index," was the most powerful prognostic determinant in their patient series. Depending on whether they were "low-risk" or "high-risk" patients, several other factors alone or in combination influenced prognosis. These were ulceration, vascular invasion, lesion diameter, and anatomical location of the lesion.

PROGNOSTIC FACTORS IN PATIENTS WITH METASTATIC MELANOMA IN REGIONAL LYMPH NODES (STAGE II)

Twelve prognostic features of melanoma were examined in a series of 551 patients with nodal metastases who were treated at the two institutions (UAB and SMU) during the past 20 years. For the purposes of designation, these patients were subgrouped into three categories: IIA patients had synchronous nodal metastases with the primary melanoma; IIB patients had subsequent (delayed) nodal metastases after primary melanoma treatment; and IIC patients had nodal metastases from an unknown primary site. The UAB data contained all three substages, whereas the SMU data did not include substage IIB. The overall survival curves for all stage II patients were virtually the same for the two institutions, with differences not exceeding 6% at any point in the survival curves calculated out to 15 years, where it was 25% at SMU and 20% at UAB. A data base comparing some stages of melanoma patients and their distribution of prognostic factors is shown in Table 19-5. As previously de-

TABLE 19–4
A COLLABORATIVE STUDY OF MELANOMA—UNIVERSITY OF ALABAMA IN BIRMINGHAM AND UNIVERSITY OF SYDNEY:
Analysis of Prognostic Factors in Subgroups of Patients with Clinical Stage I Melanoma and Summary of Multifactorial Analyses

	Number of Patients	Dominant Factors Within Subgroups								
		Tumor Thickness	Ulceration	Level of Invasion	Regression	Primary Melanoma Site	Sex	Surgical Treatment	Pathologic Stage	Other Factors
Overall	(2151)	<0.00001	<0.00001	0.0026	0.0327	<0.00001	0.0029	<0.00001	<0.00001	—
Year of First Definitive Treatment										
≤1970	(444)	<0.00001	0.0003	—†	—	0.0557	0.0018	0.0003	—	—
>1970	(1707)	<0.00001	<0.00001	0.0090	0.0156	<0.00001	—	<0.00001	<0.00001	Age p = 0.0129
Tumor Thickness (mm)										
<0.76	(556)	—	0.0088	—	—	0.0024	—	—	—	
0.76–1.49	(618)	—	0.0001	0.0228	0.0181	0.0004	0.0211	0.0509	0.0721	
1.50–2.49	(445)	—	0.0393	—	—	0.0079	—	<0.00001	0.0939	
2.50–3.99	(305)	—	—	—	—	0.0001	—	0.0025	0.0006	
4.00–5.99	(146)	—	0.0002	—	—	—	—	0.0346	—	
≥6.0	(81)	—	0.0102	—	—	0.0205	—	0.0144	0.0364	
Primary Melanoma Site										
Extremity	(730)	0.0001	<0.00001	0.0198	—	0.0435	0.572	<0.00001	—	—
Head/neck	(266)	0.00003	0.0289	—	—	0.021	—	—	—	—
Trunk	(789)	<0.00001	0.0002	0.0027	—	0.0171	—	0.0002	—	
Sex										
Male	(1039)	<0.00001	0.0021	0.0078	—	0.0052	—	<0.00001	0.0001	
Female	(1112)	<0.00001	<0.00001	—	—	<0.00001	—	0.0036	0.0855	Lymphocyte Infiltration p = 0.0148
Surgical Treatment										
WLE only	(1421)	<0.00001	<0.00001	0.0008	—	0.0046	0.0007	—	—	
WLE & RND‡	(730)	<0.00001	0.0046	—	0.0872	<0.00001	—	—	0.0001	Growth Pattern p = 0.0032
Ulceration										
Absent	(1428)	<0.00001	—	0.0090	—	<0.00001	0.0163	0.00003	0.0299	
Present	(433)	0.0004	—	0.0360	0.0849	0.0044	—	<0.000001	0.0002	Age p = 0.0635
Regression										
No	(1043)	<0.000001	<0.000001	0.0129	—	<0.00001	0.0103	<0.000001	—	
Yes	(895)	<0.000001	0.0495	—	—	0.0037	0.0533	0.0001	0.0391	—

† The dash indicates factors that were not statistically significant within that subgroup.
‡ Wide local excision plus elective regional node dissection.

TABLE 19–5
DATA BASE FOR MELANOMA PATIENTS WITH NODAL METASTASES (STAGE II)

	Simultaneous Nodal Metastases (Stage IIA)	Delayed Nodal Metastases (Stage IIB) (UAB only)	Nodal Metastases from Unknown Primary Site (Stage IIC)
Number of Patients	328	82	141
Primary Lesion Site			
Lower extremity	31%	21%	
Upper extremity	12%	13%	
Head and neck	17%	28%	
Trunk	38%	34%	
Other	2%	4%	
Median Age	44 yr	50 yr	43 yr
Sex			
Male	69%	54%	70%
Female	31%	46%	30%
Tumor Thickness			
<1.5 mm	11%	21%	
1.5 mm–4 mm	40%	48%	
>4 mm	49%	31%	
Median	3.6 mm	3.2 mm	
Level of Invasion			
II/III	28%	37%	
IV/V	72%	63%	
Ulceration			
Present	56%	38%	
Absent	44%	62%	
Growth Pattern			
Nodular	64%	70%	
Superficial spreading	34%	28%	
Lentigo maligna	2%	2%	
Lymphocyte Infiltration			
Absent/mild	39%	46%	
Moderate/heavy	61%	54%	
Pigmentation			
Present	87%	84%	
Minimal	13%	16%	
Number of Metastatic Nodes*			
1	34%	36%	53%
2–4	49%	34%	26%
>4	17%	30%	21%

* These data available for UAB patients only.

scribed in the UAB series,[5] it was found that the prognosis in the combined series was similar for all three substages (IIA, IIB, and IIC) as long as the survival rates were calculated from the diagnosis of the lymph node metastases. Prognosis for all stage II patients described in this chapter was determined in this manner.

CLINICAL FACTORS

Sex

The majority (69%) of patients with stage II melanomas were men, compared with a lower male proportion in stage I patients (44%). There were no differences in survival rates among male and female stage II melanoma patients, even when the data were cross-analyzed by other categories.

Anatomical location of primary lesion

The primary melanoma accompanied by nodal metastases occurred in anatomical locations that were distributed throughout the body, with 56% of melanomas arising in axial locations (trunk, head, and neck). Patients with melanomas on the trunk constituted the largest group, being 35% of the entire series. Those with head and neck melanomas had the worst survival rates, but there was no statistically significant difference in survival rates for patients with melanomas among these various anatomical locations, even when the data were cross-analyzed by substages of disease, sex, and the number of metastatic nodes.

Age

The median age of the entire stage II patient population was 44 years. Older stage II melanoma patients had a tendency to have a worse prognosis than younger patients did. For example, only 23% of patients were alive after 5 years if they were over 50 years of age at time of initial diagnosis, compared to 42% for patients who developed melanoma when they were 50 years of age or younger. This difference was not statistically significant. However,

significant differences did appear when the data were further subgrouped by gender (Fig. 19-11; $p = 0.0094$). Younger women (≤ 50 years of age) had a much higher survival rate than older women did, whereas the differences between younger and older men were not as great (Fig. 19-11).

Remission duration

The remission duration between initial diagnosis and onset of nodal metastases was examined in the cohort of 82 substage IIB patients treated at UAB. Survival rates were the same for patients who developed clinically detectable nodal metastases between 1 and 12 months and between 13 and 24 months after the initial diagnosis of nodal metastases (Fig. 19-12). There was a trend for patients who had a remission duration exceeding 2 years to have better survival rates, but the differences were not statistically significant for either of the other two subgroups.

PATHOLOGIC FACTORS

Number of metastatic nodes

This parameter could be evaluated only in the UAB data, where there was a direct correlation between the number of metastatic nodes and survival (Fig. 19-13). Patients with one metastatic node had a bet-

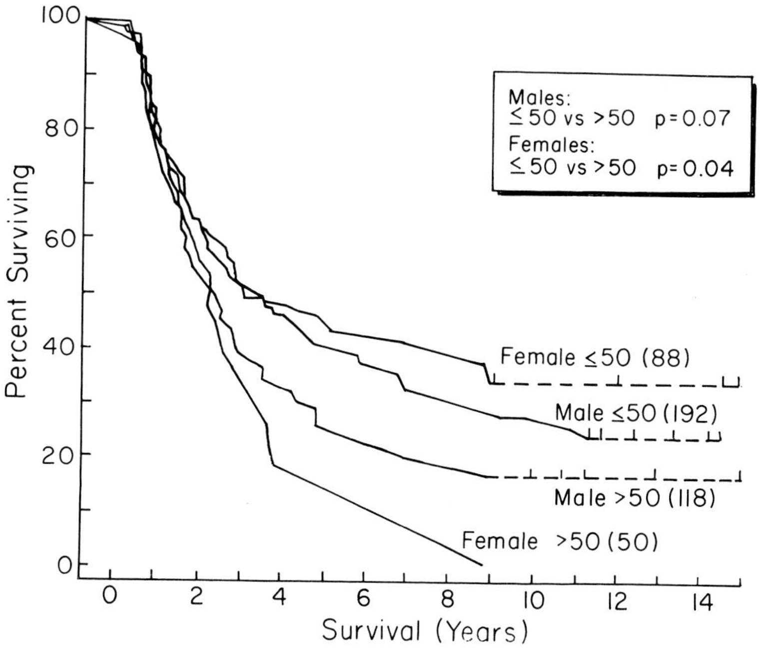

FIG. 19-11 Survival for stage II melanoma patients according to sex and age. Remission duration was determined from time of diagnosis of nodal metastases.

ter survival rate than did patients with two nodes or any multiples of metastatic nodes. All combinations of nodal metastases were analyzed for survival differences. The combination that showed the greatest differences in this series was 1 node versus 2 to 4 nodes versus ≥ 5 nodes (Fig. 19-13). Thirty-seven

percent of patients had one positive node, 41% had 2 to 4 nodes, and 22% had 5 or more metastatic nodes. Their 3-year survival rates were 65%, 43%, and 22% respectively ($p < 0.001$). Ten-year survival rates demonstrated that only patients with one positive node had a reasonable prospect of cure (40%

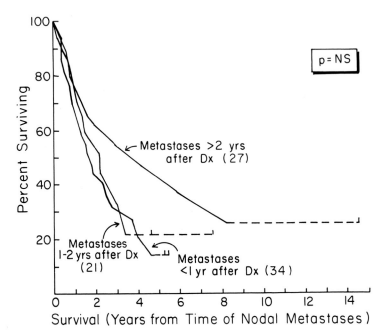

FIG. 19–12 Survival for substage IIB melanoma patients according to remission durations (Balch CM et al: A multifactorial analysis of melanoma. III. Prognostic factors in melanoma patients with lymph node metastases (stage II). Ann Surg 193:377, 1981)

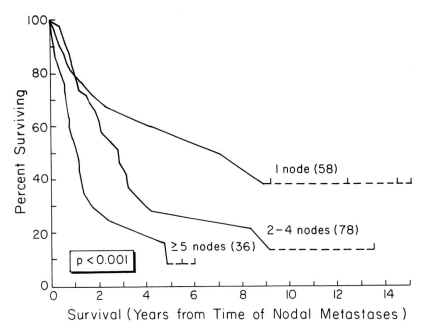

FIG. 19–13 Survival for all stage II melanoma patients according to the number of metastatic nodes (Balch CM et al: A multifactorial analysis of melanoma. III. Prognostic factors in melanoma patients with lymph node metastases (stage II). Ann Surg 193:377, 1981)

were alive at 10 years), while about 13% of patients with two or more metastatic nodes were alive at 10 years.

Ulceration

Ulceration was the most important characteristic of the primary melanoma that predicted the risk of subsequent nodal metastases in stage I patients and continued to be an important predictive factor once nodal metastases had occurred.[5,7] Thus, the 3-year survival for stage II patients with ulcerative melanomas was only 29% compared to 61% for nonulcerative melanomas (p = 0.0002; Fig. 19-14). When ulceration was cross-analyzed with the number of metastatic nodes in the UAB data, it was evident that there was some interaction between these two important prognostic factors. For each category of metastatic node, the presence of ulceration in the primary lesion implied a worse prognosis than if the melanoma had an intact overlying epithelium (Fig. 19-15). Thus, patients with one positive node and no ulceration of their primary melanoma had the most favorable prognosis of any patient group, having a 50% 10-year survival rate. In contrast, patients with five or more positive nodes *and* ulceration of the primary melanoma had an extremely poor prognosis, since none of the ten patients in this category survived more than 14 months (Fig. 19-15).

Tumor thickness

The median thickness for stage II melanomas was 3.6 mm compared with 1.5 mm for stage I lesions (p < 0.001). Of the patients with stage IIA disease, 49% had thick melanomas (< 4 mm thick), while only 31% of patients with stage IIB disease had thick melanomas. Thickness of the primary melanoma correlated with survival rates (Fig. 19-16). This correlation was much stronger in the SMU data than in the UAB data. A significant interaction was also identified between thickness and ulceration (Fig. 19-17). Nonulcerative melanomas < 4 mm thick had a relatively more favorable 5-year survival compared to those ≥ 4 mm thick (57% versus 44%, respectively), while ulcerated melanomas ≥ 4 mm thick had only an 8% 5-year survival.

Other factors

Histopathologic parameters of the primary melanoma that did not predict survival included growth pattern, degree of lymphocytic infiltration, and pigmentation, as well as level of invasion.

MULTIFACTORIAL ANALYSIS

Each of the above 12 prognostic factors was examined for its predictive value of metastatic risk and survival. Table 19-6 presents the relative importance

(*Text continues on page 346*)

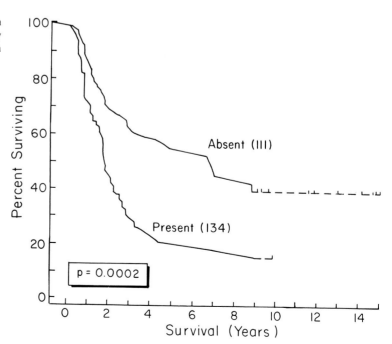

FIG. 19–14 Survival for all stage II melanoma patients according to ulceration of the primary melanoma. Presence of ulceration signified a significantly worse prognosis.

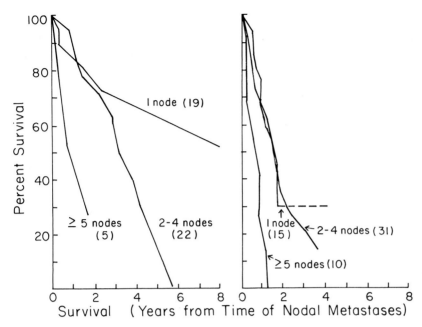

FIG. 19–15 Survival for all stage II melanoma patients according to the number of metastatic nodes and ulceration of the primary melanoma. (*Left*) ulceration absent. (*Right*) Ulceration present. The presence of ulceration had a significantly adverse prognostic effect on patients in each metastatic node category. (Balch CM et al: A multifactorial analysis of melanoma. III. Prognostic factors in melanoma patients with lymph node metastases (stage II). Ann Surg 193:377, 1981)

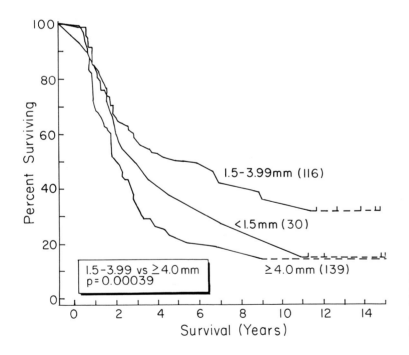

FIG. 19–16 Survival for all stage II melanoma patients according to tumor thickness. There was a significant survival difference for patients with melanomas <4.0-mm thick compared to those with melanomas ≥4.0-mm thick.

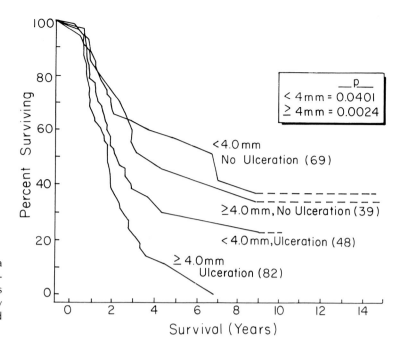

FIG. 19–17 Survival for all stage II melanoma patients according to tumor thickness and ulceration. Within each thickness group, patients with ulcerated melanomas had significantly worse prognoses than those with nonulcerated melanomas.

TABLE 19–6
PROGNOSTIC FACTORS ANALYSIS OF STAGE II MELANOMA

	UAB only	SMU only	UAB and SMU
	p Value	p Value	p Value
Single-factor Analysis			
Number of nodes	0.0002	NA	NA
Ulceration	0.0006	0.0006	<0.00001
Primary lesion location			
(extremity versus axial)	0.1213	0.7307	0.4089
Remission duration	0.1840		
Age	0.2169	0.7189	0.0369
Lymphocyte infiltration	0.3176	0.5813	0.9738
Synchronous versus			
metachronous metastases	0.3499		
Level of invasion	0.4894	0.2599	0.0953
Tumor thickness	0.5072	0.0021	0.0042
Pigmentation	0.5200	0.4358	0.6940
Growth pattern	0.5298	0.3437	0.1923
Sex	0.9719	0.5698	0.7638
Multifactorial Analysis*			
Number of nodes	0.0005	NA	NA
Ulceration	0.0019	0.0041	<0.00001
Age	NS	NS	0.0478
Tumor thickness	NS	0.0127	0.0686

* All other factors had a p > 0.10.

NS = not significant.

NA = data not available.

of single factors unadjusted for other factors. By single-factor analysis, the most significant prognostic variables were the number of nodes, the presence or absence of ulceration of the primary melanoma, tumor thickness of the primary melanoma (< 4 mm or ≥ 4 mm), and the patient's age. However, there could be other intercorrelations of these variables, such as with anatomical site of the primary melanoma and sex.

In contrast to the stage I melanoma analysis, no further dominant variables were delineated by the multifactorial analysis in the stage II patients. Thus, the multifactorial analysis confirmed that only the number of nodes ($p = 0.0005$), ulceration $p < 0.00001$), and age ($p = 0.05$) were the dominant variables, while tumor thickness had a borderline correlation ($p = 0.0686$) in the combined data but a stronger correlation in the SMU data ($p = 0.01$). All other factors had a p value greater than 0.10.

The number of metastatic nodes was first shown to be of prognostic significance in a multivariate analysis by Cohen and associates.[11] Later, both Day and associates[20] and Callery and associates[9] demonstrated that tumor thickness and the number of metastatic nodes were dominant independent variables in stage II patients. Cascinelli and colleagues[10] identified the extent of nodal metastases (*i.e.,* confined to or invading through the capsule) and the number of metastatic nodes as the most significant factors in a multifactorial analysis of 530 stage II patients (see Chap. 29).

PROGNOSTIC FACTORS IN PATIENTS WITH METASTATIC MELANOMA AT DISTANT SITES (STAGE III)

The data base for 200 patients with distant metastases treated at UAB was separated into clinical and pathologic factors (Table 19-7). The median survival for these patients was only 6 months. This data base includes some UAB patients previously analyzed under stages I and II, if they subsequently progressed into stage III disease, as well as patients who initially presented with distant metastases. All survival rates are calculated from the onset of distant metastases.[6]

CLINICAL FACTORS
Sex
Once they progressed to distant metastases, there was no correlation whatsoever with the sex of the patients and their clinical course ($p = 0.98$). Survival curves for male and female stage III melanoma patients were superimposable. Even when patients were further subgrouped according to other prognostic parameters, no difference between male and female stage III melanoma patients was discerned. When patterns of metastases were compared for men and women, there was no sex predilection to any site (*e.g.,* lung) or to combinations of metastatic sites (*e.g.,* visceral versus nonvisceral).

Anatomical location of primary lesion

Although there was a predilection for trunk melanomas to progress more commonly to distant metastases, the site of the primary melanoma was not a significant prognostic factor ($p = 0.21$).

Age

The median age of stage III melanoma patients was 51 years, which was slightly older than that for stage I patients (47 years). However, the age of the patient did not correlate with outcome for stage III disease ($p = 0.76$).

Remission duration

The length of remission was not a statistically significant factor (by single-factor analysis) in predicting the clinical course of disease when the survival rates were calculated from the onset of distant metastases ($p = 0.25$). Patients with stage I and II melanomas who relapsed within 1 year had the same survival rates as those who initially presented with stage III disease (Fig. 19-18). There was a trend for stage I and II patients with remission durations exceeding 1 year to have a slightly better survival rate, but the survival curves of different remission durations all merged after 16 months (Fig. 19-18). All stage III patients can therefore be pooled for statistical analysis, regardless of their presenting disease stage.

Site of distant metastases

The location of distant metastases was an important prognostic factor when examined by single-factor analysis ($p = 0.0001$). The skin, subcutaneous tissues, and distant lymph nodes were the most common first site of relapse. This occurred in 59% of patients (Table 19-8). In 23% of patients, these nonvisceral sites were the sole manifestation (14% for skin, 5% for subcutaneous sites, and 4% for distant lymph nodes). The median survival duration for this patient group was 7 months (see Table 19-8), whereas 25% were alive at 1 year. There was no difference in survival for any combination of these three metastatic sites. The next most common site

TABLE 19–7
CHARACTERISTICS OF PATIENTS WITH STAGE III METASTATIC MELANOMA

| | Presenting Pathologic Stage | | | | |
	I	II (Known 1°)	II (Unknown 1°)	III	Combined
Number of Patients	123 (61%)	43 (22%)	18 (9%)	16 (8%)	200
Primary Lesion Site					
Lower extremity	23%	21%		31%	21%
Upper extremity	7%	19%		12%	10%
Head and neck	26%	16%		12%	20%
Trunk	37%	44%		19%	33%
Other	7%	0%	100%	25%	16%
Age					
Median	52 yr	51 yr	46 yr	63 yr	51 yr
>65 yr	18%	16%	11%	56%	21%
Sex					
Male	54%	72%	72%	69%	61%
Female	46%	28%	28%	31%	39%
Tumor Thickness					
<1.5 mm	23%	18%		0%	20%
1.5 mm–4 mm	50%	38%		67%	42%
>4 mm	27%	44%		33%	37%
Median	2.2 mm	3.6 mm		2.8 mm	2.7 mm
Level of Invasion					
II/III	59%	13%		17%	30%
IV/V	41%	87%		83%	70%
Ulceration					
Present	51%	72%		50%	58%
Absent	49%	28%		50%	42%
Growth Pattern					
Nodular	73%	81%		83%	76%
Superficial spreading	26%	19%		17%	23%
Lentigo maligna	1%	0%		0%	1%
Lymphocyte Infiltration					
Absent/mild	51%	66%		80%	56%
Moderate/heavy	49%	34%		20%	44%
Pigmentation					
Present	82%	74%		67%	80%
Minimal	18%	26%		33%	20%
Median Duration to Distant Metastases	2.8 yr	0.9 yr			
Median Survival from Distant Metastases to Death	0.5 yr	0.4 yr		0.5 yr	0.5 yr

of first relapse was the lung (36% of patients). Patients with isolated lung metastases had the longest median survival duration for any metastatic site (11 months). Brain, liver, and bone metastases were the next most common sites of first relapse. The median duration of survival for these patients was very poor, ranging from 2 to 6 months (Table 19-8), with the 1-year survival being only 8% to 10%.

The anatomical sites of the metastases were combined into two groups: visceral (lung, brain, liver, and bone) versus nonvisceral sites (skin, sub- cutaneous tissue, and distant lymph nodes). As shown in Figure 19-19, the minority of patients who had nonvisceral metastases had a prolonged survival compared with the majority of patients who had visceral metastases, both in terms of median survival time (8 months versus 3 months) and in 1-year survival (46% versus 18%). The presence of visceral metastases had an overriding influence on survival, since those patients with combined visceral and nonvisceral sites had the same poor prognosis as those with visceral metastases alone.

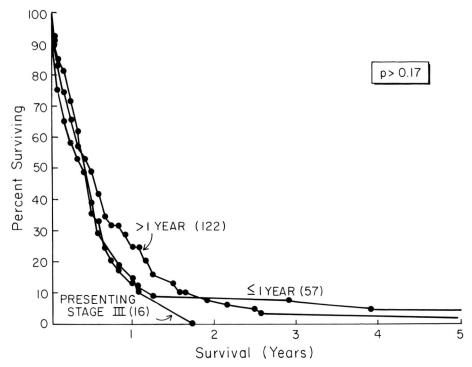

FIG. 19–18 Survival for patients with stage III melanoma according to remission duration. Survival was calculated from the onset of distant metastases. There was no significant difference in survivals (Balch CM et al: A multifactorial analysis of melanoma. IV. Prognostic factors in 200 melanoma patients with distant metastases (stage III). J Clin Oncol 1:126, 1983)

TABLE 19–8
FIRST SITE OF DISTANT METASTASES

		Site Alone		Plus Other Sites	
Site	Overall (%)	Incidence (%)	Median Survival (mo)	Incidence (%)	Median Survival (mo)
Skin, subcutaneous tissues, and distant lymph nodes	59	23	7.2	36	5.0
Lung	36	11	11.4	25	4.0
Brain	20	8	5.0	12	1.4
Liver	20	3	2.4	17	2.0
Bone	17	3	6.0	14	4.0
Other	12	2	2.2	10	2.0
Widespread	4		2.4		2.4

Number of metastatic sites

Patients with a single distant metastasis had a longer survival than did patients with two metastatic sites or a combination of three or more metastatic sites (Fig. 19-20). This was the most significant factor predicting survival in patients with distant metastases by single-factor analysis (p < 0.000001). The median survival was 7 months for one metastatic site, as against 4 months for two sites and 2 months for three or more metastatic sites. Similarly, the 1-year survival rate was 36% for one metastatic site, 13% for two sites, and 0% for three or more sites. Within the single-site grouping, patients with metastases in the lung, skin, subcutaneous tissues, or distant lymph nodes had a better survival than pa-

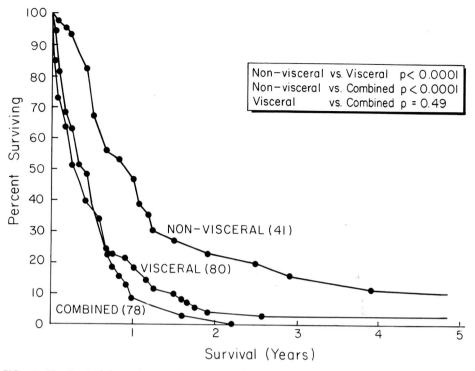

FIG. 19–19 Survival for patients with stage III melanoma according to the site of metastases. The metastases in nonvisceral sites (skin, subcutaneous tissues, and distant lymph nodes) were associated with a significantly better prognosis than those in visceral sites or a combination of visceral and nonvisceral disease (Balch CM et al: A multifactorial analysis of melanoma. IV. Prognostic factors in 200 melanoma patients with distant metastases (stage III). J Clin Oncol 1:126, 1983)

tients with metastases at any other single site (Table 19-8). When combinations of metastatic sites were examined in detail, only patients with lung plus skin, subcutaneous tissue, and distant lymph nodes fared better than patients with other combinations (median survival of 6 months versus 2 months).

PATHOLOGIC FACTORS

As with stage II patients, almost all the histopathologic parameters involving the primary melanoma were not predictive of survival in stage III patients.

MULTIFACTORIAL ANALYSIS

Each of the prognostic factors was examined for the predictive value of metastatic risk and survival rate.[6] Table 19-9 presents the relative importance of each single factor, unadjusted for other factors. Only the number of metastatic sites and the location of the

TABLE 19–9
PROGNOSTIC FACTORS ANALYSIS OF STAGE III MELANOMA

	p Value
Single-Factor Analysis	
Number of metastatic sites	<0.000001
Site of metastases	0.0001
Primary melanoma site	0.209
Remission duration	0.245
Sequence of metastases	0.300
Ulceration	0.356
Tumor thickness	0.428
Level of invasion	0.575
Lymphocyte infiltration	0.642
Pigmentation	0.708
Age	0.760
Sex	0.975
Growth pattern	0.992
Multifactorial Analysis	
Number of metastatic sites	<0.00001
Remission duration	0.0186
Site of metastases	0.0192

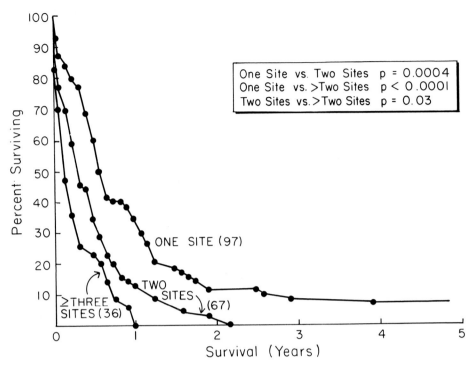

FIG. 19–20   Survival for patients with stage III melanoma according to the number of metastatic sites. There was an inverse relationship between survival and the number of sites, with each of these subgroups having a significantly different survival rate. (Balch CM et al: A multifactorial analysis of melanoma. IV. Prognostic factors in 200 melanoma patients with distant metastases (stage III). J Clin Oncol 1:126, 1983)

sites (visceral versus nonvisceral versus combined) correlated with survival rates. When all factors were analyzed in a Cox regression analysis, the dominant factors were (1) the *number of metastatic sites* (1 versus 2 versus ≥ 3; p < 0.00001); (2) the *remission duration* (< versus ≥ 12 months; p = 0.019); and (3) the *site of metastases* (visceral versus nonvisceral; p = 0.019). These results were the same even after accounting for whether palliative chemotherapy was administered or not. There were no histologic criteria of the primary melanoma that predicted the patients' clinical course once they developed distant metastases.

The only other multifactorial analysis of stage III patients was performed by Presant and Bartolucci.[32] They found that the following were all significant determinants of survival: performance (activity) status, no involvement of the liver, female sex, and bone involvement only.

CONCLUSIONS

Deciding on appropriate treatment for melanoma patients and analyzing results requires an understanding of the dominant factors that predict the risk of metastases. For example, this information has been used both to derive computerized mathematical models for categorizing patients into different risk groups and to make clinical decisions regarding the extent of surgical treatment. Furthermore, this information is important when analyzing results of surgical treatment or adjuvant therapy. Recently, preliminary evidence was presented that suggested a benefit of adjuvant *Corynebacterium parvum* immunotherapy in selected stage I melanoma patients (with tumor thickness > 3 mm–4 mm), a difference that was totally obscured when these data were analyzed for the entire population or when subdivided by any other parameter available in this study.[2]

For patients with clinically localized (stage I) melanoma, there were three pathologic factors (tumor thickness, ulceration, and pathologic stage) and two clinical factors (anatomical location of primary lesion and type of initial surgical management) that were the dominant prognostic variables in a multifactorial analysis. The sex of the patient may contribute some additional information, even after accounting for these factors, especially for extremity melanomas.

In patients with nodal metastases (stage II), the two dominant prognostic variables were the number of metastatic nodes and the presence or absence of ulceration in the primary lesion. The patient's age and tumor thickness also correlated with survival, although to a much lesser degree. Calculation of survival curves in patients with stage II melanoma should be made from the onset of nodal metastases. The only difference between patients with simultaneous and delayed metastatic melanoma is that the latter patients are first diagnosed at a relatively earlier stage in the natural history of their disease; hence, their prognosis is better when calculated from the diagnosis of their primary melanoma.

In patients with distant metastases (stage III), there were no parameters of the primary melanoma that predicted the patient's clinical course. The dominant prognostic variables in the multifactorial analysis were (1) the anatomical site of the metastases (visceral versus nonvisceral); (2) the number of sites of metastases (1 versus 2 versus ≥ 3); and (3) the remission duration (<versus ≥ 12 months). The sex and age of the patient did not influence survival rates significantly.

Although there are still some facets of melanoma behavior that are unpredictable, it is becoming increasingly possible to define the various stages and substages of melanoma with considerable precision. Additional refinements will be made when the influence of the patient's immunologic and genetic factors can be accounted for in predicting the clinical course of melanoma.

REFERENCES

1. Balch CM, Murad TM, Soong S-j, Ingalls AL, Halpern NB, Maddox WA: A multifactorial analysis of melanoma: Prognostic histopathological features comparing Clark's and Breslow's staging methods. Ann Surg 188:732, 1978
2. Balch CM, Smalley RV, Bartolucci AA, Burns D, Presant CA, Durant JR, Southeastern Cancer Study Group: A randomized prospective clinical trial of adjuvant *C. parvum* immunotherapy in 260 patients with clinically localized melanoma (stage I): Prognostic factors analysis and preliminary results of immunotherapy. Cancer 49:1079, 1982
3. Balch CM, Soong S-j, Milton GW, Shaw HM, McGovern VJ, Murad TM, McCarthy WH, Maddox WA: A comparison of prognostic factors and surgical results in 1,786 patients with localized (stage I) melanoma treated in Alabama, USA, and New South Wales, Australia. Ann Surg 196:677, 1982
4. Balch CM, Soong S-j, Murad TM, Ingalls AL, Maddox WA: A multifactorial analysis of melanoma. II. Prognostic factors in patients with stage I (localized) melanoma. Surgery 86:343, 1979
5. Balch CM, Soong S-j, Murad TM, Ingalls AL, Maddox WA: A multifactorial analysis of melanoma. III. Prognostic factors in melanoma patients with lymph node metastases (stage II). Ann Surg 193:377, 1981
6. Balch CM, Soong S-j, Murad TM, Smith JW, Maddox WA, Durant JR: A multifactorial analysis of melanoma. IV. Prognostic factors in 200 melanoma patients with distant metastases (stage III). J Clin Oncol 1:126, 1983
7. Balch CM, Wilkerson JA, Murad TM, Soong S-j, Ingalls AL, Maddox WA: The prognostic significance of ulceration of cutaneous melanoma. Cancer 45:3012, 1980
8. Breslow A: Thickness, cross-sectional areas and depth of invasion in the prognosis of cutaneous melanoma. Ann Surg 172:902, 1970
9. Callery C, Cochran AJ, Roe DJ, Rees W, Nathanson SD, Benedetti JK, Elashoff RM, Morton DL: Factors prognostic for survival in patients with malignant melanoma spread to the regional lymph nodes. Ann Surg 196:69, 1982
10. Cascinelli N, Morabito A, Bufalino R, van der Esch EP, Preda F, Vaglini M, Rovini D, Orefice S: Prognosis of stage I melanoma of the skin. Int J Cancer 26:733, 1980
11. Cohen MH, Ketcham AS, Felix EL, Li S-H, Tomaszewski M-M, Costa J, Rabson AS, Simon RM, Rosenberg SA: Prognostic factors in patients undergoing lymphadenectomy for malignant melanoma. Ann Surg 186:635, 1977
12. Cox DR: Regression model and life tables. J Royal Stat Soc B34:187, 1972
13. Cox EB: Prognostic factors in malignant melanoma. In Seigler HF (ed): Clinical Management of Melanoma, p 279. The Hague, Nijhoff, 1982
14. Day CL Jr, Lew RA, Mihm MC Jr, Harris MN, Kopf AW, Sober AJ, Fitzpatrick TB: The natural break points for primary-tumor thickness in clinical stage I melanoma. N Engl J Med 305:1155, 1981
15. Day CL Jr, Mihm MC Jr, Lew RA, Harris MN, Kopf AW, Fitzpatrick TB, Harrist TJ, Golomb FM, Postel A, Hennessey P, Gumport SL, Raker JW, Malt RA, Cosimi AB, Wood WC, Roses DF, Gorstein F, Rigel D, Friedman RJ, Mintzis MM, Sober AJ: Prognostic factors for patients with clinical stage I melanoma of intermediate thickness (1.51–3.99 mm): A conceptual model for tumor growth and metastasis. Ann Surg 195:35, 1982
16. Day CL Jr, Mihm MC Jr, Lew RA, Kopf AW, Sober AJ, Fitzpatrick TB: Cutaneous malignant melanoma: Prognostic guidelines for physicians and patients. CA, A Journal for Clinicians 32:113, 1982
17. Day CL Jr, Sober AJ, Kopf AW, Lew RA, Mihm MC Jr, Golomb FM, Hennessey P, Harris MN, Gumport SL, Raker JW, Malt RA, Cosimi AB, Wood WC,

Roses DF, Gorstein F, Fitzpatrick TB, Postel A: A prognostic model for clinical stage I melanoma of the lower extremity: Location on foot as independent risk factor for recurrent disease. Surgery 89:599, 1981

18. Day CL Jr, Sober AJ, Kopf AW, Lew RA, Mihm MC Jr, Golomb FM, Postel A, Hennessey P, Harris MN, Gumport SL, Raker JW, Malt RA, Cosimi AB, Wood WC, Roses DF, Gorstein F, Fitzpatrick TB: A prognostic model for clinical stage I melanoma of the trunk: Location near the midline is not an independent risk factor for recurrent disease. Am J Surg 142:247, 1981

19. Day CL Jr, Sober AJ, Kopf AW, Lew RA, Mihm MC Jr, Hennessey P, Golomb FM, Harris MN, Gumport SL, Raker JW, Malt RA, Cosimi AB, Wood WC, Roses DF, Gorstein F, Postel A, Grier WRN, Mintzis MN, Fitzpatrick TB: A prognostic model for clinical stage I melanoma of the upper extremity: The importance of anatomic subsites in predicting recurrent disease. Ann Surg 193:436, 1981

20. Day CL Jr, Sober AJ, Lew RA, Mihm MC Jr, Fitzpatrick TB, Kopf AW, Harris MN, Gumport SL, Raker JW, Malt RA, Golomb FM, Cosimi AB, Wood WC, Casson P, Lopransi S, Gorstein F, Postel A: Malignant melanoma patients with positive nodes and relatively good prognoses: Microstaging retains prognostic significance in clinical stage I melanoma patients with metastases to regional nodes. Cancer 47:955, 1981

21. Drzewiecki KT, Andersen PK: Survival with malignant melanoma: A regression analysis of prognostic factors. Cancer 49:2414, 1982

22. Eldh J, Boeryd B, Peterson LE: Prognostic factors in cutaneous malignant melanoma in stage I: A clinical, morphological and multivariate analysis. Scand J Plast Reconstr Surg 12:243, 1978

23. Gromet MA, Epstein WL, Blois MS: The regressing thin malignant melanoma: A distinctive lesion with metastatic potential. Cancer 42:2282, 1978

24. Hacene K, Le Doussal V, Brunet M, Lemoine F, Guerin P, Hebert H: Prognostic index for clinical stage I cutaneous malignant melanoma. Cancer Res 43:2991, 1983

25. Kaplan EL, Meier P: Nonparametric estimation from incomplete observation. J Am Stat Assoc 53:457, 1958

26. McGovern VJ, Shaw HM, Milton GW, Farago GA: Cell type and pigment content as prognostic indicators in cutaneous malignant melanoma. In Ackerman AB (ed): Pathology of Malignant Melanoma, p 327. New York, Masson, 1981

27. McGovern VJ, Shaw HM, Milton GW, Farago GA: Lymphocytic infiltration and survival in malignant melanoma. In Ackerman AB (ed): Pathology of Malignant Melanoma, p 341. New York, Masson, 1981

28. McGovern VJ, Shaw HM, Milton GW: Prognosis in patients with thin malignant melanoma: Influence of regression. Histopathology 7:673, 1983

29. McGovern VJ, Shaw HM, Milton GW, Farago GA: Is malignant melanoma arising in a Hutchinson's melanotic freckle a separate disease entity? Histopathology 4:235, 1980

30. Paladugu RR, Yonemoto RH: Biologic behavior of thin malignant melanomas with regressive changes. Arch Surg 118:41, 1983

31. Prade M, Bognel C, Charpentier P, Gadenne C, Duvillard P, Sancho-Garnier H, Petit J-Y: Malignant melanoma of the skin: Prognostic factors derived from a multifactorial analysis of 239 cases. Am J Dermatopathol 4:411, 1982

32. Presant CA, Bartolucci AA, the Southeastern Cancer Study Group: Prognostic factors in metastatic malignant melanoma: The Southeastern Cancer Study Group experience. Cancer 49:2192, 1982

33. Schmoeckel C, Bockelbrink A, Bockelbrink H, Braun-Falco O: Low- and high-risk malignant melanoma. II. Multivariate analyses for a prognostic classification. Eur J Cancer Clin Oncol 19:237, 1983

34. Schmoeckel C, Bockelbrink A, Bockelbrink H, Koutsis J, Braun-Falco O: Low- and high-risk malignant melanoma. I. Evaluation of clinical and histological prognosticators in 585 cases. Eur J Cancer Clin Oncol 19:227, 1983

35. Shaw HM, McGovern VJ, Milton GW, Farago GA, McCarthy WH: Histologic features of tumors and the female superiority in survival from malignant melanoma. Cancer 45:1604, 1980

36. Shaw HM, McGovern VJ, Milton GW, Farago GA, McCarthy WH: Malignant melanoma: Influence of site of lesion and age of patient in the female superiority in survival. Cancer 46:2731, 1980

37. Smith JL Jr, Stehlin JS Jr: Spontaneous regression of primary malignant melanomas with regional metastases. Cancer 18:1399, 1965

38. Trau H, Rigel DS, Harris MN, Kopf AW, Friedman RJ, Gumport SL, Bart RS, Grier RN: Metastases of thin melanomas. Cancer 51:553, 1983

39. Urist MM, Balch CM, Soong S-j, Milton GW, Shaw HM, McGovern VJ, Murad TM, McCarthy WH, Maddox WA: Head and neck melanoma in 536 clinical stage I patients: A prognostic factors analysis and results of surgical treatment. Ann Surg (in press)

40. van der Esch EP, Cascinelli N, Preda F, Morabito A, Bufalino R: Stage I melanoma of the skin: Evaluation of prognosis according to histologic characteristics. Cancer 48:1668, 1981

SENG-JAW SOONG

A Computerized Mathematical Model and Scoring System for Predicting Outcome in Melanoma Patients

20

Prognostic factors applicable to melanoma patients can now be identified more accurately using the multifactorial analysis technique based on regression models developed for survival data analysis. The results of such a study involving 4000 patients are described in Chapter 19. The majority of studies applying this statistical approach have used these mathematical models primarily as a tool for identifying dominant prognostic factors. However, the actual use of these models for predicting the clinical course of melanoma patients and for other potential applications, such as in the design and analysis of clinical trials, has never been fully addressed. This chapter describes the derivation and validation of a mathematical model for predicting the risks for metastases and survival outcome in patients with localized (stage I) melanoma. The potential clinical applications of this model and the scoring system derived from it are also presented.

DESCRIPTION OF THE DATA

SOURCES OF DATA

The patients used for developing the mathematical model were selected from two independent melanoma series: The University of Alabama in Birmingham (UAB) series, and the Sydney Melanoma Unit (SMU) series of patients. These two melanoma patient populations are remarkably similar in their composition, and the dominant prognostic factors identified were virtually identical.[3] Detailed descriptions of these two series can be found in Chapters 19, 21, and 24. The mathematical model was developed from a data base consisting of 1069 patients from both series for whom every piece of clinical and pathologic information was available for all prognostic factors being studied.

An additional group of 176 patients with localized melanoma was separately analyzed from the Southeastern Cancer Study Group. They were included in this study for validating the model and for illustration of the model applications. These patients received either adjuvant *Corynebacterium parvum* immunotherapy or surgical treatment alone in a previously reported clinical trial.[2]

DEFINITION AND CODING OF PROGNOSTIC VARIABLES

Four clinical factors (age, sex, lesion location, and initial surgical treatment) and seven pathologic factors (tumor thickness, level of invasion, ulceration,

growth pattern, lymphocyte infiltration, pigmentation, and pathologic stage) were examined in this study. The detailed definition and the prognostic significance of each of these eleven factors have been described.[1,3]

For mathematical manipulation and model development, all prognostic variables were transferred to numerical codes, as is shown in Table 20-1. For example, the factor *sex* is represented by X_2, which takes value 0 if the patient is female and 1 if the patient is male.

DESCRIPTION OF MATHEMATICAL MODEL

The derived mathematical model for predicting survival rates in patients with localized melanoma is based on the proportional model proposed by Cox.[7] The introduction of the Cox model represents the most important new methodologic development in the area of survival data analysis. The Cox model permits nonparametric assessment of survival data and allows the statistical inference to be restricted to the effect of concomitant information (such as prognostic factors) without knowledge of the form of survival distribution. The Cox model can be expressed in terms of (1) a hazard function, or (2) a survival function, as described below.

THE HAZARD FUNCTION

The hazard function at time t, denoted by $\lambda(t)$, is defined as the instantaneous risk of death or failure at time t, providing that death or failure has not already occurred. Roughly, it can be interpreted as the rate of death or failure per unit time. In the multifactorial analysis of survival data, the hazard is often expressed as a function of the concomitant information related to survival times of patients. Cox's model[7] describes this relationship in terms of the following mathematical form:

$$\lambda(t) = \lambda_0(t)\exp[\beta_1(X_1 - \overline{X}_1) + \beta_2(X_2 - \overline{X}_2) + \cdots + \beta_p(X_p - \overline{X}_p)]$$

where (i) $X_1, X_2, \ldots, X_p$ are p measured patient characteristics (or prognostic factors), and $\overline{X}_1, \overline{X}_2, \ldots, \overline{X}_p$ are mean values of these variables; (ii), $\beta_1, \beta_2, \ldots, \beta_p$ are regression coefficients to be estimated from data; (iii) $\lambda_0(t)$ is an arbitrary baseline hazard function where all prognostic variables are at their average values.

Cox's model can also be written in terms of

TABLE 20–1
CODING OF PROGNOSTIC VARIABLES FOR THE MODEL DERIVATION

Factor	Defined Covariate (X_i) In the Model	Coding for the Covariate X_i
Clinical Factors		
Age	X_1	In years
Sex	X_2	0 = female; 1 = male
Lesion location	X_3	0 = extremity; 1 = axial
Surgical treatment	X_4	0 = WLE only; 1 = WLE + RND
Pathologic Factors		
Tumor thickness	X_5	1 = <0.76 mm
		2 = 0.76 mm–1.49mm
		3 = 1.50 mm–2.49 mm
		4 = 2.50 mm–3.99 mm
		5 = 4.00 mm–5.99 mm
		6 = ≥6.00 mm
Level of invasion	X_6	2 = II; 3 = III; 4 = IV; 5 = V
Ulceration	X_7	0 = absent; 1 = present
Growth pattern	X_8	0 = nodular
		1 = superficial spreading
Lymphocyte infiltration	X_9	0 = absent or mild
		1 = moderate or heavy
Pigmentation	X_{10}	0 = yes; 1 = no
Pathologic stage	X_{11}	1 = stage I; 2 = stage II
		3 = stage III
Institution Comparison		
Institution	X_{12}	0 = University of Alabama in Birmingham
		1 = University of Sydney

the relative risk as defined by $\lambda(t)/\lambda_0(t)$. It is noted that the relative risk, as defined, is equal to $\exp[\beta_1(X_1 - \overline{X}_1) + \beta_2(X_2 - \overline{X}_2) + \cdots + \beta_p(X_p - \overline{X}_p)]$ and is the ratio of the risk of death per unit time for a patient with a given set of characteristics (prognostic values) to the risk for a patient when all characteristics were at their average values. Thus, the relative importance of each patient characteristic can be assessed by considering favorable and unfavorable values of that characteristic, assuming that other characteristics were at their average values.

THE SURVIVAL FUNCTION

Given the specification of the hazard function, the Cox's model can be described in terms of the survival function:

$$S(t) = \{S_0(t)\}^{\exp[\beta_1(X_1 - \overline{X}_1) + \beta_2(X_2 - \overline{X}_2) + \cdots + \beta_p(X_p - \overline{X}_p)]}$$

where $S_0(t)$ is a baseline survival function to be estimated from data. The survival function $S(t)$ denotes the probability of a patient with a given set of characteristics $X_1, X_2, \ldots, X_p$ surviving at least to time t.

Since the primary emphasis of this chapter is the prediction of a patient's survival, unless otherwise specified all mathematical models are described in terms of survival function.

The Cox model has been extensively studied both in its theoretical considerations and in its practical applications during the past decade. The model has been widely accepted as a generally useful model for analyzing survival data. However, the validity of applying this model should be carefully assessed, especially in situations where the hazard function may be nonproportional.

FITTING THE MODEL TO THE DATA

In this section, a mathematical model based on Cox's formulation is developed for the UAB and the SMU data, both as separate and combined data sets. The validity of each model is assessed not only by testing it back on the original data from which the model is developed but also on the other data set independently.

THE UNIVERSITY OF ALABAMA IN BIRMINGHAM (UAB) MODEL AND ITS VALIDATION

The eleven clinical and pathologic parameters described earlier were simultaneously compared for their relative prognostic strength using a multifactorial analysis based on the Cox model. The influence of these factors on survival was examined using a cohort of 293 stage I patients from the UAB series for whom information was available for all eleven factors being analyzed.

A stepwise procedure was used to select a subset of factors that best predicted survival rates. The dominant factors selected included: tumor thickness ($p < 0.00001$), ulceration ($p = 0.0077$), anatomical site ($p = 0.091$), surgical treatment ($p = 0.0002$), and pathologic stage ($p < 0.00001$) (Table 20-2). The mathematical model (expressed in terms of the estimated survival function) obtained through this procedure was:

$$\hat{S}(t) = [\hat{S}_0(t)]^{\exp(x\hat{\beta})}$$

where $x\hat{\beta} = 0.4844 \cdot$ (Tumor Thickness $- 2.8020$) $+ 0.8524 \cdot$ (Ulceration $- 0.3611$) $- 1.2708 \cdot$ (Surgical Treatment $- 0.4983$) $+ 0.5004 \cdot$ (Lesion Location $- 0.5188$) $+ 1.8476 \cdot$ (Pathologic Stage $- 1.0614$)

and $\hat{S}_0(t) =$ the estimated baseline survival function.

A patient's survival experience can be estimated using this equation. However, the validity of the model should be verified first. Several approaches can be used to assess the "goodness of fit" of the model. These include the examination of (1) the closeness of observed and fitted survival distributions (curves), (2) the fit via the methods of residual analysis following the methods of Kay[11] and Cox and Snell,[8] and (3) the relationship between the observed and predicted average survival times as described by Carter and associates.[5] In this chapter, only the first procedure will be discussed.

The adequacy of the UAB model was first examined on the UAB data set from which it was derived. The survival curves predicted by the model and observed survival curves as calculated by the Kaplan and Meier method[10] demonstrated that the model provides a reasonable fit to the observed data. The observed and predicted 10-year survival rates subgrouped by tumor thickness are compared in Table 20-3.

The UAB model was then applied to the SMU data to assess the predictability of this model on an independent data set. As shown in Figure 20-1, the predicted and observed survival curves for patients

TABLE 20–2
MULTIFACTORIAL ANALYSIS

Dominant Factors	UAB (n=293)		SMU (n=776)		UAB+SMU (n=1069)	
	X^2	p value	X^2	p value	X^2	p value
Tumor Thickness	22.8	< 0.00001	15.8	0.0001	25.2	< 0.00001
Ulceration	7.1	0.0077	26.1	< 0.00001	32.4	< 0.00001
Surgical treatment	13.4	0.0002	18.7	< 0.00001	31.6	< 0.00001
Anatomical site	2.9	0.0910	21.3	< 0.00001	20.4	< 0.00001
Pathologic stage	18.4	< 0.00001	1.4	NS*	15.4	0.0001
Level of invasion	2.5	NS	10.8	0.0010	15.1	0.0001

*NS = not significant with $p > 0.10$.

TABLE 20–3
OBSERVED AND PREDICTED 10-YEAR SURVIVAL RATES FOR PATIENTS WITH LOCALIZED (STAGE I) MELANOMA

Tumor Thickness	UAB		SMU		UAB+SMU	
	Observed	Predicted	Observed	Predicted	Observed	Predicted
<0.76 mm	89%	93%	87%	87%	87%	88%
0.76 mm–1.49 mm	74%	78%	73%	79%	75%	78%
1.50 mm–2.49 mm	58%	65%	61%	68%	60%	66%
2.50 mm–3.99 mm	44%	48%	45%	44%	45%	46%
≥4.00 mm	32%	20%	26%	26%	28%	26%

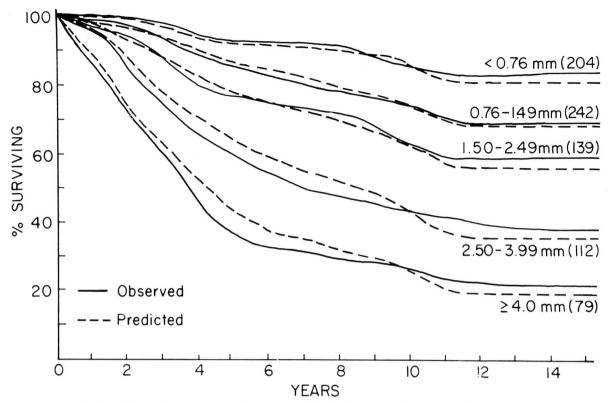

FIG. 20–1 Predicted and observed survival curves for patients with localized (stage I) melanoma treated at Sydney Melanoma Unit (SMU) using the UAB model.

with localized melanoma treated at the University of Sydney using the UAB model were almost super-imposable.

THE SYDNEY MELANOMA UNIT (SMU) MODEL AND ITS VALIDATION

In the Sydney series of 776 patients for whom all information can be assessed, the most important factors in the multifactorial analysis were tumor thickness (p = 0.0001), ulceration (p < 0.00001), surgical treatment (p < 0.00001), anatomical site (p < 0.00001), and level of invasion (p = 0.001) (Table 20-2). The model derived from this series not only fitted its original data very well (Table 20-3) but also was highly predictive in the UAB data set (data not shown). Both this and the UAB models strongly indicated that Cox's proportional hazard model formulation could be successfully applied to the development of a predictive model for evaluating patients with stage I melanoma.

THE COMBINED SERIES

The two data sets were merged because the UAB and SMU melanoma patient populations were remarkably similar and the dominant factors identified were almost the same. In addition, the uniformity in data collection, patient management, and the overall duration of patient follow-up were virtually the same. This large data base from the combined series not only permitted the development of a more powerful and accurate mathematical model but also enabled us to evaluate the model within patient subgroups.

Using the combined data set of 1069 patients, the six dominant factors affecting survival were tumor thickness (p < 0.00001), ulceration (p < 0.00001), anatomical site (p < 0.00001), level of invasion (p = 0.0001), pathologic stage (p = 0.0001), and surgical treatment (p < 0.00001). The model developed from analysis was:

$$\hat{S}(t) = [\hat{S}_0(t)]^{\exp(\underline{x}\underline{\beta})}$$

where $x\hat{\beta} = 0.3216 \cdot$ (Tumor Thickness -2.6164) $+$
$0.9013 \cdot$ (Ulceration $- 0.2561$) $-$
$0.9408 \cdot$ (Surgical Treatment $-$
$\quad 0.3826$) $+$
$0.6455 \cdot$ (Lesion Location $- 0.5210$) $+$
$1.1370 \cdot$ (Pathologic Stage $- 1.0346$) $+$
$0.4399 \cdot$ (Level of Invasion $- 3.3592$)

and $\hat{S}_0(t) =$ the estimated baseline survival function.

It has been well established that tumor thickness is the single most important prognostic parameter in stage I melanoma (see Chap. 36). However, it is possible that the dominant factors included in the UAB–SMU model may not be equally important among patients subgrouped by tumor thickness. For example, it was shown previously that the results of the initial surgical treatment varied among patients according to their tumor thickness.[1,3] Therefore, the UAB–SMU model was further examined within the following five subgroups: <0.76 mm, 0.76 mm to 1.49 mm, 1.50 mm to 2.49 mm, 2.50 mm to 3.99 mm, and ≥ 4 mm. The multifactorial analysis was performed within each subgroup and the results are shown in Table 20-4. Ulceration and anatomical site remained significant in all subgroups, with the exception of patients with tumor thickness ≥ 4 mm for whom anatomical site was not significant. Surgical treatment was significant only in the three intermediate subgroups (0.76 mm–3.99 mm), although some indication of difference existed even in patients with tumor thickness ≥ 4 mm. Level of invasion was significant only in two subgroups (0.76 mm–1.49 mm, and ≥ 4 mm), confirming the results that level of invasion was much less important after adjusting for tumor thickness (see Chap. 19). Pathologic stage was found to be significant only in patients with tumor thickness ranging from 1.50 mm to 3.99 mm. That this factor

was not significant in the other groups is probably caused by the small number of patients in these groups. Thus, there were only minor variations within the subgroups as to the relative importance of the major factors included in the UAB–SMU model, especially with regard to initial surgical treatment.

The UAB–SMU model was further stratified to incorporate the results of the above subgroup analyses. The new stratified UAB–SMU model was first tested on the data from which this model was derived, and the observed and predicted survival curves subgrouped by tumor thickness were closely in agreement (Fig. 20-2). This model was also tested on an independent data set using 176 patients with stage I melanoma from a Southeastern Cancer Study Group trial. These patients were not used in the model derivation and thus provided an important group to validate the predictive capability of this statistical approach. The closeness of the observed and the predicted survival curves as shown in Figure 20-3 demonstrated a high degree of predictability of this model in an independent group of patients.

DEVELOPMENT OF A COMPUTER PROGRAM FOR USING THE PREDICTIVE MODEL

Computer software for the stratified UAB–SMU model, which consists of five submodels, has been developed. This program has been routinely used by surgical oncologists at the UAB Comprehensive Cancer Center for making patient management decisions. The software is written in BASIC language and can be run interactively on a microcomputer or a mainframe through time-sharing options (TSO). The program prompts the user to input the patient's characteristics required by the model. After execution, estimated risks for metastases and survival for that patient can be displayed either on a

TABLE 20-4
MULTIFACTORIAL ANALYSIS OF 1069 STAGE I MELANOMA PATIENTS WITHIN TUMOR THICKNESS SUBGROUPS*

Thickness Subgroup	Number of Patients	Ulceration	Anatomical Site	Surgical Treatment	Clark's Level	Pathologic Stage
<0.76 mm	272	0.0020	0.0223	—[†]	—	—
0.76 mm–1.49 mm	313	0.0063	0.0194	0.0042	0.0055	—
1.50 mm–2.49 mm	203	0.0006	0.0258	<0.00001	—	0.0519
2.50 mm–3.99 mm	160	0.0099	0.0003	0.0175	—	0.0037
≥ 4.0 mm	121	0.0227	—	0.0626	0.0158	—

* All entries represent p values.

† Dash indicates factors that are not statistically significant.

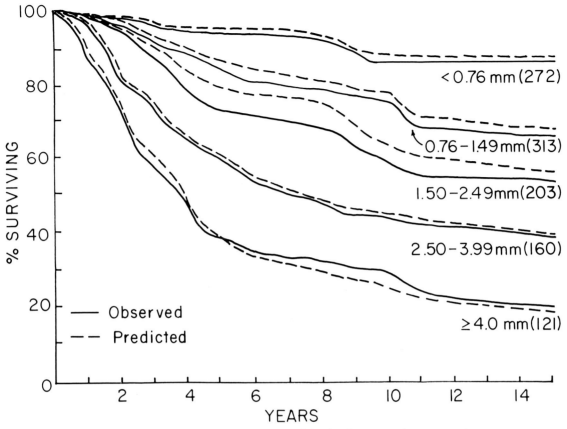

FIG. 20–2   Predicted and observed survival curves for patients with localized (stage I) melanoma treated at UAB and SMU using the combined UAB–SMU model.

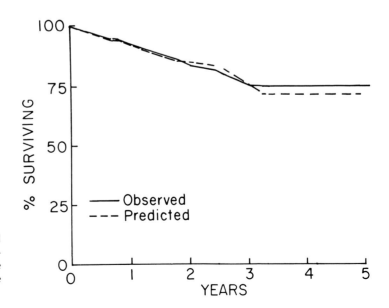

FIG. 20–3 Predicted and observed survival curves for patients with localized (stage I) melanoma enrolled in a clinical trial conducted by the Southeastern Cancer Study Group using the UAB–SMU model.

terminal screen or a line printer. A sample output of this computer program is shown in Table 20-6. In addition, an individual patient's survival plots can be generated (see Fig. 20-4 as an example).

THE CLINICAL SCORING SYSTEM

Various scoring systems have been proposed for evaluating patients with a variety of diseases. An outstanding example is the Karnofsky Performance Score for evaluating cancer patient's performance status. Scoring systems have also been proposed for melanoma[4,6,12]; however, none have been widely used. A useful clinical scoring system should meet at least the following criteria: (1) close reflection of the patient's clinical course of disease (*i.e.*, prognosis); (2) high reproducibility; and (3) easy interpretation.

On the basis of the mathematical model described earlier in this chapter, a new clinical scoring system for stage I melanoma was developed. In this system, a patient was scored according to the 10-year survival rate predicted by the model based on this patient's characteristics; for example, a patient received a score of 80 if this patient's predicted 10-year survival rate was 80%. The projected 10-year survival rate was proposed as a score because in stage I melanoma, 8 to 10 years of follow-up is considered essential for adequate patient evaluation.[3] Furthermore, a patient's conditional probability of dying from disease if he is alive at 10 years after diagnosis is relatively small.[3] Thus, the proposed clinical score could be considered as a composite prognostic indicator of several dominant prognostic factors in stage I melanoma and represents a probability of a patient's long-term survival. As a result of the high predictability of the mathematical model that generated the score, the scoring system was highly reproducible. It was also easy to remember, since the score simply reflected a patient's predicted 10-year survival rate. Examples of clinical scores for selected patients are presented in Table 20-5, and the various applications of this scoring system are presented in the following section.

FIG. 20–4 Estimated survival by treatment methods (WLE alone and WLE + ELND) and overall survival disregarding treatment for a hypothetical melanoma patient with the following characteristics: sex, male; age, 50; stage, I; lesion site, extremity; tumor thickness, 1.2 mm; ulceration, present; level of invasion, III. Survival projections were made based on the computerized UAB–SMU model.

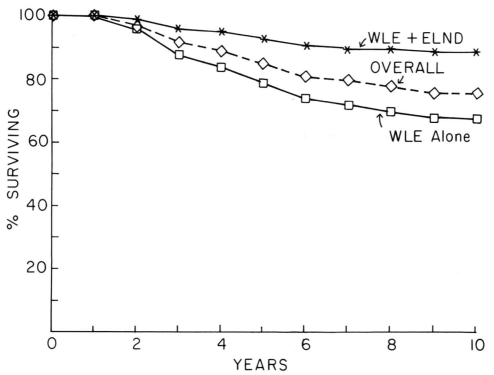

TABLE 20–5
CLINICAL SCORES FOR SELECTED PATIENTS WITH STAGE I MELANOMA

	Prognostic Characteristics				
Patient	Tumor Thickness	Ulceration	Anatomical Site	Level of Invasion	Clinical Score
1	0.5 mm	No	Arm	II	97
2	1.2 mm	Yes	Leg	III	76
3	2.3 mm	No	Neck	IV	65
4	4.5 mm	Yes	Chest	IV	22

CLINICAL APPLICATIONS OF THE MODEL AND SCORING SYSTEM

PATIENT MANAGEMENT DECISIONS

One of the most important facets of the mathematical model described in this chapter is its usefulness in a clinical setting. Prediction of the clinical course of disease and treatment outcome is an essential part of medical practice. Physicians who treat patients face daily decisions as to the selection of an "optimal" treatment for a particular patient. The requirements for follow-up evaluation may also vary according to a patient's prognosis.

As described above, the computer program for the mathematical model generates a prognostic summary analysis for an individual patient based on this patient's presenting characteristics. This summary analysis includes (1) the estimated risk for isolated metastatic melanoma in the regional nodes; (2) the estimated risk for metastatic melanoma at distant sites; and (3) estimated survival rates by year for 10 years following surgery. Estimated survival rates are given for wide local excision surgery (WLE) alone, WLE with elective lymph node dissection (ELND), and overall, disregarding treatment. A physician can use these projections in the selection of a surgical treatment in conjunction with other factors, including morbidity associated with surgery.

To illustrate this application, four hypothetical cases are presented in Tables 20-6 to 20-9. In all four cases, stage (I), tumor thickness (1.2 mm), and level of invasion (Clark's level III) are the same. Ulceration and primary site vary from patient to patient to demonstrate different prognostic results and different management decisions that might be made based on these results. In Case 1 (Table 20-6), the patient's primary lesion is on an extremity and is not ulcerated. Estimated rates for survival 10 years after surgical treatment show a 7% difference between WLE and WLE with ELND: 89% versus 96%.

Overall survival disregarding treatment is projected to be 92%. After consideration of the morbidity associated with surgery, the physician may decide that the small difference in 10-year survival rates between treatments does not warrant selection of ELND. In Case 2 (Table 20-7), all characteristics are the same as in Case 1 with the exception of the presence of ulcerated lesions. Projected 10-year survival rates are markedly different for this case: 68% for WLE alone, 89% for WLE with ELND, and 76% overall. The change in just one factor—ulceration—may then affect the physician's judgment in the selection of a treatment. In this case, ELND has a 21% better survival rate than WLE and may be the optimal treatment for this patient. Both Cases 3 and 4 (Tables 20-8 and 20-9) have an axial primary site, but Case 3's lesion is not ulcerated whereas Case 4's lesion is ulcerated. Projected survival rates differ, although WLE with ELND is probably the treatment of choice for both patients. As can be seen in these four cases, changes in just one or two important prognostic characteristics can affect the projected survival rates and the physician's selection of an optimal treatment.

STAGING PATIENTS

The importance of classification of melanoma patients and current staging systems are described in Chapter 4. Current systems are simple and easy to use, but because they do not incorporate all important prognostic factors associated with the disease, they may not accurately reflect uniform groups of patients,[9] especially in localized melanoma. A comprehensive staging system for localized melanoma, although more difficult to use, would allow for more accurate and reliable patient classification. The clinical scoring system generated from the mathematical model can be considered as a summary index of all important prognostic factors and can provide a comprehensive disease classification. In

(*Text continues on page 364*)

TABLE 20–6

PROGNOSTIC FACTORS ANALYSIS FOR METASTATIC MELANOMA: Surgical Oncology Service and Cancer Biostatistics Unit, Comprehensive Cancer Center, University of Alabama in Birmingham

Patient Name: Case 1

ID Number: 1

Patient Characteristics

Stage: 1   Primary lesion site: Extremity
Age: 26   Tumor thickness: 1.2 mm
Sex: F   Ulceration: No
                    Clark's Level: III

Risk for Metastases and Survival Rates

1. The estimated risk for isolated metastatic melanoma in regional nodes in this patient is **7%**.
2. The estimated risk for metastatic melanoma at distant sites in this patient is **4%**.
3. Estimated survival rates:

Year After Surgery	Overall	Wide Local Excision	
		Alone	With Regional Node Dissection
0	100%	100%	100%
1	100	100	100
2	99	99	100
3	97	96	99
4	96	95	98
5	95	93	98
6	94	91	97
7	93	90	97
8	93	90	97
9	92	89	96
10	92	89	96

TABLE 20–7

PROGNOSTIC FACTORS ANALYSIS FOR METASTATIC MELANOMA: Surgical Oncology Service and Cancer Biostatistics Unit, Comprehensive Cancer Center, University of Alabama in Birmingham

Patient Name: Case 2

ID Number: 2

Patient Characteristics

Stage: 1   Primary lesion site: Extremity
Age: 50   Tumor thickness: 1.2 mm
Sex: M   Ulceration: Yes
                    Clark's Level: III

Risk for Metastases and Survival Rates

1. The estimated risk for isolated metastatic melanoma in regional nodes in this patient is **21%**.
2. The estimated risk for metastatic melanoma at distant sites in this patient is **11%**.
3. Estimated survival rates:

Year After Surgery	Overall	Wide Local Excision	
		Alone	With Regional Node Dissection
0	100%	100%	100%
1	100	100	100
2	97	96	99
3	92	88	96
4	89	84	95
5	85	79	93
6	81	74	91
7	80	72	90
8	78	70	90
9	76	68	89
10	76	68	89

TABLE 20–8
PROGNOSTIC FACTORS ANALYSIS FOR METASTATIC MELANOMA: Surgical Oncology Service and Cancer Biostatistics Unit, Comprehensive Cancer Center, University of Alabama in Birmingham

Patient Name: Case 3
ID Number: 3

Patient Characteristics

Stage: 1	Primary lesion site: Axial
Age: 37	Tumor thickness: 1.2 mm
Sex: F	Ulceration: No
	Clark's Level: III

Risk for Metastases and Survival Rates

1. The estimated risk for isolated metastatic melanoma in regional nodes in this patient is **18%**.
2. The estimated risk for metastatic melanoma at distant sites in this patient is **9%**.
3. Estimated survival rates:

Year After Surgery	Overall	Wide Local Excision	
		Alone	With Regional Node Dissection
0	100%	100%	100%
1	100	100	100
2	98	96	99
3	93	90	97
4	91	87	96
5	88	83	94
6	85	79	93
7	84	77	92
8	82	76	92
9	81	73	91
10	81	73	91

TABLE 20–9
PROGNOSTIC FACTORS ANALYSIS FOR METASTATIC MELANOMA: Surgical Oncology Service and Cancer Biostatistics Unit, Comprehensive Cancer Center, University of Alabama in Birmingham

Patient Name: Case 4
ID Number: 4

Patient Characteristics

Stage: 1	Primary lesion site: Axial
Age: 60	Tumor thickness: 1.2 mm
Sex: M	Ulceration: Yes
	Clark's Level: III

Risk for Metastases and Survival Rates

1. The estimated risk for isolated metastatic melanoma in regional nodes in this patient is **36%**.
2. The estimated risk for metastatic melanoma at distant sites in this patient is **27%**.
3. Estimated survival rates:

Year After Surgery	Overall	Wide Local Excision	
		Alone	With Regional Node Dissection
0	100%	100%	100%
1	100	100	100
2	92	89	96
3	80	72	90
4	74	64	87
5	65	54	83
6	59	46	79
7	56	43	77
8	54	40	76
9	50	37	73
10	50	37	73

addition, the computer program for the model can simplify the staging process. The proliferation of microcomputers and the use of the CANSUR program developed by the American College of Surgeons and other cancer data management software packages make possible the incorporation of a simple algorithm of this comprehensive staging system to be used by physicians and tumor registry personnel. Table 20-10 presents a practical staging system based on clinical scores generated from the model for the subclassifications of localized melanoma.

Application of this scoring system to the combined UAB and SMU data base can be seen in Figure 20-5. This figure shows the marked difference in survival rates for patients subgrouped by the clinical scores defined in Table 20-10.

PLANNING CLINICAL TRIALS

In clinical trials, the purpose of stratification prior to treatment allocation is to ensure the balance of prognostic factors between treatment groups. However, in a disease such as melanoma, where there are many important prognostic factors, stratification becomes

TABLE 20–10
A PRACTICAL STAGING SYSTEM FOR LOCALIZED MELANOMA BASED ON CLINICAL SCORE GENERATED FROM THE MATHEMATICAL MODEL

Proposed Stage	Clinical Score
IA	80–100
IB	60–79
IIA	40–59
IIB	0–39

impractical as numerous subgroups are created with small numbers of patients in each subgroup. In large multi-institution trials, such stratification may inhibit patient accrual and create imbalances rather than prevent them. The mathematical model may be applied to rectify this situation. The clinical scoring system generated from the model can be used to assign patients to risk groups based on the mix of their prognostic factors. This allows for an overall balance of factors with a minimum number of statistical groups. For example, if a clinical trial of adjuvant immunotherapy for localized melanoma considered a combination of tumor thickness (three

FIG. 20–5   Survival curves for patients with localized melanoma in the UAB–SMU data base grouped by the proposed clinical scoring system defined in Table 20-10.

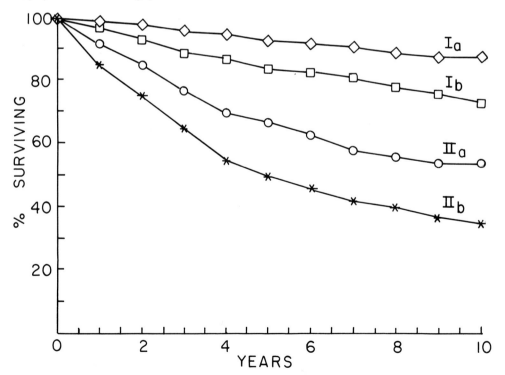

categories), ulceration (two categories), anatomical location (two categories), Clark's level of invasion (four categories), and initial surgical treatment (two categories) for stratification, patients would be stratified into 96 subgroups for randomization. However, these 96 subgroups can be summarized into three or four groups according to the clinical scoring system. Figure 20-6 is an example of the application of the scoring system in stratification.

ANALYSIS OF CLINICAL STUDIES

The mathematical model may be useful in several areas of analyses of clinical trials:

1. *Assessment of treatment outcome after adjusting for disparities in prognostic factors.* For clinical trials not employing prerandomization stratification, or employing stratification with improper prognostic factors, the mathematical model can be used to determine whether any differences in outcome are caused by treatment or by an imbalance in prognostic factors. As an example, in a clinical trial conducted by the Southeastern Cancer Study Group, patients were randomized to receive either adjuvant *Corynebacterium parvum* immunotherapy (regimen A) or surgical treatment

alone (regimen B). In an interim analysis, a 15% difference in 3-year survival rates in favor of *C. parvum* was observed (80% versus 65%). However, after applying the mathematical model separately to each treatment group, the predicted 3-year survival rate for the *C. parvum* group was 83% versus 60% for the surgery-only group. This 23% difference was caused by the imbalance of prognostic factors between these two groups, regardless of treatment regimen (Table 20-11). Therefore, the observed 15% difference could not be attributed to treatment difference. A final analysis of the data (with a larger patient sample and longer follow-up period) showed that the anticipated differences were no longer significant (see Chap. 11). This suggests that the initial differences were indeed the result of imbalance of prognostic factors, not the treatment itself.

2. *Subgroup analysis.* In analysis of clinical trials, treatments are often compared within various subgroups. These subgroups are mostly defined as combinations of important prognostic factors. A well-known limitation of this statistical analysis is the difficulty in extending analysis beyond two or three variables unless a very large sample is available. In analysis of survival data, this is further complicated by the possibility of varied censoring pattern and duration of patient follow-

FIG. 20–6 An example of planning a stratified randomized trial with stratification based on the clinical score.

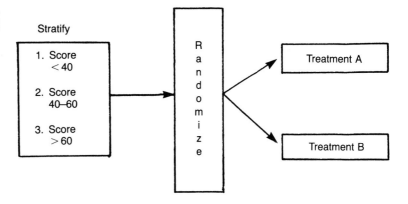

TABLE 20–11
PREDICTED AND OBSERVED SURVIVAL RATES: An Interim Analysis of Southeastern Cancer Study Group Protocol 77 MEL 313

Group	2 Year		3 Year	
	Observed	Predicted	Observed	Predicted
Overall	83%	83%	75%	76%
Regimen A	85%	87%	80%	83%
Regimen B	80%	75%	65%	60%

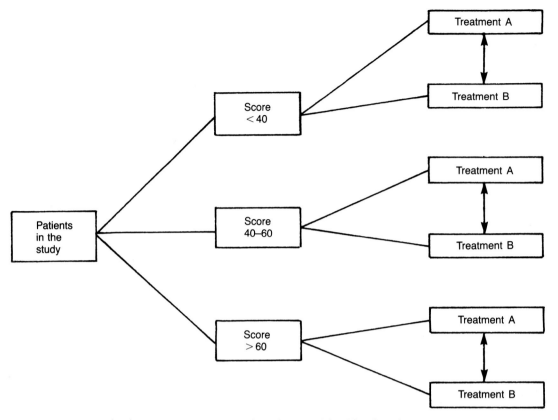

FIG. 20–7 An example of treatment comparisons within subgroups defined by clinical scores.

up within different subgroups. It is important to note that no adequate statistical inferences can be drawn from "overstretched" subgroup analyses. As in prerandomization stratification, the clinical scoring system can be used to classify patients into an adequate number of subgroups for analysis after completion of the study. For example, patients enrolled in a study can be separated into three groups according to their clinical scores (Fig. 20-7), and treatment comparisons can then be made within these subgroups.

3. *Including clinical scores as a variable multifactorial analysis of clinical trials.* Regression models incorporating important prognostic factors (including treatment comparisons) are often used in analysis of clinical studies. Treatment outcome can be assessed after adjusting for pertinent factors included in the model. The clinical score can be used as an additional variable in the regression analysis, further enhancing assessment of treatment outcome.

CONCLUSIONS

Prognostic factors in malignant melanoma have been studied intensively in the past few years. With the aid of newly developed multivariate statistical methods, the relative importance of prognostic factors in melanoma can now be assessed more accurately. Virtually all these studies focused primarily on the identification of dominant factors that characterize the outcome of melanoma. Very few have discussed the important issue of constructing a mathematical model for predicting a clinical course of disease in a future patient based on that patient's characteristics. Even in those studies that have mentioned the issue of prediction, the validity of predictive models and their clinical applications have never been addressed.

This chapter has described the development of a mathematical model for predicting outcome in patients with localized melanoma. The predictive model was derived from a well-known formulation of the proportional hazard model proposed by Cox.[7] The validity of this model was tested not only on the data from which it was developed but also on other independent data sets. The model's high degree of predictability ensures its usefulness in many clinical applications. This computerized mathematical model has already been successfully applied in a clinical setting for patient evaluation and treatment planning, especially when alternative treatment approaches are being considered for an individual patient. In addition, it has been shown to be useful in patient staging and in planning and analysis of clinical studies.

REFERENCES

1. Balch CM, Murad TM, Soong S-j, Ingalls AL, Halpern NB, Maddox WA: A multifactorial analysis of melanoma: Prognostic histopathological features comparing Clark's and Breslow's staging methods. Ann Surg 188:732, 1978
2. Balch CM, Smalley RV, Bartolucci AA, Burns D, Presant CA, Durant JR: A randomized prospective clinical trial of adjuvant *C. parvum* immunotherapy in 260 patients with clinically localized melanoma (stage I): Prognostic factors analysis and preliminary results of immunotherapy. Cancer 49:1079, 1982
3. Balch CM, Soong S-j, Milton GW, Shaw HM, McGovern VJ, Murad TM, McCarthy WH, Maddox WA: A comparison of prognostic factors and surgical results in 1,786 patients with localized (stage I) melanoma treated in Alabama, USA, and New South Wales, Australia. Ann Surg 196:677, 1982
4. Barclay TL, Crockett DJ, Eastwood DS, Eastwood J, Giles GR: Assessment of prognosis in cutaneous malignant melanoma. Br J Surg 64:54, 1977
5. Carter WH, Wampler GL, Stablein DM: Regression Analysis of Survival Data in Cancer Chemotherapy, p 39. New York, Marcel Dekker, 1983
6. Cochran AJ: Method of assessing prognosis in patients with malignant melanoma. Lancet 2:1062, 1968
7. Cox DR: Regression models and life tables (with discussion). J Royal Stat Soc B34:187, 1972
8. Cox DR, Snell E: A general definition of residuals. J Royal Stat Soc B30:248, 1968
9. Cox EB, Laszlo J, Freiman A: Classification of cancer patients: Beyond TNM. JAMA 242:2691, 1979
10. Kaplan EL, Meier P: Nonparametric estimations from incomplete observations. J Am Stat Assoc 53:457, 1958
11. Kay R: Proportional hazard regression models and the analysis of censored survival data. Applied Statistics 26:227, 1977
12. Polk HC, Linn BS: Selective regional lymphadenectomy for melanoma: A mathematical aid to clinical judgment. Ann Surg 174:402, 1971

Part V
Prognosis and Treatment Results Worldwide

WILLIAM H. McCARTHY
HELEN M. SHAW
GERALD W. MILTON
VINCENT J. McGOVERN

Melanoma in New South Wales, Australia: Experience at the Sydney Melanoma Unit

21

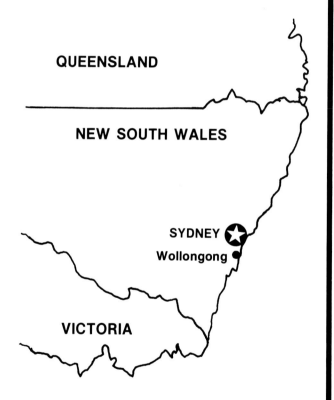

Epidemiology
  Incidence
  Changing Trends in the Characteristics of
      Melanoma
Prognostic Factors
  Patient Factors
  Tumor Factors
Treatment
  Primary Lesion Excision
  Regional Lymph Node Dissection
  Metastatic Melanoma

Between January 1950 and November 1982, the Sydney Melanoma Unit (SMU) treated 3391 patients at Royal Prince Alfred Hospital, St. Vincent's Hospital, and Sydney Hospital, Sydney, New South Wales, Australia. Their characteristics and survival rates are shown in Tables 21-1 and 21-2.

New South Wales is one of the federated states of Australia and is situated between the 28°S and 38°S latitude and between 141°E and 154°E longitude and is entirely in the temperate zone. The area of New South Wales is 801,000 square kilometers, and the population is 5.1 million. The population distribution is largely coastal, 73% being in Sydney, Newcastle, and Wollongong, with 89% of the population being urban and 11% rural. With a population of 3.4 million, Sydney is the largest city in Australia and is situated at 34°S, 151°E of Greenwich. Persons of aboriginal descent constitute 0.3% of the population of Sydney and 0.7% of the population of New South Wales. Eighty-one percent of the persons in New South Wales were born in Australia, 8% in the United Kingdom or Ireland, 3% in southern Mediterranean countries, and the remainder in northern European countries and elsewhere.

The climatic conditions in the Sydney Metropolitan Area are conducive to regular sunbathing and other outdoor activities almost throughout the entire year. There is an average of 6.7 hours of bright sunlight daily (range 5.2–7.6), and although the annual rainfall is quite high (1215 mm), cloud cover is sporadic since rainfall is restricted to an average of 148 days per year.

Prior to 1964, all patients received their first definitive treatment for melanoma at Royal Prince Alfred Hospital, and all data on these patients were collected retrospectively. Nearly all these patients were drawn from the Sydney Metropolitan Area (12,407 square kilometers). Since 1964, nearly all first definitive surgical treatment at the SMU, at St. Vincent's Hospital, and Sydney Hospital has been performed by one of two surgeons, and all histologic slides have been reviewed by the one pathologist, Professor V. J. McGovern.

Nearly three fourths of the patients on the SMU records have been seen in the last decade (Table 21-1). In 1982, 300 patients were entered on the records. This represents about 25% of all patients diagnosed as having malignant melanoma in New South Wales that year. About two thirds of these 300 patients received their first definitive treatment for melanoma at the SMU. The remaining one third were referred to the SMU either with metastatic melanoma or for routine follow-up.

TABLE 21–1
CLINICAL AND PATHOLOGIC DATA FOR MELANOMA PATIENTS TREATED AT THE SYDNEY MELANOMA UNIT, SYDNEY, AUSTRALIA

	Presenting Pathologic Stage	
	Stage I	Stage II
Clinical Characteristics		
Number of patients	3025	366
Year of diagnosis		
≤1960	6%	10%
1961–1965	7%	8%
1966–1970	12%	17%
1971–1975	25%	25%
1976–1980	50%	40%
Age (median)	44 yr	44 yr
Sex		
Male	47%	70%
Female	53%	30%
Primary Lesion Site		
Female lower extremity	24%	15%
Male lower extremity	9%	18%
Female upper extremity	10%	3%
Male upper extremity	5%	9%
Female head and neck	7%	4%
Male head and neck	8%	13%
Female trunk	11%	7%
Male trunk	24%	28%
Other	2%	3%
Pathologic Characteristics		
Breslow's tumor thickness		
<0.76 mm	27%	6%
0.76 mm–1.49 mm	28%	5%
1.50 mm–2.49 mm	20%	25%
2.50 mm–3.99 mm	14%	16%
≥4.00 mm	11%	48%
Median tumor thickness	1.3 mm	3.6 mm
Levels of invasion		
II	24%	5%
III	25%	25%
IV	45%	52%
V	6%	18%
Ulceration		
Yes	21%	50%
No	79%	50%
Growth pattern		
Nodular	30%	57%
Superficial spreading	67%	40%
Lentigo maligna	3%	3%

EPIDEMIOLOGY

INCIDENCE

Statutory notification of cancer in New South Wales has been compulsory only since 1972, when the incidence of melanoma in this state was 10.1 per 10^5 for men and 12.1 per 10^5 for women. In 1976, these incidence figures rose to 20.4 per 10^5 for men and

TABLE 21–2
ACTUARIAL SURVIVAL DATA FOR MELANOMA
PATIENTS TREATED AT THE SYDNEY MELANOMA UNIT, SYDNEY, AUSTRALIA

	Survival Rates	
	5-Year	10-Year
Stage I		
Overall survival	79%	68%
Sex		
Male	69%	55%
Female	84%	76%
Primary lesion site		
Lower extremity	84%	78%
Upper extremity	82%	73%
Head and neck	72%	66%
Trunk	71%	57%
Other	66%	
Tumor thickness		
<0.76 mm	95%	90%
0.76 mm–1.49 mm	84%	77%
1.50 mm–2.49 mm	73%	60%
2.50 mm–3.99 mm	64%	48%
≥4.00 mm	37%	25%
Level of invasion		
II	96%	92%
III	78%	72%
IV	74%	61%
V	52%	40%
Ulceration		
Yes	57%	49%
No	88%	78%

	1-Year	3-Year	5-Year
Stage II			
Overall survival	80%	48%	37%
Tumor thickness			
<1.50 mm	86%	60%	46%
1.50 mm–3.99 mm	90%	64%	53%
≥4.0 mm	70%	31%	23%
Ulceration			
Yes	75%	33%	23%
No	86%	62%	55%

24.5 per 10^5 for women.[2,3] Mortality from melanoma over this time period remained steady (4.4 versus 4.8 per 10^5 for men and 2.7 versus 2.8 per 10^5 for women). No statutory notification is required in New South Wales for either *in situ* or lentigo maligna melanoma (LMM). Thus, no data exist in this state on the incidence of these disease entities.

CHANGING TRENDS IN THE CHARACTERISTICS OF MELANOMA

Through the collaboration of the Queensland Melanoma Project, the SMU, and the New South Wales State Cancer Council, an active education program for both the medical profession and the public has been operating in Eastern Australia. As a result, melanoma in both Queensland and New South Wales has been diagnosed and treated at a much earlier and more curable stage of disease. At the SMU, the proportion of patients presenting with asymptomatic lesions has increased from 5% in 1960 to 32% in 1980. The main reasons given by patients for seeking treatment were that either they noticed the mole themselves or their attention was drawn to it by their local medical officer, friend, or spouse. Thus, the proportion of patients presenting with localized disease (*i.e.,* clinical stage I/pathologic stage I) has increased over this period. The median tumor thickness on presentation has decreased from 2.5 mm prior to 1960 to 0.8 mm in 1982 (see Chap. 18). Associated with this, a substantial increase in the proportion of *in situ* melanomas has been recorded. It is therefore not surprising that there has been no concomitant rise in mortality rate from melanoma, despite its increased incidence. Thus, the great majority of patients diagnosed with melanoma today can be cured of their disease.

PROGNOSTIC FACTORS

PATIENT FACTORS

At the SMU, considerable interest has centered around delineating those factors responsible for the overall female superiority in survival. Initially, it was shown that several endocrine factors, including puberty, menopause, estrogen administration, and parity had no influence on prognosis in women, but that there was a statistically significant sex difference in prognosis.[18] Two factors probably contributing to this better prognosis in women were that women first presented at an earlier clinical stage of the disease and had primary lesions confined to more prognostically favorable anatomical sites than men did (Table 21-1). Subsequently, it was established that in clinical stage I patients, women had significantly thinner lesions than men did (Fig. 21-1).[14] However, even in men and women with lesions of equivalent thickness, prognosis was still better in women than in men.[14] Further studies revealed that in clinical stage I patients matched by tumor thickness, anatomical site of primary lesion, and age, women with very thick tumors still survived longer.[15] Age of patient *per se* did not appear to be of prognostic significance, because associated with the decline in prognosis with increasing age in both men and women was a decline in the proportion of thin lesions.[15]

In contrast to the situation in clinical stage I patients, overall 5-year survival rates were similar in men and women with nodal metastases from melanoma (clinical stage II, pathologic stage II).[16] However, it was found that this overall survival rate in women was markedly reduced because of an extremely poor prognosis for postmenopausal women. In contrast to the situation existing in stage I patients, stage II women had significantly thicker tumors than men did (Fig. 21-2). In clinical stage II men and women matched by age and thickness of

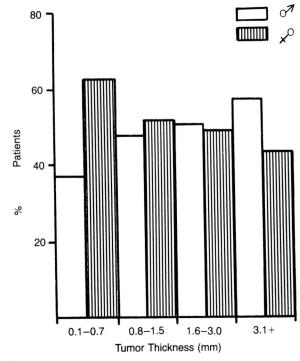

FIG. 21–1 Tumor thickness distribution in 780 clinical stage I melanoma patients according to sex.

their primary tumor, a female superiority in survival did exist for women with very thick lesions.

With the establishment of ulceration as an independent prognostic variable,[10] the female superiority in survival for both clinical stage I and stage II patients was reassessed. It was found that the overall incidence of ulceration was considerably higher in men than in women, although this sex difference in ulceration disappeared in patients matched by tumor thickness. In both sexes, there was a highly significant trend for the incidence of ulceration to increase with age. In patients matched by primary lesion site, tumor thickness, and ulceration, no female superiority existed for either patients with localized or metastatic disease.[*]

Recognition and survival from melanoma were also influenced by the occupational category of patients.[13] Unskilled patients had a markedly worse prognosis than more skilled patients, a finding attributable, at least in part, to earlier presentation in the latter. Young patients who smoked were also more

---

[*] Shaw HM, et al: manuscript in preparation

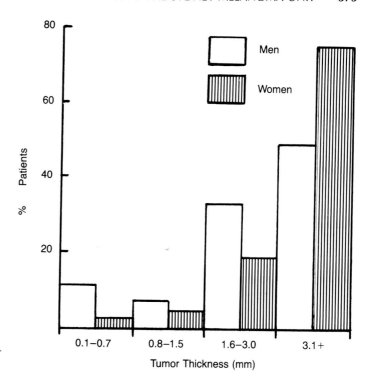

FIG. 21–2 Tumor thickness distribution in 209 clinical stage II melanoma patients according to sex.

susceptible to developing metastases than were nonsmoking patients.[17,19]

TUMOR FACTORS

Two independent and seven dependent variables were major predictors of the clinical course of SMU patients with clinical stage I disease (see Chap. 19 for details). The most important factor was tumor thickness.[6] Although ulceration drew some of its prognostic significance from its close association with tumor thickness, it has also been proven to be an independent prognostic determinant.[10] Seven other histologic features derived most, if not all, of their prognostic significance from their close correlation with tumor thickness. These were growth pattern, mitotic activity and regression,[6] cell type and pigment content,[8] lymphocytic infiltration,[9] and tumor configuration.[4] Thus, no further prognostic information could be derived from time-consuming measurements of these seven subjective and variable parameters. Tumor thickness also proved to be valuable in predicting the time and site of first recurrence from melanoma.[11] Thick lesions recurred frequently, mostly in the vicinity of the scar of primary excision, and the disease-free interval was short. On the other hand, if very thin lesions did recur, they did so much later at either regional lymph nodes or at remote sites. Despite the fact that they tended to be thick, LMM rarely metastasized; and, thus, at the SMU, this disease is treated as an entity separate from melanoma.[7] Melanomas ≤0.7 mm thick were capable of metastasizing, but only slightly more regressed than unregressed lesions metastasized (8% versus 5%, respectively). All but one of the recurrences from regressed lesions developed within 5 years, but recurrences from unregressed lesions still continued to develop after this time. Regression in these thin tumors was thus not an unfavorable prognostic sign, since it was found that in patients with long-term follow-up, survival rates were similar, irrespective of whether their lesion displayed or did not display evidence of regression (Fig. 21-3).[5] This emphasizes the importance of long-term follow-up in assessing prognosis.

In patients with nodal metastases (stage II), a multifactorial analysis showed that the two parameters that were the most important variables predicting survival were the presence of ulceration (p = 0.004) and the measured thickness of the primary melanoma (p = 0.01). The number of metastatic nodes was not available as a parameter for analysis. Further details are found in Chapter 19.

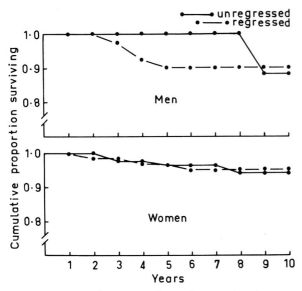

FIG. 21–3 Cumulative survival rates for 353 clinical stage I melanoma patients with lesions ≤0.7 mm thick according to whether their lesions did or did not display histologic evidence of regression.

TREATMENT

The treatment for an individual melanoma patient seen at the SMU takes into account the following considerations: (1) the type of melanoma—superficial spreading melanoma (SSM), nodular melanoma (NM), or lentigo maligna melanoma (LMM); (2) the site of the primary tumor; (3) the extent of the primary tumor (*i.e.,* thickness and ulceration); (4) the presence or absence of metastases and the type of spread; (5) the sex and age of the patient; and (6) the general condition of the patient and his wishes for treatment.

Since LMM is considered to be a disease distinct from SSM or NM, it is treated with conservative surgery or with cryotherapy (Chap. 6). Lymph node dissection (LND) is never performed as an elective procedure for LMM patients. The anatomical site of the primary tumor influences the extent of the excision. For example, SSM or NM on the face are not excised as widely as those on the back or the leg.

In situ melanomas are treated with minimal surgery (narrow excision and primary closure of the wound). It should be emphasized, however, that re-excision of the biopsy site is important to minimize the risk of local recurrence.

The policy relating to biopsy at the SMU is as follows: (1) No patient is treated for melanoma without a tissue diagnosis. (2) The biopsy consists of removing the whole tumor with a narrow margin (2 mm–3 mm) all around and deep to it. (3) Punch or incision biopsies are done only for the unusual case with a very large lesion, the excision of which would be a major procedure (*e.g.,* some LMM and some acral lentiginous melanoma). (4) The diagnosis is usually established by frozen-section examination; however, if the pathologist has the slightest doubt, a paraffin section is done. (5) Care is taken to ensure that the excision of the biopsy and the definitive excision do not encroach on each other because of the possible risk of seeding.

PRIMARY LESION EXCISION

The thickness of the lesion is the most important criterion when considering primary lesion excisions. For lesions <1 mm in thickness, excision is usually 1 cm to 2 cm wide of the lesion. For lesions ≥1 mm in thickness, the excision is 3 cm or more and consists of removal of the subcutaneous tissue down to and, on the limbs, including the deep fascia. Ulceration and level of invasion are used as additional criteria in selection of those patients to have elective lymph node dissection (ELND) but do not greatly influence the extent of excision of primary tumor.

REGIONAL LYMPH NODE DISSECTION

The evidence for disease dissemination profoundly affects treatment. As most patients present at an early stage of disease, evidence of dissemination is uncommon. Palpable and clinically involved lymph nodes automatically involve LND, provided that there is no evidence of central dissemination and the patient's general health is adequate for the operation. Evidence of central dissemination indicates that minimal surgery for palliative reasons only will be undertaken.

Because overall prognosis appears worse in men than in women, the sex of the patient has been considered to be relevant to treatment. Consequently, in the past, treatment had tended to be rather more extensive in men than in women. However, as mentioned above, recent studies from the SMU have revealed that men tended to have a high incidence of thick, ulcerated primary lesions located on the trunk—a prognostically unfavorable anatomical site. In men and women matched carefully by these three prognostic factors, survival rates were similar. Thus, differing degrees of surgery for men and women with equivalent disease are not now performed.

ELND is carried out only in patients who are less than 70 years of age and in good health. At the SMU, in both men and women with extremity lesions, ELND has been recommended for tumors greater than 2 mm thick. On the other hand, ELND is more liberally recommended for patients with axial lesions with a thickness as low as >1 mm to 1.5 mm. If the tumor is ulcerated, ELND is indicated for the thinner lesions in these ranges, while for nonulcerated tumors ELND is considered only for the thicker lesions in these ranges. However, over the past 25 years at the SMU, indications for all forms of surgery have inevitably changed as more has been learned about the behavior of the disease and more ELNDs are currently recommended for lesions between 1.5 mm and 2 mm.

Although figures from the SMU[12] and those of Balch and colleagues[1] demonstrated no enhanced survival in men who had tumors >4 mm thick, ELND is still performed at the SMU in young patients for the following reasons. (1) Local or regional recurrence (*i.e.,* at the primary lesion scar, intransit to or at regional lymph nodes) is the most common site of the first recurrence of a thick melanoma (see Chaps. 6 and 12). (2) The vast majority of patients who develop local recurrent disease do so within the first 3 years after treatment of the primary tumor. (3) Central and fatal recurrent disease most frequently occurs after the disease has recurred locally. Hence, if one takes two patients with a 3-mm tumor, their chance of survival when they present at the SMU is already determined by the thickness of their primary tumor. If one patient has only a local excision, it is highly probable that some time between 6 and 8 months after excision of the primary lesion, he will develop local recurrence for which surgery and hospitalization would be necessary. Not long after this treatment is complete, he will develop symptoms of central disease and will eventually die. The second patient who has had thorough local surgery (including ELND) will remain disease-free until the central metastases become symptomatic. Hence, ELND for thick tumors is a form of anticipatory palliative surgery. This procedure is not performed in elderly patients or those who prefer not to have such dissection.

Bilateral groin ELNDs are not advised for the rare case of low posterior or anterior trunk lesions. However, in young and otherwise fit patients, bilateral axillary ELNDs are occasionally performed for serious, centrally placed tumors. The reason for the difference is that, in the young and fit person, the morbidity for bilateral groin ELND is considerable, while it is not great for bilateral axillary ELND.

The age and general condition of the patient are other expressions of the life expectancy. In any patient whose life expectancy is less than 5 years, extensive surgery is not often performed. The wishes of the patient are taken seriously, because there is a good deal of controversy about both the extent of the primary tumor excision and of the value of ELND. Accordingly, as detailed an explanation as possible is given to the patient, and no extensive surgery is carried out without this understanding (Chap. 8).

METASTATIC MELANOMA

The following is a brief summary of the SMU policy for advanced disease (discussed in much more detail in Chaps. 12 and 13). (1) As long as the disease is surgically resectable, without excess morbidity, surgical excision is the treatment of choice in most patients <60 years of age. (2) Amputation is occasionally offered as a method of treatment if there are intractable local recurrences not responding to other forms of treatment (*e.g.,* isolated perfusion) and the patient has no evidence of central dissemination. The introduction of intra-arterial cisplatinum as a method of avoiding amputation is currently being investigated. (3) It is now felt that the use of neither adjuvant chemotherapy nor immunotherapy is practical, since no convincing evidence has been brought forward to demonstrate their effectiveness. In addition, most forms of chemotherapy have considerable morbidity, and their use does not appear justified in the symptom-free patient. (4) Either chemotherapy or immunotherapy, or a combination of both, are used when a patient has measurable disease for which surgical excision is contraindicated, one method being tried after the other, depending on the circumstances. (5) Other methods of local treatment, such as cryotherapy, diathermy curettage, or intralesional chemotherapy or immunotherapy, are used for locally advanced disease (Chap. 13).

REFERENCES

1. Balch CM, Murad TM, Soong S-j, Ingalls AL, Richards PC, Maddox WA: Tumor thickness as a guide to surgical management of clinical stage I melanoma patients. Cancer 43:883, 1979

2. McCarthy WH, Black AL, Milton GW: Melanoma in New South Wales: An epidemiologic survey 1970–1976. Cancer 46:427, 1980

3. McCarthy WH, Martyn AL, Roberts G, Dobson AJ: Melanoma in New South Wales 1970–1976: Confirmation of increased incidence. Med J Aust 2:137, 1980

4. McGovern VJ, Shaw HM, Milton GW: Prognostic significance of a polypoid configuration in malignant melanoma. Histopathology 7:663, 1983

5. McGovern VJ, Shaw HM, Milton GW: Prognosis in patients with thin malignant melanoma: Influence of regression. Histopathology 7:673, 1983

6. McGovern VJ, Shaw HM, Milton GW, Farago GA: Prognostic significance of the histological features of malignant melanoma. Histopathology 3:385, 1979

7. McGovern VJ, Shaw HM, Milton GW, Farago GA: Is malignant melanoma arising in a Hutchinson's melanotic freckle a separate disease entity? Histopathology 4:235, 1980

8. McGovern VJ, Shaw HM, Milton GW, Farago GA: Cell type and pigment content as prognostic indicators in cutaneous malignant melanoma. In Ackerman AB (ed): Pathology of Malignant Melanoma, p 327. New York, Masson, 1981

9. McGovern VJ, Shaw HM, Milton GW, Farago GA: Lymphocytic infiltration and survival in malignant melanoma. In Ackerman AB (ed): Pathology of Malignant Melanoma, p 341. New York, Masson, 1981

10. McGovern VJ, Shaw HM, Milton GW, McCarthy WH: Ulceration and prognosis in cutaneous malignant melanoma. Histopathology 6:399, 1982

11. Milton GW, Shaw HM, Farago GA, McCarthy WH: Tumour thickness and the site and time of first recurrence in cutaneous malignant melanoma (stage I). Br J Surg 67:543, 1980

12. Milton GW, Shaw HM, McCarthy WH, Pearson L, Balch CM, Soong S-j: Prophylactic lymph node dissection in clinical stage I cutaneous malignant melanoma: Results of surgical treatment in 1319 patients. Br J Surg 69:108, 1982

13. Shaw HM, McGovern VJ, Milton GW, Farago GA: Cutaneous malignant melanoma: Occupation and prognosis. Med J Aust 1:37, 1981

14. Shaw HM, McGovern VJ, Milton GW, Farago GA, McCarthy WH: Histologic features of tumors and the female superiority in survival from malignant melanoma. Cancer 45:1604, 1980

15. Shaw HM, McGovern VJ, Milton GW, Farago GA, McCarthy WH: Malignant melanoma: Influence of site of lesion and age of patient in the female superiority in survival. Cancer 46:2731, 1980

16. Shaw HM, McGovern VJ, Milton GW, Farago GA, McCarthy WH: The female superiority in survival in clinical stage II cutaneous malignant melanoma. Cancer 49:1941, 1982

17. Shaw HM, Milton GW: Smoking and the development of metastases from malignant melanoma. Int J Cancer 28:153, 1981

18. Shaw HM, Milton GW, Farago GA, McCarthy WH: Endocrine influences on survival from malignant melanoma. Cancer 42:669, 1978

19. Shaw HM, Milton GW, McCarthy WH, Farago GA, Dilworth P: Effect of smoking on the recurrence of malignant melanoma. Med J Aust 1:208, 1979

G. RODERICK McLEOD
NEVILLE C. DAVIS
JOHN H. LITTLE
ADELE GREEN
DAVID CHANT

Melanoma in Queensland, Australia: Experience of the Queensland Melanoma Project

22

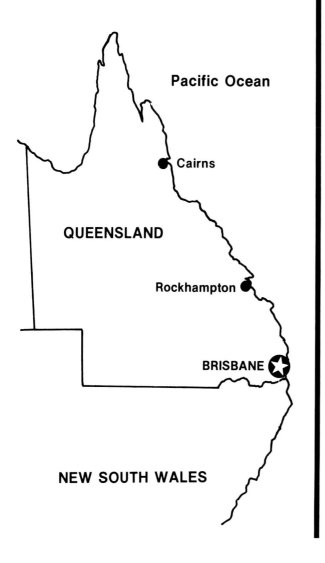

Pacific Ocean

QUEENSLAND

Cairns

Rockhampton

BRISBANE

NEW SOUTH WALES

Epidemiology
　　Overall Incidence
　　Changing Trends
　　Possible Etiologic Factors
Prognostic Factors
Treatment
　　Level I Melanomas
　　Invasive Melanomas
　　　　Primary lesion
　　　　Regional lymph nodes
　　　　Other treatment
Conclusion

This report from the Queensland Melanoma Project (QMP) describes results from a prospective, population-based registry of 1441 melanoma patients treated in Queensland between July 1963 and December 1969 (Tables 22-1 and 22-2). All patients were followed for a minimum of 10 years from first treatment, and only 3% were lost to follow-up.

The northeastern Australian state of Queensland is divided by the Tropic of Capricorn into roughly equal tropical and subtropical zones, lying between the 10th and 29th parallels of south latitude and the 138th and 154th meridians of east longitude. Although Queensland occupies 1.7 million square kilometers, approximately half of its population of 2.2 million live in the capital city of Brisbane and adjacent areas in the southeast corner, while most of the remainder live along the coast. For the majority of the Queenslanders, sunlight exposure is recreational and, because of the favorable climate, outdoor leisure activities are frequent. Many beaches are readily accessible to the majority of the population. In the southeast corner of Queensland, there is an average of 7 to 8 hours of sunlight daily. Most of the remainder of the eastern half of the state has an average of 8 to 9 hours of sunlight throughout the year, while the sparsely populated western half has an average of 9 to 10 hours of sunlight daily.

The QMP was established in 1963 and has been

TABLE 22–1
CLINICAL AND PATHOLOGIC DATA FOR MELANOMA PATIENTS TREATED IN QUEENSLAND

| | Presenting Pathologic Stage | | | |
	Stage I	Stage II	Stage III	Total
Clinical Characteristics				
Number of patients	1174	64	10	1248
Year of diagnosis				
≤1960	0%	0%	0%	0%
1961–1965	43%	45%	40%	43%
1966–1970	57%	55%	60%	57%
1971–1975	0%	0%	0%	0%
1976–1980	0%	0%	0%	0%
Median age	47 yr	53 yr	61 yr	47 yr
Sex				
Male	42%	69%	70%	43%
Female	58%	31%	30%	57%
Primary lesion site				
Female lower extremity	22%	14%	0%	22%
Male lower extremity	8%	19%	10%	8%
Female upper extremity	14%	14%	0%	14%
Male upper extremity	7%	6%	0%	6%
Female head and neck	10%	3%	30%	10%
Male head and neck	8%	8%	10%	8%
Female trunk	11%	0%	0%	11%
Male trunk	20%	36%	50%	21%
Other	0%	0%	0%	0%
Pathologic Characteristics				
Breslow's tumor thickness				
<0.76 mm	32%	5%	10%	30%
0.76 mm–1.49 mm	25%	6%	10%	24%
1.50 mm–2.49 mm	20%	13%	10%	19%
2.50 mm–3.99 mm	14%	28%	20%	14%
≥4.00 mm	10%	48%	50%	13%
Median tumor thickness	1.2 mm	3.7 mm	3.7 mm	1.3 mm
Ulceration				
Yes	26%	69%	40%	28%
No	74%	31%	60%	72%
Growth Pattern				
Nodular	23%	70%	50%	25%
Superficial spreading	68%	25%	40%	66%
Lentigo maligna	9%	5%	10%	9%

supported through the years by the Queensland Cancer Fund. Its objective was to establish a population-based registry of melanoma patients treated throughout Queensland. Entry of patients into the registry was initiated by pathologists throughout the state who notified the QMP of each melanoma diagnosis. General practitioners and specialists treating these patients cooperated by providing personal and clinical details of the patients. All pathology specimens were examined by a panel of three pathologists, and before the case was included in the registry, all three independently confirmed the diagnosis. Although there was no Cancer Registry in Queensland prior to 1982, the cooperation by pathologists and clinicians was exceptional, since nearly every case in Queensland was recorded. The histologic material has been updated using level of invasion and tumor thickness measurements. Since 1977, epidemiologic studies from the Queensland Institute of Medical Research and the Queensland Melanoma Project have been used to obtain incidence figures and other data. Similar cooperation by

TABLE 22–2
ACTUARIAL SURVIVAL DATA FOR MELANOMA PATIENTS TREATED IN QUEENSLAND

	Survival Rates	
	5-Year	*10-Year*
Stage I		
Overall survival	85%	80%
Sex		
Male	79%	72%
Female	90%	86%
Primary lesion site		
Lower extremity	90%	86%
Upper extremity	90%	89%
Head and neck	83%	76%
Trunk	79%	71%
Other	75%	75%
Tumor thickness		
<0.76 mm	97%	95%
0.76 mm–1.49 mm	92%	87%
1.50 mm–2.49 mm	83%	76%
2.50 mm–3.99 mm	77%	63%
≥4.00 mm	48%	40%
Ulceration		
Yes	68%	60%
No	91%	87%

	1-Year	*3-Year*	*5-Year*
Stage II			
Overall survival	70%	32%	27%
Tumor thickness			
<1.50 mm	71%	43%	29%
1.50 mm–3.99 mm	62%	42%	38%
≥4 mm	77%	20%	16%
Number of positive nodes			
1	82%	43%	33%
2–4	62%	21%	21%
>4	38%	25%	25%
Ulceration			
Yes	72%	29%	24%
No	65%	39%	34%

	6-Month	*1-Year*	*2-Year*
Stage III			
Overall survival	60%	40%	40%

the pathologists from 1977 to the present has permitted the collection of these additional epidemiologic data.

EPIDEMIOLOGY

OVERALL INCIDENCE

Over the past 15 years, the reported incidence of primary cutaneous melanoma in Queensland has been increasing, when results from three studies in 1963 to 1968,[1] 1977,[16] and 1979 to 1980[8] are compared. The crude annual incidence of level I melanoma was 1.4×10^5 inhabitants in 1966, rising to 8.1 in 1977 and to 11.2×10^5 in 1979 to 1980. For invasive melanoma, the crude rates rose from 15.1×10^5 in 1966 to 25 in 1977, and in 1979 to 1980 the annual rate was 28.4×10^5.

Age-specific and age-standardized data according to level of invasion were not available for the 1963 to 1969 study but have been calculated for the 1979 to 1980 data. When standardized to the age distribution of the European population,[6] the annual incidence rate for level I melanoma is 13.2×10^5 and for invasive melanoma, 30.6×10^5. These are the highest rates of cutaneous melanoma reported anywhere in the world.

An increase in the proportion of thin melanomas accounts for some of this observed rise in incidence. Although quantitation in melanoma has been very valuable, there are problems in subjective estimations that have resulted in some disagreement among pathologists. A small survey[13] among Brisbane pathologists and an international survey showed that one pathologist in three or four will disagree on quantitation. This is particularly important in the case of lentigo maligna melanoma (LMM).[8,16] The possibility of misclassification or overdiagnosis of LMM lesions has been considered,[9] and although diagnostic variation exists, it does not seem sufficient to explain the rising trend.

CHANGING TRENDS

Because of intensive public education campaigns, Queenslanders are aware of pigmented lesions and seek medical advice at an early stage of the disease.[8] This may also have been responsible for the increased incidence, especially for level I lesions. Level I melanoma is considered by the QMP to be an important stage in the development of invasive melanoma, so this entity is separately included in this report. The designation of "level I" melanoma instead of other terminology has probably contributed in part to the increasing proportion of level I melanomas diagnosed in Queensland. Prior to 1970, the proportion was 7% but rose to 24% in 1977 and further to 28% in 1979 to 1980. Earlier diagnosis was also reflected in the increasing proportion of lesions with small diameter and flatter profile.

There is now no statistically significant difference in incidence rates of melanoma between the sexes, in contrast to the female preponderance of both level I and invasive melanoma observed in the 1960s.[1] In 1979 to 1980, the annual incidence of level I lesions was 12×10^5 population for men and 11.4 for women. For invasive tumors, annual incidence rate among men was 26.7×10^5 compared with the female rate of 30.1×10^5.

Age distribution varies according to the gender of the patient and to the growth pattern of the melanoma. The age-specific incidence rates for 1979 to 1980 are shown in Tables 22-3 and 22-4 for each type of growth pattern. In women, superficial spreading melanoma (SSM) occurred predominantly in younger age groups, whereas nodular melanomas (NM) predominated in older age groups. Nodular melanoma in men showed a similar age pattern to that of women, whereas the peak incidence of SSM in men occurred at an older age than in women. An age-dependent incidence pattern was seen in both sexes for LMM.

The distribution of level I and invasive melanomas for the 1979 to 1980 data are shown in Tables 22-5 and 22-6, subgrouped according to anatomical site and growth pattern of the primary melanoma. Tumors of the LMM variety, classically seen on the head and neck, were seen on other sites in over one third of the 247 patients reported for this time period.[8] For other growth patterns, site distributions generally resembled those reported for previous decades, where the male trunk and the female lower limb were the predominant sites.[1,16] An exception to these patterns was seen for SSM in women, which appeared as frequently on the trunk as on the lower limb.

POSSIBLE ETIOLOGIC FACTORS

The high incidence of melanoma in Queensland was examined from the perspective of latitude and geographical terrain. A higher frequency of melanoma in subtropical rather than tropical areas has been reported previously.[1,11,16] However, in a recent study of incident cases during one year

TABLE 22–3
AGE-SPECIFIC ANNUAL INCIDENCE RATES OF INVASIVE MELANOMA $\times 10^5$ IN QUEENSLAND 1979-1980 ACCORDING TO GROWTH PATTERN—MEN

Age (years)	Growth Pattern				
	SSM	NM	LMM	IND	ALM
0–9	0.0	0.0	0.0	0.0	0.0
10–19	4.9	0.0	0.0	0.0	0.0
20–29	9.9	2.1	0.0	0.0	0.0
30–39	12.8	5.5	0.0	3.1	0.0
40–49	25.2	5.0	0.8	0.8	0.8
50–59	37.1	13.3	3.5	1.8	0.9
60–69	47.9	19.8	7.0	8.2	1.2
70+	33.8	37.0	8.1	3.2	0.0
All ages	16.3	6.6	1.5	1.5	0.3

SSM = superficial spreading melanoma; NM = nodular melanoma; LMM = lentigo maligna melanoma; IND = indeterminate; ALM = acral lentiginous melanoma.

TABLE 22–4
AGE-SPECIFIC ANNUAL INCIDENCE RATES OF INVASIVE MELANOMA $\times 10^5$ IN QUEENSLAND 1979–1980 ACCORDING TO GROWTH PATTERN—WOMEN

Age (years)	Growth Pattern				
	SSM	NM	LMM	IND	ALM
0–9	0.0	0.0	0.0	0.0	0.0
10–19	1.0	0.5	0.0	0.0	0.0
20–29	27.3	2.7	0.0	1.1	0.0
30–39	33.2	2.6	0.0	1.9	0.0
40–49	40.0	8.9	2.7	2.7	0.0
50–59	28.9	9.0	5.4	5.4	0.0
60–69	25.4	9.5	15.9	5.3	1.1
70+	15.3	17.6	12.9	1.2	0.0
All ages	19.5	4.8	3.2	1.8	0.9

SSM = superficial spreading melanoma; NM = nodular melanoma; LMM = lentigo maligna melanoma; IND = indeterminate; ALM = acral lentiginous melanoma.

TABLE 22–5
DISTRIBUTION OF 247 LEVEL I MELANOMAS BY GROWTH PATTERN AND SITE*

Anatomical Location	Growth Pattern (%)					
	SSM		LM		IND	
	Men (36)	Women (60)	Men (84)	Women (64)	Men (2)	Women (1)
Head and neck	8	10	62	63	50	0
Trunk	56	35	24	5	50	0
Upper extremity	8	23	10	19	6	0
Lower extremity	25	30	2	9	0	100
Unknown	3	2	2	5	0	0

* Figures in parentheses indicate numbers of patients.

SSM = superficial spreading melanoma; LMM = lentigo maligna melanoma; IND = indeterminate.

TABLE 22–6
DISTRIBUTION OF 624 INVASIVE MELANOMAS BY GROWTH PATTERN AND SITE*

Anatomical Location	Growth Pattern (%)									
	SSM		NM		LMM		IND		ALM	
	Men (184)	Women (218)	Men (74)	Women (54)	Men (17)	Women (36)	Men (17)	Women (20)	Men (3)	Women (1)
Head and Neck	14	5	18	15	53	64	27	25	0	0
Trunk	58	34	47	18	35	6	53	50	0	0
Upper extremity	7	20	15	17	6	14	7	25	0	0
Lower extremity	16	39	16	44	0	14	13	0	100	100
Unknown	5	2	4	6	6	2	0	0	0	0

* Figures in parentheses indicate numbers of patients.

SSM = superficial spreading melanoma; NM = nodular melanoma; LMM = lentigo maligna melanoma; IND = indeterminate; ALM = acral lentiginous melanoma.

(1979), there was no association with latitude,[10] but there was significantly increased incidence for patients living in coastal areas (where there are more outdoor activities) than in the inland regions. The ultraviolet (UV) light levels in tropical and subtropical Queensland are similar in the long summer, during which outdoor activities are especially popular. This may explain the observed geographic distribution of melanoma.

It has been suggested that persons of Celtic origin have an increased susceptibility to melanoma.[12] To test this hypothesis, a random sample of persons on the electoral rolls of the state was studied to determine origins during the 1979 to 1980 survey. Based on the place of birth of parents and grandparents, those with origins in Ireland and Scotland were classified as Celts, while those persons of other British and North European origin were not. According to this definition of "Celticity," 63% of the sample had no Celtic origin, 28% had moderate Celticity (one half of the family), and 9% had strong Celticity (both sides of the family). A similar distribution of Celticity was found among melanoma patients. Also, no melanomas had been documented in Queensland aboriginals (comprising 2% of the state's population) until the recent 1979 to 1980 series, when one black-skinned patient was reported to have a melanoma on the sole of the foot.

The inherited risk of developing melanoma in Queensland has been estimated to be 10%.[21] In a study of patients in 42 kindreds affected by melanoma, a pattern suggestive of polygenic inheritance was found.[20] Familial patients tended to be younger and prone to multiple primary melanomas. An investigation of this group is now being conducted.

PROGNOSTIC FACTORS

Clinical and histologic features of melanoma were analyzed for prognostic significance by single-factor analysis. Although the early data did not include tumor thickness, the series has since been completely reviewed so that thickness measurements could be analyzed.

Significant prognostic features were (1) the presence or absence of tumor in the lymph nodes; (2) the diameter of the lesion (greater or less than 20 mm); (3) profile of the tumor (divided into flat, convex, or pedunculated profiles); (4) height of the lesion above the skin surface; (5) level of invasion; (6) presence of ulceration and also its width; (7) mitotic rate; and (8) presence of plasma cells. Less

valuable features were cell type, degrees of cell pleomorphism, and inflammatory infiltrate. Although level of invasion was a useful prognostic indicator in patients with level IV or V melanomas, it was less helpful in predicting the clinical course of patients with level II or III melanomas. Tumor thickness measurement has now been found to be the most useful guide to prognosis.

For stage I lesions, 5- and 10-year survival rates were better for women than for men, with the differences being more pronounced for extremity lesions than for trunk and head and neck lesions (Table 22-7). When results were analyzed according to lesion thickness, the female superiority in survival was most pronounced for lesions 1.5 mm to 3.99 mm thick (Table 22-8). Patients with lesions displaying histologic evidence of ulceration had a poorer prognosis than those patients with non-ulcerated lesions (Table 22-9).

The number of pathologic stage II lesions in the Queensland series is small (44 men and 20 women). In these patients, the number of histologic positive nodes appeared to be the best indicator of prognosis. Women with a single metastatic node had a far better prognosis than other subgroups, where the survival rates were poor regardless of the extent of lymph node involvement (Table 22-10).

TREATMENT

LEVEL I MELANOMAS

Most level I melanomas can be diagnosed clinically, though occasionally a lesion thought to be a level II melanoma will prove to be level I on histologic examination. When a patient is first seen with what clinically appears to be a level I lesion, surgical excision with about 1 cm of surrounding normal skin is performed using a "no-touch" technique. Lesser margins are acceptable where there are anatomical limitations. When a patient is referred after a biopsy excision of a level I lesion, re-excision is usually performed if it is considered to be indicated (depending on the biopsy margins and other factors). The QMP prefers to excise the wound beyond the stitch holes so as to minimize the risk of local recurrence from residual tumor or implantation. Follow-up of patients with level I melanoma is arranged mainly to examine the patient for any other lesions that may subsequently appear. In addition, the patients are taught to recognize such lesions, rather than just to examine themselves for recurrent dis-

TABLE 22–7
SURVIVAL RATES IN CLINICAL STAGE I PATIENTS ACCORDING TO ANATOMICAL LOCATION OF PRIMARY LESION

| | Survival Rate (%) | | | | | |
| | 5-Year | | | 10-Year | | |
Anatomical Location	*Men*	*Women*	*Total*	*Men*	*Women*	*Total*
Head and neck	80	85	83	73	78	76
Trunk	78	81	79	68	74	71
Upper extremity	83	93	90	77	93	89
Lower extremity	79	94	90	75	90	86
Unknown	0	75	75	0	75	75

TABLE 22–8
SURVIVAL RATES IN CLINICAL STAGE I PATIENTS ACCORDING TO TUMOR THICKNESS

| | Survival Rate (%) | | | | | |
| | 5-Year | | | 10-Year | | |
Tumor Thickness (mm)	*Men*	*Women*	*Total*	*Men*	*Women*	*Total*
<0.76	95	97	97	92	97	95
0.76–1.49	89	94	92	83	91	87
1.50–2.49	71	90	83	63	83	76
2.50–3.99	65	88	77	49	76	63
≥4.00	52	44	48	41	39	40

TABLE 22–9
SURVIVAL RATES IN CLINICAL STAGE I PATIENTS ACCORDING TO ULCERATION OF THE PRIMARY LESION

| | Survival Rate (%) | | | | | |
| | 5-Year | | | 10-Year | | |
Ulceration	*Men*	*Women*	*Total*	*Men*	*Women*	*Total*
Present	60	76	68	50	69	60
Absent	87	91	91	81	91	87

TABLE 22–10
SURVIVAL RATES IN PATHOLOGIC STAGE II PATIENTS ACCORDING TO NUMBER OF POSITIVE LYMPH NODES

| | Survival Rate (%) | | | | | |
| | 1-Year | | 3-Year | | 5-Year | |
Number of Positive Nodes	*Men*	*Women*	*Men*	*Women*	*Men*	*Women*
1	85	75	40	49	25	49
2–4	54	75	18	25	18	25
>4	43		29		29	

ease. No recurrence of a level I lesion has been seen in any of 105 patients in whom the pathologist reported the lesion to be totally excised.

INVASIVE MELANOMAS

The extent of treatment for invasive melanomas used by the surgical authors has changed considerably during the 20-year history of the QMP, varying from a wide excision of the primary lesion and elective lymph node dissection (ELND) in the earlier years to a much more limited surgical excision of the melanoma at present, with ELND restricted to a few carefully selected patients.[17,18] This change in policy has not been accompanied by an increase in local recurrence or a reduction in survival rates.

Primary lesion

The treatment policy used by the surgical authors is based on the clinical and histologic assessment of the primary melanoma. It is usual to treat the lesion on the basis of clinical assessment and to consider whether further excision is indicated after the histologic findings become available. Clinical observations that are considered when making patient treatment decisions include the diameter and profile of the melanoma, its anatomical location, any evidence of ulceration or regression, and its apparent growth pattern. A naked-eye assessment of the thickness of the lesion can also be done with reasonable accuracy by experienced physicians. The histologic features used in subsequent treatment decisions are tumor thickness and, to a lesser extent, level of invasion, mitotic rate, round cell infiltration, and any evidence of lymphatic or vascular invasion.[14]

The problem of how widely and how deeply to excise a melanoma remains controversial. There is no uniformity of opinion about the required margins of excision, even among the members of the QMP. As the consequences of undertreatment may be fatal, the surgical authors recommend a slight bias toward what may be regarded as overtreatment. The aim is to treat the patient adequately at the first operation. In all cases, a "no-touch" technique is favored. If there is doubt about the diagnosis, the lesion is excised with a narrow margin (2 mm-3 mm) and a frozen-section examination is obtained. The pathologists at Princess Alexandra Hospital are experienced with this technique, and their reporting is reliable.[4,15]

In situations where the clinical diagnosis is evident and the clinical findings suggest a favorable prognosis, the melanoma is excised incorporating at least a 1-cm margin of skin. Where the diagnosis has been established by frozen-section examination of the excisional biopsy, the operation continues with a re-excision of the initial wound with an additional 1-cm surgical margin. In those patients with clinically advanced lesions, a wider margin is used. The very wide excisions practiced up to 10 years ago are not recommended. The aim is to remove only enough tissue to permit primary closure, without the need for a skin graft. There is no evidence that more extensive excisions improve the prognosis for patients, even those with advanced lesions. The site of the primary lesion may also influence the margins of excision, where anatomical limitations and possible deformity may result from extensive surgical excisions. The depth of excision is down to, but not necessarily including, the deep fascia. The authors have shown that removal of the deep fascia does not alter the prognosis and believe that some benefits may actually be gained by its preservation.

A histologic report of an unexpectedly thick lesion, extensive lymphatic invasion, or satellite lesions in the dermis may lead to a further surgical excision, although this is rarely necessary.

Regional lymph nodes

Originally, ELND was performed in clinical stage I patients with lesions on the extremities. This was largely abandoned in 1965, except for advanced lesions,[5] because less than 10% of these stage I patients had detectable histologic evidence of nodal metastases.[19]

With further analysis of results, the QMP now believes that there is a small subgroup of patients who may benefit from ELND, since stage I patients exhibit an inverse correlation between tumor thickness and survival (Table 22-8). The patients considered for ELND are those with tumors 1.5 mm to 3.99 mm thick. Those patients with tumors <1 mm thick rarely have ELND, and those with tumors 1 mm to 1.5 mm thick are occasionally advised to have ELND.[18] Other factors, such as the sex and age of the patient, anatomical site of the lesion and its mitotic rate, and patient preference are also taken into consideration when making this clinical decision. Using this careful selection process, improved survival might be expected in those patients with thicker lesions, while unnecessary operations can be avoided in those with thinner lesions.

When the regional lymph nodes are clinically involved, they are excised by block dissection, usually in continuity with the primary lesion, if anatomically feasible. Ilioinguinal lymphadenectomy is not performed unless there is evidence of involvement of the lower iliac nodes. The QMP has some long-term survivors after this procedure.

Other treatment

Isolated regional perfusion is used for the management of patients with intransit metastases on the limb, but never as a primary or adjuvant treatment.[7] Radiotherapy is of use where surgery is not possible, especially for painful areas of bone metastases and for inoperable lymph node metastases.[2] Chemotherapy and immunotherapy are used in some cases of advanced or recurrent melanoma, but not where surgical treatment is possible and never as adjuvant therapy.[3]

CONCLUSION

Although melanoma incidence has increased at a rapid pace, melanoma is being diagnosed earlier in its natural history. We are convinced that public and professional education about melanoma and consequently presentation for treatment at an early biologic stage of disease have contributed to the improved survival rates.

REFERENCES

1. Beardmore GL: The epidemiology of malignant melanoma in Australia. In McCarthy WH (ed): Melanoma and Skin Cancer, p 39. Sydney, Blight, 1972
2. Bourne RC: Radiotherapeutic treatments. In Emmett AJ, O'Rourke MG (eds): Malignant Skin Tumours, p 160. Edinburgh, Churchill Livingstone, 1982
3. Clunie GH: Chemotherapy and immunotherapy. In Emmett AJ, O'Rourke MG (eds): Malignant Skin Tumours, p 176. Edinburgh, Churchill Livingstone, 1982
4. Davis NC, Little JH: The role of frozen section in the diagnosis and management of malignant melanoma. Br J Surg 61:505, 1974
5. Davis NC, McLeod GRC: Elective lymph node dissection for melanoma. Br J Surg 58:820, 1971
6. Doll R: Comparison between registries, age-standardized rates. In Waterhouse J, Muir C, Correa P, Powell J (eds): Cancer Incidence in Five Continents, Vol III, p 453. Lyon, International Agency for Research in Cancer, 1976
7. Egerton W: Regional cytotoxic arterial perfusion for recurrent malignant melanoma in limbs. In Emmett AJ, O'Rourke MG (eds): Malignant Skin Tumours, p 183. Edinburgh, Churchill Livingstone, 1982
8. Green A: Incidence and reporting of cutaneous melanoma in Queensland. Aust J Dermatol 23:105, 1982
9. Green A, Little JH, Weedon D: The diagnosis of Hutchinson's melanotic freckle (lentigo maligna) in Queensland. Pathology 15:33, 1983
10. Green A, Siskind V: Geographic distribution of cutaneous melanoma in Queensland. Med J Aust 1:407, 1983
11. Herron J: The geographical distribution of malignant melanoma in Queensland. Med J Aust 2:892, 1969
12. Lane-Brown M, Sharpe CAB, Macmillan DS, McGovern VJ: Genetic predisposition to melanoma and other skin cancers in Australia. Med J Aust 1:852, 1971
13. Larsen TE, Little JH, Orell JR, Prade M: International pathologists congruence survey on quantitation of malignant melanoma. Pathology 12:245, 1980
14. Little JH: Histology and prognosis in cutaneous malignant melanoma. In McCarthy WH (ed): Melanoma and Skin Cancer, p 122. Sydney, Blight, 1972
15. Little JH, Davis NC: Frozen section diagnosis of suspected malignant melanoma of the skin. Cancer 34:1163, 1974
16. Little JH, Holt J, Davis N: Changing epidemiology of malignant melanoma in Queensland. Med J Aust 1:66, 1980
17. McLeod GRC: Malignant melanoma: Primary treatment. In Emmett AJ, O'Rourke MG (eds): Malignant Skin Tumours, p 122. Edinburgh, Churchill Livingstone, 1982
18. McLeod GRC: Malignant melanoma: Elective and therapeutic lymph node dissection. In Emmett AJ, O'Rourke MG (eds): Malignant Skin Tumours, p 130. Edinburgh, Churchill Livingstone, 1982
19. McLeod GRC, Davis NC, Herron JJ, Caldwell RA, Little JH, Quinn RL: A retrospective survey of 498 patients with malignant melanoma. Surg Gynecol Obstet 126:99, 1968
20. Wallace DC, Beardmore GL, Exton LA: Familial malignant melanoma. Ann Surg 177:15, 1973
21. Wallace DC, Exton LA, McLeod GR: The genetic factor in malignant melanoma. Cancer 27:1262, 1971

CHARLES M. BALCH
CURTIS METTLIN

Melanoma in the United States: A National Survey of 4800 Patients

23

COMMISSION ON CANCER SURVEY

In 1981, a survey on cutaneous melanoma was undertaken by the American College of Surgeon's Commission on Cancer in collaboration with tumor registries from hospital cancer programs approved by the American College of Surgeons. A total of 614 hospitals from 48 states and the District of Columbia reported on 4545 melanoma cases. This total represents 32% of the 14,100 cases of melanoma estimated to have been diagnosed in the United States in 1980. The purpose of this report is to describe some survey results with regard to patient symptoms and clinical features, characteristics of the melanoma itself, and the types of surgical treatment employed. Characteristics of an additional 255 patients with melanoma in situ are also described.

Survey forms were sent to tumor registries of approved cancer programs throughout the United States. Institutions were asked to submit case records of patients with histologically confirmed melanoma of the skin diagnosed during the calendar year 1980. Hospitals with more than 25 eligible admissions were instructed to include at least 25 consecutively admitted patients. Those admitting fewer than 25 patients were to include all cases meeting selection criteria. No patient received prior definitive therapy. Patients excluded from this study were those with a melanoma from an unknown primary site, melanomas of the eye or mucous membrane, or melanomas diagnosed only at autopsy.

Only the initial definitive treatment was recorded. Planned combined treatment modalities of any type initiated within 4 months from the date of diagnosis were interpreted as part of the initial treatment. Patients receiving no cancer-directed treatment were included in this study and categorized as having "no treatment."

The survey results on computerized forms were received from 48 states, Puerto Rico, and the District of Columbia. A total of 614 hospitals reported on 4800 cases of invasive and noninvasive melanoma. All data were coded and processed by the Department of Cancer Control and Epidemiology at Roswell Park Memorial Institute.

SYMPTOMS OF MELANOMA

A change in a mole is the most common presenting symptom of melanoma.[7] In 81% of the 4545 melanoma patients, a change in the physical character-istics of the mole was described in terms of either size, elevation, or color. The most common presenting symptom was a change in size of a mole (41%). Itching around the mole was described in 8% of patients, and 15% complained of a discharge from the mole.

CLINICAL FEATURES

Characteristics of the patient population are summarized in Table 23-1. The majority of patients presented with clinically localized melanoma (87%) without evidence of metastatic disease (stage I). Clinical evidence of regional node metastases (stage II) was found in 10% of patients, and another 3% presented with distant metastases (stage III).

SEX AND SITE

Melanoma occurred equally in both sexes. Overall, the melanomas were distributed rather uniformly throughout the body. This was true even when the data were subgrouped by thickness, level of invasion, and age. There was a predominance of men with stage II (63%) and stage III melanomas (60%).

When the site distribution of melanoma was examined in men and women, significant differences were apparent (Fig. 23-1). The 2147 melanomas in men were predominantly located on the trunk (53%) and head and neck area (24%). The distribution of the melanomas in 2287 women was different. Only 31% were located on the trunk, while 50% of the melanomas occurred on the upper and lower extremities. These differences in site distribution were highly significant (p < 0.001).

AGE

Melanoma occurred in adult age groups, with the median age in the fifth decade of life. Eleven percent of patients were >30 years of age. Eleven patients were children or adolescents ranging in age from 3 to 14 years. Patients over 50 years of age had thicker and more invasive melanomas than younger patients did. For example, 40% of older patients (>50 years) had a melanoma >1.5 mm thick compared with 27% of patients under the age of 50 (p < 0.0001). Similarly, 42% of patients over 50 years of age had a level IV or V melanoma, compared with 28% of patients under age 50 years. There was no discernible difference when the younger age population was further subdivided into those less than 20

TABLE 23–1
CHARACTERISTICS OF 4545 PATIENTS WITH CUTANEOUS MELANOMA

Presenting Stage	
I (localized disease)	87%
II (regional metastases)	10%
III (distant metastases)	3%
Sex	
Female	48%
Male	52%
Race	
White-skinned	98%
Black-skinned	1%
Other (Hispanic, Latin, Oriental)	1%
Median Age	53 years
Growth Pattern (Available for 3272 Patients)	
Superficial spreading	56%
Nodular	30%
Lentigo maligna	14%
Tumor Thickness (Available for 2045 Patients)	
<0.76 mm	39%
0.76 mm–1.5 mm	27%
1.51 mm–3.00 mm	22%
>3.00 mm	12%
Level of Invasion (Available for 4046 Patients)	
II	30%
III	34%
IV	30%
V	6%
Ulceration	
Present	9%
Absent or not stated	91%

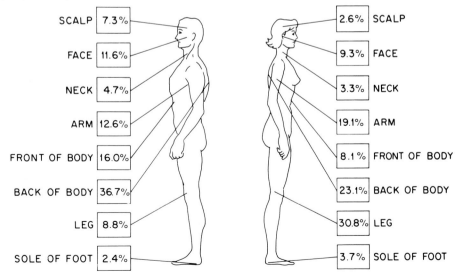

FIG. 23–1 The site distribution of cutaneous melanoma in men and women. There was significant disparity, with a predominance of trunk melanomas in men and extremity melanomas in women.

	MEN			WOMEN	
SCALP	7.3%			2.6%	SCALP
FACE	11.6%			9.3%	FACE
NECK	4.7%			3.3%	NECK
ARM	12.6%			19.1%	ARM
FRONT OF BODY	16.0%			8.1%	FRONT OF BODY
BACK OF BODY	36.7%			23.1%	BACK OF BODY
LEG	8.8%			30.8%	LEG
SOLE OF FOOT	2.4%			3.7%	SOLE OF FOOT

years of age compared with those aged 20 to 49 years.

RACE

Melanoma occurs more often in white-skinned persons who have a tendency to sunburn rather than tan.[4] This was evidenced by the fact that 98% of the patients in the survey were white-skinned, and less than 1% were black-skinned. Another 1% were designated as "other" (Hispanic, Oriental, and so forth). This distribution is significant, since over 20% of Americans are dark-skinned. There were significant differences in the site distribution and type of melanoma among these ethnic groups, with black-skinned individuals tending to have prognostically unfavorable lesions.

Melanoma among the 37 black-skinned patients in this survey had an approximately equal sex distribution. However, 79% of their melanomas were thicker than 1.5 mm, compared to 34% in white-skinned patients and 31% in other patients. Similarly, 78% of the black-skinned patients had a level IV or V melanoma, compared to 36% for those with white skin and 31% for others. A higher frequency of ulcerating melanomas was also noted, being present in 32% of black-skinned patients, 9% of white-skinned patients, and 9% of other patients. The majority (66%) of melanomas in black-skinned patients were located on the extremities and were equally distributed between men and women. Melanomas in these patients usually occurred in less pigmented areas of skin. For example, 49% of their melanomas were located on the sole of the foot, compared with only 3% for white-skinned patients and 4% for other ethnic groups.

PATHOLOGIC FEATURES

GROWTH PATTERN

The growth pattern of melanoma was recorded for 72% of the patients. The most common growth pattern identified in the survey was superficial spreading melanoma (56%), followed by nodular melanoma (30%) and lentigo maligna melanoma (14%). The primary reason nodular melanomas are associated with the worst prognosis is that they are generally thicker lesions than the superficial spreading growth pattern (51% of superficial spreading lesions measured <0.76 mm compared to only 8% for nodular lesions). Lentigo maligna melanomas occurred most frequently on the head and neck area (61% of

patients) and were thinner (60% were <0.76 mm) and less invasive (54% were level II).

LEVEL OF INVASION

Ninety percent of the patients surveyed had measurements of the level of invasion. The most common level of invasion was to the papillary reticular dermal interface (level III) occurring in 34% of patients (Table 23-1). Thirty percent of patients had prognostically favorable lesions invading into the papillary dermis (level II). There was significant heterogeneity within each level of invasion when the data were subdivided by tumor thickness (Table 23-2).

TUMOR THICKNESS

Tumor thickness was reported for only 45% of the patients surveyed. In those patients for whom data were available, it was noteworthy that more than one third of patients with localized melanoma had a "thin" lesion measuring <0.76 mm (Table 23-1). These patients have an extremely favorable prognosis, with an estimated cure rate exceeding 95%.[1,2] Only one third of the patients had melanomas >1.5 mm thick, where the risk of regional and distant metastases is increased. Only 12% of the melanomas were thick (i.e., >3 mm in vertical height), where the risk of distant metastases is quite high.[1,2,5]

ULCERATION

Ulceration of a melanoma is another important histopathologic feature that reflects a more biologically aggressive tumor.[3,6] Ulcerative melanomas occurred in only 9% of the patients where the data were available and usually occurred in thicker lesions. For example, 60% of patients with ulcerative melanomas had a tumor thickness ≥ 2.26 mm compared with nonulcerative melanomas, where only 31% exceeded 2.26 mm in thickness (p < 0.0001). The presence or absence of ulceration in a melanoma was reported in only a small fraction of patients, presumably because it has only recently been recognized as an important prognostic factor.

SURGICAL TREATMENT

The majority of patients (61%) in the survey had their primary melanoma excised with a 3-cm or larger margin of skin. About 22% had a 1-cm or smaller margin of excision. There was no clear correlation of surgical margin with either thickness or level of invasion (Table 23-3). This finding probably reflects the lack of objective data concerning the optimal margins of excision, though several prospective clinical trials are now under way to address this issue. Another debated topic is whether to remove the underlying muscular fascia as part of the primary melanoma excision. In this survey, 57% of the patients with thinner melanomas and 64% of the patients with thicker melanomas had fascial excision as part of their surgical treatment (Table 23-3).

There were 454 patients diagnosed as having enlarged regional nodes suspicious of metastases (stage II). A therapeutic lymphadenectomy was performed in 85% of these patients, and the pathologic diagnosis of nodal metastases was confirmed in 56% of these patients. The yield of pathologically confirmed nodal metastases correlated with the tumor thickness: 38% for melanomas ≤1.5 mm in thickness, 48% for tumors 1.5 mm to 3 mm in thickness, and 69% for melanomas >3 mm in thickness. The yield of metastatic nodes in clinical stage III patients also correlated with the level of invasion (data not shown). Presumably, the 15% of patients who did

not undergo lymphadenectomy within 4 months after the diagnosis (the time limit for inclusion in the survey) were followed and underwent a later surgical procedure.

The efficacy of elective lymph node dissection for melanoma patients with clinically normal nodes is still controversial (see Chap. 8). Since it is clear that not all melanoma patients benefit from this procedure, the debate centers around whether a subgroup of patients exists who may have improved survival rates with elective lymphadenectomy compared with those whose initial management of the lymph nodes is observation. The results of this melanoma survey demonstrated that some patients undergo an elective lymph node dissection, especially those with melanomas >0.76 mm thick or those with level III, IV, or V melanomas (Table 23-3). Twenty-seven percent of patients surveyed with melanomas measuring 0.76 mm to 1.5 mm in thickness had elective lymph node dissections, while 38% of patients with melanomas >1.5 mm thick underwent elective lymphadenectomy as part of their initial surgical management. When the data were analyzed by Clark's level, only 28% of patients

TABLE 23–2
DISTRIBUTION OF PATIENTS WITH CUTANEOUS MELANOMA BY CLARK'S LEVEL OF INVASION AND TUMOR THICKNESS ACCORDING TO BRESLOW MICROSTAGING*

Tumor Thickness (mm)	Level of Invasion				
	II	*III*	*IV*	*V*	*Total*
<0.1–0.76	85%	29%	6%	3%	38% (751)
0.76–1.50	11%	43%	27%	8%	27% (525)
1.51–2.25	1%	16%	27%	8%	14% (288)
2.26–3.0	0%	5%	17%	9%	7% (149)
>3.0	1%	4%	22%	69%	12% (234)
Total %	100% (596)	100% (668)	100% (579)	100% (104)	100% (1947)

* Figures in parentheses indicate numbers of patients.

TABLE 23–3
SURGICAL TREATMENT OF STAGE I MELANOMA

	Tumor Thickness (mm)		
	<0.76	*0.76–1.5*	*>1.5*
Skin margins (cm)			
≤1	20%	18%	17%
1–3	40%	34%	32%
>3	40%	48%	51%
Fascia			
Removed	52%	59%	64%
Not removed	48%	41%	36%
Lymph nodes			
Observed only	94%	72%	62%
Electively removed	6%	28%	38%

with levels III, IV, or V melanomas had an elective lymph node dissection.

NONSURGICAL TREATMENT

Nonsurgical treatments were offered to a minority of patients in this survey. This probably reflects the disappointing results that have been obtained so far in clinical trials involving chemotherapy and immunotherapy.

Adjuvant immunotherapy was administered to 3% of the patients with stages I and II melanoma. The proportion of patients receiving immunotherapy ranged from 1% of patients with melanomas <0.76 mm in thickness to 6% of those with melanomas >3 mm thick. Four percent of patients had adjuvant chemotherapy, while another 2% had regional chemotherapy, perfusion or infusion, as part of their initial treatment. Less than 1% of patients received radiation therapy. Stage III patients were treated with chemotherapy (24%), immunotherapy (1%), radiation therapy (10%), excision without lymph node dissection (36%), or excision with lymph node dissection (18%). The treatments listed in the survey were restricted to those initiated within 4 months of diagnosis, so it is possible that palliative treatments for patients with metastatic disease were instituted later in the patient's clinical course.

MELANOMA *IN SITU*

A separate group of 255 patients who had a noninvasive melanoma was analyzed. These lesions have also been termed Clark's level I melanomas, melanoma *in situ,* or atypical melanocytic hyperplasia. In contrast to invasive melanomas, they do not metastasize. Step-sectioning of such lesions is important to ensure that the lesion has not invaded into the papillary dermis or beyond. Compared to invasive melanomas, the *in situ* lesions occurred in a slightly older population and more commonly on the head and neck area (Table 23-4).

SUMMARY

In the American College of Surgeons Melanoma Survey of 4800 melanoma patients diagnosed during 1980, the typical melanoma was relatively thin

TABLE 23–4
COMPARISON OF NONINVASIVE *(IN SITU)* AND INVASIVE (MALIGNANT) MELANOMAS

	Noninvasive Melanomas	Invasive Melanomas
Patients	255	3819
Women	57%	52%
Age >50 years	66%	55%
Anatomical Location		
Head and neck	31%	17%
Trunk	35%	43%
Extremities	34%	40%

(<1.5 mm), not ulcerated (except in 9%), and did not invade into the reticular dermis or beyond (level IV or V). The melanomas were most commonly located on the trunk in men and on the lower extremity in women. Eighty-seven percent of patients had no clinical evidence of metastases to regional nodes or to distant sites at the time of initial diagnosis. Only a small proportion (1%) of surveyed patients were dark-skinned, and in most of these patients, their melanoma was located on the feet or hands.

The treatment of melanoma was surgical in 93% of patients, with the majority of patients undergoing a wide excision of the melanoma as the initial form of treatment. Only one fifth of the patients underwent elective regional node dissection for suspected micrometastases, and most of these patients had a tumor thickness >1.5 mm or a lesion invading to the reticular dermis (level III, IV, or V). Although tumor thickness is now recognized as the most important criterion that predicts the patient's clinical course, this parameter was reported in only 45% of patients in the survey.

Melanoma is an important malignancy for surgeons, since it can be cured with surgical treatment if diagnosed at an early stage. The results of this survey showed a great heterogeneity of surgical approaches, both with respect to margins of excision, removal of the underlying fascia, and elective lymph node dissection. The findings probably reflect the lack of objective data concerning the optimal margins of excision and whether or not the fascia should be included. Several prospective surgical trials are being initiated to address these important questions, especially for those patients with lesions of intermediate thickness (1 mm–4 mm) as described in Chapter 8.

REFERENCES

1. Balch CM, Soong S-j, Milton GW, Shaw HM, McGovern VJ, Murad TM, McCarthy WH, Maddox WA: A comparison of prognostic factors and surgical results in 1,786 patients with localized (stage I) melanoma treated in Alabama, USA, and New South Wales, Australia. Ann Surg 196:677, 1982
2. Balch CM, Soong S-j, Murad TM, Ingalls AL, Maddox WA: A multifactorial analysis of melanoma. II. Prognostic factors in patients with stage I (localized) melanoma. Surgery 86:343, 1979
3. Balch CM, Wilkerson JA, Murad TM, Soong S-j, Ingalls AL, Maddox WA: The prognostic significance of ulceration of cutaneous melanoma. Cancer 45:3012, 1980
4. Beral V, Evans S, Shaw H, Milton G: Cutaneous factors related to the risk of malignant melanoma. Br J Dermatol 109:165, 1983
5. Day CL Jr, Lew RA, Mihm MC, Sober AJ, Harris MJ, Kopf AW, Fitzpatrick TB, Harrist TJ, Golomb FM, Postel A, Hennessey P, Gumport SL, Raker JW, Malt RA, Cosimi AB, Wood WC, Roses DF, Gorstein F, Rigel D, Friedman RJ, Mintzis MM, Grier RW: A multivariate analysis of prognostic factors for melanoma patients with lesions ≥3.65 mm in thickness: The importance of revealing alternative Cox models. Ann Surg 195:44, 1982
6. McGovern VJ, Shaw HM, Milton GW, McCarthy WH: Ulceration and prognosis in cutaneous malignant melanoma. Histopathology 6:399, 1982
7. Wick MM, Sober AJ, Fitzpatrick TB, Mihm MC Jr, Kopf AW, Clark WH Jr, Blois MS: Clinical characteristics of early cutaneous melanoma. Cancer 45:2684, 1980

CHARLES M. BALCH
MARSHALL M. URIST
WILLIAM A. MADDOX
SENG-JAW SOONG

Melanoma in the Southern United States: Experience at the University of Alabama in Birmingham

24

SOUTHERN UNITED STATES

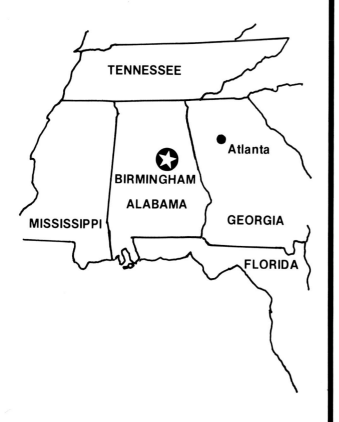

This chapter describes the experience of the Surgical Oncology Service at the University of Alabama in Birmingham (UAB) in treating over 1000 melanoma patients during the past 27 years. Patients have been referred primarily from the State of Alabama, with some patients coming from the surrounding states of Florida, Mississippi, Tennessee, and Georgia. This geographic area is situated between the 31° and 35° parallels of north latitude and the 85° and 88° meridians of west longitude. The climate is temperate throughout most of the year.

The State of Alabama has a population of over 3.9 million, with almost one million people living in the Birmingham metropolitan area. Birmingham has an average temperature of 80°F (27°C) in summer months and 47°F (8°C) in winter months. It is situated in the north central part of the state at an altitude of 630 feet above sea level.

Clinical and pathologic data about 919 melanoma patients treated from 1955 to 1980 at UAB are shown in Tables 24-1 and 24-2. All patients were treated by one of three surgeons (CMB, WAM,

TABLE 24–1
CLINICAL AND PATHOLOGIC DATA FOR MELANOMA PATIENTS TREATED AT THE UNIVERSITY OF ALABAMA IN BIRMINGHAM

	Presenting Pathologic Stage			
	Stage I	Stage II	Stage III	Total
Clinical Characteristics				
Number of patients	783	119	17	919
Year of diagnosis				
≤1960	6%	5%	6%	6%
1961–1965	10%	5%	18%	9%
1966–1970	14%	13%	29%	14%
1971–1975	18%	24%	6%	18%
1976–1980	52%	53%	41%	52%
Median age	48 yr	51 yr	65 yr	49 yr
Sex				
Male	48%	66%	71%	51%
Female	52%	34%	29%	49%
Primary lesion site				
Female lower extremity	18%	14%	6%	17%
Male lower extremity	5%	14%	24%	6%
Female upper extremity	11%	5%	0%	10%
Male upper extremity	8%	11%	12%	8%
Female head and neck	11%	6%	6%	10%
Male head and neck	17%	9%	6%	15%
Female trunk	10%	9%	6%	10%
Male trunk	18%	31%	18%	19%
Other	2%	1%	24%	6%
Pathologic Characteristics				
Breslow's tumor thickness				
<0.76 mm	31%	5%	0%	27%
0.76 mm–1.49 mm	24%	7%	0%	21%
1.50 mm–2.49 mm	17%	24%	57%	18%
2.50 mm–3.99 mm	14%	17%	14%	15%
≥4.00 mm	13%	46%	29%	18%
Median tumor thickness	1.1 mm	2.8 mm	2.8 mm	1.2 mm
Levels of invasion				
II	27%	3%	0%	24%
III	30%	17%	16%	28%
IV	36%	58%	68%	39%
V	7%	22%	16%	9%
Ulceration				
Yes	35%	65%	50%	39%
No	66%	35%	50%	61%
Growth pattern				
Nodular	45%	75%	83%	49%
Superficial spreading	50%	25%	17%	46%
Lentigo maligna	5%	0%	0%	5%

MMU), and all the pathology slides were reviewed by either Dr. T. M. Murad or, since 1982, Dr. S. Kheir. The surgery for more than 90% of the patients was performed by these three surgeons, and the remainder were referred for follow-up evaluations or for participation in adjuvant therapy trials. The 30-day operative mortality rate was 0.1%. The single patient in the UAB series who died had an unrelated cardiopulmonary arrest 2 weeks after an uneventful surgical procedure.

All data for patients diagnosed after 1975 were entered into this computerized registry on a prospective basis, and the data concerning patients diagnosed prior to 1975 were accumulated retrospec-

TABLE 24–2
ACTUARIAL SURVIVAL DATA FOR MELANOMA PATIENTS TREATED AT THE UNIVERSITY OF ALABAMA IN BIRMINGHAM

| | Survival Rates | |
	5-Year	10-Year
Stage I		
Overall survival	77%	66%
Sex		
Male	74%	62%
Female	76%	70%
Primary lesion site		
Lower extremity	73%	69%
Upper extremity	93%	85%
Head and neck	72%	62%
Trunk	70%	59%
Other	39%	39%
Tumor thickness		
<0.76 mm	98%	92%
0.76 mm–1.49 mm	87%	77%
1.50 mm–2.49 mm	76%	62%
2.50 mm–3.99 mm	73%	64%
≥4.00 mm	55%	42%
Level of invasion		
II	93%	93%
III	81%	70%
IV	77%	66%
V	50%	33%
Ulceration		
Yes	69%	58%
No	85%	78%

	1-Year	3-Year	5-Year
Stage II			
Overall survival	75%	46%	28%
Tumor thickness			
<1.50 mm	80%	40%	40%
1.50 mm–3.99 mm	60%	43%	43%
≥4.0 mm	66%	44%	33%
Number of positive nodes			
1	78%	66%	57%
2–4	72%	39%	31%
>4	22%	15%	15%
Ulceration			
Yes	57%	28%	24%
No	82%	72%	62%

	6-Month	1-Year	2-Year
Stage III			
Overall survival	56%	25%	8%

tively from the personal records of one of the authors (WAM). The 1000 melanoma patients entered into this registry represent 99% of all patients treated for melanoma at UAB (see Tables 24-1 and 24-2). Follow-up information is available for over 96% of these patients.

EPIDEMIOLOGY

Incidence data for cutaneous melanoma is not available for Alabama. However, the mortality rate for melanoma was known to be among the highest in the United States for white-skinned men (2.2×10^5) and women (1.7×10^5) when the data were last tabulated by the National Cancer Institute in 1970.[15] The surrounding states in the Southern United States (Georgia, Mississippi, and South Carolina) are ranked next highest in mortality rates for melanoma. The annual age-adjusted incidence rate for the Birmingham Standard Metropolitan Statistical Area (SMSA) during the 1969 to 1971 period was 5.6×10^5 for the white population and is comparable to the Atlanta SMSA in the neighboring state of Georgia (Table 24-3). It is interesting to note that only 3% of the UAB melanoma patients were blacks, despite the fact that 35% of the UAB Hospital patients are black and 26% of the general population in Alabama are blacks. This implies that melanoma occurs preferentially in white-skinned persons. The preponderance of UAB melanoma patients (and the general population in Alabama) are of Scottish, Irish, or English ancestry.[2] Over 90% of

TABLE 24-3
AVERAGE ANNUAL AGE-ADJUSTED INCIDENCE OF MELANOMA PER 10^5 POPULATION (1969–1971)

	Birmingham SMSA*	Atlanta SMSA
All Races	4.4	5.5
White	5.6	6.6
Male	6.1	6.5
Female	5.2	6.6
Black	0.9	1.0
Male	1.4	1.3
Female	0.6	0.8

(Data from the Third National Cancer Survey published by the National Cancer Institute, Washington, D.C.)

* SMSA = Standard Metropolitan Statistical Area.

UAB patients had either light-colored hair (*e.g.*, red, blond, auburn) or blue eyes, or some combination of these physical features. There appear to be several reproducible genetic markers associated with melanoma outcome.[1] In a case control study of 98 melanoma patients and 135 matched controls from Alabama, those with DR-4 histocompatibility tissue antigens or the Bf-S genotype of a serum complement factor (properdin) have a twofold to sixfold increased risk for developing melanoma.[12,13] In contrast, those with a DR-3 phenotype or a Bf-F genotype of the properdin factor B had a significantly decreased incidence of melanoma and a lower risk set of prognostic factors if they developed melanoma.[12,13] Finally, persons with blond or red hair were more prone to develop more aggressive melanomas (Table 24-4).

TABLE 24-4
PATHOLOGIC AND GENETIC FACTORS IN MELANOMA PATIENTS*

	Hair Color		
Factor	Blond, red	Light brown	Medium or dark brown, black
Tumor Thickness (Average ± SE)	2.63 mm ± 0.36 mm	2.16 mm ± 0.42 mm	1.91 mm ± 0.26 mm
Ulceration	37%	33%	28%
DR-3			
Patient	17%	23%	21%
Control	37%	23%	32%
DR-4			
Patient	66%	43%	30%
Control	41%	18%	18%

* Analysis of 116 melanoma patients and 116 controls who were matched for ethnic origin and eye and hair color. The DR-3 antigen is associated with a protective influence, while the DR-4 antigen is associated with a higher risk and more aggressive type of melanoma.[12] Note that patients with blond or red hair have thicker, more ulcerative melanomas, with a higher frequency of DR-4 and lower incidence of DR-3 histocompatibility type.

This chapter only concerns patients with cutaneous melanoma. At UAB, only 1.4% of all patients had melanoma involving mucous membranes[3] and 3% of patients had ocular melanoma.

PROGNOSTIC FACTORS

Melanoma has many prognostic factors that influence outcome. These data are reviewed in detail in Chapter 19, so only the salient points will be summarized here.

STAGE OF DISEASE

Whether or not patients present with clinically localized or metastatic disease is one of the most important predictors of their subsequent clinical course.[5,10] The majority of patients (85%) presented with

localized disease (stage I). The 5-year survival rate for patients with stage I disease was 77% but was reduced to 28% in patients with stage II disease (Table 24-2). Only 8% of patients who presented with stage III disease lived more than 2 years. A previously published analysis of survival rates and their recurrence patterns according to the clinical stage is shown in Figure 24-1. A summary of the dominant prognostic variables for each disease stage is listed in Table 24-5.

PROGNOSIS IN PATIENTS WITH LOCALIZED MELANOMA (STAGE I)

Patient factors

The anatomical site of the melanoma is the most important clinical feature predicting the patient's clinical course in the UAB experience.[5,7,8] Patients with extremity melanomas (42% of the UAB series,

FIG. 24–1   Patterns of metastases in 850 cutaneous melanoma patients treated at this institution during a 25-year period. The majority of patients (82%) presented with localized melanomas (stage I); 15% of these patients subsequently developed nodal metastases (stage II) after 16 months, while another 15% progressed directly to stage III disease after 34 months. (Balch CM et al: A multifactorial analysis of melanoma. IV. Prognostic factors in 200 melanoma patients with distant metastases (stage III). J Clin Oncol 1:126, 1983)

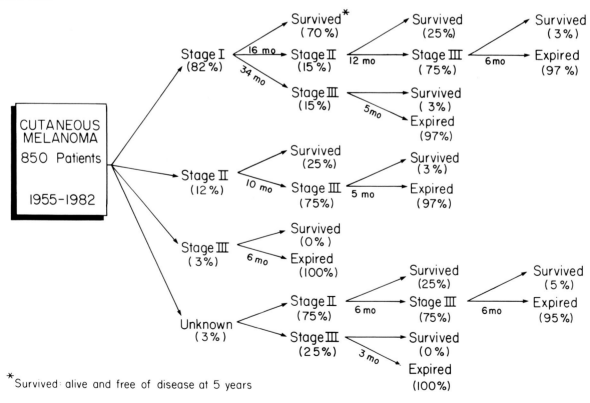

*Survived: alive and free of disease at 5 years

TABLE 24–5
A MULTIFACTORIAL PROGNOSTIC FACTORS ANALYSIS OF MELANOMA
PATIENTS USING THE COX REGRESSION MODEL

	p Value
Localized Melanoma (stage I)[7,8]	
Tumor thickness	<0.00001
Surgical treatment (± elective node dissection)	0.0077
Tumor ulceration (present or absent)	0.0002
Anatomical site (extremity versus axial)	0.0910
Nodal Metastases (stage II)[9]	
Number of metastatic nodes (1 versus 2 to 4 versus >4)	0.0005
Ulceration of the primary melanoma (present or absent)	0.0019
Distant Metastases (stage III)[10]	
Number of metastatic sites (1 versus 2 versus ≥3)	<0.000001
Remission duration (< or >12 mo)	0.0186
Site of metastases (visceral versus nonvisceral)	0.0192

*Other factors examined that did not independently correlate with survival were level of invasion, pigmentation, lymphocyte infiltration, growth pattern, lesion regression, sex, and age.[7,8]

†Other factors examined that did not independently correlate with survival are those listed in the first footnote *plus* tumor thickness and substage of metastatic disease (synchronous versus metachronous).[9]

‡Other factors examined that did not independently correlate with survival are those listed in the first footnote *plus* tumor thickness, tumor ulceration, and the sequence of metastases.[10]

of which 65% are in women) had the best prognosis. In contrast, patients with melanomas located on the trunk (28% in the series, of which 66% are men) had the worst prognosis (Tables 24-1 and 24-2). Patients with head and neck melanomas could be further subdivided into those with scalp and neck melanomas that had a worse prognosis than those with face and ear melanomas.[17] Men had more head and neck melanomas than women did (61% versus 39%), especially in the scalp and neck subsites (Fig. 24-2). It appears from these data that the reason men have a worse prognosis than women is that they have lesions located on more unfavorable anatomical sites, rather than some inherent (or hormonal) differences between sexes. Age was not an important prognostic parameter in the UAB experience, since the increased risk of metastatic disease in older persons probably resulted from their having thicker tumors.[5,8] An exception to this was lentigo maligna melanoma that occurred in older persons and had a more favorable prognosis.

Pathologic factors

Tumor thickness and ulceration were the most important predictors of survival in the UAB melanoma patients.[7,8] Tumor thickness was the most objective and quantitative prognostic feature of melanoma, with a p value of correlation that is <0.00001. More than half the patients had a melanoma measuring <1.5 mm in thickness, which was associated with a very good prognosis (Table 24-2). Level of invasion also delineated different risk groups but required more subjective interpretation that limited its reproducibility. A direct comparison of these two parameters demonstrated that tumor thickness was the more accurate prognostic indicator.[5,7]

Ulceration of a melanoma reflected a more aggressive, infiltrating property of the tumor and was therefore associated with a worse prognosis.[5,8,11] When present, it was one of the dominant predictors of survival even after matching for tumor thickness.[7,8,11] Thirty-nine percent of all UAB patients had an ulcerated melanoma (Table 24-1), but the incidence has decreased in recent years to less than 33% (see Chap. 18). This incidence is still higher than that reported from other institutions and may reflect a more aggressive form of the disease that arises in the Alabama population of patients.

Nodular and superficial spreading melanomas were distinctive biologic growth patterns, but they were not so important prognostically. Ten-year survival rates were similar in patients with nodular and superficial spreading melanoma of comparable

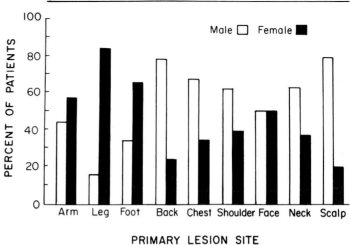

SEX DISTRIBUTION BY PRIMARY LESION SITE

FIG. 24–2 Distribution of melanoma at different anatomical sites in men and women. Men had a higher proportion of melanomas arising in unfavorable anatomical locations, such as back, chest, and scalp. (Balch CM, Soong S-j: Characteristics of melanoma that predict the risk of metastases. In Costanzi JJ (ed): Malignant Melanoma 1, p 117. The Hague, Martinus Nijhoff Publishers, 1982)

thickness (see Chap. 19). Polypoid melanomas represented a special configuration (usually with a nodular growth pattern) with an especially poor prognosis.[14] Overall, the majority (49%) of UAB melanoma patients were listed as having a nodular growth pattern (Table 24-1), although the incidence has decreased in recent years (1981–1982), so that only 33% were nodular, 62% were superficial spreading, and 5% were lentigo maligna melanomas (see Chap. 18). These changes are unlikely to be the result of differences in pathologic interpretation, since all slides were reviewed by only two pathologists. Lentigo maligna melanoma occurred in an older population (mean age, 61 years) and appeared to have a less aggressive clinical course with an 85% 10-year survival rate.[17] Acral lentiginous melanoma has only been recognized as a distinct pathologic entity recently and has not yet been analyzed in the UAB patient series.

In summary, tumor thickness, ulceration, and, to a lesser extent, growth pattern were the dominant prognostic factors in the UAB patients. Other pathologic features of the primary melanoma are secondarily associated with the above features. Collectively, these parameters may reflect different grades of tumor differentiation. For example, a poorly differentiated tumor may be amelanotic, may have a paucity of lymphocyte infiltration, and may exhibit angioinvasion, a high mitotic index, microsatellites, or some combination thereof. However, such tumors are usually thick or ulcerated, so that in a practical sense only the latter two variables need to be taken into account. Although the other

histopathologic aspects of melanoma are certainly useful in understanding the biology of the disease, they are probably not important in making patient management decisions.

Multifactorial analysis

Dominant prognostic variables in a Cox regression analysis were limited to features of the tumor itself (thickness and ulceration) and the anatomical site of the melanoma. Whether or not an elective lymph node dissection (ELND) was performed also significantly influenced survival rates of these patients. Because of this finding, the multifactorial analysis within each of the two initial surgical treatments (wide local excision [WLE] alone versus WLE plus ELND) was separately analyzed.[8] For the patient group having WLE alone, the only significant parameters were tumor thickness ($p < 10^{-8}$) and ulceration ($p = .01$). Tumor thickness had a less significant correlation in those patients who had a WLE plus ELND ($p = 0.038$), whereas ulceration and location were not significant factors in this subgroup. The diminished level of statistical significance in this last patient subgroup suggests that the predictive value of thickness measurements for the entire patient population was derived in part from a correlation with the risk of regional node micrometastases. Presumably, the residual statistical correlation with survival in the WLE plus ELND group was a result of the risk of micrometastases at distant sites, especially in patients with melanoma ≥ 4 mm in thickness. In the UAB patient series, the sex of the patient was not a dominant prognostic variable once other parameters, particularly anatomical location, were accounted for. A detailed account of these analyses is found in Chapter 19.

PROGNOSIS IN PATIENTS WITH NODAL METASTASES (STAGE II)

About 13% of the UAB melanoma patients first presented with regional node metastases. Not surprisingly, they had many of the prognostic features associated with a poor survival (Table 24-1). Thus, 66% of these patients were men and 40% of primary lesions were located on the trunk, and the median thickness was 2.8 mm. As in stage I patients, ulceration of the primary melanoma was an ominous prognostic sign. This occurred in 65% of the patients, and only 24% of these were alive at 5 years (Table 24-2). One of the most important prognostic parameters was the number of metastatic lymph nodes.[9] Patients with one positive node (37% of the patients) had a 57% 5-year survival rate, while the 22% of patients with more than four metastatic nodes had a 5-year survival rate of only 15%. Another small subgroup of patients with a relatively favorable prognosis consisted of those with clinically occult metastatic nodes identified at the time of ELND; these patients had a 48% 5-year survival rate.[9]

Patients who presented with delayed (metachronous) nodal metastases had a better overall survival rate than those with simultaneous (or synchronous) nodal metastases. However, these differences can be explained on the basis of tumor burden (microscopic versus macroscopic) at the time of initial diagnosis. Since the survival curves were identical between these two groups of patients, their survival was calculated from the onset of detectable nodal metastases. Patients with nodal metastases from an unknown primary site had the same prognosis as those whose primary melanoma was present, when the survival rates were calculated from the onset of nodal metastases.[9]

In a multifactorial analysis of stage II melanoma patients, ulceration was the only feature of the primary tumor that continued to predict the biologic risk of distant metastases once the patients had documented metastases in regional lymph nodes (Table 24-5). The actual number of metastatic nodes (1 versus 2 to 4 versus >4 nodes) was the only other dominant prognostic factor. Tumor thickness was not a significant predictive factor. Further details are described in Chapter 19.

PROGNOSIS IN PATIENTS WITH DISTANT METASTASES (STAGE III)

There were only 17 patients in the UAB series whose first presentation was distant metastatic melanoma (stage III). These patients had a grim prognosis, with a median survival of only 6 months (see Fig. 24-1). Details about prognostic factors in all 200 UAB patients who developed distant metastases at any time in their clinical course have been published.[10] Details are described in Chapter 19.

In a multifactorial analysis of the 200 patients with stage III melanoma, the three most dominant prognostic variables were the number of metastatic sites, the actual location of metastases, and the remission duration. (Table 24-5)[10] There were no histologic criteria of the primary melanoma that predicted the patient's clinical course once distant metastases developed clinically.

PROGNOSIS IN BLACKS

Thirty patients (3%) of the entire series were black-skinned. The histologic characteristics and anatomical distribution of their primary melanomas were strikingly different from that of white-skinned melanoma patients. Melanomas on the foot occurred in 73% of black patients compared to 6% for white patients. Mucosal melanomas occurred in 10% of the black patients (one each on the anus, nasal cavity, and genitalia) compared to 1% in white patients. Compared with whites having melanoma, black-skinned patients had a higher incidence of metastatic disease at initial diagnosis (40% versus 17%), a higher incidence of ulcerated melanomas (62% versus 37%), thicker melanomas (median thickness of 3.5 mm versus 1.4 mm) and a lower overall 5-year survival rate (38% versus 67%). It is of interest to note that melanoma occurred on pigmented skin in only two patients, while the remainder were on low pigmentation sites (*e.g.,* soles, palms, subungual).

It seems likely that the poorer prognosis in blacks was primarily caused by the fact that their lesions were located at unfavorable anatomical sites, rather than by neglect or delay in diagnosis.

SURGICAL MANAGEMENT

In stage I patients, the prognostic factors described above are used for defining the probability of local control of the primary melanoma and for defining the risk of microscopic metastases in regional nodes and at distant sites.[4] The operative risk itself is also taken into account for each patient.[18] More than 80% of those patients are cured. In patients with nodal metastases (stage II), the operation is indicated primarily for palliation, although some patients are cured. Surgical treatment can also be important palliative therapy in carefully selected stage III patients with limited and surgically accessible metastatic disease as described in Chapter 13. The clinical, radiologic and laboratory evaluation for metastases in the preoperative and postoperative melanoma patient is described in Chapter 12.

SURGERY FOR THE PRIMARY MELANOMA

The primary melanoma is widely excised with a margin of normal-appearing skin around the biopsy site. The skin margins vary according to the risk of local recurrence (see Chap. 6). It is now clear that this risk correlates more with tumor thickness than it does with the actual surgical margins.[6] Thin melanomas (<0.76 mm) have only a minimal risk for local recurrence. At the present time, these lesions are excised with a 1-cm to 2-cm skin margin, using an elliptical incision and a primary skin closure. For patients with intermediate and thick melanomas (*i.e.,* those >0.76 mm in thickness), a 2-cm to 3-cm margin is employed as standard treatment. The skin margins are reduced in anatomical sites such as the face or distal extremities, where a wide excision is not feasible. The underlying fascia is generally incorporated into the surgical resection, although the evidence showing a potential benefit for this procedure is sparse. Patients with lentigo maligna melanomas are treated more conservatively than those with other growth patterns.[17] Their surgery usually consists of a 1-cm margin of excision around the primary tumor if anatomically possible.

SURGERY FOR REGIONAL LYMPH NODES

A standard radical lymphadenectomy (LND) is performed in all patients with enlarged nodes suspicious of metastatic disease (stage II) as described in Chapter 7. A partial LND or simple excision of nodal metastases is not sufficient treatment for patients with metastatic melanoma. Two thirds or more of these patients have metastatic disease present in multiple lymph nodes.[9] Since it is impossible for the surgeon to detect microscopic nodal metastases, a philosophy of limited excision for only clinically detectable nodes will often compromise both

the palliative and curative goals of this surgical treatment.

There is considerable controversy about the benefit of ELND in patients with clinically normal regional lymph nodes (see Chap. 8). Since it is clear that not all melanoma patients benefit from this procedure, the debate centers around finding the subgroup of patients that has improved survival rates with ELND compared with the subgroup whose initial management of the lymph nodes is observation only. In the UAB experience, there is a subgroup of patients that can be defined by such prognostic factors. The most important factors are tumor thickness and ulceration, although the anatomical site of the melanoma and the sex of the patient are also considered in this estimation.[4,6,7,8,18] In general, those patients with intermediate-thickness melanomas (0.76 mm–4 mm) have an increasing risk (up to 50%) of harboring occult regional metastases, but a relatively low risk (less than 10%–20%) of distant metastases. The patient's gender and the anatomical site of the melanoma are also taken into account. In general, ELND is performed more liberally for melanomas located on the trunk, head, and neck and is performed more conservatively for extremity melanomas (especially in women). This is because the greatest risk for lymphedema after inguinal dissection occurs in obese older women, but the morbidity is quite low in patients undergoing a modified cervical dissection or axillary neck dissection.[17,18] An ELND is not considered in patients with lentigo maligna melanoma because of their low biologic risk for metastases.

Melanomas located on the trunk can potentially have multiple directions of lymphatic drainage. This makes it difficult for the surgeon to assess accurately which nodal basins are at risk for harboring microscopic metastases in patients who may be considered candidates for ELND. In these circumstances, a radionuclide cutaneous scan (see Chap. 9) is an accurate and reproducible test for determining the lymphatic drainage of trunk melanomas.[16]

Isolated whole limb perfusion for regional chemotherapy and hyperthermia is probably beneficial in selected patients with extremity melanomas (see Chap. 10). In a comparison of patients undergoing isolated limb perfusion at other institutions with the patients not undergoing perfusion at UAB, the primary benefit of this procedure was in those with extremity melanomas exceeding 4 mm to 5 mm in thickness.*

* Unpublished data

NONSURGICAL MANAGEMENT

The treatment approach for patients with metastatic disease is described in Chapters 11, 13, and 15.

REFERENCES

1. Acton RT, Balch CM, Barger BO, Budowle B, Go RCP, Soong S-j, Roseman JM: The occurrence of melanoma and its relationship with host, lifestyle and environmental factors. In Costanzi JJ (ed): Malignant Melanoma, p 151. The Hague, Nijhoff, 1983
2. Acton RT, Balch CM, Budowle B, Go RCP, Roseman JM, Soong S-j, Barger BO: Immunogenetics of melanoma. In Reisfeld RA, Ferrone S (eds): Melanoma Antigens and Antibodies, p 1. New York, Plenum, 1982
3. Balch CM: Oral and cutaneous melanoma: Clinical recognition, pathological features, and prognostic factors. Ala J Med Sci 17:51, 1980
4. Balch CM: Surgical management of regional lymph nodes in cutaneous melanoma. J Am Acad Dermatol 3:511, 1980
5. Balch CM, Murad TM, Soong S-j, Ingalls AL, Halpern NB, Maddox WA: A multifactorial analysis of melanoma: Prognostic histopathological features comparing Clark's and Breslow's staging methods. Ann Surg 188:732, 1978
6. Balch CM, Murad TM, Soong S-j, Ingalls AL, Richards PC, Maddox WA: Tumor thickness as a guide to surgical management of clinical stage I melanoma patients. Cancer 43:883, 1979
7. Balch CM, Soong S-j, Milton GW, Shaw HM, McGovern VJ, Murad TM, McCarthy WH, Maddox WA: A comparison of prognostic factors and surgical results in 1,786 patients with localized (stage I) melanoma treated in Alabama, USA, and New South Wales, Australia. Ann Surg 196:677, 1982
8. Balch CM, Soong S-j, Murad TM, Ingalls AL, Maddox WA: A multifactorial analysis of melanoma. II. Prognostic factors in patients with stage I (localized) melanoma. Surgery 86:343, 1979
9. Balch CM, Soong S-j, Murad TM, Ingalls AL, Maddox WA: A multifactorial analysis of melanoma. III. Prognostic factors in melanoma patients with lymph node metastases (stage II). Ann Surg 193:377, 1981
10. Balch CM, Soong S-j, Murad TM, Smith JW, Maddox WA, Durant JR: A multifactorial analysis of melanoma. IV. Prognostic factors in 200 melanoma patients with distant metastases (stage III). J Clin Oncol 1:126, 1983
11. Balch CM, Wilkerson JA, Murad TM, Soong S-j, Ingalls AL, Maddox WA: The prognostic significance of ulceration of cutaneous melanoma. Cancer 45:3012, 1980
12. Barger BO, Acton RT, Soong S-j, Roseman J, Balch CM: Increase of HLA-DR4 in melanoma patients from Alabama. Cancer Res 42:4276, 1982
13. Budowle B, Barger BO, Balch CM, Go RCP, Roseman JM, Acton RT: Associations of properdin factor B with melanoma. Cancer Genet Cytogenet 5:247, 1982
14. Manci EA, Balch CM, Murad TM, Soong S-j: Polypoid melanoma, a virulent variant of the nodular growth pattern. Am J Clin Pathol 75:810, 1981
15. Mason TJ, McKay FW: U.S. Cancer Mortality by County: 1950–1969. DHEW Publ No (NIH) 74-615, 1974
16. Meyer CM, Lecklitner ML, Logic JR, Balch CM, Bessey PQ, Tauxe WN: Technetium-99m sulfur-colloid cutaneous lymphoscintigraphy in the management of truncal melanoma. Radiology 131:205, 1979
17. Urist MM, Balch CM, Soong S-j, Milton GW, Shaw HM, McGovern VJ, Murad TM, McCarthy WH, Maddox WA: Head and neck melanoma in 536 clinical stage I patients: A prognostic factors analysis and results of surgical treatment. Ann Surg (in press, 1985)
18. Urist MM, Maddox WA, Kennedy JE, Balch CM: Patient risk factors and surgical morbidity after regional lymphadenectomy in 204 melanoma patients. Cancer 51:2152, 1983

EDWIN B. COX
ROBIN T. VOLLMER
HILLIARD F. SEIGLER

Melanoma in the Southeastern United States: Experience at The Duke Medical Center

25

SOUTHEASTERN UNITED STATES

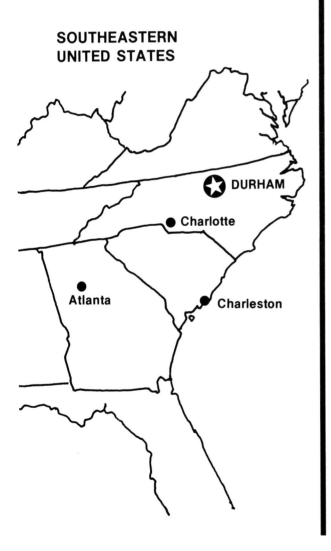

DURHAM

Charlotte

Atlanta

Charleston

Melanoma is a relatively common neoplasm in the southeastern United States. Over 3000 patients have been treated at the Duke Medical Center (DMC) Comprehensive Cancer Center during the past 10 years. This large volume of patients is partly a result of its increased frequency in this geographic area, as well as an active referral to the DMC because of its melanoma research programs and a vigorous multimodal treatment approach. Six percent of these patients received their initial evaluation and surgical treatment at this center, while the remainder were referred postoperatively for adjuvant therapy or treatment for either recurrent or metastatic disease. For all patients, the data were stored in the Time-Oriented Record for Oncology System.[4] Information about 2949 patients with complete records is analyzed in this chapter (Tables 25-1, 25-2). Patients excluded from this analysis include 34 patients with mucosal melanoma, 49 with ocular melanoma, and 124 with unknown primary lesion

TABLE 25–1
CLINICAL AND PATHOLOGIC DATA FOR MELANOMA PATIENTS TREATED AT THE DUKE MEDICAL CENTER

| | Presenting Pathologic Stage | | | |
	Stage I	Stage II	Stage III	Total
Clinical				
Number of patients	2470	418	61	2949
Year of diagnosis				
≤1960	—	—	—	—
1961–1965	1%	1%	—	1%
1966–1970	5%	3%	3%	5%
1971–1975	20%	28%	31%	22%
1976–1980	52%	48%	56%	51%
1981–1982	22%	20%	10%	21%
Age (median)	47 yr	49 yr	53 yr	
Sex				
Male	50%	61%	66%	51%
Female	50%	39%	34%	49%
Primary lesion site				
Female lower extremity	18%	15%	5%	18%
Male lower extremity	6%	5%	1%	6%
Female upper extremity	9%	4%	2%	8%
Male upper extremity	6%	5%	2%	5%
Female head and neck	6%	4%	2%	5%
Male head and neck	9%	11%	11%	10%
Female trunk	15%	8%	3%	14%
Male trunk	27%	22%	13%	26%
Other*	4%	26%	61%	8%
Pathologic				
Breslow's tumor thickness				
<0.76 mm	22%	10%		21%
0.76 mm–1.49 mm	36%	16%	29%	34%
1.50 mm–2.49 mm	21%	21%		21%
2.50 mm–3.99 mm	12%	23%		13%
≥4.00 mm	9%	30%	71%	11%
Median tumor thickness	1.8 mm	3.3 mm	4.3 mm	
Level of invasion				
II	11%	8%	7%	11%
III	48%	26%	20%	45%
IV	36%	47%	40%	37%
V	5%	19%	33%	7%
Ulceration				
Yes	35%	55%	67%	38%
No	65%	45%	33%	62%
Growth pattern				
Nodular	25%	46%	75%	27%
Superficial spreading	71%	49%	25%	69%
Lentigo maligna	4%	5%		4%

*Most of these patients had metastases from an unknown primary melanoma

site. The clinical management, treatment results, and prognosis of these patients have been published.[9,11]

EPIDEMIOLOGY

The southeastern United States has four seasons but has a shorter winter period than the northern United States. It is unusual to have snow in most of these states. The majority of patients referred to the DMC are from the state of North Carolina. North Carolina has a population of 6 million, of which 76% are white-skinned and 24% are black-skinned. There is no dominant country of origin for the white-skinned persons living in North Carolina.

There is a relatively high incidence of melanoma in the white population of the 11 states comprising the southeastern United States. These 11 states are also among the 12 states having the highest

TABLE 25–2
ACTUARIAL SURVIVAL DATA FOR MELANOMA PATIENTS TREATED AT THE DUKE MEDICAL CENTER

Survival Data	Survival Rates	
	5-year	7-year
Stage I		
Overall survival	81%	73%
Sex		
Male	76%	66%
Female	85%	82%
Primary lesion site		
Lower extremity	86%	82%
Upper extremity	93%	88%
Head and neck	67%	63%
Trunk	80%	70%
Other	—	—
Tumor thickness		
<0.76 mm	93%	88%
0.76 mm–1.49 mm	85%	79%
1.50 mm–2.49 mm	74%	66%
2.50 mm–3.99 mm	68%	68%
≥4.00 mm	54%	47%
Level of invasion		
II	93%	86%
III	87%	79%
IV	68%	63%
V	54%	54%
Ulceration		
Yes	61%	54%
No	85%	82%

	1-year	3-year	5-year
Stage II			
Overall survival	81%	53%	42%
Tumor thickness			
<1.50 mm	86%	60%	55%
1.50 mm–3.99 mm	72%	98%	24%
>4.0 mm	75%	47%	47%
Number of positive nodes			
1	87%	59%	55%
2–4	88%	69%	58%
>4	65%	16%	16%
Ulceration			
Yes	69%	46%	35%
No	84%	63%	52%

	6-month	1-year	2-year
Stage III			
Overall survival	62%	27%	23%

mortality from melanoma reported in the period from 1950 to 1969.* The mortality rates for melanoma in the white population of the 11 states range from 1.18 to 2.29 deaths $\times 10^5$ population (Table 25-3). This is higher than the rate of 1.31×10^5 for the entire United States. No further clustering of melanomas within smaller geographic locales in the southeastern United States was identified.

Similarly, there was no clustering of patients by occupational status or for any particular time periods. As in other series, a very low incidence of melanoma was found in the black-skinned population in this region.[7] They comprised only 1.2% of patients, while at other cancer sites in the Duke Tumor Registry, the ratio of white-skinned to black-skinned persons was 4:1 during the same time frame. Thus, a preferential incidence for white persons of 20:1 was estimated, their mortality ratio being somewhat lower. This observation might well result from the tendency for black-skinned persons to have acral lentiginous lesions or melanoma involving the mucous membranes, sites with an especially poor survival.

PROGNOSTIC FACTORS

STAGE OF DISEASE

Anatomical extent of disease is clearly the predominant factor determining prognosis in melanoma. Eighty-four percent of patients were stage I at

* Mason TJ, McKay FW: US cancer mortality by county: 1950–1969. DHEW Publication no. (NIH)74-615, 1974

presentation, and 14% presented with stage II disease. Survival data are shown in Figure 25-1. However, clinical staging is an imperfect reflection of the true extent of disease. Because the true stage of disease can only be estimated roughly by current methods, an important role of prognostic analysis is to identify factors that can be used to predict the true biologic state of metastases. These prognostic factors may be identified only retrospectively and on a statistical, not an individual, basis. Much of the significance of level of invasion and thickness, for example, is attributable to their prediction of stage. The definition of stage in this series encompasses pathologic data, in addition to clinical data, when they are available. Some high-risk stage I and stage II patients received active specific immunotherapy as described below, and this may have influenced their prognosis.

PROGNOSIS IN PATIENTS WITH LOCALIZED MELANOMA (STAGE I)

Patient factors

One of the most intriguing aspects of melanoma is the difference in survival between men and women. The survival curves for men and women diverged to a difference of 9% at 5 years and 16% at 7 years.

Melanomas occurred in all areas of the integument (see Table 25-1). Trunk melanomas made up 42% of the overall series, while 15% of patients had head and neck primary lesions. For women, there was a predominance of lesions on the limbs, whereas in men, there was a preponderance on the trunk, head, and neck. Thus, leg melanomas occurred three times more often in women, while

TABLE 25–3
AGE-ADJUSTED MELANOMA MORTALITY RATES ($\times 10^5$) FOR THE SOUTHERN UNITED STATES FOR THE YEARS 1950–1969

State	White		Nonwhite	
	Male	Female	Male	Female
Alabama	2.19	1.72	0.32	0.42
Arkansas	1.70	1.42	0.23	0.16
Florida	1.97	1.18	0.43	0.21
Georgia	2.14	1.57	0.44	0.33
Louisiana	1.90	1.34	0.54	0.27
Mississippi	2.07	1.56	0.29	0.25
North Carolina	1.99	1.46	0.44	0.35
Oklahoma	1.82	1.41	0.51	0.19
South Carolina	1.78	1.50	0.38	0.19
Tennessee	1.86	1.43	0.26	0.31
Texas	2.29	1.57	0.49	0.34

(U.S. Cancer Mortality by County: 1950–1969. HEW, NIH, Government Printing Office, 1974)

trunk melanomas were twice as frequent in men. Stage I patients with upper extremity lesions fared best of all (Fig. 25-2). Patients with lower extremity and truncal lesions had an intermediate and similar outcome. Patients with head and neck lesions had significantly worse survival rates than those with extremity lesions.

Pathologic factors

Tumor thickness and level of invasion were found to be important prognostic variables (p ≤ 0.005). The level of invasion was used exclusively by the pathologists at the DMC for expressing degree of penetration for several years before tumor thickness was added to the protocol. A larger number of patients was therefore available for determining prognosis according to the level of invasion than for tumor thickness, and these patients have, on the average, also been followed longer. Nevertheless, in 1021 patients, both values were available for assessing the relative significance of the two factors. There was a progressive decrement in survival with each thickness subgroup up to 4 mm. Patients with lesions ≥4 mm thick did not have a worse prognosis than those with lesions 2.5 mm to 3.99 mm thick (Fig. 25-3). No difference in survival was found between level II and level III patients. Level IV patients had a distinctly poorer prognosis than level II and level III

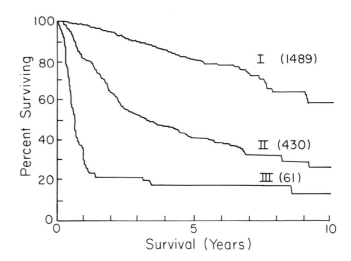

FIG. 25–1 Actuarial survival curves for melanoma patients according to stage of disease at diagnosis. Number of patients is shown in parentheses.

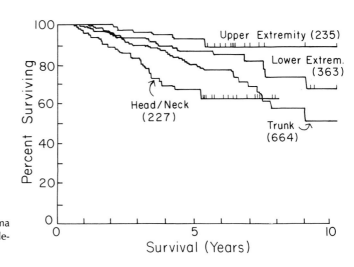

FIG. 25–2 Actuarial survival curves for stage I melanoma patients according to anatomical location of primary lesion.

patients, but a substantially better prognosis than level V patients. Ulcerated melanomas occurred more frequently in thicker melanomas. Nevertheless, ulceration of the melanoma as evaluated histologically was also found to be an important independent prognostic factor (Fig. 25-4).

There are four major growth patterns in melanoma: superficial spreading melanoma (SSM, 71% of these data), nodular melanoma (NM, 25%), lentigo maligna melanoma (LMM, 4%), and acral lentiginous melanoma (ALM, only recently used at DMC). Patients with NM had a poorer survival rate than those with either SSM or LMM, and in stage I patients, growth pattern was the dominant prog-

nostic factor (Fig. 25-5). Compared with patients with SSM or LMM, patients with NM had a relative mortality risk of 2.8. To delineate the significance of growth patterns further, patients were grouped according to thickness and the presence of ulceration. Nodular growth pattern was only rarely observed in the thinnest melanomas and became increasingly frequent as thickness increased. In each of the thickness ranges up to 1.5 mm, patients with NM fared significantly worse, with a trend toward poorer survival for those with lesions 1.5 mm to 2.25 mm thick (p = 0.09). In lesions thicker than 2.25 mm, patients with all growth patterns had equally poor survival rates.

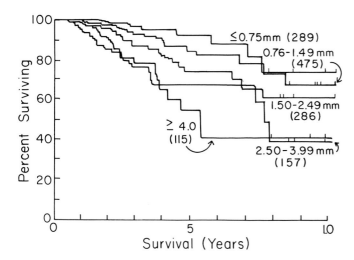

FIG. 25–3 Actuarial survival curves for stage I melanoma patients according to tumor thickness.

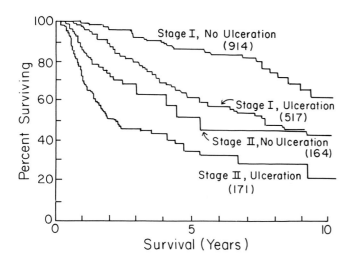

FIG. 25–4 Actuarial survival curves for stage I and stage II melanoma patients according to presence or absence of ulceration.

Multifactorial analysis

Four different models were used to evaluate prognostic factors in stage I patients.[3] The model presented in Table 25-4 is based on 1489 patients, including those with the longest follow-up. Unfortunately, the number of factors available for study in the larger group had more limited histopathologic data until recent years. Only level of invasion and growth pattern were recorded in the earlier period. A second model that also incorporates tumor thickness and ulceration was analyzed in 1021 patients (where all information was available), as shown in

Table 25-5. The independent prognostic factors in stage I patients with cutaneous melanoma included (1) sex, (2) primary lesion site, (3) level of invasion, (4) tumor thickness, (5) ulceration, and (6) growth pattern. After adjustment for these factors, elective lymph node dissection (ELND) also conveyed a significant survival benefit, as described in the next section.

In the first model (see Table 25-4), sex was found to be an independent factor after adjustment for site, level, and growth pattern. Tumor thickness and ulceration, however, were not included in this

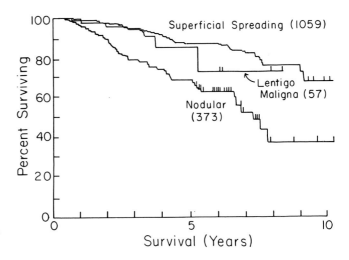

FIG. 25–5 Actuarial survival curves for stage I melanoma patients according to growth pattern.

TABLE 25–4
MULTIFACTORIAL ANALYSIS OF 1489 STAGE I MELANOMA PATIENTS*

Variable	Single-factor Analysis	Multifactorial Analysis	Relative Risk†
Growth pattern	<0.0001	<0.0001	2.78
Nodular vs others	(46.7‡)	(37.5)	
Level of invasion	<0.0001	<0.0001	1.81
Clark	(37.9)	(27.0)	
Primary tumor site	0.0003	0.004	0.31
Upper extremity vs others	(14.1)	(8.6)	
Sex	0.002	0.005	1.61
Male vs female	(10.8)	(8.1)	
Primary tumor site	0.0003	0.02	1.60
Head/neck vs others	(14.5)	(5.5)	

*Thickness and ulceration data are not available for some patients.

†The risk that a patient with the first characteristic will die compared with a patient who has the second characteristic (e.g., a patient with a nodular melanoma has a 2.78 times greater risk for dying than one with the other two growth patterns, superficial spreading and lentigo maligna melanoma).

‡Chi-square with 1 d.f. overall model chi-square 105.8 (d.f. = 5, p < 0.0001).

evaluation. There was a substantially better prognosis for patients with upper extremity lesions, the death rate being only one third that of patients with lower extremity and trunk lesions (see Table 25-4). Patients with head and neck lesions had a relative death rate 1.6 times that of the trunk/lower extremity group. Evidence will be presented in the section on surgical treatment implicating treatment and sex as primary variables. The anatomical site of the primary melanoma appeared to be significant through its association with these variables.

The level of invasion and tumor thickness are two correlated measures of tumor proliferation that may represent a composite of more fundamental biologic tumor factors. For example, the importance of the growth patterns, mitotic rate, lymphocyte infiltrate, regression, and pigmentation for survival is reduced when either level of invasion or thickness is included in the multivariate analysis.

In the subgroup of stage I patients for whom both level of invasion and tumor thickness were recorded, thickness provided additional prognostic information even after the prognostic significance of level of invasion was accounted for (p = 0.002). In contrast, level of invasion provided no additional significant information once thickness was taken into account (p = 0.14). That is, thickness provided all the information contained in level of invasion and a significant amount of additional information besides. In the second model, which incorporated thickness and ulceration, both level of invasion and sex were dropped because they failed to provide significant additional prognostic information after the other five factors were accounted for (Table 25-5).

In stage I patients, ulceration was more common in NM, but adjustment for growth pattern in the Cox model did not remove the significant contribution of ulceration entirely. The nodular growth pattern itself was a strong additional risk factor when ulcerated primary lesions (p = 0.004) and nonulcerated lesions (p = 0.0005) were considered separately. This growth pattern was highly significant (p = 0.0002) on entry into a Cox model after adjusting for both thickness and ulceration. While NM was strongly associated with both increasingly thick and ulcerated lesions, growth pattern remained a major independent prognostic factor in this series.

In summary, a major finding in these two models was the significance of the nodular growth pattern. Patients with NM had a death rate nearly three times that of patients with other growth patterns. Level of invasion was the next most significant factor. The death rate nearly doubled with a one-step change in Clark's level. Primary lesion site was next in relative importance, with patients with upper extremity lesions having only one third of the mortality rate of patients with trunk and lower extremity lesions. Head and neck lesions had a hazard rate 1.6 times that of other primary lesion sites. The final factor identified was sex, with men having a relative mortality rate of 1.6 once all other factors were accounted for. Tumor thickness and ulceration were also very important prognostic variables when considered in the second model (see Table 25-5).

TABLE 25–5
MULTIFACTORIAL ANALYSIS OF 1021 STAGE I MELANOMA PATIENTS*

Variable	Single-factor Analysis	Multifactorial Analysis	Relative Risk[†]
Growth pattern	0.0001	<0.0004	2.68
Nodular vs others	(28.2[‡])	(13.5)	
Thickness	0.0001	0.02	1.09
Breslow	(16.7)	(5.6)	
Ulceration	0.0009	0.04	1.33
Present vs absent	(11.6)	(4.5)	
Primary tumor site	0.08	0.009	2.13
Trunk vs others	(3.0)	(6.9)	
Primary tumor site	0.35	0.08	1.99
Head/neck vs others	(0.9)	(3.1)	

* This data includes thickness and ulceration.
[†] See footnote for relative risk in Table 25-4.
[‡] Chi-square with 1 d.f. overall model chi-square 45 (d.f. = 5, p < 0.0001).

PROGNOSIS IN PATIENTS WITH NODAL METASTASES (STAGE II)

Prognosis in these patients was poor, with a 10-year survival rate of only 25% (see Fig. 25-1). Those patients with metastatic nodes at the time of their original diagnosis had no better survival from the time of node positivity than those who subsequently relapsed with nodal metastases. Accordingly, the two groups were combined to evaluate the significance of other factors. The actual number of metastatic nodes correlated with survival (Fig. 25-6). Those with more than four nodes had a median survival of only 16 months, while those with four or fewer nodes had much better survival rates.

Most of the features of melanoma that were of prognostic significance in stage I patients had little or no role in determining survival in node-positive (stage II) patients. Ulceration of the primary melanoma was the only feature that remained as an independent prognostic factor in stage II patients. Survival for women was slightly higher than for men when taken from the diagnosis of nodal disease. Level of invasion, thickness, and growth pattern did not provide any additional prognostic information regarding long-term survival.

PROGNOSIS IN BLACK-SKINNED PATIENTS

There was a low incidence of melanoma in black-skinned patients, as compared to white-skinned patients, and a striking difference in primary lesion site distribution. In this series, survival was distinctly worse in the former (31 months median survival from diagnosis) than in the latter (104 months). On the average, black-skinned patients had a more advanced stage of disease on presentation—36% with stage II and stage III melanoma compared with 16% of white-skinned patients. Thirty-six percent of their primary lesions were Clark's level V, and 52% were level IV, compared with 7% and 37% in white-skinned patients, respectively. After univariate adjustments for stage, level of invasion, sex, growth pattern, and treatment, there remained a highly significant difference in survival between the two races.[7]

Melanoma is thus an aggressive, highly lethal malignancy in black-skinned persons. Largely responsible are the more deeply invasive primary lesions with which these patients present, the more advanced stage of disease, and the predominance of mucosal, acral, and unknown primary lesions. Adjustment for inequalities in all these dominant prognostic factors resulted in a suggestion that there was still an additional unfavorable prognosis for black-skinned persons compared with white-skinned persons (p = 0.11).

SURGICAL MANAGEMENT

Surgical management of patients with melanoma at DMC has traditionally consisted of a conventional surgical approach using wide local excision of the primary lesion and lymph node dissection where indicated for clinically positive regional nodes and used electively in those judged to be at high risk for microscopic metastasis to the regional nodes.[9,10] The treatment program is individualized for unusual

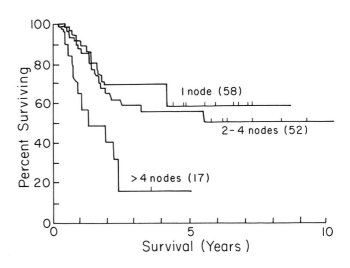

FIG. 25–6 Actuarial survival curves for stage II melanoma patients according to number of involved nodes.

presentations requiring special consideration of tissue conservation or compartmental spread, such as facial or digital lesions.

The indications for and benefit of ELND have long been subjects of controversy. In the hope that the DMC experience might shed some light on this issue, a recent review was made of recurrence rates among those patients who did and did not have ELND.[6] The study was based on the subset of patients for whom values were available for all the prognostically significant variables, including thickness, ulceration, primary lesion site, sex, and age. The majority of patients referred to DMC had their primary surgery, including nodal dissections, performed in their community hospitals. Surgical treatment varied considerably. Of particular interest was the rate of ELND performed in clinical stage I patients with intermediate-thickness primary lesions. This procedure was performed in 125 of 305 (41%) patients with an extremity primary lesion and in 62 of 308 (20%) patients with a primary lesion on the trunk. Patients with a more deeply invasive primary lesion were more likely to have nodal dissections that those with a less invasive primary lesion (Table 25-6). Cox-model analysis was used to adjust for prognostic factor inequalities between the two groups (Table 25-7).

After adjusting for thickness and ulceration, the two most important factors in this subset, ELND was the next most significant factor and appeared to convey significant benefit in delaying disease recurrence ($p = 0.02$). A confounding factor in the inter-

TABLE 25–6
DISTRIBUTION OF PROGNOSTIC FACTORS IN 613 STAGE I MELANOMA PATIENTS WITH INTERMEDIATE-THICKNESS (0.76 mm–4 mm) MELANOMAS

Variable	Elective Lymph Node Dissection (n=187)	No Elective Lymph Node Dissection (n=426)
Tumor thickness (mm; mean ± SD)*	1.81 ± 0.80	1.60 ± 0.73
Ulceration:		
Yes	36%	31%
No	64%	69%
Number dead	5%	12%
Sex:		
Male	45%	45%
Female	55%	55%
Primary site:		
Trunk	33%	58%
Extremity	67%	42%
Mean age (years)	45.7	45.5

* SD = standard deviation

TABLE 25–7
MULTIFACTORIAL ANALYSIS OF 487 STAGE I PATIENTS WITH INTERMEDIATE-THICKNESS (0.76 mm–4 mm) MELANOMA*

Variable	Single-factor Analysis	Multifactorial Analysis	Relative Risk[†]
Ulceration	0.0002	0.0008	1.89
Present vs absent	(15.6[‡])	(11.7)	
Thickness	0.003	0.008	1.77
Breslow	(9.6)	(7.0)	
Elective node	0.06	0.06	0.309
dissection	(3.6)	(3.6)	
Yes vs no			
Primary site	0.14	0.22	1.57
Trunk vs others	(2.2)	(1.5)	

* Ulceration data are not available for some patients.
[†] See footnote for relative risk in Table 25-4.
[‡] Chi-square with 1 d.f. overall model chi-square 28.8 (d.f. = 4, $p = 0.00002$).

pretation of the significance of ELND is the fact that ELND was performed more frequently for extremity primary lesions. Patients with extremity lesions may themselves have a better prognosis, either inherently or by virtue of the fact that most of these patients are women. Indeed, after adjusting first for primary lesion site in a stepwise analysis of this group, the significance of ELND was diminished.

In order to determine whether the prognostic significance of primary site was due to the more favorable location (extremity lesions) or sex (female patients) rather than to the benefit of ELND, another model was set up on the 371 patients who did not have ELND. In this model, neither primary lesion site nor sex was found to be a significant factor, singly or in combination with other factors. This finding indicates that ELND was the prime factor in survival and that primary lesion site was involved only secondarily through its correlation with choice of treatment. The small population size and the relatively short follow-up of this group underscore the tentative status of these results. Whether these results will translate into long-term difference in disease-free survival can be ascertained only by further follow-up of the patient population. However, this study is particularly interesting, because it reflects the results of treatment given by community surgeons, not that of a single surgeon's or cancer center's experience. Its results should therefore be a more relevant guide to treatment planning. Although the significance level is marginal, owing mainly to the small number of total failures observed, it should be emphasized that the estimated death rate for the untreated group is more than twice that for the ELND group.

SPECIFIC ACTIVE IMMUNOTHERAPY

Over the past 10 years, all patients referred to DMC judged to be at significant risk of harboring microscopic disease have been entered into a protocol using specific active immunization in an adjuvant mode. This study was designed to determine whether immune responses directed against the tumor-associated antigen present on melanoma cell membranes could be elicited in patients.[10] Additionally, the study was designed to evaluate whether stage, sex, and other factors modulate the immune response and whether these responses were of any prognostic significance.

The immunization regimen has consisted of four subcutaneous injections of approximately 2.5×10^7 x-irradiated melanoma cells if the patient had documented stage I disease only, and seven total immunizations if the patient had stage II disease. No patient with stage III disease was included in the study. The adjuvant immunization treatment regimen has been demonstrated to be virtually devoid of any toxicity. Comparisons with reported series of melanoma cases stratified by stage and level of invasion show a favorable pattern of survival through the first 5 years, especially in patients with stage I Clark's level III and level IV disease (see Chap. 11 for details). At every level, the immunized patients have experienced survival apparently better than the best reported outcomes in the literature. Follow-up is relatively short; therefore, no firm conclusions have been made concerning this mode of adjuvant therapy at the present time.

METASTATIC MELANOMA

The diagnosis and clinical management of patients with metastatic melanoma treated at DMC have been published.[1,2,5,8–14] Most patients with distant metastases are treated with a four-drug-combination (BOLD) chemotherapy.[12]

Supported in part by PHS Grants CA–11265, CA–20364, 1 PO 1 CA–32672, CA–21192, and CA–14236.

The technical assistance of Ms. Nancy Anderson is gratefully acknowledged.

REFERENCES

1. Bullard DE, Cox EB, Seigler HF: Central nervous system metastases in malignant melanoma. Neurosurgery 8:26, 1981
2. Chen JTT, Dahmash NS, Ravin CE, Heaston KD, Putman CE, Seigler HF, Reed JC: Metastatic melanoma to the thorax: Report of 130 patients. Am J Roentgenol 137:293, 1981
3. Cox EB: Prognostic factors in malignant melanoma. In Seigler HF (ed): Clinical Management of Melanoma, p 279. The Hague, Nijhoff, 1982
4. Cox EB, Stanley W: Schema driven time-oriented record on a minicomputer. Comput Biomed Res 12:503, 1979
5. Oddson RA, Rice RP, Seigler HF, Thompson WM, Kelvin FM, Clark WM: The spectrum of small bowel melanoma. Gastrointest Radiol 3:419, 1978

6. Reintgen DS, Cox EB, McCarty KS Jr, Vollmer RT, Seigler HF: Efficacy of elective lymph node dissection in patients with intermediate thickness primary melanoma. Ann Surg 198:379, 1983

7. Reintgen DS, McCarty KS Jr, Cox E, Seigler HF: Malignant melanoma in black American and white American populations: A comparative review. JAMA 248:1856, 1982

8. Reintgen DS, McCarty KS Jr, Woodard B, Cox E, Seigler HF: Metastatic malignant melanoma with an unknown primary. Surg Gynecol Obstet 156:335, 1983

9. Seigler HF (ed): Clinical Management of Melanoma. The Hague, Nijhoff, 1982

10. Seigler HF, Cox E, Mutzner F, Shepherd L, Nich-olson E, Shingleton WW: Specific active immunotherapy for melanoma. Ann Surg 190:366, 1979

11. Seigler HF, Fetter BF: Current management of melanoma. Ann Surg 186:1, 1977

12. Seigler HF, Lucas VS Jr, Pickett NJ, Huang AT: DTIC, CCNU, bleomycin and vincristine (BOLD) in metastatic melanoma. Cancer 46:2346, 1980

13. Stewart WR, Gelberman RH, Harrelson JM, Seigler HF: Skeletal metastases of melanoma. J Bone Joint Surg 60A:645, 1978

14. Sullivan DC, Croker BP Jr, Harris CC, Deery P, Seigler HF: Lymphoscintigraphy in malignant melanoma: ^{99m}Tc antimony sulfur colloid. Am J Roentgenol 137:847, 1981

DONALD L. MORTON
DENISE J. ROE
ALISTAIR J. COCHRAN

Melanoma in the Western United States: Experience with Stage II Melanoma at the UCLA Medical Center

26

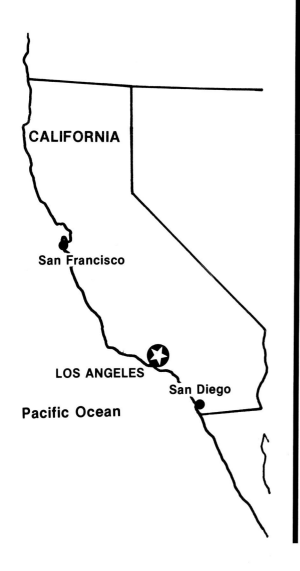

The annual age-adjusted incidence of melanoma in the county of Los Angeles for white, non-Hispanic men is approximately 14 per 100,000 and for white, non-Hispanic women is approximately 11 per 100,000.[27] The Tumor Registry at the University of California at Los Angeles (UCLA) has maintained records of the incidence of melanomas treated at the Medical Center since 1955. Los Angeles is located 34° north of the equator on the coast of the Pacific Ocean. The 1980 census showed that the city itself had a population of 3.5 million. The county had a population of 7.5 million, of which 60% were Caucasians, 25% were Hispanics, 12.5% were blacks, and the remaining 3%, Orientals and native Americans. Los Angeles County measures 50 miles from north to south and 30 miles from the San Gabriel Mountains to the sea. Its altitude varies from sea level to 2800 feet. Average temperatures range from a daytime low of 51°F in January to 74°F in July.

The studies described in this report resulted from a discrepancy in the results of two clinical trials. Patients whose melanoma is localized to the primary site (stage I) have a 5-year survival rate of 75% to 90%.[9,12] However, when tumor spreads to regional nodes (stage II), survival drops to 14% to 51%.[2,9,12,17] Because the stage II patient is more likely to develop recurrence of his disease and die of it, he is a candidate for experimental immunotherapeutic or chemotherapeutic adjuvant trials. To maximize the validity of such trials, the patient population under study must be as homogeneous as possible and should be stratified by those factors related to the stage of the disease that are of prognostic importance.

An early simultaneously controlled, but nonrandomized, trial reported in 1976[13] showed that patients whose stage II melanoma was treated with surgical resection, lymphadenectomy, and BCG (Bacillus Calmette Guérin) had fewer early postoperative recurrences and prolonged survival. Encouraged, we began a second prospective clinical trial in which all patients with stage II melanoma had surgical resection and lymphadenectomy and were then randomized to three groups: operation only; operation plus BCG; and operation, BCG, and tumor cell vaccine.[28] This trial was completed in 1978, and the results were not nearly so impressive as those of its predecessor, except for one finding. In the second trial, 60% of the operation-only group were alive at 2 years compared with 38% in the first trial; 50% were alive at 3 years versus 28% in the first group. The operation-only group did so well

that we could not demonstrate a significant effect for adjuvant therapy. This finding led us to a retrospective study of the natural history of melanoma metastatic to lymph nodes treated at UCLA by surgery.[6]

We assessed the effect of various histologic and clinical features on the survival of 150 patients with stage II melanoma who were treated with surgical resection and lymphadenectomy, but who did not receive chemotherapy or immunotherapy until development of detectable recurrent disease. These patients were seen at UCLA between January 1954 and June 1976 and were representative of a population that would constitute a stage II adjuvant therapy trial. Their clinical course up to the point of development of postlymphadenectomy metastases would represent the natural history of the disease in patients treated by operation only. To determine the prognostic factors important for predicting clinical outcome, multivariate statistical analyses were used.

PROGNOSTIC FACTORS IN STAGE II MELANOMA

PATIENT FACTORS

Clinical records were reviewed of all melanoma patients with histologically proven regional lymph node metastases (stage II) who were treated between January 1954 and June 1976 (Tables 26-1, 26-2). Reasons for exclusion from the study included presence of soft-tissue invasion at lymphadenectomy site or indication of disseminated melanoma at the time of lymphadenectomy. Satellitosis or intransit metastases were not exclusion indications. Patients who initially presented with localized melanoma but whose disease had progressed regionally were entered into the study if the later disease had been treated at UCLA and if the nodal disease was diagnosed before systemic involvement. All told, 150 stage II patients, 90 men and 60 women, between 14 and 79 years of age (median age, 48 years) were found. This group represented the 22-year UCLA experience with patients whose stage II melanoma was treated by operation only.

Factors to be statistically analyzed were selected from the investigator's clinical experience, an examination of published literature, and a preliminary review of the results of the study. Sufficient clinical and histologic data were available for valid statistical analysis of age, sex, parity, site of primary lesion, presence of satellitosis, clinical status of nodes, number of histologically positive lymph nodes, and

TABLE 26–1
CLINICAL AND PATHOLOGIC DATA FOR MELANOMA PATIENTS TREATED AT UCLA—STAGE II MELANOMA NATURAL HISTORY STUDY

Characteristics	Presenting Pathologic Stage
	Stage II
Clinical	
Number of patients	150
Year of diagnosis of stage II disease*	
≤ 1960	7%
1961–1965	26%
1966–1970	13%
1971–1975	39%
1976–1977	15%
Age	48 yr
Sex	
Male	60%
Female	40%
Primary Lesion Site	
Lower extremity	32%
Upper extremity	7%
Head and neck	17%
Trunk	36%
Other (unknown primary)	7%
Pathologic	
Breslow's tumor thickness	
< 0.76 mm	10%
0.76 mm–1.49 mm	18%
1.50 mm–2.49 mm	33%
2.50 mm–3.99 mm	24%
≥ 4.00 mm	14%
Median tumor thickness	2.1 mm
Level of invasion	
II	4%
III	30%
IV	59%
V	7%
Ulceration	
Yes	53%
No	47%
Growth Pattern	
Nodular	25%
Superficial spreading	73%
Lentigo maligna	1%

* Year of lymphadenectomy

histologic characteristics of the primary lesion. Survival was computed as the interval between lymphadenectomy and last follow-up visit or death. Of the patients who died, all but two had clinically detectable or autopsy-confirmed melanoma as the cause of death. Because autopsy was not performed on the two patients, statistical analysis treated them as having died with disease.

Survival curves were calculated by the Kaplan-Meier estimate.[21] Cox's[11] proportional hazards model was used to test for differences in the survival of patients within different subcategories of each factor. When only one factor was considered, the procedure was similar to the Mantel-Haenszel, or log-rank, test of differences during the entire period of the survival curve. Thus, 5-year survival rates are given for illustrative purposes only.

Adequate histologic information was unavailable for some patients. At each step in the step-up Cox analysis, data from all patients with complete information for each factor were used. Thus, the total number of patients in the analysis decreased as the number of steps increased. To verify the results of the step-up analysis, all patients were selected who had complete information for the factors found to be prognostic when analyzed individually. A reanalysis of this limited number of patients yielded conclusions similar to those of the Cox analysis of the larger, though less complete, group of patients.

The stepwise procedure included an assessment of the statistical significance of the interaction (cross-product terms) between the factors in the Cox model. The interaction was significant if the effect of a factor on survival was significantly different among patients with varying levels of another factor. For example, the interaction between tumor thickness and number of tumor-positive nodes showed increased survival when the primary tumor was less than 1 mm thick but decreased survival when the primary tumor was more than 4 mm thick. However, this was not true in this analysis.

Characteristics of patients with and without available histopathologic material were compared to assess possible sources of bias. Differences in demographic and clinical characteristics and in survival were not detected between these groups.

PATHOLOGIC FACTORS

Histologic and clinical data collected from patient charts, local physicians, or family members included demographic information, location and gross description of the primary lesion, treatment of the lesion and any associated complications, clinical assessment of lymph nodes, chronology of disease, timing and extent of complications after lymphadenectomy, and clinical or autopsy status at last visit or death. Histologic slides of the primary melanoma were available for 97 (70%) of 139 patients who had identifiable primary tumors. Eleven patients had regional nodal metastases from unknown primary melanomas (7%).

Histologic evaluation of the slides by one pa-

TABLE 26–2
ACTUARIAL SURVIVAL DATA FOR MELANOMA PATIENTS TREATED AT UCLA—STAGE II MELANOMA NATURAL HISTORY STUDY

Survival Data	Actuarial Survival Rates (after Lymphadenectomy)		
	1-Year	3-Year	5-Year
Stage II			
Overall survival	73%	46%	37%
Tumor thickness			
< 1.50 mm	80%	56%	49%
1.50 mm–3.99 mm	78%	53%	43%
≥ 4.0 mm	58%	0%	0%
Number of positive nodes			
1	81%	58%	45%
2–4	72%	46%	43%
≥ 4	65%	28%	15%
Ulceration			
Yes	65%	34%	34%
No	91%	62%	47%

thologist (A.J.C.) who had no knowledge of any patient's clinical course, confirmed the nature of the primary tumor for the 97 patients whose slides were available for review. The recorded histologic features included tumor profile,[23] the presence and micrometer-measured width of ulceration,[3] the growth pattern,[24] the level of invasion,[7] the tumor thickness as measured by micrometer,[1,4,5,14] the presence or absence of lymphatic or blood vascular invasion, the mitotic rate using the intervals established by McGovern and colleagues,[24] and the extent of any associated lymphoreticular infiltrate. After the histologic evaluation, 10% of the slides were coded and reviewed again by the same pathologist. The results of the two readings were virtually identical. The total number of positive and negative lymph nodes identified in each lymphadenectomy specimen was obtained from pathology reports. When slides of the nodes were available, the actual node profiles were verified.

The Cox procedure analyzed both continuous and categorizable variables and identified those factors most related to survival in a stepwise manner. The number of tumor-containing nodes was analyzed first as a continuous variable and then by dividing the overall range into intervals based on experience and on results found in published literature. For example, the effect of the number of positive nodes on survival was analyzed by subcategories—1 positive node versus 2 to 4 positive nodes versus 5 or more positive nodes, or 3 or fewer positive nodes versus 4 or more positive nodes. The subcategories

were revised if preliminary analysis suggested that patients in two or more original subcategories could be combined on the basis of similar survival. For each factor, the subcategory arrangement that maximally separated the subgroups and yielded the greatest statistical significance was used in the final analyses. Statistical analyses with the continuous factors yielded results similar to those obtained when the factors were satisfactorily categorized.

STATISTICAL ANALYSIS

Univariate analysis

The Kaplan-Meier estimates of survival after lymphadenectomy for 150 patients with stage II melanoma were 73%, 55%, 37%, and 34% for 1, 2, 5, and 10 years (Fig. 26-1). When age, sex, parity, lymph node status, site of the primary lesion, satellitosis, biopsy type (excisional or incisional), growth pattern, and level of invasion or frequency of mitoses were analyzed separately, there were no statistically significant differences in survival among patients in the different subcategories (Table 26-3).

The number of nodes containing tumor on histopathologic examination was recorded for 122 patients but was not available for the other 28 patients. The number of tumor-positive nodes was prognostic for survival after lymphadenectomy—the more nodes involved, the shorter the life span (Fig. 26-2). The greatest statistical significance was observed when the 95 patients who had one to three positive

STAGE II MELANOMA

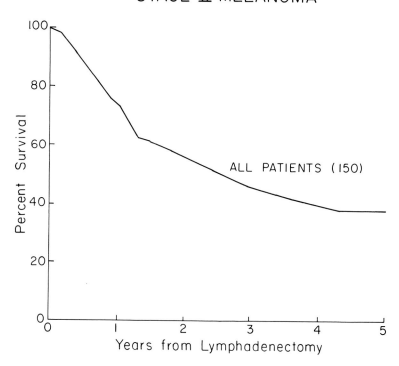

ALL PATIENTS (150)

FIG. 26–1 Actuarial survival for all 150 surgically treated stage II melanoma patients, none of whom received adjuvant therapy. *Parentheses* indicate the number of patients.

nodes were compared with the 27 who had four or more positive nodes (p = 0.026). The measured thickness of the vertically invasive component of primary melanomas was strongly and directly correlated with survival (Fig. 26-3). There was a statistically significant difference in survival when tumors ≤0.99 mm (n = 13), 1 mm to 2.99 mm (n = 46), 3 mm to 3.99 mm (n = 16), and ≥4 mm (n = 12)(p < 0.001) were compared. The presence or absence of ulceration involving the primary melanoma was also a significant prognostic variable by univariate analysis (p = 0.003; Fig. 26-4).

Multivariate analysis

Multivariate analysis with the use of the Cox procedure showed that thickness of the primary melanoma (p < 0.001) and the number of melanoma-involved lymph nodes (p = 0.04) were the statistically significant prognostic factors. The statistical tests of the interaction between thickness and number of melanoma-involved lymph nodes (the multiplicative effect of these two variables on survival) yielded a p value of 0.10. None of the other

factors analyzed in the univariate analysis achieved significance in the multivariate analysis. The presence and width of ulceration of the primary lesion, which were statistically significant factors when analyzed separately, were not significant in the multivariate analysis (p = 0.21 and p = 0.19, respectively) because of the strong association between thickness categories and the width of ulceration categories (Table 26-3). For example, of the 13 patients with tumor thickness less than 1 mm, 10 (83%) had no ulceration, 2 (17%) had ulceration 6 mm wide or less, and none had ulceration greater than 6 mm. Conversely, of the 12 patients with thickness 4 mm or greater, 1 (8%) had no ulceration, 5 (42%) had ulceration 6 mm wide or less, and 6 (50%) had an ulceration greater than 6 mm. This strong association was largely the result of our success in choosing subcategories of thickness and width of ulceration because the correlation coefficient between these two characteristics (considered as continuous variables) was 0.35, largely because of the wide scatter of values observed.

(*Text continues on page 426*)

TABLE 26–3
PROGNOSTIC FACTORS BY UNIVARIATE ANALYSIS OF CLINICAL AND HISTOLOGIC DATA IN STAGE II MELANOMA PATIENTS*

Factors	Number of Patients	5-year Survival	p Value
Thickness (Breslow's)			
≤ 0.99 mm	13	62%	< 0.001
1.00 mm–2.99 mm	46	46%	
3.00 mm–3.99 mm	16	31%	
≥ 4.00 mm	12	0%	
Width of ulceration			
None	42	49%	0.003
≤ 6 mm	30	36%	
> 6 mm	13	0%	
Number of positive nodes			
≤ 3	95	45%	0.026
> 3	27	21%	
Ulceration			
Yes	49	34%	0.029
No	43	47%	
Sex			
Male	90	35%	0.13
Female	60	41%	
Biopsy type			
Excision	116	40%	0.13
Incision	17	24%	
Parity			
No children	15	53%	0.17
One or more children	41	38%	
Node status			
Negative	29	48%	0.20
Positive	119	36%	
Age			
≤ 40	42	46%	0.20
> 40	108	34%	
Growth pattern			
Superficial spreading	58	41%	0.35
Nodular	20	21%	
Clark's level			
II	4	50%	0.36
III	27	46%	
IV	53	37%	
V	6	0%	
Location primary			
Extremity	63	42%	0.43
Axial	76	32%	
Satellitosis			
Present	14	29%	0.53
Absent	106	39%	
Slide availability			
Yes	97	39%	0.78
No	53	35%	
Frequency of mitoses			
Many	24	35%	0.93
Moderate	44	42%	
Minimal	21	41%	

* Results are presented for each postulated prognostic factor tested in univariate analysis. Continuous variables were tested using a variety of cutoff points, and only the most significant result for each variable is shown. Statistical significance for each univariate comparison was derived from the entire Kaplan-Meier life-table curve for each factor. Figures for 5-year survival after lymphadenectomy were derived from the Kaplan-Meier estimates and are presented for illustrative purposes only.

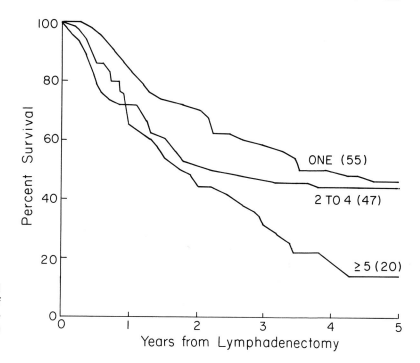

FIG. 26–2 Actuarial survival of stage II melanoma patients according to number of metastatic lymph nodes. *Parentheses* indicate the number of patients. The correlation with survival was significant (P = 0.04).

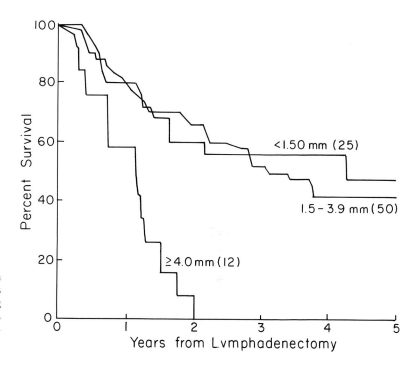

FIG. 26–3 Prognosis of stage II melanoma patients according to tumor thickness. This was the most significant feature predicting survival in the multifactorial analysis (P = 0.001). The number of patients is indicated in *parentheses*.

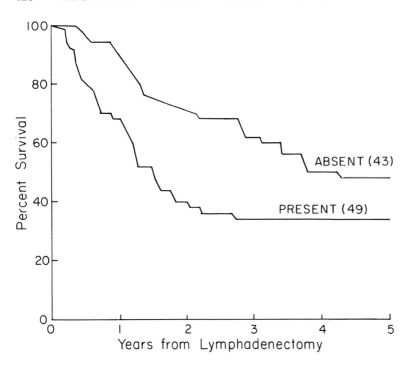

FIG. 26–4   Prognosis of stage II melanoma patients according to ulceration of the primary melanoma. Although this was a significant feature by univariate analysis, it was not by multivariate analysis. The number of patients is shown in *parentheses*.

When all the factors were analyzed, the number of tumor-containing nodes was of greatest predictive value. The greatest difference in survival was between patients with three or fewer positive nodes and those who had four or more nodes containing tumor. In the univariate analysis, three characteristics of the primary tumor—thickness, absence of ulceration, and micrometric measurement of ulceration—were prognostic for survival. In the multivariate analysis, only thickness was of independent prognostic importance; the presence and extent of ulceration were closely related to the measurement of thickness. Of interest is the fact that *characteristics of the primary tumor can predict survival after therapeutic lymphadenectomy* just as much, if not more, than the time-honored parameter of the tumor burden of the nodes.

The prognostic factors identified, number of tumor-containing nodes, and thickness of the primary, should be the stratification criteria of future trials of therapy for stage II melanoma. If these individual factors could be combined into a score or index, such as the index devised for primary melanoma by Cochran[8] and MacKie and associates,[25] prognosis could be assigned more accurately and the number of stratification factors could be reduced in future randomized clinical trials.

TREATMENT FOR NODAL METASTASES

SURGICAL TREATMENT

For the patient with clinically suspicious or pathologically proven metastases to regional lymph nodes, regional lymphadenectomy is indicated. Therapeutic lymphadenectomy was carried out in 119 of 148 patients (80%) and elective (or prophylactic) lymphadenectomy for clinically negative, histologically positive nodes in the remaining 20%. Cohen,[10] Das Gupta,[12] and others[19,22,26] reported that node palpability prior to operation in nodes subsequently found to contain tumor on histology is an unfavorable prognostic sign. Although the group of patients in our study who had negative nodes on preoperative clinical assessment survived better than those with clinically positive nodes, the difference in survival was not statistically significant in either the univariate or multivariate analysis with the number of patients available for study.

Although patients who have occult regional node metastases and elective lymph node dissection have not demonstrated a significantly improved survival over those who have palpable disease, it is clear that a regional lymphadenectomy is the only available staging procedure. Patients with primary melanoma without regional lymph node metastases enjoy an 80% to 90% survival rate, whereas at least 50% of patients with metastases to the lymph nodes have recurrent disease within 2 years of their surgical procedure. Therefore, therapeutic advantage or disadvantage becomes a moot point because lymphadenectomy is the only method for achieving adequate pathologic staging. Without lymphadenectomy, the clinician can neither inform the patient of his or her general prognosis nor identify those patients at high risk (positive nodes) for recurrence in order to include them in possibly beneficial postoperative adjuvant therapy trials. We suggest that patients with melanoma invasive to 0.65 mm or deeper, and Clark's level III to V, be considered for regional lymphadenectomy.[20] This thickness was chosen because some of our patients with lesions between 0.65 mm and 0.76 mm developed regional node metastases.

Furthermore, it is evident that, if this procedure is done for staging, the entire chain of nodes in the region must be dissected. Although Sappey[30] showed many years ago that the lymphatic system of the forehead, cheek, and anterior ear drained first to the parotid lymph nodes, this fact seems to have escaped common clinical recognition. These parotid nodes are within the capsule of the parotid gland, and when a melanoma of the head or neck is located in this area, a regional lymphadenectomy must, of necessity, include parotidectomy.

A second area of controversy concerns the lymphatic areas of the trunk from which lymph shed is equivocal. Sappey[30] defined a 2-cm-wide line that encircles the trunk, above which lesions generally drain to the axillary nodes and below which they drain to the inguinal nodes (Fig. 26-5).[26,31] However, there are a number of patients in whom midline lesions drain to all four nodal areas, particularly those with primaries of the umbilical area or midline back. Although this group of patients is in a minority, they present a very difficult and perplexing problem. We have described a technique using injectable colloidal gold(^{198}Au) or technetium sulfur colloid (^{99}Tc) scanning to demonstrate the lymph shed in these marginal areas.[15,29] Only six patients of 182

FIG. 26–5 Sappey's line defining lymph drainage. The area above the line drains to axillary nodes, below to inguinal nodes. (Grabb WC, Smith JW (eds): Plastic Surgery—A Concise Guide to Clinical Practice. Boston, Little, Brown & Co, 1979)

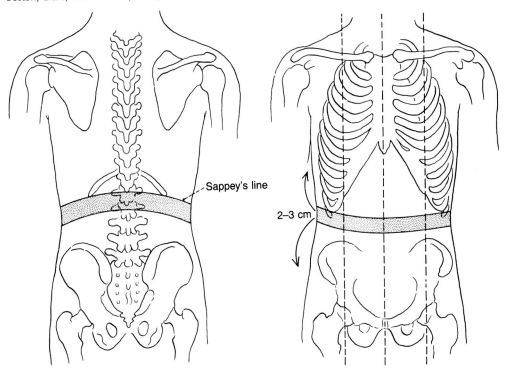

studied have developed microscopic or clinically apparent lymph node metastases in an area not identified by this scanning technique.[18]

One of the major reasons regional lymphadenectomies have been controversial is their attendant morbidity. Our group[16,20] has described a modified technique for inguinal lymph node dissection that appears to reduce the morbidity associated with this procedure markedly to less than 10%. Only the inguinal lymph nodes are removed routinely. The iliohypogastric nodes are dissected only if the inguinal nodes are involved with melanoma. Furthermore, our experience with cervical lymph node dissections has shown that a modified neck dissection, one that preserves the sternocleidomastoid muscle, is possible in patients with nonpalpable metastases to the neck.

At UCLA, current practice is to perform lymph node dissections on all patients with clinically suspicious or pathologically positive regional nodes. Elective node dissections are advocated for all patients with Clark's level IV and V melanoma and for selected level III patients whose lesions have invaded to a depth greater than 0.65 mm.

ADJUVANT THERAPY

Patients with metastases to regional nodes have a high rate of treatment failure despite lymphadenectomy. This failure is seldom the result of uncontrolled primary or regional disease, but of distant metastases. Nearly 60% of these metastases become apparent within 2 years of the initial surgical treatment, and it is probable that this disease was present at the time of the patient's first evaluation. Therefore, to improve treatment results, some form of systemic adjuvant therapy is necessary. We have chosen immunotherapy for patients with stage II melanoma because it is relatively nontoxic and has been effective for treatment of clinically evident disease.[13]

The patients in our second clinical trial, completed in 1978, were randomized into one of three groups: operation only (48 patients); operation and BCG (49 patients); and operation, BCG, and tumor-cell vaccine (TCV) (52 patients). Ten patients were excluded from the analysis for protocol violations. Analysis was performed on 139 patients at a median follow-up of 62 months. Patients randomized to receive BCG were started on immunotherapy during the early postoperative period. The patients in each treatment group were followed monthly by physical examination, complete blood count, liver chemistries, and chest radiographs. Patients who developed disease recurrence continued to receive adjuvant therapy if assigned to an adjuvant group, but also received chemotherapy consisting of dacarbazine (DTIC) in combination with carmustine (BCNU) or lomustine (CCNU) or high-dose methotrexate. Patients in the control group who had disease recurrence were placed on the same chemotherapy.

The recurrence rates were essentially the same for the three groups of stage II patients. For example, the 2-year rates of the control, BCG, and BCG and TCV groups were 48%, 49%, and 52%, respectively. There appeared to be a difference in survival early in the trial, but this disappeared as time went on. By 4 years, there was no significant difference in survival among the three groups. However, once recurrence had taken place, patients in the BCG group survived substantially longer (p = 0.01 by the Mantel-Haenszel test). There were marked differences in the median times from recurrence to death for controls (5.2 months) and the tumor-cell vaccine group (6.8 months) compared to the BCG group (14.4 months). Three patients in the BCG group survived for 82 ± 8.5 months after recurrence (median 74 months), and one patient in the BCG-TCV group survived for 51 months.

Tumor recurrences locally and in regional lymph nodes were more common in the BCG and BCG-TCV groups than in the control group. The control patients had more initial recurrences in viscera. The most striking difference was in the frequency of brain metastases in the control group—6 out of 28 compared with 1 out of 28 in the BCG group and none in the BCG-TCV group (p < 0.05). Initial recurrences in the immunotherapy group occurred more frequently in surgically manageable sites and less often in therapeutically inaccessible and vital organs. The longer survival of these patients after disease recurrence resulted, in part, from the favorable distribution of the recurrent disease from a management standpoint. The immunotherapy did not cure these patients, but it did ameliorate the gravity of recurrent disease by confining the disease to surgically manageable sites, thus permitting a prolongation of survival for many patients.

Because it became clear that BCG immunotherapy was of benefit to patients with stage II melanoma, the randomized trial was terminated, and BCG immunotherapy was advocated by our group for all patients with stage II melanoma. The amount of benefit cannot be established because it is anticipated that more of these stage II patients will die of their disease over the next 2 to 3 years. Nonetheless, it is apparent that BCG immunotherapy does have activity as an adjuvant in patients with melanoma metastatic to regional lymph nodes. However, the treatment failure rate for melanoma remains excessively high, and better programs must be developed for this disease.

Supported by grants CA–12582, CA–29605, and CA–09010, awarded by the National Cancer Institute, DHHS.

REFERENCES

1. Balch CM, Murad TM, Soong S-j, Ingalls AL, Halpern NB, Maddox WA: A multifactorial analysis of melanoma: Prognostic histopathological features comparing Clark's and Breslow's staging methods. Ann Surg 188:732, 1978
2. Balch CM, Soong S-j, Murad TM, Ingalls AL, Maddox WA: A multifactorial analysis of melanoma. III. Prognostic factors in melanoma patients with lymph node metastases (stage II). Ann Surg 193:377, 1981
3. Balch CM, Wilkerson JA, Murad TM, Soong S-j, Ingalls AL, Maddox WA: The prognostic significance of ulceration of cutaneous melanoma. Cancer 45:3012, 1980
4. Breslow A: Thickness, cross-sectional areas and depth of invasion in the prognosis of cutaneous melanoma. Ann Surg 172:902, 1970
5. Breslow A: Prognostic factors in the treatment of cutaneous melanoma. J Cutan Pathol 6:208, 1979
6. Callery C, Cochran AJ, Roe DJ, Rees W, Nathanson SD, Benedetti JK, Elashoff RM, Morton DL: Factors prognostic for survival in patients with malignant melanoma spread to the regional lymph nodes. Ann Surg 196:69, 1982
7. Clark WH Jr, From L, Bernardino EA, Mihm MC Jr: The histogenesis and biologic behavior of primary human malignant melanomas of the skin. Cancer Res 29:705, 1969
8. Cochran AJ: Method of assessing prognosis in patients with malignant melanoma. Lancet 2:1062, 1968
9. Cochran AJ: Malignant melanoma: A review of 10 years' experience in Glasgow, Scotland. Cancer 23:75, 1969
10. Cohen MH, Ketcham AS, Felix EL, Li SH, Tomaszewski MM, Costa J, Rabson AS, Simon RM, Rosenberg SA: Prognostic factors in patients undergoing lymphadenectomy for malignant melanoma. Ann Surg 186:635, 1977
11. Cox DR: Regression models and life tables (with discussion). J Royal Stat Soc B 34:187, 1972
12. Das Gupta TK: Results of treatment of 269 patients with primary cutaneous melanoma: A five-year prospective study. Ann Surg 186:201, 1977
13. Eilber FR, Morton DL, Holmes EC, Sparks FC, Ramming KP: Adjuvant immunotherapy with BCG in treatment of regional-lymph-node metastases from malignant melanoma. N Engl J Med 294:237, 1976
14. Eldh J, Boeryd B, Peterson L: Prognostic factors in cutaneous malignant melanoma in stage I: A clinical, morphological and multivariate analysis. Scand J Plast Reconstr Surg 12:243, 1978
15. Fee HJ, Robinson DS, Sample WF, Graham LS, Holmes EC, Morton DL: The determination of lymph shed by colloidal gold scanning in patients with malignant melanoma: A preliminary study. Surgery 84:626, 1978
16. Finck SJ, Giuliano AE, Mann BD, Morton DL: Results of ilioinguinal dissection for stage II melanoma. Ann Surg 196:180, 1982
17. Fortner JG, Booher RJ, Pack GT: Results of groin dissection for malignant melanoma in 220 patients. Surgery 55:485, 1964
18. Gallagher WJ, Bennett LR, Morton DL: Lymphoscintigraphy for management of malignant melanoma. Submitted to Surgery
19. Goldsmith HS, Shah JP, Kim D: Prognostic significance of lymph node dissection in the treatment of malignant melanoma. Cancer 26:606, 1970
20. Holmes EC, Moseley HS, Morton DL, Clark W, Robinson D, Urist MM: A rational approach to the surgical management of melanoma. Ann Surg 186:481, 1977
21. Kaplan EL, Meier P: Nonparametric estimation from incomplete observations. J Am Stat Assoc 53:457, 1958
22. Karakousis CP, Seddiq MK, Moore R: Prognostic value of lymph node dissection in malignant melanoma. Arch Surg 115:719, 1980
23. Little JH: Histology and prognosis in cutaneous malignant melanoma. In McCarthy WH (ed): Melanoma and Skin Cancer, p 107. Sydney, Blight, 1972
24. McGovern VJ, Mihm MC Jr, Bailly C, Booth JC, Clark WH Jr, Cochran AJ, Hardy EG, Hicks JD, Levene A, Lewis MG, Little JH, Milton GW: The classification of malignant melanoma and its histologic reporting. Cancer 32:1446, 1973
25. MacKie RM, Carfrae DC, Cochran AJ: Assessment of prognosis in patients with malignant melanoma. Lancet 2:455, 1972
26. McNeer G, Das Gupta T: Routes of lymphatic spread of malignant melanoma. In Malignant Melanoma. New York, American Cancer Society, 1965
27. Mack TM, personal communication
28. Morton DL, Eilber FR, Weisenburger TH, Liu P-Y: Multimodality therapy of malignant melanoma, skeletal and soft-tissue sarcomas using immunotherapy, chemotherapy, and radiation therapy. In Salmon SE,

Jones SE (eds): Adjuvant Therapy of Cancer III, p 241. New York, Grune & Stratton, 1981

29. Rees WV, Robinson DS, Holmes EC, Morton DL: Altered lymphatic drainage following lymphadenectomy. Cancer 45:3045, 1980

30. Sappey MPC: Traite d'anatomie descriptive. In Anatomie, Physiologie, Pathologie des Vaisseaux Lymphatiques Considéres Chez l'Homme et les Vertebres, 4th ed. Paris, A Delahaye and Lecrosnier, 1888

31. Sugarbaker EV, McBride CM: Melanoma of the trunk: The results of surgical excision and anatomic guidelines for predicting nodal metastasis. Surgery 80:22, 1976

FRANKLIN H. SIM
WILLIAM F. TAYLOR
EDWARD T. CREAGAN
JOHN E. WOODS
EDWARD H. SOULE

Melanoma in the Midwestern United States: Experience at the Mayo Clinic

27

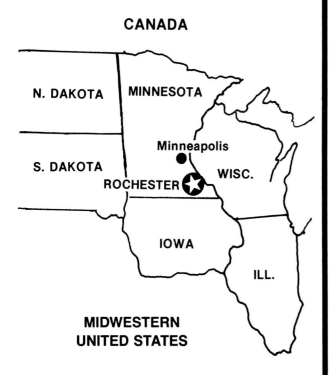

CANADA

N. DAKOTA

MINNESOTA

S. DAKOTA

Minneapolis

ROCHESTER

WISC.

IOWA

ILL.

MIDWESTERN
UNITED STATES

Epidemiology
Prognostic Factors in Melanoma
  Pathologic Features
  Clinical Features
Surgical Treatment of Stage I Patients
  Primary Lesions
  Regional Lymph Node Dissection
Surgical Treatment of Stage II Patients
Nonsurgical Treatment

From 1971 through 1980, 1259 patients were treated for malignant melanoma at the Mayo Clinic (MC), as reported by the Mayo Cancer Patient Data System (MCPDS). The Mayo Clinic is located in Rochester, Minnesota, which has a population of 60,000. It is situated at 44°N, 93°E of Greenwich. Minnesota's state population is over 4 million. The average summer temperature is 69.7°F, and the average winter temperature is 16.1°F. Only 35 days a year (8-year record) have subzero temperatures. Five days have temperatures of 90°F or above. The average date of the first snowfall is September 28, and the average date of the last frost in the spring is May 13. More than 52% of days have sunshine.

For this report, the MC has analyzed the MCPDS data, which have been augmented by special data on level of invasion, tumor thickness, and growth patterns. In many instances, the first biopsy was done elsewhere, and the pathologic data were not available. The referral area for the MC patients with melanoma is widespread geographically, but 90% of the MC patients come from Minnesota and the surrounding six-state area (Illinois, Wisconsin, South Dakota, Iowa, Nebraska, and Michigan). The patients were primarily Caucasians with a mixed ethnic background, although a high proportion of these were of German or Scandinavian descent.

EPIDEMIOLOGY

The incidence of malignant melanoma of the skin in the population of Rochester, Minnesota, was studied through use of a countywide diagnostic indexing system at the Mayo Clinic.[8] Within the 25-year period from 1950 to 1974, 42 cases of melanoma of the skin were found in the resident population (Table 27-3). The mean annual incidence rate was 4.0 per 100,000 among males and 3.9 per 100,000 among females. The standardized rate adjusted to the age structure of the United States 1950 population for comparison with the Third National Cancer Survey was 4.2 for the total population (4.5 for males, 4.1 for females). This was similar to other locations in the United States at the approximate latitude of Rochester. The incidence rates for males increased steadily with age. The relationship between age and incidence was less clear for females. Six of the 19 (32%) skin melanomas in male patients were on the limbs as compared with 14 of 23 (61%) among female patients. This difference is marginally significant (p = 0.056). The incidence of cutaneous mela-

noma was determined for three approximately equal periods in order to examine trends in time (Table 27-4). Unlike reports from other studies, no significant change in incidence rate during the 25 years from 1950 to 1974 was detected in Rochester. Probability of survival for 5 years after diagnosis was 0.66, compared with 0.9 expected (relative survival, 73%). At 10 years, it was 0.49, compared with 0.81 expected (relative survival, 60%).

PROGNOSTIC FACTORS IN MELANOMA

Prognostic factors were examined for 777 stage I patients and 209 stage II patients (Table 27-1). Most of the patients with stage II disease received their initial melanoma treatment elsewhere, and the number of positive nodes was not known, so a detailed prognostic factors analysis could not be performed.

PATHOLOGIC FEATURES

The superficial spreading growth pattern was more than three times as common as the nodular growth pattern. Lentigo maligna was relatively rare (see Table 27-1). In those patients in whom the level of invasion was known, level IV melanomas were the most frequent occurrence (41% of patients). The majority of melanomas were thin (60% were 1.5 mm or less), while only a small minority (8%) were very thick (4 mm or more, some exceeding 10 mm). Ulceration was not evaluated. Five-year survival rates for patients with stage I melanoma are shown in Table 27-2. The strongest association was noted between survival and thickness of the lesion; shorter survival occurred with thicker lesions. The level of invasion was also significantly associated with survival, but not as strongly as thickness.

CLINICAL FEATURES

All patients were adults (age 20 to 79 years; median, 51 years) and half were women. The four primary lesion sites (upper and lower extremities, trunk, head, and neck) were nearly equally represented, the frequency varying from 20% to 29% (see Table 27-1). Patients with head and neck involvement had a considerably poorer survival than those with lesions on the trunk or extremities, while men had only a slightly shorter survival than women (see Table 27-2).

Thus, aside from thickness and level of inva-

TABLE 27–1
CLINICAL AND PATHOLOGIC DATA FOR MELANOMA PATIENTS TREATED AT MAYO CLINIC

Characteristics	Presenting Pathologic Stage	
	Stage I	Stage II
Clinical		
Number of Patients	777	209
Median age	51 yr	54 yr
Sex		
Male	50%	52%
Female	50%	48%
Primary lesion site		
Female lower extremity	22%	12%
Male lower extremity	6%	
Female upper extremity	12%	15%
Male upper extremity	8%	
Female head and neck	9%	23%
Male head and neck	14%	
Female trunk	9%	29%
Male trunk	20%	
Other		21%
Pathologic		
Breslow's tumor thickness		
<0.76 mm	35%	8%
0.76 mm–1.49 mm	25%	16%
1.50 mm–2.49 mm	20%	28%
2.50 mm–3.99 mm	13%	26%
≥4.00 mm	8%	21%
Median tumor thickness	1.2 mm	2.4 mm
Level of invasion		
II	23%	4%
III	34%	19%
IV	41%	64%
V	2%	13%
Growth pattern		
Nodular	21%	49%
Superficial spreading	74%	50%
Lentigo maligna	5%	1%

sion, there was little variation when the data were subgrouped by other available clinical or pathologic features. This may result in part from restricting the analysis to stage I patients, for whom survival is generally good. Additional studies are under way.

SURGICAL TREATMENT OF STAGE I PATIENTS

PRIMARY LESION

Because of the dogma passed down in the literature that incisional or punch biopsies might increase the hazard of metastatic spread or local recurrence, an excisional biopsy has been favored. However, no one has clearly documented that incisional biopsies actually increase this hazard. However, an excisional biopsy is performed at the MC so that the pathologist has the entire specimen for representative sampling.

The primary lesion is generally excised with a 5-cm margin, including the deep muscular fascia. The excision is usually an elliptical one made along an axis oriented toward the regional lymphatic flow 8 cm or 10 cm proximally. However, the concept of arbitrary wide margins may not be justified for all melanomas.

Lesions of the head and neck that are 1.5 mm or less in thickness are excised with margins of 1.5 cm to 2 cm, with perhaps a larger margin longitudinally in an ellipse extending toward the area drained by lymph nodes. Lesions thicker than 1.5 mm are excised with margins of 1.5 cm to 3 cm when facial features allow, except on the scalp, where margins of up to 4 cm may be achieved in thick lesions.

TABLE 27–2
ACTUARIAL SURVIVAL DATA FOR MELANOMA PATIENTS TREATED AT MAYO CLINIC

	Survival Rate
Stage I	5-Year
Overall survival	83%
Sex	
Male	80%
Female	87%
Primary lesion site	
Lower extremity	86%
Upper extremity	91%
Head and neck	70%
Trunk	84%
Tumor thickness	
<0.76 mm	98%
0.76 mm–1.49 mm	93%
1.50 mm–2.49 mm	78%
2.50 mm–3.99 mm	61%
≥4.00 mm	45%
Level of invasion	
I and II	98%
III	89%
IV	77%
V	—

Excision is usually performed well into the subcutaneous tissue for lesions less than 0.76 mm in thickness that are over the distribution of the facial nerve and in other instances is carried down to fascia, muscle, or periosteum.

Lesions on the hands and feet may pose specific problems. While the margin of excision will necessarily be smaller, closure of the defect may need to be modified to include a rotation flap in order to provide weight-bearing function and sensation. Patients who have melanomas of the digits are treated by ray resection.

REGIONAL LYMPH NODE DISSECTION

Since the preliminary analysis of the MC prospective randomized study[9] showed no significant benefit to the patient from immediate or delayed lymphadenectomy in the trunk and extremities, the regional nodes in these areas are now treated expectantly, and a therapeutic dissection is performed at the earliest suspicion of node involvement (see Chap. 8 for additional discussion). Although the MC study and a similar study by the World Health Organization Melanoma Group[10] suggested that this was the best approach, because the issue remains unsettled without a clear consensus of opinion, a national prospective study on a larger number of patients should be encouraged so that firm treatment guidelines can be established.

Unlike the surgical policy with respect to melanomas on the trunk and extremity, elective lymph node dissection (ELND) is commonly performed when melanomas involve the head and neck. These ELND are usually performed for melanomas exceeding 0.75 mm in thickness, especially when they are immediately over a node-bearing area or within 4 cm to 5 cm of such an area. For lesions greater than 3 mm in thickness, even if they are situated more than 5 cm from regional nodes, ELND is performed if the lymphatic drainage site is predictable. ELND is not performed for lesions within 3 cm of the midline. In our experience, the morbidity with such procedures in the head and neck region is extremely low.

For lesions draining to the parotid region, a superficial parotidectomy and excision of only the upper jugular nodes is performed; further cervical node dissection is considered only if the upper nodes are clinically positive. It has been the MC experience that with melanoma of the facial area draining to the neck, if the upper neck nodes are negative, skip nodes or positive nodes lower in the neck are extremely uncommon.

Currently, modified radical cervical dissections are usually performed at the MC even when cervical nodes contain detectable metastases, as long as they are small (i.e., <2 cm). For more advanced nodal disease, a classic radical cervical dissection is used.

SURGICAL TREATMENT OF STAGE II PATIENTS

Patients with clinically suspicious regional nodes undergo a therapeutic lymph node dissection. This early detection of clinically suspicious nodes, as advocated by the World Health Organization Melanoma Group, may be an important factor in improving outcome compared with situations in which patients present with advanced nodal disease, especially with multiple nodes involved. In the prospective randomized study involving lymphadenectomy,[9] 12 of the 62 patients whose nodes were left intact subsequently required therapeutic lymphadenectomy. Of this group, six are long-term survivors.

Patients with local recurrences involving an extremity are considered for regional perfusion with chemotherapy or innovative regimens involving hyperthermia. Although these investigational ap-

TABLE 27–3
INCIDENCE OF MALIGNANT MELANOMA OF THE SKIN IN ROCHESTER, MINNESOTA, 1950 THROUGH 1974, BY AGE AND SEX

Age (Yr)	Number of Cases			Average Annual Incidence Per 100,000 Population		
	Total	Male	Female	Total	Male	Female
0–19	5	1	4	1.2	0.5	1.9
20–39	9	3	6	2.9	2.2	3.4
40–59	16	7	9	7.8	7.5	8.0
60 +	12	8	4	8.8	15.5	4.7
Total	42	19	23	4.0	4.0	3.9

(Resseguie LJ, Marks SJ, Winkelmann RK, Kurland LT: Malignant melanoma in the resident population of Rochester, Minnesota. Mayo Clin Proc 52:191, 1977)

TABLE 27–4
DISTRIBUTION OF CASES OF MALIGNANT MELANOMA OF THE SKIN OVER TIME

Years	Crude Incidence Per 100,000 Person-Years	Observed Number	Expected Number* for Age and Sex Composition of Population
1950–1958	4.4	13	12.2
1959–1966	3.5	12	13.1
1967–1974	4.0	17	16.6

*Calculated by applying the age- and sex-specific incidence rates of Table 27-3 to the age and sex composition of the population for each time period. The assumption is that there was no secular trend in incidence.

proaches have produced some tumor regression, they have technical limitations and attendant morbidity. Perhaps more important, randomized trials of regional therapy have provided no evidence of enhanced survival. In a noninvestigational setting, local excision of the local recurrence or intransit lesions has been performed without concomitant regional or systemic chemotherapy. Usually the regional lymph nodes are excised as well. For the patient in whom multiple local recurrences cannot technically be removed, systemic therapy or radiation therapy is recommended.

NONSURGICAL TREATMENT

During the past decade, 647 patients with advanced melanoma have been treated in 26 prospective clinical drug trials of single agents, multiple drugs, and additive hormonal therapies. Only 19 patients (3%) demonstrated some objective regression from treatment, with a median survival of approximately 5 months from the onset of therapy. Almost all of these patients received no prior chemotherapy. The relative futility of secondary chemotherapy in our experience is consistent with the findings from other

centers. Among single agents in the MC studies, methyl-CCNU as a primary therapy produced a response rate of 26% (5/19).[1] Among similarly treated patients, the combinations of dacarbazine with either methyl-CCNU or vincristine achieved response rates of 28% and 21%, respectively.[2,3] The responses were characteristically transient and made little, if any, substantive impact on survival. The combination vinblastine-bleomycin-cisplatin has recently been evaluated because of data from other investigators[7] indicating a response rate of 72%. However, among 18 MC patients (17 without prior chemotherapy), a response rate of only 11% was achieved coincident with substantial gastrointestinal and hematologic toxicity.[4]

In light of these disappointing results, every reasonable effort should be made to enroll patients into phase II studies of potentially promising agents. However, this option is realistically not viable for all patients. When standard treatment is employed, dacarbazine or a nitrosourea may offer some possibility of palliation, although this is infrequent. Objective response rates are approximately 15% to 20% for either dacarbazine or a nitrosourea. Methyl-CCNU offers some advantage over dacarbazine, since the former can be conveniently administered on a 1-day oral schedule every 6 weeks whereas dacarbazine is usually administered intravenously on a 5-day schedule each month.

Currently at the MC, all patients with stage I primary lesions thicker than 1.5 mm and also patients with nodal involvement are considered for randomized clinical trials involving megestrol acetate versus observation. In the overall group, 209 patients had stage II disease. However, most had been treated elsewhere, and the sample size was too small for survival analysis at present. Patients with measurable, biopsy-proven advanced melanoma can participate in a phase II study of recombinant leukocyte A interferon.

Melanoma generally has been considered not to be radiosensitive. This impression was confirmed in a clinical trial conducted at the MC in which patients treated with irradiation for either gross or residual melanoma involving the head and neck had no therapeutic advantage over patients described in the literature with comparable lesions treated only with surgical excision.

The radiation dose was 5000 rad administered by split-course technique (2500 rad given in 15 fractions), each separated by a 3-week rest interval.[5] Although results from some clinical studies, including the one from the MC, have been disappointing, experimental data indicate that melanoma cells are not inherently radioresistant. A dose of 600 rad/week for 6 weeks is now considered for the palliation of osseous or soft-tissue metastatic disease. For patients with disease of the central nervous system or lesions contiguous with radiosensitive viscera, a dose of 600 rad/week for 4 weeks is considered.

A prospective randomized clinical trial (5000 rad administered by split-course technique) involving adjuvant radiation therapy has also been evaluated in 56 stage II melanoma patients.[6] Although the initial results appeared to show some survival benefit from adjuvant radiation therapy, the final statistical analysis demonstrated that radiation to the resected area of regional nodes conferred no real advantage after the impact of age, sex, and number of involved lymph nodes was accounted for.

REFERENCES

1. Ahmann DL: Nitrosoureas in the management of disseminated malignant melanoma. Cancer Treat Rep 60:747, 1976
2. Ahmann DL, Bisel HF, Edmonson JH, Hahn RG, Eagan RT, O'Connell MJ, Frytak S: Clinical comparison of Adriamycin and a combination of methyl-CCNU and imidazole carboxamide in disseminated malignant melanoma. Clin Pharmacol Ther 19:821, 1976
3. Ahmann DL, Hahn RG, Bisel HF: Evaluation of 1-(2-chloroethyl-3-4-methyl-cyclohexyl)-1-nitrosourea (methyl-CCNU, NSC 95441) versus combined imidazole carboxamide (NSC 45388) and vincristine (NSC 67574) in palliation of disseminated malignant melanoma. Cancer 33:615, 1974
4. Creagan ET, Ahmann DL, Schutt AJ, Green SJ: Phase II study of the combination of vinblastine, bleomycin, and cisplatin in advanced malignant melanoma. Cancer Treat Rep 66:567, 1982
5. Creagan ET, Cupps RE, Ivins JC, Pritchard DJ, Sim FH, Soule EH, O'Fallon JR: Adjuvant radiation therapy for regional nodal metastases from malignant melanoma: A randomized, prospective study. Cancer 42:2206, 1978
6. Creagan ET, Woods JE, Cupps RE, O'Fallon JR: Radiation therapy for malignant melanoma of the head and neck. Am J Surg 138:604, 1979
7. Nathanson L, Kaufman SD, Carey RW: Vinblastine-bleomycin-platinum (VBD): A high response rate regimen in metastatic melanoma. Proc Am Soc Clin Oncol 21:479, 1980
8. Resseguie LJ, Marks SJ, Winkelmann RK, Kurland LT: Malignant melanoma in the resident population of Rochester, Minnesota. Mayo Clin Proc 52:191, 1977
9. Sim FH, Taylor WF, Ivins JC, Pritchard DJ, Soule EH: A prospective randomized study of the efficacy of routine elective lymphadenectomy in management of malignant melanoma: Preliminary results. Cancer 41:948, 1978
10. Veronesi U, Adamus J, Bandiera DC, Brennhovd IO, Caceres E, Cascinelli N, Claudio F, Ikonopisov RL, Javorskj VV, Kirov S, Kulakowski A, Lacour J, Lejeune F, Mechl Z, Morabito A, Rodé I, Sergeev S, van Slooten E, Szczygiel K, Trapenznikov NN, Wagner RI: Inefficacy of immediate node dissection in stage I melanoma of the limbs. N Engl J Med 297:627, 1977

ARTHUR J. SOBER
CALVIN L. DAY, Jr.
HOWARD K. KOH
ROBERT A. LEW
MARTIN C. MIHM, Jr.
ALFRED W. KOPF
THOMAS B. FITZPATRICK

Melanoma in the Northeastern United States: Experience of the Melanoma Clinical Cooperative Group

28

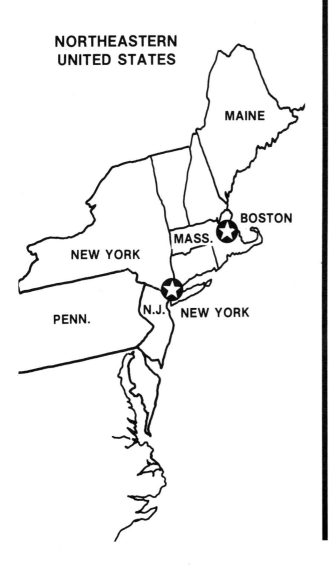

NORTHEASTERN
UNITED STATES

The results described in this chapter represent a special prospective study of 634 patients conducted by the Melanoma Clinical Cooperative Group (MCCG) from 1972 to 1977 at two of its member institutions: Massachusetts General Hospital, Boston, Massachusetts, and New York University Medical Center, New York, New York.

Boston (42°N) is a seaport located on the Atlantic Ocean with a total population of 2.6 million. New York City (40°N), encompassing 505 square kilometers, has a total population of 9.5 million. It is also located on the Atlantic seacoast. Both cities have four changes of season, with temperatures ranging from 0°F to 100°F. The inhabitants of Boston and New York derive primarily from immigrants from England, Ireland, Italy, and Eastern Europe. By surname, patients in both our series are heavily weighted toward persons of Celtic, Italian, and Jewish extraction, with less than 2% of patients having Hispanic or Oriental surnames. Boston has a substantial black and Hispanic community that exceeds 10% of the population. New York City has an even larger black and Hispanic community.

Patients enrolled in these two series were initially referred from a relatively wide metropolitan area because of the established reputations of each institution. As greater local publicity about the study was achieved, community physicians, especially dermatologists, referred patients directly to pigmented lesion clinics that had been established at each institution to provide comprehensive care for melanoma patients and to study the disease in a prospective manner.

The major goal of the MCCG was to evaluate the natural history and developmental biology of cutaneous melanoma. To achieve this aim best, patients were enrolled in the study within 30 days of the diagnosis. No patient was enrolled in the study unless sufficient histopathologic materials were available. All patients in the series had invasive disease, while those with *in situ* melanomas were excluded. In most cases (in all when the primary tumor was removed at New York University Medical Center [NYU] or the Massachusetts General Hospital [MGH]), serially sectioned blocks of the primary tumor were available for study. In approximately half of the cases at each institution, the primary tumors were still present on initial examination. All histopathology was reviewed by a single dermatopathology fellow (C.L.D.) and a single pathologist (M.C.M.). The vast majority of patients enrolled in this study had clinical stage I melanoma

(94%). The bulk of this data analysis has therefore been confined to this stage (Tables 28-1 and 28-2).

Because this is a specialized prospective study, it is heavily weighted toward stage I melanoma. However, it is thought to be reasonably representative of early melanoma for this region. Major efforts were directed at maintaining adequate follow-up on this group. To date only one of 234 cases followed at MGH has been lost, and 32 of 400 from NYU, giving an overall lost to follow-up rate of 5%.

EPIDEMIOLOGY

During the enrollment period of the MCCG from 1972 to 1977, there were no population-based tumor registries in either New York or Massachusetts to give accurate melanoma incidence figures for this region. However, the Connecticut Tumor Registry, located geographically between the two areas of enrollment, continuously monitored melanoma incidence in that state. Connecticut Tumor Registry data for 1980 indicate an incidence rate for invasive melanoma of approximately 9×10^5 a year for Caucasians.

We did not record ethnic origins of the patient population, having been advised at the outset by epidemiologists at Harvard School of Public Health that meaningful data on ethnic origin is nearly impossible to obtain. The present series is composed almost entirely of Caucasians currently living in the northeastern United States. Ninety-four percent of patients in the MGH portion of the study were residents of Massachusetts, 4% were residents of other New England states, and a few were from outside the Northeast. Ninety-eight percent of patients in the NYU series were residents of New York or New Jersey. Sex ratio was near unity throughout the period of study (318 men, 316 women).[19] Eye color and hair color on a subset of the overall group were compared with a control group of friends of similar age (± 5 years) and sex (Table 28-3). Thirty-three percent of patients had blond or red hair and 36% had blue eyes. No statistical differences were noted between cases and controls for eye or hair color.

PROGNOSTIC FACTORS IN STAGE I MELANOMA

Analysis of the MCCG data has depended heavily on the use of multivariate analysis.[3,4] In each of these

(Text continues on page 441)

TABLE 28–1
CLINICAL AND PATHOLOGIC DATA FOR MELANOMA PATIENTS TREATED BY THE MELANOMA CLINICAL COOPERATIVE GROUP

Characteristics	Presenting Clinical Stage			
	Stage I	Stage II	Stage III	Total
Clinical				
Number of patients	598	33*	3	634
Year of diagnosis				
1972–1977	100%	100%	100%	100%
Median age	50 yr	51 yr	71 yr	50 yr
Sex				
Male	49%	70%	67%	50%
Female	51%	30%	33%	50%
Primary lesion site				
Female lower extremity	20%	3%	33%	19%
Male lower extremity	6%	9%	0%	6%
Female upper extremity	10%	6%	0%	10%
Male upper extremity	8%	3%	0%	8%
Female head and neck	5%	6%	0%	5%
Male head and neck	8%	15%	0%	8%
Female trunk	16%	15%	0%	16%
Male trunk	27%	43%	67%	28%
Other	0%	0%	0%	0%
Pathologic				
Breslow's tumor thickness				
<0.76 mm	28%	6%	0%	26%
0.76 mm–1.49 mm	30%	12%	0%	30%
1.50 mm–2.49 mm	17%	6%	33%	17%
2.50 mm–3.99 mm	13%	18%	0%	13%
≥4.00 mm	12%	58%	67%	14%
MCCG thickness criteria				
<0.85 mm	34%	6%	0%	32%
0.85 mm–1.69 mm	28%	12%	0%	27%
1.70 mm–3.64 mm	25%	15%	33%	25%
≥3.65 mm	13%	67%	67%	16%
Median tumor thickness	1.3 mm	4.5 mm	5.0 mm	1.3 mm
Level of invasion				
II	25%	9%	0%	24%
III	33%	12%	0%	32%
IV	35%	49%	67%	36%
V	7%	30%	33%	8%
Ulceration				
Yes	31%	76%	33%	33%
No	69%	24%	67%	67%
Growth pattern				
Nodular	15%	27%	0%	16%
Superficial spreading	71%	58%	100%	71%
Lentigo maligna	4%	0%	0%	4%
Acral lentiginous and				
unclassified	10%	15%	0%	10%
Microscopic satellites				
Yes	16%			
No	84%			

*Five patients had histologically negative nodes.

TABLE 28–2
ACTUARIAL SURVIVAL DATA FOR MELANOMA PATIENTS TREATED BY THE MELANOMA CLINICAL COOPERATIVE GROUP

	Survival Rates	
	5-Year	7-Year
Stage I		
Overall survival	85%	82%
Sex		
Male	81%	75%
Female	90%	87%
Primary lesion site		
Lower extremity	92%	88%
Upper extremity	89%	86%
Head and neck	82%	74%
Trunk	80%	78%
Both extremities		
except hands and feet	95%	92%
Hands and feet	63%	58%
Tumor thickness		
< 0.76 mm	99%	99%
0.76 mm–1.49 mm	95%	94%
1.50 mm–2.49 mm	84%	77%
2.50 mm–3.99 mm	70%	51%
≥ 4.00 mm	44%	39%
MCCG tumor thickness intervals		
< 0.85 mm	99%	99%
0.85 mm–1.69 mm	94%	93%
1.70 mm–3.64 mm	78%	66%
≥ 3.65 mm	42%	38%
Level of invasion		
II	99%	99%
III	95%	91%
IV	75%	69%
V	39%	34%
Ulceration		
Yes	68%	63%
No	93%	90%
Microscopic satellites		
Yes	52%	42%
No	91%	89%

	1-Year	3-Year	5-Year
Clinical Stage II (33 patients)*			
Overall survival	73%	52%	30%
Tumor thickness			
< 1.50 mm (6 patients)	83%	67%	50%
1.50 mm–3.99 mm (8 patients)	75%	63%	50%
≥ 4.00 mm (19 patients)	68%	42%	16%
Ulceration			
Yes (25 patients)	68%	48%	24%
No (8 patients)	88%	63%	50%
Clinical Stage I,			
Pathologic Stage II (46 patients)			
Overall survival			42%[†]
Tumor thickness			
≤ 3.5 mm			59%[†]
> 3.5 mm			22%[†]
Number of positive nodes			
1–3			48%[†]
≥ 4			17%[†]
Ulceration			
Yes			41%[†]
No			46%[†]

*Five patients had histopathologic negative nodes.
[†]Disease-free survival

TABLE 28–3
HAIR AND EYE COLOR FOR 111 MELANOMA PATIENTS AND 107 CONTROLS

	Patients (%)	Controls (%)
Hair Color		
Black	5	6
Dark brown	31	41
Light brown	32	33
Blond	21	15
Red	12	6
Eye Color		
Blue	36	37
Brown	20	32
Green	15	13
Hazel	29	18

TABLE 28–4
FACTORS STUDIED IN MULTIVARIATE ANALYSES OF PROGNOSIS BY THE MELANOMA CLINICAL COOPERATIVE GROUP*

Clinical Variables
  Sex
  Age
  Location of primary lesion
  Adjuvant therapy
  Surgical treatment (wide local excision only versus wide local excision and elective regional lymph node dissection)

Histologic Variables
  Histologic type
  Level of invasion (Clark)
  Thickness (Breslow)
  Ulceration width determined histologically
  Mitotic rate
  Lymphocytic response
  Histologic regression
  Microscopic satellites
  Pathologic stage

Regional Node Variables
  Number of positive nodes
  Node metastases size (mm)
  Percentage positive nodes

*Not all factors were used in all analyses.

studies, between 13 and 15 clinical and histopathologic variables were studied simultaneously for their possible effect on prognosis (listed in Table 28-4). While many of these factors correlate with prognosis when studied as single variables, some are simply alternative ways of measuring the same phenomenon. The multivariate analysis tends to select complementary factors. Thus, in selecting a set of prognostic factors, a factor that correlates with prognosis, such as level of invasion, will be eliminated by a factor that more strongly correlates (*e.g.,* thickness), since both factors reflect tumor volume.

PATIENT FACTORS

These studies suggested that once thickness was controlled, anatomical subsite of the primary lesion was the second most important factor in determining outcome (Table 28-5).[8,9,12,14,15,16] The effect of location on prognosis in melanoma has traditionally been studied as follows: (1) axial versus extremity; (2) head and neck versus trunk versus extremities; or

(3) head and neck versus trunk versus upper extremity versus lower extremity. A multivariate analysis of melanoma prognostic factors indicated that these location groupings do not accurately reflect the differences in regional behavior of this neoplasm.[5] Rather, the risk of metastases and death varies by "subsites" within each of the above broad location groupings even after correcting for the dominant prognostic variable in clinical stage I melanoma; namely, primary tumor thickness. The subsite concept for metastases in clinical stage I melanoma is based on the following clinical observations: (1) patients with melanomas located on the

TABLE 28–5
PROBABILITY OF DEATH FROM CLINICAL STAGE I MELANOMA AT INTERVALS OF 2.5 YEARS AFTER DIAGNOSIS BY PRIMARY TUMOR THICKNESS*

Tumor Thickness	Number of Patients	Percent Dead		
		2.5 Years	5 Years	7.5 Years
< 0.85 mm	190	1%	1%	1%
0.85 mm–1.69 mm	178	3%	6%	7%
1.70 mm–3.64 mm	151	12%	24%	31%
≥ 3.65 mm	79	43%	59%	62%

* Determined by life-table analysis of 598 clinical stage I patients from the Massachusetts General Hospital and New York University Medical Center.

scalp, the posterior neck, and the lateral neck have worse prognoses than those patients with equally thick lesions located on the face and anterior neck[5]; (2) patients with melanomas of the upper trunk of the same thickness have worse prognoses than those whose tumor is located on the lower trunk[5]; (3) patients with lesions located on the hands and feet have worse prognoses than those patients with melanomas of equal thickness located on the thigh, leg, arm, and forearm.[5] The difference in prognosis between a highly favorable site, such as the extremities, excluding hands and feet (95% 5-year survival), and that noted for hands and feet (63% 5-year survival), is striking (see Table 28-2). While these observations are highly significant in the MCCG patients, confirmation in other series will be necessary to determine the general practicality of this concept. When multivariate analysis was used, neither sex nor age appeared to be important in the models, since both were replaced by subsite. Location on the extremities appears to account for the more favorable overall prognosis noted for women, while the

relatively less favorable prognosis noted with age can be accounted for in part by a disproportionately higher percentage of lesions on hands and feet occurring in older persons.[14]

Overall subsite distribution was different in men and women (Fig. 28-1). The back was by far the most frequent site in men (34%), with relative sparing of the lower extremities (13%). In women, the lower leg was most frequently involved (39%), while the back was still a common site (23%); the abdomen was usually spared.

For superficial spreading melanoma, which represented 71% of the tumors, there was a direct correlation of increasing mean age with increasing level of invasion (42 years for level II, 57 years for level V).[23]

PATHOLOGIC FACTORS

As in other series, thickness was the dominant variable determining progress. Not only did thickness correlate directly with likelihood of death, but it also

FIG. 28–1 Anatomical distribution of primary cutaneous melanoma by sex (Courtesy Melanoma Clinical Cooperative Group).

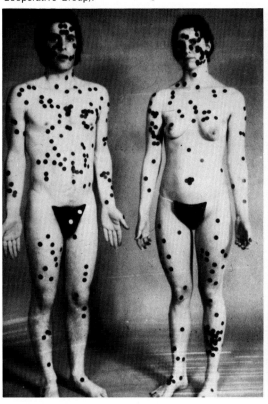
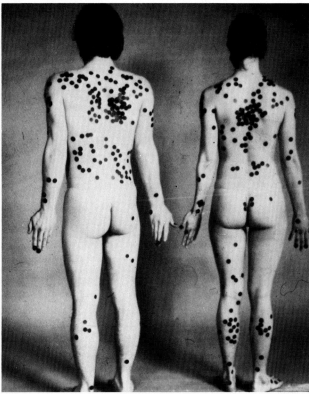

seemed to correlate with rate of death. There appeared to be an inverse relationship between thickness and time to death; those patients with the thickest tumors die soonest.[13,20,21] One half of patients with level V tumors were dead within 24 months of diagnosis, whereas among persons free of disease after 5 years of follow-up, only patients in the intermediate thickness category, 1.70 mm to 3.64 mm, died from melanoma (see Table 28-6).[13] Hence, the concept that 5-year survival is roughly equivalent to cure may not be valid for this subgroup.

Various groups have used different thickness ranges to assess prognosis. The findings of the MCCG group indicated that the risk of death did not change in an exactly linear pattern with thickness, but moved upward in a stair-step pattern marked by breakpoints where risk increased more rapidly.[7] A computer algorithm designed to select those breakpoints in which risks accelerated significantly could delineate four thickness intervals: < 0.85 mm, 0.85 mm to 1.69 mm, 1.70 mm to 3.64 mm, and ≥ 3.65 mm. Since these four groups differ somewhat from those set out by Breslow, we have presented our data using both these and the Breslow intervals for comparison (see Table 28-1). Similar analyses on several pooled series would be of interest to determine the possibility of establishing "universal" values that would best divide the data for all groups.

In this series, there was a close correlation between level of invasion and prognosis (see Table 28-2). Overall, levels of invasion were nearly as valuable as thickness in determining prognosis. However, level III patients can be subdivided further according to thickness into two groups, one with low and one with intermediate-to-high risk.

There was also a very close correlation between ulceration and prognosis; this feature complemented the significance of thickness in the prognostic analyses. In this series, ulceration width was more useful than simply noting the presence or absence of an ulcer.[6] Patients with tumors having ulcer widths ≤ 3 mm had no worse prognosis than patients with nonulcerated tumors, while those with tumors having ulcer widths > 3 mm had substantially worse prognoses.[6]

The MCCG has also pointed out the prognostic significance of *microscopic satellites* (presence of discrete tumor nests > 0.05 mm in diameter that are separated from the main body of tumor by normal reticular dermal collagen or subcutaneous fat).[6] In this series, the 5-year survival was 52% when microscopic satellites were present and 91% when they were absent. For patients with level IV tumors, this was an additional prognostic factor. In this series, microscopic satellites added more to thickness in prognostic value than did ulceration.

Several prognostic factors appear to be highly intercorrelated; namely, ulceration, microscopic satellites, and mitotic rates. The dominant factor appearing in any particular analysis varied from subgroup to subgroup.

In many instances, significant prognostic information could be obtained from the gross examination of the primary tumor. If the patient has perceived an increase in the height of his tumor, the tumor is most likely level III or greater (36% frequency level II versus 60% level III to V) and less likely to be < 0.85 mm (36% versus 51% to 82% for lesions ≥ 0.85 mm).[22,23] Patients with tumors displaying plaquelike configurations had highly favorable prognosis (metastatic rate of 11% at 7.5 years), whereas those with major ulceration clinically (> 80% of surface) had a very poor prognosis (metastatic rate 85% at 7.5 years).[11] Nodule location (central or marginal; 33% versus 66% metastatic

TABLE 28-6
PROBABILITY OF DEATH FROM CLINICAL STAGE I MELANOMA IN THE FIRST 7.5 YEARS AFTER DIAGNOSIS BY PRIMARY TUMOR LOCATION AND THICKNESS*

Tumor Thickness	BANS[†]	Non-BANS Locations			
		Extremities[‡]	Hands and Feet	Head and Neck	Trunk
< 0.85 mm	2%	0%	0%	0%	0%
0.85 mm–1.69 mm	22%	0%	0%	0%	3%
1.70 mm–3.64 mm	42%	14%	40%	36%	23%
≥ 3.65 mm	67%	17%	100%	35%	78%

* Determined by life-table analysis of 598 clinical stage I patients from the Massachusetts General Hospital and New York University Medical Center.

† BANS = upper back, posterolateral arm, posterior and lateral neck, and posterior scalp.

‡ excluding hands and feet.

rates at 7.5 years respectively) and nodule diameter were also of prognostic consequence.[11]

Surprisingly, in the present data primary tumor thickness was still the major determinant of prognosis in patients with microscopic nodal metastases (clinical stage I, pathologic stage II).[17] Primary tumor thickness ≤ 3.5 mm and less than four metastatic nodes (or less than 20% of involved nodes) had a 5-year disease-free survival of 80%, whereas for primary tumors > 3.5 mm had the 5-year disease-free survival was about 20%.

SURVIVAL RATES

Survival rates by stages can be seen in Table 28-2. Overall 5-year survival for clinical stage I melanoma was quite high (85%). Since approximately 60% of this series was composed of low-risk patients (5-year survival 95% or greater), the overall favorable prognosis is not surprising. In spite of this relatively favorable prognosis, the subgroup of clinical stage I patients with primary tumors ≥ 3.65 mm in thickness has a 5-year survival of only 42%.

It is vital to distinguish between patients with microscopic nodal metastases (clinical stage I, pathologic stage II) and those with macroscopic disease (clinical stage II, pathologic stage II). These two groups should be analyzed separately to compare results accurately. The prognosis at 5 years was somewhat worse for clinical stage II patients (30%) than for clinical stage I, pathologic stage II (42% overall). This difference is increased further, since 5 of 33 clinical stage II patients had negative lymph node dissections and should have been classified as stage I patients. When these five are eliminated, the 1-, 3-, and 5-year survival rates of the remaining 28 clinical stage II, pathologic stage II patients were 68%, 43%, and 18% respectively. The relatively favorable prognosis for clinical stage I, pathologic stage II patients with primary tumors ≤ 3.5 mm and fewer than four nodes or $< 20\%$ of nodes involved has already been discussed. A similar favorable prognosis in a comparable group of patients has also been reported from UCLA.[1]

TREATMENT

The majority of patients in this series were treated by a small group of surgeons at NYU and MGH. These surgeons had previously developed a surgical treatment protocol based on level of invasion of the primary tumor.

MARGINS OF PRIMARY TUMOR EXCISION

For tumor types except lentigo maligna melanoma (LMM), wide local excision of 4 cm to 5 cm down to or including fascia was performed. Split-thickness skin graft closure was used when primary closure was impossible. For LMM, a margin or at least 1 cm was recommended. More recently, we have recommended smaller treatment margins for primary tumors.[2,10] At present, tumors < 0.85 mm in thickness are excised with margins of 1.5 cm and closed primarily when possible. Margins not exceeding 3 cm are used for tumors ≥ 0.85 mm.[10] So far, no increase in the frequency of local recurrence has been detected using these surgical margins.[2]

ELECTIVE REGIONAL LYMPH NODE DISSECTION (ELND)

During the study period (1972–1977), patients for ELND were selected according to level of invasion. These dissections were recommended for patients whose tumors were level III or greater and in whom a single lymph node drainage area could be delineated. Elective nodal dissection was not used for patients with LMM.

Although the MCCG suggested in April, 1979 that patients with melanomas 2 mm to 3.5 mm in thickness might benefit from ELND,[18] subsequent analysis showed no significant differences in survival rates between patients who had an ELND and those who did not, irrespective of the thickness range examined. In addition, ELND was examined as a prognostic factor in all analyses of clinical stage I patients, but it never appeared as an independent variable. As discussed in detail elsewhere, ELND prolongs survival for only 5% to 15% of patients with melanomas of intermediate risk.[9,12] A series much larger than the MCCG one would be required to detect a benefit at the 0.05 level of statistical significance.

At the present time the policy of ELND rests with the individual surgeon, is quite variable, and is based on thickness of the primary tumor. Minimum thickness for consideration of ELND for the MGH group currently ranges from 1.7 mm to 2 mm depending on the surgeon. For patients with truncal melanomas in anatomical locations with potential ambiguous drainage, lymphoscintigraphy has been performed to delineate drainage pathways. In many of these patients, drainage to more than one nodal area was demonstrated, and bilateral ELND were not performed. The current policy on ELND at

NYU is somewhat different from that at MGH, since it is used more liberally. Some surgeons at NYU recommend ELND at 1 mm; most, however, use 1.5 mm as the minimum thickness.

ADJUVANT THERAPY

Adjuvant therapy with BCG and DTIC was evaluated at MGH from 1975 to 1982 for patients with high-risk primary melanoma (level III > 1.5 mm, or level IV or V) and for stage II patients rendered surgically disease-free. This approach seemed beneficial when compared with a control arm of BCG alone.[24] However, since several other series have failed to demonstrate a benefit from this combination, adjuvant therapy is not recommended at the present time.

Supported in part by the National Cancer Institute Grant R-10-CA-13651-01, the Marion Gardner Jackson Trust, NIH Research Training Grant No. 5 T 32 AM 07190-05; National Institute of Occupational Safety and Health Grant No. R01 0H00915; National Cancer Institute Grant No. 2 RIO CA 1366-05; The Rudolf L. Baer Foundation for Diseases of the Skin; the Skin Cancer Foundation; and Department of Energy Grant No. EY-76-C-02-3077.

This is a publication of the Melanoma Clinical Cooperative Group. The following persons are or were members of the Melanoma Clinical Cooperative Group at Massachusetts General Hospital or New York University Medical Center:

REFERENCES

1. Callery C, Cochran AJ, Roe DJ, Rees W, Nathanson SD, Benedetti JK, Elashoff RM, Morton DL: Factors prognostic for survival in patients with malignant melanoma spread to the regional lymph nodes. Ann Surg 196:69, 1982
2. Cosimi AB, Sober AJ, Mihm MC Jr, Fitzpatrick TB: Conservative surgical management of superficially invasive cutaneous melanoma. Cancer 53:1256, 1984
3. Cox DR: Analysis of Binary Data. London, Chapman & Hall, 1970
4. Cox DR: Regression model and life tables. J Royal Stat Soc B34:187, 1972
5. Day CL Jr: Subsite concept for metastases in clinical stage I melanoma. Lancet 2:154, 1982

6. Day CL Jr, Harrist TJ, Gorstein F, Sober AJ, Lew RA, Friedman RJ, Pasternack BS, Kopf AW, Fitzpatrick TB, Mihm MC Jr: Malignant melanoma: Prognostic significance of "microscopic satellites" in the reticular dermis and subcutaneous fat. Ann Surg 194:108, 1981

7. Day CL Jr, Lew RA, Mihm MC Jr, Harris MN, Kopf AW, Sober AJ, Fitzpatrick TB: The natural break points for primary-tumor thickness in clinical stage I melanoma. N Engl J Med 305:1155, 1981

8. Day CL Jr, Lew RA, Mihm MC Jr, Sober AJ, Harris MN, Kopf AW, Fitzpatrick TB, Harrist TJ, Golomb FM, Postel A, Hennessey P, Gumport SL, Raker JW, Malt RA, Cosimi AB, Wood WC, Roses DF, Gorstein F, Rigel D, Friedman RJ, Mintzis MM, Grier WR: A multivariate analysis of prognostic factors for melanoma patients with lesions ≥ 3.65 mm in thickness: The importance of revealing alternative Cox models. Ann Surg 195:44, 1982

9. Day CL Jr, Mihm MC Jr, Lew RA, Harris MN, Kopf AW, Fitzpatrick TB, Harrist TJ, Golomb FM, Postel A, Hennessey P, Gumport SL, Raker JW, Malt RA, Cosimi AB, Wood WC, Roses DF, Gorstein F, Rigel D, Friedman RJ, Mintzis MM, Sober AJ: Prognostic factors for patients with clinical stage I melanoma of intermediate thickness (1.51 mm–3.99 mm): A conceptual model for tumor growth and metastasis. Ann Surg 195:35, 1982

10. Day CL Jr, Mihm MC Jr, Sober AJ, Fitzpatrick TB, Malt RA: Narrower margins for clinical stage I malignant melanoma. N Engl J Med 306:479, 1982

11. Day CL Jr, Mihm MC Jr, Sober AJ, Fitzpatrick TB, Malt RA, Kopf AW, Lew RA, Harrist TJ: Skin lesions suspected to be melanoma should be photographed: Gross morphological features of primary melanoma associated with metastases. JAMA 248:1077, 1982

12. Day CL Jr, Mihm MC Jr, Sober AJ, Harris MN, Kopf AW, Fitzpatrick TB, Lew RA, Harrist TJ, Golomb FM, Postel A, Hennessey P, Gumport SL, Raker JW, Malt RA, Cosimi AB, Wood WC, Roses DF, Gorstein F, Rigel D, Friedman RJ, Mintzis MM: Prognostic factors for melanoma patients with lesions 0.76 mm–1.69 mm in thickness: An appraisal of "thin" level IV lesions. Ann Surg 195:30, 1982

13. Day CL Jr, Mihm MC Jr, Sober AJ, Harris MN, Kopf AW, Fitzpatrick TB, Lew RA, Harrist TJ, Golomb FM, Postel A, Hennessey P, Gumport SL, Raker JW, Malt RA, Cosimi AB, Wood WC, Roses DF, Gorstein F, Rigel D, Friedman RJ, Mintzis MM: Predictors of late deaths among patients with clinical stage I melanoma who have not had bony or visceral metastases within the first five years after diagnosis. J Am Acad Dermatol 8:864, 1983

14. Day CL Jr, Sober AJ, Kopf AW, Lew RA, Mihm MC Jr, Golomb FM, Hennessey P, Harris MN, Gumport SL, Raker JW, Malt RA, Cosimi AB, Wood WC, Roses DF, Gorstein F, Fitzpatrick TB, Postel A: A prognostic model for clinical stage I melanoma of the lower extremity: Location on foot as independent risk factor for recurrent disease. Surgery 89:599, 1981

15. Day CL Jr, Sober AJ, Kopf AW, Lew RA, Mihm MC Jr, Golomb FM, Postel A, Hennessey P, Harris MN, Gumport SL, Raker JW, Malt RA, Cosimi AB, Wood WC, Roses DF, Gorstein F, Fitzpatrick TB: A prognostic model for clinical stage I melanoma of the trunk: Location near the midline is not an independent risk factor for recurrent disease. Am J Surg 142:247, 1981

16. Day CL Jr, Sober AJ, Kopf AW, Lew RA, Mihm MC Jr, Hennessey P, Golomb F, Harris MN, Gumport SL, Raker JW, Malt RA, Cosimi AB, Wood WC, Roses DF, Gorstein F, Postel A, Grier WR, Mintzis MM, Fitzpatrick TB: A prognostic model for clinical stage I melanoma of the upper extremity: The importance of anatomic subsites in predicting recurrent disease. Ann Surg 193:436, 1981

17. Day CL Jr, Sober AJ, Lew RA, Mihm MC Jr, Fitzpatrick TB, Kopf AW, Harris MN, Gumport SL, Raker JW, Malt RA, Golomb FM, Cosimi AB, Wood WC, Casson P, Lopansri S, Gorstein F, Postel A: Malignant melanoma patients with positive nodes and relatively good prognoses: Microstaging retains prognostic significance in clinical stage I melanoma patients with metastases to regional nodes. Cancer 47:955, 1981

18. Day CL Jr, Sober AJ, Lopansri S, Mihm MC Jr, Kopf AW, Fitzpatrick TB: Primary tumor thickness is the major determinant for recurrence in clinical stage I malignant melanoma patients with histologically positive lymph nodes. Clin Res 27:383A, 1979

19. Sober AJ, Blois MS, Clark WH Jr, Fitzpatrick TB, Kopf AW, Mihm MC Jr: Primary malignant melanoma of the skin—1130 cases from the Melanoma Clinical Cooperative Group. In Proceedings of the XV International Congress of Dermatology, Mexico, October 1977. Amsterdam, Excerpta Medica, 1979

20. Sober AJ, Day CL Jr, Fitzpatrick TB, Lew RA, Kopf AW, Mihm MC Jr: Early death from clinical stage I melanoma. J Invest Dermatol 80:50S, 1983

21. Sober AJ, Day CL Jr, Fitzpatrick TB, Lew RA, Kopf AW, Mihm MC Jr: Factors associated with death from melanoma from 2 to 5 years following diagnosis in clinical stage I patients. J Invest Dermatol 80:53S, 1983

22. Sober AJ, Day CL Jr, Kopf AW, Fitzpatrick TB: Detection of "thin" primary melanomas. CA 33:160, 1983

23. Wick MM, Sober AJ, Fitzpatrick TB, Mihm MC Jr, Kopf AW, Clark WH Jr, Blois MS: Clinical characteristics of early cutaneous melanoma. Cancer 45:2684, 1980

24. Wood WC, Cosimi AB, Carey RW, Kaufman SD: Randomized trial of adjuvant therapy for "high risk" primary malignant melanoma. Surgery 83:677, 1978

NATALE CASCINELLI
MAURIZIO NAVA
MAURIZIO VAGLINI
RAFFAELE MAROLDA
MARIO SANTINAMI
DARIO ROVINI
CLAUDIO CLEMENTE

Melanoma in Italy: Experience at the National Cancer Institute of Milan

29

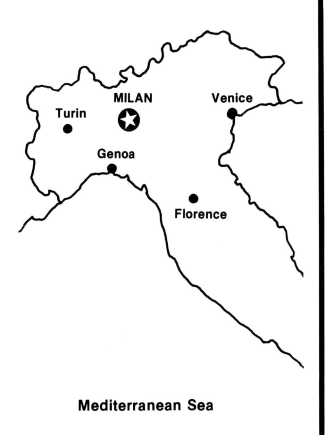

Epidemiology
Prognostic Factors
  Stage I
  Stage II
  Stage III
Treatment
  Stage I
    Primary lesion surgery
    Surgery of regional lymph nodes
    Surgery of local tumor recurrence
  Stage II
    Regional lymph nodes
    Role of adjuvant therapy
    Treatment of intransit metastases
  Distant Metastases

Over 1683 melanoma patients were treated at the National Cancer Institute of Milan (NCIM) between January 1967 and December 1979. Milan is the second largest city in Italy and is situated at 45°N, 9°E of Greenwich. It has a population of 1.7 million. The population density in this highly industrialized part of Italy is 649 inhabitants per square kilometer. Milan has three winter months with an average temperature of 0°C and three summer months with an average temperature of 23°C to 25°C. According to the Meteorologic Observatory of Brera in Milan, the sun shines from a minimum of 8 hours and 42 minutes during the winter to a maximum of 15 hours and 41 minutes during the summer. No information on ethnic groups is available from the Milan area.

Of the entire 1683 patients treated at the NCIM, 70% resided in the Milan area, while the other 30% were referred to the NCIM from all parts of Italy. Fifteen percent of these patients were referred with their melanoma intact, while the remaining patients had had a previous biopsy. A computerized data base of all patients treated at the NCIM has been sorted on the IBM-4331 computer using the MFS-MEDIC System implemented at the NCIM.[12]

EPIDEMIOLOGY

The mortality rate for melanoma in Italy is 1.6×10^5 inhabitants per year according to the latest available data.[1] No differences were observed according to sex. In the north of Italy, a population-based registry collecting epidemiologic data from the Province of Varese (located 50 kilometers from Milan) showed that the death rate per year for melanoma was 1.1×10^5 for men and 1.4×10^5 for women. The observed incidence in 1976 to 1977 was 2.4×10^5 for men and 5.4×10^5 for women.[3]

PROGNOSTIC FACTORS

Of the entire 1683 patients treated at the NCIM, 967 (57%) had localized melanoma (stage I), 566 (34%) had regional lymph node metastases (stage II), and the remaining 150 (9%) had distant metastases (stage III) when first referred for treatment.

A detailed analysis was conducted on a selected group of 282 melanoma patients who met the following criteria: (1) they had not been treated or biopsied before undergoing definitive treatment at the NCIM, and (2) good quality and representative slides of the primary melanoma were available. The patients were otherwise unselected. They were all treated between 1967 and 1979. Review of the pathologic material was performed by a single pathologist, who was unaware of the patient's clinical course.

The use of a selected group may be questionable. However, it was thought more useful to deal with this group of patients, since the distribution by site of origin, age, and sex of this group compared with the total series was very similar and all prognostic criteria were fully evaluable. Distribution by melanoma thickness of the selected group was quite similar to the one reported by the WHO Melanoma Group: the mean melanoma thickness of the WHO patients was 3.6 mm; 24% of patients had a primary less than 1.5 mm in thickness; 29% had a primary more than 4 mm in thickness. This feature was not evaluable for those patients who were treated after excisional biopsy of primary melanoma performed elsewhere, since pathologic slides were not available for the present review. Clinical and pathologic information for the 282 patients who met these requirements is shown in Table 29-1.

STAGE I

The 234 stage I patients had a median age of 49 years. Almost two thirds were women. The most common anatomical sites of the melanomas were the lower extremities in women (36% of patients) and the trunk in men (21%). These melanomas were thinner than in other series, with a median thickness of 3.2 mm, 27% being less than 1.5 mm in thickness (Table 29-1). Fifty-one percent were level III, 52% were ulcerated, and 75% had a superficial spreading growth pattern. No level I melanomas were considered.

With regard to survival, 67% of patients were alive at 5 years and 57% at 10 years. Sex and site of primary tumor were not related to survival at a statistically significant level (Table 29-2), but patients with lower extremity melanomas had by far the best survival rate (Fig. 29-1). Tumor thickness (Fig. 29-2) and level of invasion were significantly correlated with survival. None of the patients with a primary melanoma thinner than 0.76 mm died, while only 30% of patients with thick melanomas (≥ 4 mm) were alive 5 years after surgical treatment ($p = 10^7$). Patients with ulcerated melanomas had a worse prognosis than those with nonulcerated melanomas, but the difference was not statistically sig-

TABLE 29–1
CLINICAL AND PATHOLOGIC DATA FOR MELANOMA PATIENTS TREATED AT THE NATIONAL CANCER INSTITUTE OF MILAN, ITALY (This is a subgroup of the 1683 total patients for whom all data were available)

Characteristics	Presenting Pathologic Stage			
	Stage I	Stage II	Stage III	Total
Clinical				
Number of patients	234	45	3	282
Year of Diagnosis				
≤ 1960	0%	0%	0%	0%
1961–1965	0%	0%	0%	0%
1966–1970	11%	7%	0%	10%
1971–1975	51%	49%	100%	51%
1976–1980	38%	46%	0%	39%
Median age	49yr	49yr	49yr	49yr
Sex				
Male	39%	58%	67%	42%
Female	61%	42%	33%	58%
Primary lesion site				
Female lower extremity	36%	9%	33%	32%
Male lower extremity	11%	13%	0%	11%
Female upper extremity	7%	9%	0%	8%
Male upper extremity	3%	5%	0%	3%
Female head and neck	9%	5%	0%	8%
Male head and neck	3%	16%	33%	5%
Female trunk	9%	20%	0%	10%
Male trunk	21%	24%	33%	22%
Other	2%	0%	0%	2%
Pathologic				
Breslow's tumor thickness				
< 0.76 mm	7%	10%	0%	8%
0.76 mm–1.49 mm	20%	5%	0%	17%
1.50 mm–2.49 mm	20%	13%	0%	20%
2.50 mm–3.99 mm	28%	13%	0%	25%
≥ 4.00 mm	25%	59%	100%	31%
Median tumor thickness	3.2 mm	5.8 mm	7.0 mm	4.0 mm
Level of invasion				
II	12%	7%	0%	11%
III	51%	40%	33%	49%
IV	32%	24%	67%	31%
V	6%	29%	0%	10%
Ulceration				
Yes	52%	66%	100%	56%
No	48%	34%	0%	46%
Growth Pattern				
Nodular	20%	51%	33%	25%
Superficial spreading	75%	49%	67%	71%
Lentigo maligna	5%	0%	0%	4%

nificant (Fig. 29-3; p = 0.10). Patients with nodular melanoma had a significantly lower 5-year survival rate than patients with superficial spreading and lentigo maligna melanomas (Fig. 29-4; p = 0.02).

The overall survivals observed in the total series of patients were almost identical to those obtained in the small selected group (5-year survival rate was 66% and the 10-year survival rate was 56%). These values were the same as the ones reported by the WHO Melanoma Group. The nonsignificant differences observed in the 234 patients when survival was evaluated according to ulceration and sex were probably owing to the relatively small number of patients. As regards ulceration, the observed survival rate of patients with nonulcerated melanoma was 72% at 5 years compared with 59% in patients

TABLE 29–2
ACTUARIAL SURVIVAL DATA FOR MELANOMA PATIENTS TREATED AT THE NATIONAL CANCER INSTITUTE OF MILAN, ITALY

	Survival Rates	
	5-Year	10-Year
Stage I		
Overall survival	67%	57%
Sex		
Male	62%	54%
Female	70%	59%
Primary lesion site		
Lower extremity	78%	68%
Upper extremity	47%	33%
Head and neck	64%	40%
Trunk	53%	53%
Other	100%	100%
Tumor thickness		
<0.76 mm	100%	100%
0.76 mm–1.49 mm	86%	86%
1.50 mm–2.49 mm	78%	58%
2.50 mm–3.99 mm	70%	70%
≥4.00 mm	30%	27%
Level of invasion		
II	96%	96%
III	72%	56%
IV	57%	52%
V	27%	0%
Ulceration		
Yes	59%	49%
No	72%	65%

	1-Year	3-Year	5-Year
Stage II			
Overall survival	55%	31%	27%
Tumor thickness			
<1.50 mm	100%	50%	50%
1.50 mm–3.99 mm	30%	20%	0%
≥4.0 mm	64%	27%	21%
Ulceration			
Yes	55%	38%	21%
No	52%	44%	35%

with ulcerated melanoma. The same finding was observed in a larger series published by the WHO Melanoma Group: in this case the difference was significant even when adjusted by maximum tumor thickness (Table 29-3). The same may be said for the sex difference in survival, where men had a lower 5-year survival rate than women did (62% and 70%, respectively). In a larger series, there was a significant superiority in survival whether adjustment was made for maximum tumor thickness or not (Table 29-3).

A multivariate analysis was carried out taking into consideration the four criteria that were found to be significantly associated with survival of stage I melanoma patients. The Cox's linear regression model was used by means of a step-down procedure of selection of variables. Table 29-4 shows that the dominant prognostic variable of this series was tumor thickness. Growth pattern and anatomical site had a borderline significance ($p = 0.05$).

STAGE II

There were only 45 patients whose data were available according to the strict criteria described above. Their characteristics and survival rates are shown in

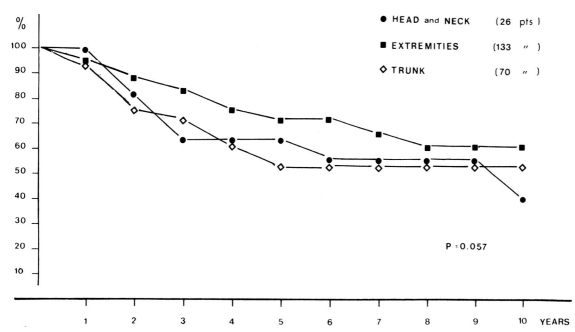

FIG. 29–1 Survival according to anatomical site in 229 stage I melanoma patients treated at the National Cancer Institute of Milan; *P* value refers to overall correlation.

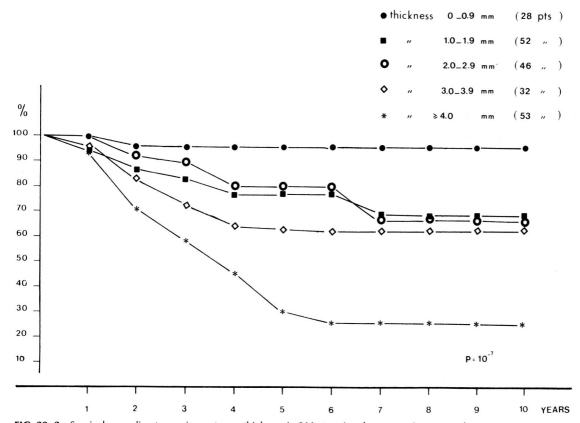

FIG. 29–2 Survival according to maximum tumor thickness in 211 stage I melanoma patients treated at the National Cancer Institute of Milan; *P* value refers to overall correlation.

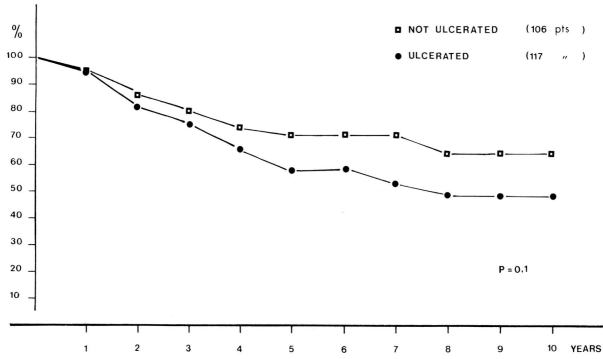

FIG. 29–3 Survival according to tumor ulceration (on microscopic section) in 223 patients from the National Cancer Institute of Milan; *P* value refers to overall correlation.

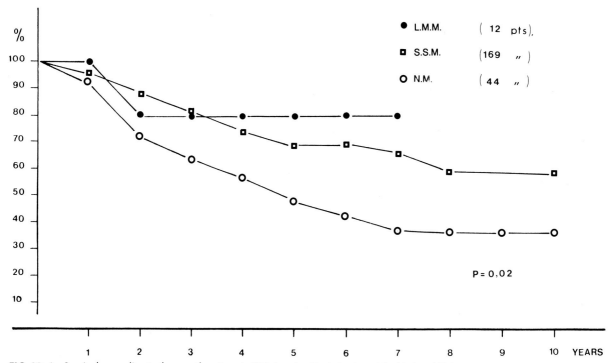

FIG. 29–4 Survival according to the growth pattern in 225 stage I patients treated at the National Cancer Institute of Milan; *P* value refers to overall correlation.

452

TABLE 29–3
INFLUENCE OF SEX OF PATIENT AND ULCERATION OF THE PRIMARY LESION ON SURVIVAL OF STAGE I MELANOMA PATIENTS—DATA FROM THE WHO MELANOMA GROUP REGISTRY

	Number of Patients	5-year Survival	p* Value	p† Value
Sex				
Men	261	54%	10^{-4}	10^{-4}
Women	599	71%		
Ulceration				
Present	264	53%	10^{-9}	10^{-2}
Absent	352	80%		

* Not adjusted

† Adjusted by tumor thickness

TABLE 29–4
MULTIVARIATE ANALYSIS OF STAGE I MELANOMA PATIENTS

Variables	X^2	d.f.	p Value
Anatomical site of primary lesion			
(thickness, level, growth pattern)*	5.78	2	0.055
Tumor thickness			
(site of primary lesion, level, growth pattern)	11.99	5	0.03
Clark's level			
(site of primary lesion, thickness, growth pattern)	4.23	3	0.2
Growth pattern			
(site of primary lesion, thickness, level)	5.84	2	0.053

* Adjustments in parentheses

Tables 29-1 and 29-2. Patients with melanomas measuring less than 1.5 mm had a better 5-year survival rate than patients with tumors 4 mm thick (50% versus 21%). Also, patients with ulcerated melanomas had a worse 5-year survival rate than those with nonulcerated melanomas (21% versus 35%). However, the small number of patients precluded any meaningful statistical evaluation, so a separate evaluation of the entire group of 530 stage II patients treated at the NCIM was performed. The characteristics of these patients are shown in Table 29-5. These data show that stage II melanoma was equally divided among men and women, that the most common site of the primary melanoma was the lower extremity, and that only one third of patients had a single metastatic node. The key prognostic factors in these patients are those relating to regional lymph nodes,[5] while the characteristics of primary melanoma play a secondary role. In the NCIM experience, the level of invasion correlated significantly when considered as a single factor,[5] but

this significance disappeared when adjustment was made for other variables.

Two characteristics of regional node metastases had a significant impact on survival ($p < 10^{-9}$): the extent of nodal metastases and the number of positive nodes. As to the extent of nodal metastases, three categories could be delineated with different survival rates: (1) lymph node(s) not completely replaced by metastatic tumor, (2) complete replacement of regional node(s) but still confined within lymph node capsule, and (3) nodal metastases extending beyond the lymph node capsule (Fig. 29-5). The patients with a single metastatic node had a 45% 10-year survival rate compared with 18% for those with three or more nodes (Fig. 29-6).

In a multifactorial analysis of 530 stage II patients, the extent of nodal metastases was found to be the most important criterion ($p < 10^4$). The number of metastatic nodes was the only other significant prognostic factor in the NCIM experience ($p = 0.05$). The number of positive nodes and the

TABLE 29–5
CHARACTERISTICS OF 530 STAGE II MELANOMA PATIENTS TREATED AT THE NATIONAL CANCER INSTITUTE OF MILAN, ITALY

	Number of Patients	*Percent*
Sex		
Men	267	50
Women	263	50
Anatomical Site of Primary Lesion		
Head and neck	70	13
Lower extremities	221	42
Upper extremities	44	8
Trunk	195	37
Number of Positive Nodes*		
One	179	35
Two	112	22
Three or more	223	43
Extent of Metastases*		
Embolic	41	8
Massive	270	52
Beyond capsule	203	40

*Information not available in 16 patients.

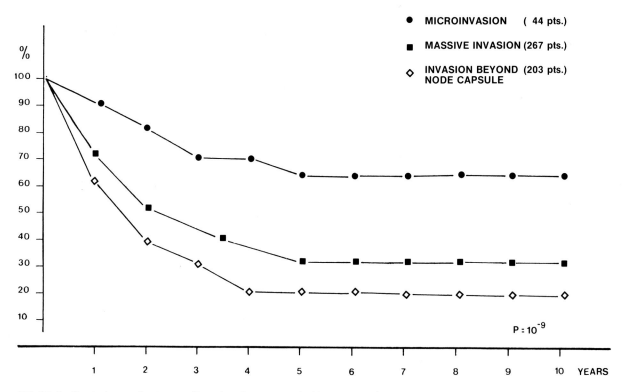

MICROINVASION (44 pts.)

MASSIVE INVASION (267 pts.)

INVASION BEYOND (203 pts.)
NODE CAPSULE

$P = 10^{-9}$

FIG. 29–5 Survival according to type of lymph node metastases in 514 stage II melanoma patients treated at the National Cancer Institute of Milan; *P* value refers to overall correlation.

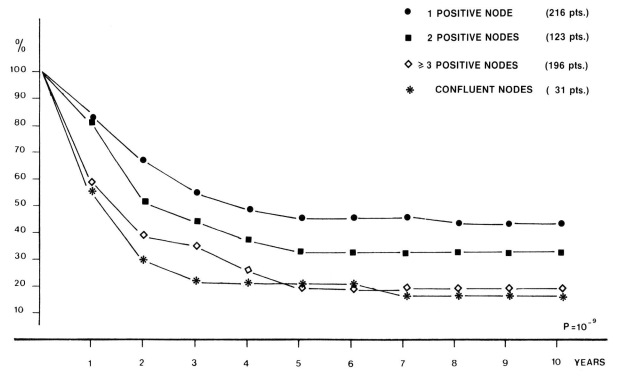

FIG. 29–6 Survival according to the number of metastatic lymph nodes in 566 stage II melanoma patients treated at the National Cancer Institute of Milan; P value refers to overall correlation.

extent of nodal metastases are closely correlated. Thus, patients with metastasis confined within the lymph nodes more frequently have one metastatic node (64%), while patients with invasion beyond the lymph node capsule more frequently have three or more positive nodes (43%). This trend is statistically significant (p < 0.001).

STAGE III

The appearance of distant metastases at any site portended a very bad prognosis. Practically all patients died within 2 years. Unpublished data from the WHO Melanoma Group Register demonstrates this (Fig. 29-7). The median survival varies from 9 months when the first distant metastases are localized at superficial sites (skin and distant lymph nodes) to 1 month in patients with brain metastases (Fig. 29-7).

TREATMENT

The policy of treatment of melanoma is strictly dependent on the stage of the disease. In general, stage I and stage II patients are primarily considered for

surgical treatment, while stage III patients are considered for chemotherapy. The current treatment policies at NCIM are described below and are summarized in Table 29-6.

STAGE I

Primary lesion surgery

Wide excision of the melanoma is the treatment of choice irrespective of tumor thickness. The skin is excised with a margin of 3 cm to 5 cm in all directions from the visible edge of the tumor, together with a somewhat larger area of subcutaneous fat and muscular fascia. The rate of local recurrence in clinical stage I melanoma of the limbs is around 2%,[8] irrespective of whether or not an elective lymph node dissection (ELND) is performed. When melanomas arise on the face, the extent of the resection is reduced appropriately.

The question about how wide a margin of skin to excise is an important but unresolved one.[10] According to the WHO Melanoma Group Register,[4] the size of resection margins did not influence the mortality rate. The evaluation of the frequency of local recurrences is rather difficult because this num-

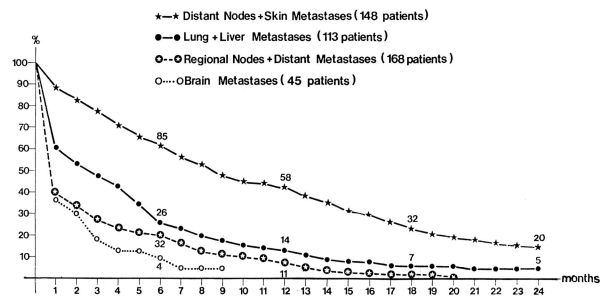

FIG. 29–7 Survival of 474 melanoma patients with distant metastases from the WHO Melanoma Group Registry according to the site of the metastases; *P* value is not significant.

TABLE 29–6
TREATMENT POLICY AT THE NATIONAL CANCER INSTITUTE OF MILAN

	Supported Treatment	Treatment Under Evaluation
Stage I		
Head and Neck	Wide excision, margins compatible with the possibility of reconstructive surgery	
Trunk		
< 2 mm	Wide excision	Wide vs narrow excision (WHO Clinical Trial No. 10)
≥ 2 mm	Wide excision	Immediate vs delayed node dissection (WHO Clinical Trial No. 14)
Extremities		
< 2 mm	Wide excision	Wide vs narrow excision (WHO Clinical Trial No. 1)
≥ 2 mm	Wide excision	
Local Recurrence (or Intransit Metastases)		
Any site	Wide excision and node dissection (if possible)	
Extremities	Hyperthermic perfusion	
Stage II		
Any site	Wide excision and node dissection	Evaluation of the efficacy of Poly A-Poly U (WHO Clinical Trial No. 13)
Stage III		
Any site	DTIC 300 mg/m^2 per 5 days every 4 weeks	CCP, Vindesine, Etoposide (VP-16) vs CLP, Vindesine CCNU

ber is limited if only stage I patients are used. If one uses data for both stage I and stage II patients, the correlation between thickness and the local recurrence rate is very close and is highly significant.

Surgery of regional lymph nodes

The most important problem in the surgical treatment of lymph nodes concerns dissection of clinically uninvolved regional lymph nodes. Routine ELND was performed at NCIM until 1967, when a randomized clinical trial was begun to address this issue. The results of this protocol conducted by the WHO Melanoma Group indicated that immediate node dissection did not improve survival rates.[7,8] Since these studies provided evidence that ELND was not of proven value in the treatment of patients with stage I melanoma, this additional surgical procedure is no longer performed. The patient is closely followed, and a node dissection is performed later if the nodes become clinically involved with metastases. It should be emphasized that a radical lymph node dissection is not a minor surgical procedure, since the incidence of postoperative complications is not negligible in the NCIM experience. Inguinal dissections in particular are associated with more complications than axillary or cervical dissections.

One might ask whether the results obtained in the WHO Melanoma Group prospective study, which included only melanoma of the extremities, should be applicable to melanomas of the whole skin surface of the head and neck or trunk. In principle, there are no essential biologic reasons for melanomas at other sites to behave differently. Nevertheless, the WHO Melanoma Group is now conducting a randomized clinical trial to evaluate the efficacy of ELND in patients with trunk melanomas exceeding 2 mm in thickness.

Surgery of local tumor recurrence

A local recurrence can arise at the site of the primary tumor excision, or in the immediate area (*i.e.,* within 5 cm of it). Surgery is the treatment of choice when melanoma recurs locally as a single cutaneous or subcutaneous nodule.[10] The incidence is relatively low in stage I patients (2% in the NCIM experience), but it occurs more frequently in stage II patients. In the Register of the WHO Collaborating Centres for Evaluation of Methods of Diagnosis and Treatment of Melanoma, there are 2066 surgically treated patients, of whom 48 (2%) had a documented local recurrence. It is interesting to note that 26 of these patients relapsed during the first 3 years.

Wide excision of skin recurrences with margins similar to those usually applied to primary lesions are advocated by the NCIM, especially if the nodes are not clinically involved. In selected cases with bulky recurrences on the extremities or multiple intransit metastases not suitable for hyperthermic perfusion, or with involvement of nerves or major blood vessels, major amputative surgery (*i.e.,* shoulder or interscapulothoracic amputation for upper extremities and hip disarticulation for lower limbs) may be indicated.

STAGE II

Regional lymph nodes

There is no controversy about the need to excise obviously involved nodal areas when no other signs of dissemination are present. The regional lymph node dissection is sometimes performed in continuity with the primary melanoma if the primary lesion site is not too far from the lymph node area. However, in the NCIM experience, the incidence of intransit metastases was not affected by en bloc node dissection. In a series of 83 stage II patients with melanoma of the extremities, intransit metastases appeared in 4 of 52 patients treated by en bloc dissection and in 1 of 31 treated by discontinuous lymph node dissection.[11]

Results of surgery for stage II melanoma patients were poor, since only 33% of patients were alive 5 years after adequate surgical procedure. A high percentage of patients developed distant spread of their disease in spite of the fact that surgery was more than satisfactory.

Role of adjuvant therapy

The NCIM was one of the major participants in a clinical trial involving adjuvant therapy conducted by the WHO Melanoma Group.[6] The aim of the study was to compare four treatment modalities: dacarbazine (DTIC) alone, Bacillus Calmette-Guerin (BCG) alone, DTIC plus BCG, or a control without treatment following the initial surgery. All patients had documented nodal metastases (stage II). The results showed that neither disease-free nor overall survival was modified by adjuvant treatment (Fig. 29-8). The failure of this treatment was probably due to the low antitumor activity of both agents. Any action in the field of adjuvant treatments has to be considered experimental, and no adjuvant treatment can be justified as a substitute for radical surgery, which is the only proven treatment for this stage of melanoma.

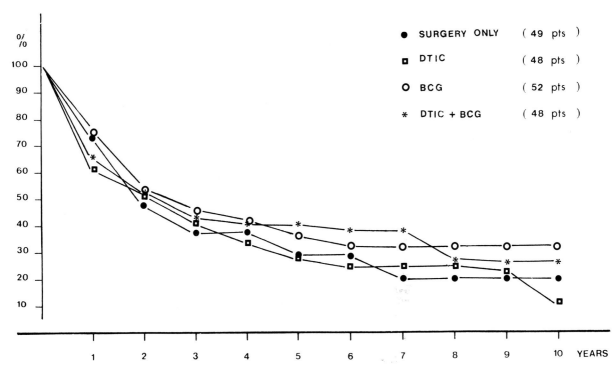

FIG. 29–8 Survival in 197 melanoma patients from the WHO Melanoma Group Trial treated with adjuvant therapy; *P* value is not significant.

Treatment of intransit metastases

The choice of treatment depends on the site of origin of melanoma. In general, chemotherapy is used unless intransit metastases appear at the extremities. In the latter situation, hyperthermic perfusion and chemotherapy in extracorporeal circulation are the treatment of choice, as described in Chapter 10. The drug used at the NCIM is melphalan (1.2 mg/kg–1.5 mg/kg) at a temperature of 40°C to 41°C perfused for 1 hour.

DISTANT METASTASES

Distant metastases can be treated with systemic chemotherapy. A single drug regimen (DTIC) given at a dosage of 300 mg/m² intravenously for 5 consecutive days every 4 weeks is used at the NCIM. Although a great number of multiple drug regimens have been tested, the therapeutic results have failed to show a definite superiority of any combination over DTIC alone in advanced melanoma.[2] This was also confirmed by a study carried out by the WHO Collaborating Centres for Evalua-tion of Methods of Diagnosis and Treatment of Melanoma.[2]

In another randomized prospective clinical trial conducted by the WHO Melanoma Group, the combination of DTIC chemotherapy with either *Corynebacterium parvum* or BCG immunotherapy was studied. There were 196 evaluable patients with advanced disease treated between 1976 and 1980. The results indicated that there were no significant differences between these three treatment groups. Twenty-five patients (13%) responded with complete tumor regression and 18 (9%) with partial regression, giving an overall response of 22% in evaluable patients.[9]

REFERENCES

1. Annuario di statistiche sanitarie, Istituto Centrale di Statistica, Vol XXII. Rome: Edizione 1977
2. Bajetta E, Beretta G, Bonadonna G, Canetta R, Veronesi U: A review of the W.H.O. Trials for the treatment of the patients with advanced melanoma. In Kumar S (ed): Advances in Medical Oncology Re-

search and Education, p 91. New York, Pergamon Press, 1979

3. Berrino F, Crosignani P, Riboli E, Vigano C: Epidemiologia dei tumori maligni: Incidenze e mortalita in provincia di Varese. Notizie Sanita 31:1, 1981

4. Cascinelli N, van der Esch EP, Breslow A, Morabito A, Bufalino R: Stage I melanoma of the skin: The problem of resection margins. Eur J Cancer 16:1079, 1980

5. Nava M, Santinami M, Bajetta E, Marolda R, Vaglini M, Clemente C, Cascinelli N: II melanoma cutaneo con metastasi ai linfonodi regionali (stadio II): Diagnosi, terapia, prognosi. Argomenti di Oncologia 3:119, 1982

6. Veronesi U, Adamus J, Aubert C, Bajetta E, Beretta G, Bonadonna G, Bufalino R, Cascinelli N, Cocconi G, Durand J, DeMarsillac J, Ikonopisov RL, Kiss B, Lejeune F, MacKie R, Madej G, Mulder H, Mechl Z, Milton GW, Morabito A, Peter H, Priario J, Paul E, Rumke P, Sertoli R, Tomin R: A randomized trial of adjuvant chemotherapy and immunotherapy in cutaneous melanoma. N Engl J Med 307:913, 1982

7. Veronesi U, Adamus J, Bandiera DC, Brennhovd IO, Caceres E, Cascinelli N, Claudio F, Ikonopisov RL, Javorskj VV, Kirov S, Kulakowski A, Lacour J, Lejeune F, Mechl Z, Morabito A, Rodé I, Sergeev S, van Slooten E, Szczygiel K, Trapeznikov NN, Wagner RI: Inefficacy of immediate node dissection in stage I melanoma of the limbs. N Engl J Med 297:627, 1977

8. Veronesi U, Adamus J, Bandiera DC, Brennhovd IO, Caceres E, Cascinelli N, Claudio F, Ikonopisov RL, Javorski VV, Kirov S, Kulakowski A, Lacour J, Lejeune F, Mechl Z, Morabito A, Rodé I, Sergeev S, van Slooten E, Szczygiel K, Trapeznikov NN, Wagner RI: Delayed regional lymph node dissection in stage I melanoma of the skin of the lower extremities. Cancer 49:2420, 1982

9. Veronesi U, Aubert C, Bajetta E, Beretta G, Bonadonna G, Cascinelli N, De Marsillac J, Ikonopisov RL, Kiss B, Krementz T, Lejeune F, Mechl Z, Milton GW, Morabito A, Mulder P, Pawlicki P, Priario J, Rumke P, Sertoli R, Tomin R, Trapeznikov N, Wagner R: Controlled study with imidazole carboxamide (DTIC), DTIC + Bacillus Calmette-Guerin (BCG), and DTIC + *Corynebacterium parvum* in advanced malignant melanoma. Tumori 70:41, 1984.

10. Veronesi U, Bajetta E, Cascinelli N, Clemente C, Rilke F: New trends in the treatment of malignant melanoma. In Murphy GP (ed): International Advances in Surgical Oncology, Vol 1, p 113. New York, AR Liss, 1978

11. Veronesi U, Cascinelli N, Balzarini GP, et al: Treatment of regional node metastases. In McCarthy WH (ed): Melanoma and Skin Cancer, p 417, Sydney, Blight, 1972

12. Zonca G: "Il sistema MFS-MEDIC." Techn Inform Radioter Onc. p 75, 1982

KRZYSZTOF T. DRZEWIECKI
HENRIK POULSEN
PETER VIBE
CHRISTIAN LADEFOGED
PER KRAGH ANDERSEN

Melanoma in Denmark: Experience at the University Hospital, Odense

30

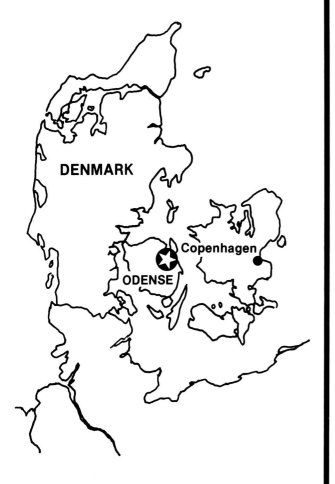

This chapter describes the prognosis and surgical results in 648 patients treated at the Department of Plastic Surgery and the Radium Station of the Odense University Hospital in Denmark between 1964 and 1982. This institution serves a well-defined geographical area of Denmark consisting of three administrative districts (*i.e.,* Fünen, Southern Jutland, and Ribe) and patients from the southern half of the administrative district of Vejle. Thus, the total population served by this hospital is just over 1 million inhabitants. The area is entirely in the temperate zone. There are four distinct seasons, each of 3 months' duration. According to the Danish Institute of Meteorology, the mean temperatures for these seasons were 0.5°C, 6.5°C, 15.9°C, and 8.9°C, and there are, on average, 1724 sunshine hours per year.

The Department of Plastic Surgery was established in mid-1964. By 1970, there was a steady influx of melanoma patients from this geographic area, so that most patients from this area have been treated by this institution since that time. Because of the centralized referral for the treatment of melanoma, it was possible to obtain quickly a special expertise that was important in promoting many educational programs to the physicians and the public in Denmark. This positive development began with Dr. Grete Olsen's pioneer work.[11]

The present report is based on a retrospective analysis of 648 case records covering the period 1964 to 1982 (Tables 30-1 and 30-2). For comparative purposes, it should be noted that in the period 1963 to 1977, 4303 new cases of melanoma were diagnosed in the whole of Denmark.[1,2] All histologic slides were reviewed, and, if necessary, new slides were made from the original paraffin blocks. The present data documented only those patients for whom it has been possible to obtain histologic slides for the revision. For this reason, 65 patients have been excluded.

A statistical analysis described in this report was concluded in February 1983 from computerized records at the Odense Hospital. The follow-up was 100%. Statistical analyses were made by the Statistical Research Unit of the Danish Medical and Social Science Research Councils.

This study is supported by a grant from the Regional Research Foundation in Odense.

The authors wish to express gratitude to Ms. Lise Hansen, Department for Computerized Registration at the University Hospital of Odense, for her help and cooperation.

EPIDEMIOLOGY

The sex distribution shows that there are more women than men in the series (61% and 39%, respectively). This sex distribution corresponds to that published for the entire Danish melanoma population between 1963 and 1977.[1,2] The anatomical location of the primary tumors in this series was also similar to that found in the entire Danish melanoma population. This series excludes level I melanomas. Previous reports on the entire Danish population included level I melanomas.[1,2] Patients with such preinvasive tumors constituted 6% of the series from Odense. Corresponding figures for the entire Danish melanoma population are not available.

INCIDENCE

A striking increase in the number of melanoma patients treated at this melanoma center has occurred during the past decade. Thus, an average of 38 new patients were seen each year during the period 1971 to 1975, but this increased to 52 patients per year from 1976 to 1980. The melanoma incidence for all of Denmark during the period 1968 to 1972 was 4.7×10^5 for men and 7×10^5 for women.[1] In the period 1973 to 1977, the incidence went up to 5.8 and 8.2, respectively.[2] Therefore, both these statistical observations reinforce the view that the incidence of melanoma is increasing in Denmark. A similar tendency is observed in the whole of Scandinavia.[10]

A report from the neighboring country of Sweden showed that in recent years an increasing number of people take vacations in the Mediterranean area.[6] Similar reports are not available for Denmark, but this travel pattern is also popular in this country. This is especially true in the autumn and winter period from September to May. A concentrated exposure to ultraviolet (UV) irradiation may be particularly important in the etiology of melanoma.[9] It is therefore postulated that the increase in incidence of melanoma in Denmark may be partially explained by an increase in UV-radiation exposure.

CHANGING TRENDS

In order to illustrate the trends in the diagnosis of thin melanomas, patients were divided into two groups: those treated up to 1973 and those treated thereafter (Table 30-3). Sixteen percent of patients in the former group had tumors ≤ 0.76 mm in thick-

TABLE 30–1
CLINICAL AND PATHOLOGIC DATA FOR MELANOMA PATIENTS TREATED IN DENMARK

Characteristics	Presenting Pathologic Stage			
	Stage I	Stage II	Stage III	Total
Clinical				
Number of patients	632	11	5	648
Year of diagnosis				
≤ 1960	0%	0%	0%	0%
1961–1965	2%	0%	0%	2%
1966–1970	16%	9%	20%	16%
1971–1975	30%	46%	60%	30%
1976–1980	40%	27%	20%	40%
1981–	12%	18%	0%	12%
Median age	53 yr	56 yr	54 yr	53 yr
Sex				
Male	38%	55%	80%	39%
Female	62%	45%	20%	61%
Primary lesion site				
Female lower extremity	32%	11%	25%	31%
Male lower extremity	7%	11%	25%	7%
Female upper extremity	10%	0%	0%	9%
Male upper extremity	3%	0%	0%	3%
Female head and neck	9%	11%	0%	10%
Male head and neck	9%	0%	0%	9%
Female trunk	11%	22%	0%	11%
Male trunk	18%	45%	50%	19%
Other	1%	0%	0%	1%
Pathologic				
Breslow's tumor thickness				
< 0.76 mm	21%	0%	0%	21%
0.76 mm–1.49 mm	24%	0%	0%	23%
1.50 mm–2.49 mm	17%	0%	0%	17%
2.50 mm–3.99 mm	19%	44%	40%	20%
≥ 4.00 mm	19%	56%	60%	19%
Median tumor thickness	1.7 mm	4.0 mm	4.4 mm	1.8 mm
Level of invasion				
II	13%	0%	0%	13%
III	44%	18%	20%	44%
IV	35%	46%	40%	35%
V	8%	36%	40%	8%
Ulceration				
Yes	38%	91%	40%	39%
No	62%	9%	60%	61%
Growth pattern				
Nodular	19%	45%	20%	19%
Superficial spreading	77%	55%	80%	76%
Lentigo maligna	4%	0%	0%	5%

ness, while 24% in the latter group had such thin tumors. The comparative data on median tumor thickness and ulceration revealed that melanomas treated after 1972 were generally thinner and less ulcerated. This is reflected by higher 5-year survival rates for this group of patients. This pronounced increase in thin, nonulcerated tumors suggests that the diagnosis of melanoma was made at an earlier stage. The comparative data also suggest an increase in the proportion of trunk lesions for both sexes, while lesions on extremities remained virtually unchanged (Table 30-3).

PROGNOSTIC FACTORS IN STAGE I PATIENTS

Almost all (98%) melanoma patients referred to this institution had clinical and pathologic stage I disease, so the prognostic factors analysis was confined

TABLE 30–2
ACTUARIAL SURVIVAL DATA FOR MELANOMA PATIENTS
TREATED IN DENMARK

	Survival Rates	
	5-Year	10-Year
Stage I		
Overall survival	82%	71%
Sex		
Male	76%	64%
Female	85%	75%
Primary lesion site		
Lower extremity	85%	75%
Upper extremity	84%	71%
Head and neck	81%	72%
Trunk	78%	74%
Tumor thickness		
<0.76 mm	98%	97%
0.76 mm–1.49 mm	91%	87%
1.50 mm–2.49 mm	78%	56%
2.50 mm–3.99 mm	73%	52%
≥4.00 mm	58%	58%
Level of invasion		
II	97%	97%
III	88%	80%
IV	73%	54%
V	57%	53%
Ulceration		
Yes	65%	51%
No	92%	84%

	1-Year	3-Year	5-Year
Stage II			
Overall survival	82%	56%	19%
Tumor thickness			
<1.50 mm	—	—	—
1.50 mm–3.99 mm	100%	50%	25%
≥4.0 mm	60%	60%	0%
Ulceration			
Yes	80%	50%	25%
No	—	—	—

	6-Month	1-Year	2-Year
Stage III			
Overall Survival	40%	0%	0%

to this stage (see Tables 30-1 and 30-2). In this series of Danish patients, elective lymph node dissection was not performed in any case. This data base is therefore uniform with respect to initial surgical treatment, in contrast to prognostic factors analyses at some other institutions where some stage I melanoma patients received an elective regional node dissection that may have influenced prognosis. Patients in whom histologic node metastases were found by clinical examination within 3 months of primary operation were classified as stage II. Likewise, pa-

tients with lymph node metastases from an unknown primary site were considered to be stage II. Stage III refers to histologically verified distant metastases that have come about within 3 months from the primary operation.

In some patients, the melanoma was previously excised with a minimum margin of skin for diagnostic purposes. A previous report from this institution[5] described the prognostic influence of the biopsy technique (excisional biopsy and later radical surgery versus immediate radical surgery) in pa-

TABLE 30–3
CHANGING TRENDS IN STAGE I MELANOMA TREATED IN DENMARK

	Year	
	1964–1972 (179 patients)	1973–1982 (453 patients)
Men		
Extremity	27%	26%
Trunk	44%	54%
Head and neck	29%	20%
Women		
Extremity	70%	66%
Trunk	10%	21%
Head and neck	20%	13%
Characteristics		
Median Tumor Thickness	2.3 mm	1.5 mm
≤0.76 mm thick	16%	24%
Ulcerated	49%	34%
5-Year Survival Rate	73%	85%

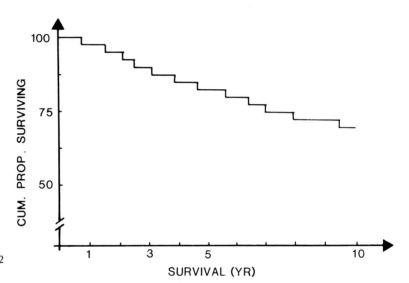

FIG. 30–1 Cumulative survival rates in 632 patients with clinical stage I melanoma.

tients treated from 1964 to 1973 (32% of the total series to date). An excisional biopsy did not influence the prognosis so long as a radical operation was performed within 3 weeks.[5] Because of this finding, all prognostic data were analyzed without subgrouping by the type of biopsy procedure.

The 5- and 10-year cumulative survival rates for all patients were 82% and 71%, respectively (Fig. 30-1). This is considerably better than previous reports from Denmark.[4,11] The former report from this institution[4] was based on the original 226

patients treated from 1964 to 1973. Their 5- and 10-year survival rates were 71% and 50%, respectively.

The prognostic factors analysis described in this report consisted of two patient groups: those treated from 1964 to 1982 and a section of this group treated before 1973. A multivariate analysis was performed only on the patient group treated before 1973. The analysis focused on the most powerful prognostic factors such as sex, tumor thickness, and ulceration.[3,7,8]

PATHOLOGIC FACTORS

Of the 632 pathologic stage I patients, 45% had tumors < 1.5 mm thick. The 5-year survival rate for these patients was about 94% (see Table 30-2). Nineteen percent of patients had tumors ≥ 4 mm in thickness, and the 5-year survival rate for them was only 58%. In patients with tumors between 1.5 and 3.99 mm thick (36% of the total series), mortality was continuous throughout the entire 10-year observation period (Fig. 30-2). Moreover, those patients had a better survival than those patients with tumors ≥ 4 mm in thickness during the first 5 years after operation. These differences were minimal in the subsequent 5-year period, but the number of patients with long-term follow-up in the latter group was small. It is possible that an intensified surgical treatment in the form of elective lymph node dissection might result in an improvement in survival rate in the group of patients with tumors of intermediate thickness.

Ulceration of the melanoma was one of the most significant prognostic parameters (Fig. 30-3). The 10-year survival rate for patients with non-ulcerated tumors was 84% and for patients with ulcerated tumors, only 51% (p < 0.0001). The level of invasion of the tumor was likewise a good prognostic factor (Fig. 30-4). A significant correlation

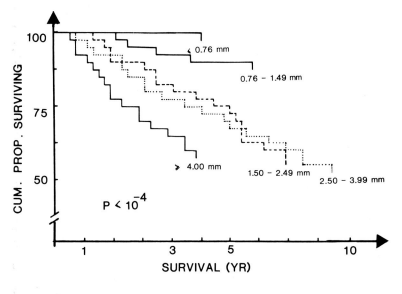

FIG. 30–2 Cumulative survival rates in 632 patients with clinical stage I melanoma according to the thickness of their primary tumor. In this and subsequent figures, the *P* value for correlation with survival is indicated.

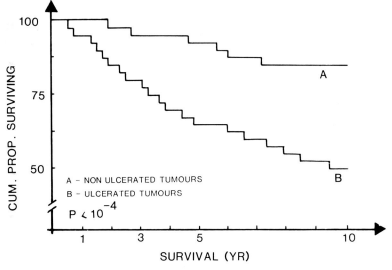

FIG. 30–3 Cumulative survival rates in 632 patients with clinical stage I melanoma according to whether their primary tumor displayed histologic evidence of ulceration.

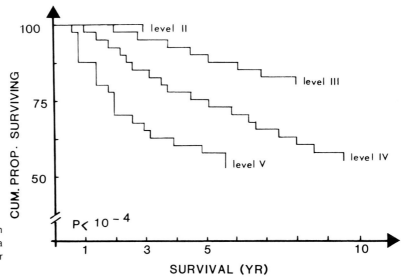

FIG. 30–4 Cumulative survival rates in 632 patients with clinical stage I melanoma according to the level of invasion of their primary tumor.

was found between survival and the four levels of invasion (p < 0.0001; see Table 30-2).

PATIENT FACTORS

Women had a better overall 10-year survival than men (75% versus 64%; p < 0.05). This was probably attributable to the fact that most melanomas in women were located on prognostically favorable sites, particularly the lower extremity (see Table 30-1). Surprisingly, however, there were minimal differences in 5- and 10-year survival rates when the data were subgrouped according to the anatomical site of the primary melanoma (see Table 30-2). Thus, the 10-year survival for all trunk melanomas was 74%, as against 75% for lower extremity melanoma.

MULTIFACTORIAL ANALYSIS

Patients treated before 1973 were analyzed in detail by application of Cox's regression model.[3] Ulceration of the tumor was the most powerful prognostic parameter (p < 0.002). Thickness of the tumor and level of invasion were also important parameters, but they were strongly correlated with each other, and therefore the regression coefficients had low p values compared with their estimated standard errors. Since both these parameters described the same characteristics (*i.e.,* the invasive capacity of the tumor), if one of them was withdrawn from the model, the other became highly significant. Women

had a significantly better prognosis than did men. The presence of epithelioid cells in the tumor indicated a poorer survival than that in patients with spindle, small ovoid, and polymorphic cells. A strong rim of inflammatory cell infiltrate in the tumor indicated a better prognosis than for those patients whose tumors had a slight infiltrate or no infiltrate at all. The analysis surprisingly showed that biopsy before the radical operation (delayed versus immediate) had a positive influence on the survival probability. Thus, a biopsy procedure performed before a radical procedure (not immediately with frozen section diagnosis) was associated with an increased survival. At present, however, this finding must be taken with reservation until confirmed on a larger population of melanoma patients.

TREATMENT

The standard treatment of cutaneous melanoma has consisted of wide excision of the primary tumor or biopsy scar with at least a 5-cm margin down to, but not including, the fascia. Since 1979, the fascia has been included as part of the dissection in all patients. The skin is excised with a margin of 5 cm from the tumor in all directions. The defects are covered by free skin graft. Melanomas on the face are excised with a margin of 2 cm wherever possible. Melanomas on the fingers or toes are generally treated by amputation at the metacarpophalangeal joint.

The surgical treatment for level I melanoma has

varied at this institution through the years. Most melanomas have been excised with a margin of 1 cm to 3 cm, but in recent years there has been a tendency toward using only 1-cm margins. Patients with clinically apparent lymph node metastases are treated with a standard radical lymphadenectomy. Elective lymph node dissections are not performed.

Systemic chemotherapy, mainly dacarbazine (DTIC) alone or combined with other agents, has yielded disappointing results. These drugs are used only for palliative purposes and even then in a minority of patients. Likewise, radiotherapy has been used only for advanced stages of disease and for palliative purposes only. Immunotherapy has not been used in any form.

CONCLUSIONS

It is considered that this series, consisting of 648 patients treated at the Department of Plastic Surgery in Odense between 1964 and 1982, constitutes a representative section of the Danish melanoma population. There was an increase in the number of patients treated, reflecting an increased incidence of disease in the whole country. At the same time, however, an increasing proportion of thin melanomas has been diagnosed. This has resulted in a considerably improved survival rate from melanoma compared with previous reports from Denmark. This may be explained by the fact that a large part of the present series consisted of patients with thin, nonulcerated tumors. Two of the most powerful prognostic factors were the thickness of the tumor and the presence or absence of ulceration. Patients with melanomas of intermediate thickness (1.50 mm–3.99 mm) will be considered for elective lymph node dissection in the future.

REFERENCES

1. Clemmesen J: Statistical studies in aetiology of malignant neoplasms V. Acta Pathol Microbiol Scand (Suppl) 261:276, 1977
2. Danish Cancer Registry: Incidence of Cancer in Denmark 1973–1977. Copenhagen, 1982, p. 94
3. Drzewiecki KT, Andersen PK: Survival with malignant melanoma: A regression analysis of prognostic factors. Cancer 49:2414, 1982.
4. Drzewiecki KT, Christensen HE, Ladefoged C, Poulsen H: Clinical course of cutaneous malignant melanoma related to histopathological criteria of primary tumour. Scand J Plast Reconstr Surg 14:229, 1980
5. Drzewiecki KT, Ladefoged C, Christensen HE: Biopsy and prognosis for cutaneous malignant melanomas in clinical stage I. Scand J Plast Reconstr Surg 14:141, 1980
6. Eklund G, Malec E: Sunlight and incidence of cutaneous malignant melanoma: Effect of latitude and domicile in Sweden. Scand J Plast Reconstr Surg 12:231, 1978
7. Eldh J, Boeryd B, Peterson LE: Prognostic factors in cutaneous malignant melanoma in stage I: A clinical, morphological and multivariate analysis. Scand J Plast Reconstr Surg 12:243, 1978
8. Liestol K, Larsen TE, Grude TH: A retrospective histological study of 669 cases of primary cutaneous malignant melanoma in clinical stage I: The relative prognostic value of various clinical and histopathological features evaluated by Cox regression model. Acta Pathol Microbiol Immunol Scand Sect A 90:449, 1982
9. MacKie RM, Aitchison T: Severe sunburn and subsequent risk of primary cutaneous malignant melanoma in Scotland. Br J Cancer 46:955, 1982
10. Magnus K: Incidence of malignant melanoma of the skin in the five Nordic countries: Significance of solar radiation. Int J Cancer 20:477, 1977
11. Olsen G: The malignant melanoma of the skin: New theories based on a study of 500 cases. Acta Chir Scand (Suppl) 365:1, 1966

JAN ELDH
BERNT BOERYD
MART SUURKÜLA
LARS-ERIK PETERSON
HANS HOLMSTRÖM

Melanoma in Sweden: Experience at the University of Göteborg

31

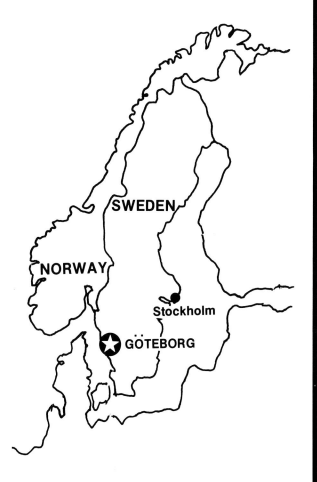

At the Plastic Surgery Unit, University of Göteborg, Sweden, 573 melanoma patients were treated between 1959 and 1980. Most of the patients were referred from the city of Göteborg (0.6 million inhabitants), with the remainder referred from the surrounding region (1.2 million inhabitants). Göteborg is the second largest city in Sweden and is situated on its western coast, 58°N and 12°E of Greenwich. Göteborg is in the northern temperate zone and has four seasons, with a long winter. The summer is only 3 months long but is sunny, which encourages outdoor life with sunbathing and sea-bathing in the North Sea since it is heated up by the Gulf Stream. The great majority of the population is of the original light-skinned Nordic race who sunburn easily.

All patients were followed up, and all data were prospectively accumulated. All patients who died were autopsied. The microscopic analysis of the melanomas was based on reviews of the histologic slides of all cases. The slides from 1959 to 1974 were reexamined earlier[2] by one pathologist (B.B.), and the slides from 1975 onward were reviewed by another (M.S.). In this study, the prognosis has been expressed as absolute survival rates; that is, the exact number of patients who did not die of melanoma within the observation time of 3 years to 23 years (average, 8 years). The survival rates described in this chapter are therefore not directly comparable with actuarial survival rates used elsewhere. The statistical analyses were performed at the Göteborg Computing Center. All correlations between melanoma survival and possible prognostic factors were analyzed by the chi-square method with Yates correction. Fisher's exact test was used in situations where there was a small sample size. Corrected survival was calculated according to the method of Kaplan and Meier.

EPIDEMIOLOGY

The source of incidence data on melanoma for the entire country is the Swedish Cancer Registry of the National Board of Health and Welfare. This registry contains detailed information based on obligatory reports from physicians and pathologists. The reliability of the registry was checked in a retrospective examination of pathologically documented cases diagnosed between 1959 and 1968. There was only a 3.7% incidence of incorrect diagnosis, a sufficiently small degree of error to render the Swedish Cancer Registry suitable for epidemiologic studies.[4] Mor-

tality data for melanoma were obtained from the National Central Bureau of Statistics of Sweden.

In Sweden, the incidence of cutaneous melanoma has increased steadily from 2.5×10^5 inhabitants in 1958 to 11.6×10^5 in 1980 (Fig. 31-1). This is the most pronounced rise in incidence for any cancer in Sweden. During the same time span, the incidence of extracutaneous melanomas (mucosal and ocular) has been constant at 1.4×10^5, and the overall proportion of extracutaneous melanomas has decreased from 34% of all melanomas in 1958 to 11% of all melanomas in 1980. These observations confirm that the striking increase in melanoma incidence overall is in fact limited to cutaneous melanomas (Fig. 31-2).

Over the last two decades, the survival rates for melanoma patients have also increased considerably. The mortality rate for cutaneous melanoma has more than doubled from 1.3×10^5 inhabitants in 1958 to 3.1×10^5 in 1980, and the incidence rate has increased nearly fivefold (2.5 to 11.6×10^5). This difference in incidence and mortality rates indicates that the cure rate for melanoma has increased. This is mainly owing to awareness about the dangers of skin cancer that has resulted in earlier diagnosis. In contrast, it is interesting to note that the incidence of ocular melanoma has not increased despite the fact that it is also easily recognizable (Fig. 31-2). Another factor that may influence the incidence rate to a minor extent is that the incidence of melanoma rises sharply in older persons and that the overall age of the Swedish population is increasing as well. Finally, overdiagnosis of melanoma by the pathologists may have contributed to an unknown degree.

The incidence data were further analyzed over time according to the patient's sex and the site of the primary melanoma. The overall melanoma incidence in 1980 was 5.4×10^5 for men and 6.2×10^5 for women. The female-to-male ratio increased through the years from 1.15:1 (1958–1960) to 1.22:1 (1968–1970) and to 1.25:1 (1978–1980). Between 1958 and 1980, melanomas on the lower extremities in women increased from 0.3 to 2.1×10^5, while melanomas on the trunk in men increased from 0.4 to 2.5 over the same period. Other anatomical locations had a less pronounced increase. Despite the increased incidence, the anatomical distribution of cutaneous melanomas has not changed substantially throughout the years of this study. Melanomas on the trunk were twice as common in men as in women, while lower extremity melanomas were three times as common in women as in men. Despite the fact that more women than men had melanomas,

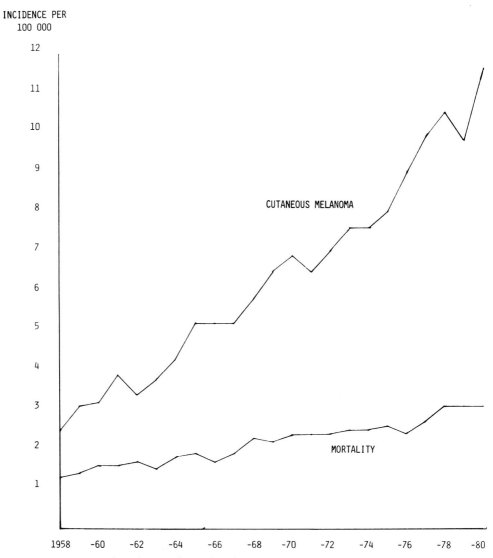

FIG. 31–1 Annual incidence and mortality of cutaneous malignant melanoma in Sweden, 1958–1980.

the mortality rate was higher in men than in women.

An increase in melanoma incidence has been observed in most countries with a predominance of white-skinned inhabitants. The increase in cutaneous melanoma incidence in Sweden was linear during the past 12 to 15 years. It seems probable, therefore, that a further increase will occur in the next decade. The same may be true for the mortality rate. The current incidence of 11.6×10^5 is, however,

much lower than the reported incidence of 32×10^5 from Queensland, Australia,[3] although the latter figure includes level I melanomas. An excess of sunlight exposure has long been suspected as an important predisposing factor in skin melanoma. Studies have been performed in Sweden that support such a hypothesis.[1] Intensified efforts should be made to gain a better understanding of these relationships and to determine what preventive measures should be taken.

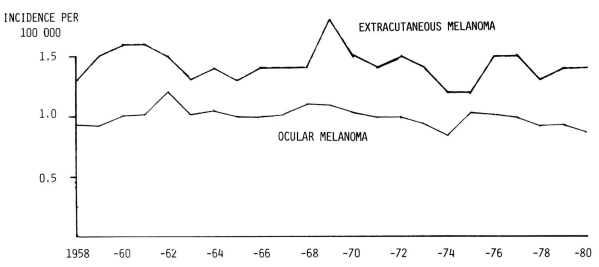

FIG. 31–2 Annual incidence of extracutaneous malignant melanoma (mucosal and ocular) in Sweden, 1958–1980. The proportion due to ocular melanomas is shown separately.

PROGNOSIS IN STAGE I PATIENTS

All patients in the present series had clinically localized disease (stage I). Patients who first presented as clinical stage II or those who subsequently developed metastases were mostly referred to another department at the hospital. In order to find those variables that exerted the greatest influence on prognosis, an Automatic Interaction Detection (AID) analysis was carried out.[2] This analysis was based on 464 patients with an observation time of at least 5 years. The following variables were tested: age and sex of the patient and location, maximum diameter, thickness, level of invasion, growth pattern, and ulceration of the tumor. Ulceration and tumor thickness were found to be the most important prognostic factors.

PATIENT FACTORS

The median age was similar for both men and women, while the anatomical location of the primary lesion occurred most frequently on the lower extremity in women and on the trunk in men (Table 31-1). The overall survival rate for all patients was 80% at 5 years and 75% at 8 years. Women had a better 5-year survival rate than men did, and patients with extremity melanomas fared better than those with truncal lesions (Table 31-2). Further subsite analysis showed a 41% mortality for melanomas on the foot, which was significantly higher than the 13% mortality for the rest of the lower extremity ($p < 0.001$; Table 31-3). Melanomas of the foot were, however, much thicker, with 55% of tumors exceeding 2.5 mm in thickness compared with 28% >2.5 mm among melanomas arising elsewhere on the lower leg ($p < 0.01$). A highly significant mortality difference among men and women was identified in the patients with head and neck melanomas (28% for men and 2% for women; $p < 0.001$). One explanation for this is that women had a higher proportion of thin melanomas in this location, since 38% of melanomas in women were <0.76 mm in thickness compared with 12% for men.

PATHOLOGIC FACTORS

Tumor diameter and thickness were similar between the sexes. Most of the tumors were Clark's level III and IV (Table 31-1), but there was no sex difference in distribution of Clark's levels, growth patterns, or presence of ulceration.

Since ulceration was found to be of such prognostic significance by the AID analysis, a cross-classification analysis of the melanoma mortality for the total series of 573 patients was made according to the presence of ulceration. These patients had an observation time between 3 years and 20 years (mean, 8 years). In the nonulcerated group, 45 out of 401 patients (11%) died of melanoma compared with 76 out of 172 patients (44%) with ulceration. This difference was highly significant ($p < 0.001$). There was also a significant sex difference in overall mortality, being 27% for men and 16% for women

TABLE 31–1
CLINICAL AND PATHOLOGIC DATA FOR MELANOMA PATIENTS TREATED AT GÖTEBORG, SWEDEN

Characteristics	Clinical Stage Stage I
Clinical	
Number of patients	573
Year of diagnosis	
≤1960	<1%
1961–1965	6%
1966–1970	18%
1971–1975	42%
1976–1980	33%
Median age	55 yr
Sex	
Male	46%
Female	54%
Primary lesion site	
Female lower extremity	23%
Male lower extremity	7%
Female upper extremity	7%
Male upper extremity	4%
Female head and neck	11%
Male head and neck	8%
Female trunk	12%
Male trunk	27%
Pathologic	
Breslow's tumor thickness	
<0.76 mm	26%
0.76 mm–1.49 mm	24%
1.50 mm–2.49 mm	21%
2.50 mm–3.99 mm	16%
≥4.00 mm	13%
Median tumor thickness	1.5 mm
Level of invasion	
II	21%
III	42%
IV	32%
V	5%
Ulceration	
Yes	30%
No	70%
Growth pattern	
Nodular	35%
Superficial spreading	40%
Lentigo maligna	24%
Unclassified	1%

TABLE 31–2
SURVIVAL DATA FOR MELANOMA PATIENTS TREATED AT GÖTEBORG, SWEDEN

	Survival Rates 5-Year	Survival Rates 8-Year
Stage I		
Overall survival	80%	75%
Sex		
Male	75%	
Female	84%	
Primary lesion site		
Lower extremity	82%	
Upper extremity	90%	
Head and neck	83%	
Trunk	75%	
Other	0%	
Tumor thickness		
<0.76 mm	96%	95%
0.76 mm–1.49 mm	90%	87%
1.50 mm–2.49 mm	80%	71%
2.50 mm–3.99 mm	73%	68%
≥4.00 mm	35%	30%
Another thickness range		
<1.00 mm	97%	96%
1.00 mm–1.99 mm	84%	75%
2.00 mm–2.99 mm	78%	78%
3.00 mm–3.99 mm	69%	59%
≥4.00 mm	35%	30%
Level of invasion		
II	96%	
III	83%	
IV	73%	
V	36%	
Ulceration		
Yes	57%	
No	90%	

TABLE 31–3
ABSOLUTE SURVIVAL RATES IN STAGE I PATIENTS SUBGROUPED BY ANATOMICAL LOCATION ULCERATION, AND SEX (MEAN OBSERVATION TIME, 8 YEARS)*

	Anatomical Location				
	Head and Neck	Upper Extremity	Trunk	Lower Extremity	Foot
Nonulcerated melanomas	88%	96%	85%	94%	72%
	♂ 72%	♂ 91%	♂ 83%	♂ 100%	
	♀ 98%	♀ 100%	♀ 89%	♀ 92%	
Ulcerated melanomas	58%	67%	47%	70%	44%
Total	81%	89%	72%	87%	59%

*Survival rates are given in percentages except when sample size is <15. The number of patients with ulcerated melanomas was too small to subgroup by sex in this and succeeding tables.

(p < 0.001). In patients with nonulcerated lesions, 30 out of 183 men (16%) died of melanoma compared with 15 out of 218 women (7%; p < 0.01). In those with ulcerated lesions, 43 out of 84 men (51%) died of melanoma, as did 33 out of 88 women (38%). The p value was not significant. Thus, in the subgroup of patients with ulcerated melanomas, the female superiority in survival was diminished (Table 31-4). Prognosis is therefore correlated to ulceration and, in the nonulcerated lesions, to the sex of the patient as well.

Besides ulceration, thickness of the tumor was the most important prognostic factor. Survival decreased with increasing thickness of the tumor from 96% (6 of 150 patients died) for patients with tumors <0.76 mm in thickness to 38% (44 of 71 patients died) in those with tumors >4 mm in thickness (Table 31-5). At each level of thickness, patients with ulcerated melanomas fared much worse than did patients with nonulcerated tumors. As would be expected, very few of the thin melanomas were ulcerated.

With increasing level of invasion, there was a progressive decrease in survival from 97% for level II lesions to 35% for level V melanomas. The subgroup of patients with the lowest survival rate in the present study were those with ulcerated level V tumors (2 of 17, or 12%; Table 31-6).

As to the maximum diameter of the tumor, the survival fell with increasing size from 86% for lesions <10 mm wide to 65% for lesions >20 mm wide (p < 0.001; Table 31-7). In nonulcerated lesions at least, this overall difference appeared to be entirely due to an increase in mortality for men.

The growth pattern of the tumors also proved to be an important determinant of mortality. Patients with nodular melanomas fared worst, with a survival rate of 65%, while those with LMM fared best, with a 90% survival rate. This difference in survival rate was entirely within patients with nonulcerated lesions. Men with nodular melanoma had an especially high mortality rate of 14 of 53 patients (26%), and women with LMM had an extremely good prognosis with only one death from metastatic

TABLE 31–4
ABSOLUTE SURVIVAL RATES IN STAGE I PATIENTS SUBGROUPED BY ULCERATION AND SEX (MEAN OBSERVATION TIME, 8 YEARS)

	Nonulcerated Lesions	Ulcerated Lesions	Total
Men	84%	49%	73%
Women	93%	62%	84%
Total	89%	55%	

TABLE 31–5
ABSOLUTE SURVIVAL RATES IN STAGE I PATIENTS SUBGROUPED BY THICKNESS, ULCERATION, AND SEX (MEAN OBSERVATION TIME, 8 YEARS)*

	Tumor Thickness (mm)				
	< 0.76	0.76–1.49	1.50–2.49	2.50–3.99	> 4.00
Nonulcerated melanomas	97%	93%	79%	86%	59%
	♂ 93%	♂ 91%	♂ 74%	♂ 79%	♂ 5/12
	♀ 99%	♀ 95%	♀ 84%	♀ 92%	♀ 73%
Ulcerated melanomas	4/5	65%	76%	56%	33%
Total	96%	89%	78%	70%	38%

*Survival rates are given in percentages except when sample size is < 15.

TABLE 31–6
ABSOLUTE SURVIVAL RATES IN STAGE I PATIENTS SUBGROUPED BY LEVEL OF INVASION, ULCERATION AND SEX (MEAN OBSERVATION TIME, 8 YEARS)*

	Clark's Level			
	II	III	IV	V
Nonulcerated melanomas	97%	89%	82%	7/9
	♂ 92%	♂ 85%	♂ 72%	♂ 3/4
	♀ 100%	♀ 92%	♀ 89%	♀ 4/5
Ulcerated melanomas	6/6	64%	53%	12%
Total	97%	80%	70%	35%

*Survival rates are given in percentages except when sample size is < 15.

melanoma among 67 patients who were treated (Table 31-8).

TREATMENT

The surgical treatment of all stage I patients in this series was a wide local excision of their primary lesion without elective regional lymph node dissection. The extent of the local excision has varied through the years, but most patients have had a margin of excision of 5 cm or more, except on the face. All the defects were covered with skin grafts. In more recent years, thinner melanomas have been treated with less radical margins. In most patients, the muscular fascia was not excised, according to the recommendations of Olsen.[5] Postoperatively, the patients were followed at the Department of Plastic Surgery at intervals of 3 months for the first 3 years and every 6 months thereafter.

Patients who first presented with clinical stage II melanoma or who subsequently developed metastases were treated with a standard therapeutic lymph node dissection. In addition, some patients had an isolated regional perfusion using a cytostatic drug.

In stage III patients, different chemotherapeutic regimens have been employed through the years, but the results have been disappointing.

CONCLUSIONS

A nearly fivefold increase in the incidence rate of cutaneous melanoma in Sweden has taken place during the past two decades. This increase has been higher in women than in men, but the mortality is higher in men than in women. Prognostic factors in 573 clinical stage I patients who had had local surgery only were analyzed in detail. Ulceration was the most important prognostic factor, which increased the mortality four times over that for patients with nonulcerated lesions. Increasing thickness, diameter, and level of invasion were also associated with an increased mortality risk. As to the anatomical site of the primary melanomas, those on the foot, the trunk, and the face in men had an especially poor prognosis. When extended surgery or additional therapy is contemplated, detailed prognostic information is essential to select the highest risk group properly.

TABLE 31–7
ABSOLUTE SURVIVAL RATES IN STAGE I PATIENTS SUBGROUPED BY MAXIMUM DIAMETER, ULCERATION, AND SEX (MEAN OBSERVATION TIME, 8 YEARS)

	Lesion Diameter (mm)		
	< 10	10–20	> 20
Nonulcerated melanomas	91%	89%	82%
	♂ 89%	♂ 83%	♂ 72%
	♀ 93%	♀ 93%	♀ 93%
Ulcerated melanomas	71%	53%	42%
Total	86%	78%	65%

TABLE 31–8
ABSOLUTE SURVIVAL RATES IN STAGE I PATIENTS SUBGROUPED BY GROWTH PATTERN, ULCERATION, AND SEX (MEAN OBSERVATION TIME, 8 YEARS)

	Growth Pattern		
	Lentigo Maligna	Superficial Spreading	Nodular
Nonulcerated melanomas	94%	92%	78%
	♂ 88%	♂ 87%	♂ 74%
	♀ 99%	♀ 95%	♀ 82%
Ulcerated melanomas	63%	57%	51%
Total	90%	85%	65%

REFERENCES

1. Eklund G, Malec E: Sunlight and incidence of cutaneous malignant melanoma: Effect of latitude and domicile in Sweden. Scand J Plast Reconstr Surg 12:231, 1978
2. Eldh J, Boeryd B, Peterson LE: Prognostic factors in cutaneous malignant melanoma in stage I: A clinical, morphological and multivariate analysis. Scand J Plast Reconstr Surg 12:243, 1978
3. Little JH, Holt J, Davis N: Changing epidemiology of malignant melanoma in Queensland. Med J Aust 1:66, 1980
4. Malec E, Eklund G, Lagerlof B: Re-appraisal of malignant melanoma diagnosis in the Swedish Cancer Registry. Acta Pathol Microbiol Scand Sect A 85:707, 1977
5. Olsen G: Removal of fascia—Cause of more frequent metastases of malignant melanomas of the skin to regional lymph nodes? Cancer 17:1159, 1964

RONA M. MacKIE
DOUGLAS H. CLARK
ALISTAIR J. COCHRAN

Melanoma in the West of Scotland, 1939–1981

32

SCOTLAND

GLASGOW

Edinburgh

This report is based on a study of 951 melanoma patients treated at various hospitals throughout the West of Scotland (WOS) between 1940 and 1969. Glasgow, the main city in the WOS, is at a latitude of 56°N, has a total population of slightly over 1 million, and acts as a melanoma referral center for over one half of the total Scottish population of 5.2 million. Over 99% of patients presenting with cutaneous melanomas are white-skinned. This has until recently accurately reflected the relatively static population. In the past 15 to 20 years, a small Asian community has established itself in Glasgow, but other racial types are rare.

The great majority of patients and their parents were born in the WOS. The lack of mobility is even reflected in holiday patterns. In a recent study, over 50% of melanoma patients had never left the British Isles, even for a brief holiday in continental Europe.[6] Over the past 200 years, there has been considerable migration to and from Northern Ireland. The Irish phenotype is more commonly represented in the WOS than in the east of the country.

There is thus a strong representation in the WOS of the fair or red-haired, fair-skinned, blue-eyed phenotype who possesses a tendency to freckle or burn on exposure to sunlight. This phenotype, common in both Scots and Irish, has been designated Celtic,[3] but because the true origin of the Celts and their phenotypic expression is debated by anthropologists, the term *Caledonian* is more precise.

Climatic conditions do not encourage frequent sunbathing. The annual rainfall is 1079 mm, and there is an average of 3.7 hours (range, 0.9–6.1) of bright sunlight daily. This type of climate results in a population that is not generally aware of the possible dangers of cutaneous exposure during unexpected and often welcome heat waves. There is therefore a strong tendency for even fair-skinned persons to expose their skin on such occasions until erythema and burning result. The use of sunscreens is a recent development. Even now, only younger people tend to use them, and then on continental holidays rather than at home.

Approximately 90% of patients described in this chapter are referred to Glasgow teaching hospitals (National Health Service) from the WOS for initial treatment of their primary lesions and for subsequent surgery, chemotherapy, and radiotherapy for advanced disease. All patients described in this chapter had invasive melanoma (Clark's level II or deeper). No accurate figures are available for level I melanoma. The figures quoted below include lentigo maligna melanoma (LMM) but not lentigo maligna. The survival rates described in this chapter are calculated as crude survival rates and therefore cannot be directly compared with actuarial survival rates described in other chapters of this book.

INCIDENCE

Cutaneous melanoma in the WOS has been a subject of review on three separate occasions in the past 30 years.[1,7,11] The work of the Scottish Melanoma Group, which has collected data on melanoma patients over all of Scotland for the past 5 years, has enabled valid comparisons to be made between incidence in Scotland and in other parts of the world.[8]

The incidence of melanoma in the WOS in 1979 was 4.9×10^5 (141 cases). Figures for 1980 and 1981 are 154 (5.3×10^5) and 137 (4.7×10^5), respectively. Figures published for earlier years almost certainly represent significant underregistration. It is therefore difficult to comment on trends over the past 10 to 20 years. Even allowing for underregistration, it seems likely that there has been a steady increase. Although cancer registration has been operative in the WOS for a considerable time, it is clear that registration prior to 1975 was far from complete and that published figures for this period almost certainly represent significant underregistration.

A feature common to Scotland, England, and Wales is the high ratio of women to men. In the WOS, there were 102 women and 39 men diagnosed in 1979, a ratio of 5:2. It has been postulated that this is due to an endocrine factor that is revealed only in areas of relatively low incidence in which prolonged and intense sun exposure is not a feature.[4]

WOS patients have a relatively high incidence of LMM (12%) relative to other reported series. Lentigo maligna lesions are not included in this study, since many elderly patients do not undergo surgical removal and histologic confirmation of their lesions. The high incidence of LMM in the WOS may reflect the fact that the area is served by a large plastic surgery unit (Canniesburn Hospital). A similar high incidence of this growth pattern is seen in other parts of Scotland, however, suggesting that LMM may well be associated with the Scottish phenotype.

As in many other series, superficial spreading melanoma (SMM) was the predominant growth pattern. There was a clear sex difference in the anatomical location of SSM, with the leg being the most common site in women and the trunk the most common site in men. Nodular melanomas (NM) appeared to be less frequent in both sexes and tended to occur on covered sites of the body. It is difficult to comment on acral lentiginous melanomas (ALM) on the palms and soles, as they have been included in growth patterns only during the last 4 to 5 years. There is no doubt that the sole is more common than the palm as a site of involvement of these lesions, but it should be emphasized that not all lesions on this site are ALM. In 1981, 25% of all primary melanomas in men were on the sole of the foot.

CHANGING SURVIVAL TRENDS

Five-year crude (not actuarial) survival figures for the three cohorts are indicated below for patients presenting with stage I disease.

	1940–1949	1950–1959	1960–1969
Women	52%	62%	63%
Men	38%	30%	40%

These trends show a slight improvement in the survival figures over the period of study and clearly indicate the better prognosis for women with melanoma. This point is further elaborated in the earliest cohort studied, in which the 5-year survival rate for women under the age of 50 years is 70%. This may be due, in large part, to the high proportion of women in this age range with prognostically favorable lesions of the lower limb. Crude 5-year survival rate for younger women with leg lesions is 85% for this cohort. Although tumor thickness figures are not available, it is likely that these good results are largely due to the fact that these lesions are relatively thin, prognostically favorable tumors.

In the 1960 to 1969 cohort of patients, the 5-year survival rate was 72% for women under 50 years compared with 46% for those older than 50 years. These results, with the striking sex difference in incidence figures, suggest a possible endocrine dependency in both the etiology of melanoma and its subsequent progression.

PROGNOSTIC FEATURES

PATIENT FACTORS

Patients with tumors on the leg had the best prognosis, with a 5-year crude survival rate of 54% in the 1950 to 1959 cohort. However, when this was corrected for tumor thickness in the 1960 to 1969 co-

hort, the improved prognosis disappeared for this anatomical site. Survival rates correlated only with tumor thickness in this patient group, and the anatomical site was not an independent variable.

PATHOLOGIC FACTORS

Five-year survival rates according to tumor thickness were available for the 223 patients registered between 1960 and 1969. There were significant differences among the thickness groups listed in Table 32-1. All patients with thin melanomas (<0.76 mm) survived 5 years. The levels of invasion delineated significant prognostic groups as well (Table 32-2). In agreement with other published results, these figures indicated that tumor thickness had a greater accuracy and reproducibility compared with the levels of invasion.[9,10]

The prognostic influence of growth pattern was also examined in the 1960 to 1969 cohort. The

TABLE 32–1
SURVIVAL DATA FOR MELANOMA PATIENTS TREATED IN THE WEST OF SCOTLAND

	Crude Survival Rates*	
	5-Year	
Stage I		
Overall survival	58%	
Sex		
Male	37%	
Female	63%	
Tumor thickness		
<0.76 mm	100%	
0.76 mm—1.49 mm	77%	
1.50 mm—2.49 mm	52%	
2.50 mm—3.99 mm	39%	
≥4.00 mm		
Level of invasion		
II	94%	
III	64%	
IV	59%	
V	29%	
Ulceration		
Yes	40%	
No	60%	

	1-Year	3-Year
Stage II		
Overall survival	71%	24%

	6-Month	1-Year
Stage III		
Overall survival	43%	11%

*These are crude survival rates, so they are not directly comparable with actuarial survival data described in other chapters.

5-year survival rate for LMM was 75%; for SSM, 69%; for NM, 41%; and for ALM, 56%. However, when the growth pattern was corrected for tumor thickness, this histologic feature was not an independent predictive variable.

Ulceration of a melanoma (microscopically defined) was recorded only for the 1960 to 1969 cohort. Patients with ulceration had a 5-year survival rate of 40% compared with 66% for those with nonulcerated tumors. However, when ulceration was corrected for tumor thickness, the prognostic significance of this feature was lost. Thus, in this series, ulceration did not appear to be an independent variable.

In addition to the variables listed in Table 32-2, three other tumor features of melanoma were found to have prognostic significance: tumor diameter, preexisting status of the melanoma (*i.e.,* any evidence of an associated nevus), and the mitotic index.

When tumor diameter was examined in the 1950 to 1959 and 1960 to 1969 cohorts, the 5-year crude survival rates were 87% and 65%, respectively, for tumors under 1 cm in diameter, 63% and 55% for tumors 1 cm to 1.99 cm in diameter, and 24% and 36% for tumors greater than 2 cm in diameter.

In the 1940 to 1949 series, 39% of all melanomas were said to arise in a preexisting nevus; in the 1950 to 1959 cohort, the rate was 50%; and in the 1960 to 1969 cohort, it was 46%. Local recurrence was less frequent in the group with a preexisting nevus. Similarly, 5-year survival rates for those with a preexisting nevus in the 1960 to 1969 cohort was 65%, compared with 51% for those without such a history.

Mitotic index was available only for the 1960 to 1969 cohort. It was low (less than one in five high power fields [1/5 HPF]) in 31%, moderately frequent (1/5 to 1/1 HPF) in 34%, and high (more than 1/HPF) in 35%. Five-year survival figures were 77%, 55%, and 44%, respectively. However, when corrected for tumor thickness, mitotic index was not an independent variable.

TREATMENT

STAGE I

Over the period of study, the treatment approach for patients with primary melanoma has changed very little. The mainstay of initial therapy for stage I disease is a wide surgical excision of the primary tumor with coverage of the defect with a split-

TABLE 32–2
CLINICAL AND PATHOLOGIC DATA FOR MELANOMA PATIENTS TREATED IN THE WEST OF SCOTLAND

Characteristics	Presenting Pathologic Stage
	Stage I
Clinical	
Number of patients	847
Year of diagnosis	
≤ 1960	31%
1961–1970	23%
1971–1980	45%
Median age	43 yr
Sex	
Male	32%
Female	67%
Primary lesion site	
Female lower extremity	35%
Male lower extremity	12%
Female upper extremity	10%
Male upper extremity	4%
Female head and neck	10%
Male head and neck	9%
Female trunk	12%
Male trunk	10%
Pathologic	
Breslow's tumor thickness	
< 0.76 mm	20%
0.76 mm–1.49 mm	21%
1.50 mm–2.49 mm	22%
2.50 mm–3.99 mm	19%
≥ 4.00 mm	17%
Median tumor thickness	
Male	3.4 mm
Female	2.5 mm
Level of invasion	
II	12%
III	31%
IV	37%
V	20%
Ulceration	
Yes	14%
No	86%
Growth pattern	
Nodular	15%
Superficial spreading	73%
Lentigo maligna	12%

thickness skin graft. In the earliest years of this study, the margins of excision were commonly 5 cm or more. During the past 20 years, this margin has decreased to around 3 cm for the majority of patients, with the exception of LMM. As LMM lesions occur on the face in over 90% of patients, the location frequently does not allow a margin exceeding 1 cm to 2 cm. Prophylactic node dissection has not been practiced in the WOS, and arterial perfusion has been performed only in a small group of patients (<10) with recurrent melanoma of the limbs.

STAGES II AND III

Patients presenting with clinically enlarged lymph nodes undergo routine surgical dissection. No patient with metastatic nodes received adjuvant chemotherapy during this period, although patients from the WOS have subsequently been entered into a randomized clinical trial in the World Health Organization Melanoma Group (Trial No. 6). Patients with generalized metastases have usually been treated symptomatically. Prior to 1970, the only cytotoxic drug used was melphalan, with poor results. Radiotherapy has been used only for palliation of advanced disease at selected sites in patients with cerebral or bony metastases.

COMMENT

The three studies quoted in this chapter provide a useful review of melanoma in the WOS over a 30-year period. Although incidence figures are not available for earlier years in the study, it is of interest to note how little the disease has changed over the years in terms of female-to-male ratio, histologic features, and survival figures.

It is particularly valuable to have an accurate incidence figure for the Scottish population in *Scotland,* since many publications discussing the Australian experience refer to the high incidence of melanoma in settlers of Scottish or Irish descent. Comparing the current incidence figure of around 5×10^5 for Scotland and 32×10^5 for Queensland, Australia,[5] would seem to suggest that environmental factors are responsible for a sixfold or greater increase in melanoma incidence, assuming that the two populations are strictly comparable in terms of genotype. In fact, it appears that the incidence in Queensland is not uniform among ethnic groups but is actually higher for those of Scottish or Irish descent and lower for those of Mediterranean extraction. The incidence figure of melanomas among Queenslanders of Scottish or Irish descent may therefore be even higher than the figures quoted above. It must be emphasized, however, that the Queensland incidence figure includes level I melanomas, while the WOS figure does not.

The particular points that appear to be unique to the Scottish population are first, the sex ratio, and second, the high incidence of LMM. The 2:1 female-to-male ratio is also seen in England, Wales, Italy, and Denmark but not in Sweden, Australia or North America, where the sex ratio is about equal, or there may be a slight preponderance of men in

some areas (see Chapter 36). Similarly, the striking female preponderance is not seen in other racial types, such as the Japanese. If lesions on the lower leg of women are excluded from the analysis, the sex ratio reverts to around unity and the improved survival advantage for women under 50 years of age is lost. It is tempting, therefore, to suggest a distinct good prognosis subset of SSM on the lower limbs of women of child-bearing age. The good prognosis in this group clearly is closely related to thickness, which in this WOS series overrides all other features such as ulceration, mitotic rate, and the level of invasion. Combining these features in an attempt to develop a more accurate prognostic index does not produce a more predictive guide than does the measurement of tumor thickness alone.

Lentigo maligna melanoma regularly comprises 10% to 15% of reported cases of malignant melanoma in Scotland. This incidence does not result from inaccurate histologic reporting but reflects the histologic type confirmed by ultrastructural examination.[2] The majority of these arise on the face of women 70 years of age and older. Comparison with geographically adjacent areas, such as Denmark, suggests that this distribution of growth pattern is unique to Scotland.[†] Lentigo maligna is fairly common on the faces of elderly people, particularly outdoor workers and inhabitants of the Scottish islands,[*] but no accurate incidence figures for this noninvasive or radial growth phase lesion are available. Therefore, the high Scottish incidence of LMM could either be caused by a high incidence of LM with a proportion proceeding to LMM, or by an incidence of LM similar to that of other countries, with a higher proportion proceeding to LMM. The first explanation seems more likely.

An important area of comparison between the elderly Scots with LMM and those in other countries is the population at risk. It may be that there is a significantly higher proportion of the Scottish population in the 60 years and older age group. If this is not the case, it must be concluded that Scottish skin has a particular tendency to develop LMM. Scots also readily tend to develop squamous and basal cell carcinoma and appear to have a higher incidence of these tumors than do other racial types. The current opinion regarding the etiology of squamous and basal cell lesions is that total cumulative lifetime sun exposure is the important factor rather

---

[†] A higher incidence of LMM lesions was reported from the University of Gotëborg in Sweden than from Scotland or Denmark (see Chapter 36)—ed.

[*] Personal observation

than the short duration, high–intensity exposures that may be more important in SSM and NM. This is further evidence for the biologic separation of LMM from the other varieties of melanoma.

REFERENCES

1. Cochran AJ: Malignant melanoma: A review of 10 years' experience in Glasgow, Scotland. Cancer 23:75, 1969
2. Hunter JAA, Zaynoun S, Paterson WD, Bleehen SS, MacKie RM, Cochran AJ: Cellular fine structure in the invasive nodules of different histogenic types of malignant melanoma. Br J Dermatol 98:255, 1978
3. Lane Brown MM, Melia DF: Celticity and cutaneous malignant melanoma in Massachusetts. In McGovern VJ, Russell P (eds): Pigment Cell: Mechanisms in Pigmentation, Vol 1, p 229. Basel, Karger, 1973
4. Lee JAH, Storer BE: Excess of malignant melanoma in women in the British Isles. Lancet 2:1337, 1980
5. Little JH, Holt J, Davis N: Changing epidemiology of malignant melanoma in Queensland. Med J Aust 1:66, 1980
6. MacKie RM, Aitchison TC: Severe sunburn and subsequent risk of primary cutaneous malignant melanoma in Scotland. Br J Cancer 46:955, 1982
7. MacKie RM, Cochran AJ, Fitzgerald B: Malignant melanoma in the West of Scotland (1960–1970). (Manuscript in preparation)
8. MacKie RM, Hunter JAA: Cutaneous malignant melanoma in Scotland. Br J Cancer 46:75, 1982
9. Prade M, Sancho-Garnier H, Cesarine JP, Cochran AJ: Difficulties encountered in the application of Clark classification and the Breslow thickness measurement in cutaneous malignant melanoma. Int J Cancer 26:159, 1980
10. Rampen F: Changing concepts in melanoma management. Br J Dermatol 104:341, 1981
11. Wright RB, Clark CH, Milne JA: Malignant cutaneous melanoma: A review. Br J Surg 150:360, 1953

JÜRGEN TONAK
PAUL HERMANEK
FRANK WEIDNER
IRENE GUGGENMOOS-HOLZMANN
ANNELORE ALTENDORF

Melanoma in Germany: Experience at the University of Erlangen–Nürnberg

33

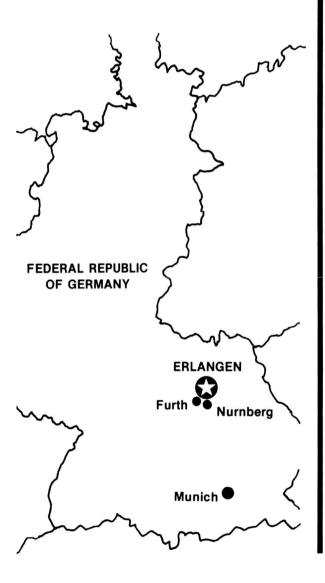

Epidemiology
**Prognostic Factors for Patients with Extremity
 and Trunk Melanomas**
    Patient Factors
    Pathologic Factors
    Multifactorial Analysis
Treatment
    Primary Melanoma
    Regional Lymph Node Dissection
    Hyperthermic Limb Perfusion
    Immunotherapy and Chemotherapy

At the University of Erlangen–Nürnberg, 662 melanoma patients were treated in the Department of Surgery between January 1967 and December 1981. The city of Erlangen is one of the three old university towns in Bavaria, along with Munich and Würzburg. Together with Nürnberg and Fürth it is part of the urban center of Northern Bavaria.

Bavaria is located between 47° and 51° N latitude and between 10° and 13° E longitude. It has an area of 70,000 square kilometers and is thereby the largest state in the Federal Republic of Germany. Bavaria has a population of 10.8 million inhabitants, which is equivalent to a population density of 153 persons per square kilometer. Despite its increasing industrialization, especially in the urban centers of Munich and Nürnberg–Erlangen, 53% of the total area is still used for farming purposes.

The Federal Republic of Germany, including Bavaria, is located in a zone of moderate climate. The average temperature in Nürnberg calculated from long-term observations is 18°C in July and −0.8°C in winter. During the summer months (May to September), the maximum daytime temperatures average 20°C to 25°C, although in July and August they sometimes exceed 30°C. The winter period (December to February) is a relatively short 3 months. In the summertime, the average daily duration of sunshine in Nürnberg is 6.7 hours (range, 5.3–8.6) and in the wintertime, 2.1 hours (range, 1.2–3.3).

The geographic area from which patients are referred to the Erlangen University Clinic corresponds approximately to the region of Northern Bavaria with about 4.5 million inhabitants. Data on patients treated from 1967 to 1973 were accumulated retrospectively, while all data were entered prospectively thereafter. Two thirds of these patients had their initial treatment here, while the remainder were referred after initial treatment elsewhere.

The data were evaluated using a specially developed computer program. The treatment and follow-up of patients were possible because of close cooperation between the Departments of Surgery and Dermatology. As long as the patients remained free of disease, they were followed up postoperatively every 3 months for 2 years, then every 6 months until the fifth year, and yearly thereafter until the tenth year. The median follow-up time was 48 months, and all patients had a minimum 1 year of follow-up. Only four patients (0.6%) were lost to follow-up.

The histologic diagnosis was made first in the Pathology Section of the Department of Surgery and then independently in the Department of Dermatology in all cases. Only invasive melanomas were considered in this study; melanoma *in situ* (level I) was excluded.

Characteristics of the 662 patients and their survival rates are shown in Tables 33-1 and 33-2. The melanomas of these patients are largely confined to the extremities and trunk. A relatively small number of patients (4%) have melanomas of the head and neck, because these are usually treated in other specialized hospitals. On the other hand, the proportion of melanoma patients with regional metastases (pathologic stage II) is rather high (28%), because of referral patterns where patients with more advanced disease stages were referred selectively to this hospital. In recent years, a better education of the public and referring physicians about the dangers of melanoma has led to a change in the composition of the Erlangen patients. This is evidenced by the steady increase in incidence of thinner melanomas (<1.5 mm) that comprised 50% of all treated cases in 1982.

EPIDEMIOLOGY

Melanoma is an uncommon cancer in West Germany, representing only about 1% of all malignant diseases. There is no national tumor registry office in West Germany, so the incidence of melanoma in Germany can only be estimated using standard mortality rates.

Wagner and Becker[12] have analyzed cancer mortality rates in Germany and nine other central European countries. In their study, the average death rate from melanoma in men increased from 0.49×10^5 inhabitants in 1956 to 1.62×10^5 by 1975, while in women it increased from 0.41 to 1.19×10^5 inhabitants per year. These increases were by far the highest for any malignant tumor (Table 33-3). The current incidence of melanoma in West Germany is estimated to be 4×10^5 inhabitants per year.

This considerable increase in melanoma incidence is reflected by an increased number of patients treated at this institution, which has more than tripled from the period 1970 to 1974 to the period 1980 to 1984 (Table 33-4). A similar increase was observed at the Hospital of Münster–Hornheide,[2] which is located in Northern Germany. In contrast, the number of patients with colorectal carci-

TABLE 33–1
CLINICAL AND PATHOLOGIC DATA FOR MELANOMA PATIENTS TREATED AT THE DEPARTMENT OF SURGERY, UNIVERSITY OF ERLANGEN, WEST GERMANY

| Characteristics | Presenting Pathologic Stage | | | |
	Stage I	Stage II	Stage III	Total
Clinical				
Number of patients	455	185	22	662
Year of diagnosis				
≤1960	0%	0%	0%	0%
1961–1965	0%	0%	0%	0%
1966–1970	11%	16%	23%	13%
1971–1975	22%	22%	14%	22%
1976–1980	67%	62%	64%	66%
Median age	50 yr	52 yr	51 yr	50 yr
Sex				
Male	35%	49%	41%	39%
Female	65%	51%	59%	61%
Primary lesion site				
Female lower extremity	39%	31%	18%	38%
Male lower extremity	11%	17%	9%	13%
Female upper extremity	15%	8%	0%	17%
Male upper extremity	5%	6%	4%	5%
Female head and neck	1%	2%	9%	1%
Male head and neck	2%	2%	14%	2%
Female trunk	9%	21%	5%	12%
Male trunk	18%	9%	14%	15%
Other	0%	4%	27%	2%
Pathologic				
Breslow's tumor thickness				
≤0.75 mm	21%	1%	0%	17%
0.76 mm–1.49 mm	23%	12%	0%	21%
1.50 mm–3.00 mm	32%	30%	33%	32%
≥3.01 mm	24%	57%	67%	30%
Level of invasion				
II	14%	0%	0%	11%
III	33%	25%	14%	31%
IV	48%	62%	43%	51%
V	5%	13%	43%	7%
Ulceration				
Yes	24%	38%	33%	27%
No	76%	62%	67%	73%
Growth pattern				
Nodular	29%	52%	83%	34%
Superficial spreading	57%	35%	17%	52%
Lentigo maligna	8%	3%	0%	7%
Acral melanoma	6%	9%	0%	7%

noma treated at Erlangen–Nürnberg Department of Surgery has only doubled (Table 33-4). Although these figures could be affected by other factors, it is believed that, since the patients of both these institutions were drawn from such a large geographic area, they are representative of the entire German population. This increase is probably restricted to cutaneous melanoma, since no increase was observed in the number of mucosal melanomas treated at this institution. The referral area of this institution, together with that of the special clinic of Münster–Hornheide (which is about twice the size of this institution), constitutes about 20% of the total population of Western Germany.

The ethnic composition of this population is extraordinarily varied and has become even more mixed since the Second World War because of immigration from Eastern Europe, and in recent years

TABLE 33–2
ACTUARIAL SURVIVAL DATA FOR MELANOMA PATIENTS TREATED AT THE DEPARTMENT OF SURGERY, UNIVERSITY OF ERLANGEN, WEST GERMANY

	Survival Rates	
	5-Year	10-Year
Stage I		
Overall survival	81%	71%
Sex		
Male	75%	61%
Female	84%	75%
Primary lesion site		
Lower extremity	83%	76%
Upper extremity	89%	70%
Head and neck	88%	0%
Trunk	69%	57%
Tumor thickness		
≤0.75	96%	99%
0.76 mm–1.49 mm	100%	79%
1.50 mm–3.00 mm	79%	78%
≥3.01 mm	67%	40%
Level of invasion		
II	89%	97%
III	84%	83%
IV	78%	60%
V	63%	36%
Ulceration		
Yes	70%	56%
No	87%	74%

	1-Year	3-Year	5-Year
Stage II			
Overall survival	68%	41%	33%
Tumor thickness			
≤1.49 mm	71%	73%	51%
1.50 mm–3.00 mm	88%	85%	72%
≥ 3.01 mm	76%	38%	22%
Number of positive nodes			
1	80%	53%	50%
2	82%	55%	52%
≥3	44%	23%	16%
Ulceration			
Yes	74%	37%	38%
No	81%	66%	49%

	6-Month	1-Year	2-Year
Stage III			
Overall survival	46%	37%	11%

TABLE 33–3
AGE-CORRECTED CANCER DEATH RATES IN CENTRAL EUROPE IN MEN AND WOMEN

	Death Rate (Per 10^5 Inhabitants/Year)					
	1956		1975		Percent Change	
	Women	Men	Women	Men	Women	Men
Lung cancer	5.75	38.27	7.62	70.86	+ 33	+ 85
Stomach cancer	34.07	57.40	18.50	37.78	− 46	− 34
Colorectal cancer	19.63	24.96	22.37	30.83	+ 14	+ 26
Malignant melanoma	0.41	0.49	1.19	1.62	+190	+230

(Abridged from Wagner G, Becker N: Die Krebssterblichkeit in Mitteleuropa. Deutsches Ärzteblatt 79:41, 1982)

TABLE 33–4
NEWLY REGISTERED PATIENTS WITH MALIGNANT MELANOMA AND COLORECTAL CARCINOMA

	1970–1974 *(N)*	*1975–1979* *(N)*	*Percent* *Increase*	*1980–1984* *(Estimated)* *(N)*	*Percent* *Increase* *(Estimated)*
Malignant melanoma (Erlangen)	152	269	+ 79	520 (1980–1982; n = 319)	+240
Malignant melanoma (Münster–Hornheide)	349	902	+158	1370 (1980–1981; n = 543)	+292
Colorectal carcinoma (Erlangen)	741	1154	+ 56	1480 (1980–1982; n = 888)	+100

(Data from the Surgical Clinic, Erlangen, and Münster–Hornheide Specialist Clinic)

because of the arrival of guest-workers from Southern Europe. Although no records of ethnic origin are kept, it is believed that the majority of melanoma patients are fair-skinned. Supporting this observation is the fact that mortality rates for melanoma are higher in North European countries with predominantly fair-skinned populations than in Southern European countries, where more of the population have a darker skin (Table 33-5).

This increased incidence of melanoma in Europe may result from increased sunlight exposure.[8] Jung[4] suggested that the anatomical location, as well as the actual incidence of malignant tumors of the skin, depends on the extent and frequency of exposure to strong sunlight. In addition, the type of pigmentation, the effectiveness of cellular repair mechanisms, and the immunologic competence of the patient influence this risk. The spontaneous and light-induced sister chromatid exchange (SCE) and the persistence of a strong erythema were significantly increased for melanoma patients compared with a control group.

PROGNOSTIC FACTORS FOR PATIENTS WITH EXTREMITY AND TRUNK MELANOMAS

There are many factors that influence prognosis in melanoma. In this analysis, those factors were analyzed that were considered to have the most prognostic significance, as listed in Table 33-6. From the entire series of 662 patients, 426 clinical stage I patients were selected for this analysis. This data base included only those patients with melanomas located on the trunk and the extremities (Fig. 33-1). Excluded were those patients with head and neck melanomas, those with multiple primary melano-

TABLE 33–5
MORTALITY FROM MELANOMA IN FOUR EUROPEAN COUNTRIES

	Mortality $\times 10^5$	
	♂	♀
Norway*	3.1	1.9
Denmark[†]	2.6	2.8
Federal Republic of Germany[†]	1.9	1.4
France[†]	0.9	0.6

* According to Magnus K: Incidence of malignant melanoma of the skin in Norway 1955–1970. Cancer 32:1275, 1973
[†] According to Wagner G, Becker N: Die Krebssterblichkeit in Mitteleuropa. Deutsches Ärzteblatt 79:41, 1982

TABLE 33–6
VARIABLES TESTED FOR THEIR VALUES IN PREDICTING SURVIVAL IN 426 CLINICAL STAGE I MELANOMA PATIENTS

Clinical Variables
  Sex (women or men)
  Site (trunk or extremities)

Histologic Variables
  Growth pattern (nodular versus superficial spreading and lentigo maligna melanoma)
  Level of invasion (Clark II, III, IV, V)
  Thickness (mm)
    ≤0.75
    0.76–1.50
    1.51–3.0
    ≥3.01
  Ulceration (present/absent)

mas, those with unknown microstaging or growth pattern, and those with acral lentiginous or unclassified growth patterns.

PATIENT FACTORS

As in other series, there was a striking sex difference in the site distribution of melanomas, with the majority of women having extremity melanomas (83%) and men having trunk melanomas (54%) (Fig. 33-1). Five-year survival rates for the 270 women patients were significantly better than for the 156 men (84% versus 72%, respectively; p<0.05) (Fig. 33-2). Patients with melanomas on the extremities had a significantly better survival rate than those with melanomas on the trunk (p<0.05) (Fig. 33-3).

PATHOLOGIC FACTORS

Tumor thickness was the most significant prognostic factor in this analysis (Fig. 33-4). The 5-year survival rate of 138 patients with melanomas <1.5 mm in thickness was nearly 100%. The worst 5-year survival rate was 61% in 99 patients with melanomas >3 mm in thickness. The differences between each of the thickness groups was statistically significant (p<0.05) (Fig. 33-4).

The presence or absence of ulceration delineated significant differences in survival rates. Thus, 85 patients with ulcerated melanomas had a 68% 5-year survival rate compared with 84% in 261 patients with nonulcerated melanomas (Fig. 33-5).

In contrast, the level of invasion did not discriminate significant differences in survival (Fig.

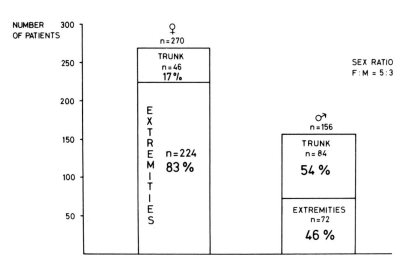

FIG. 33–1 Anatomical distribution of primary tumors in 426 clinical stage I melanoma patients according to sex.

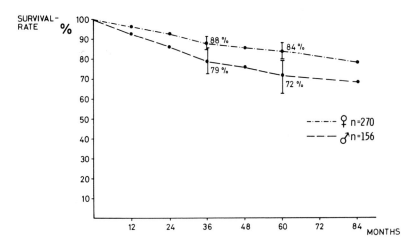

FIG. 33–2 Cumulative survival rates according to sex. *P* < 0.05. The *bars* in this figure and all subsequent figures represent SE ± 2.

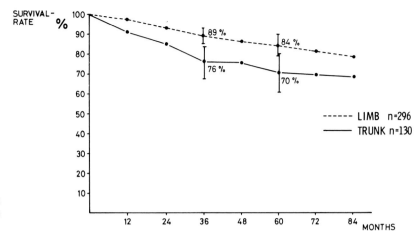

FIG. 33–3 Cumulative survival rates according to anatomical location of the primary tumor; $P < 0.05$

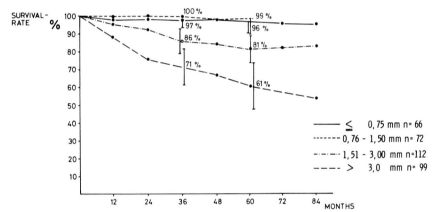

FIG. 33–4 Cumulative survival rates according to the thickness of the primary tumor; $P < 0.05$.

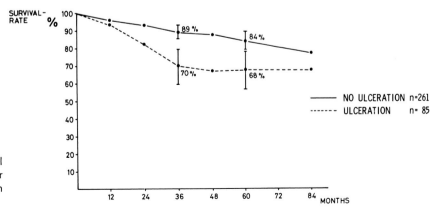

FIG. 33–5 Cumulative survival rates according to the presence or absence of histologic ulceration in the primary tumor; $P < 0.05$.

33-6). For example, the 55 patients with level II melanomas had similar 5-year survival rates to those 139 patients with level III melanomas (90% versus 86%, respectively). The only significant differences in survival rates were between patients with level II and level V melanomas (Fig. 33-6).

The prognostic significance of growth pattern was examined using the WHO classification scheme. The survival rate in 131 patients with nodular melanomas was significantly lower than the corresponding rate in 295 patients with either lentigo maligna melanoma or superficial spreading melanoma (p<0.05) (Fig. 33-7). However, these differences in survival are probably not the result of differences in biologic behavior of these growth patterns.[3] Our previous studies showed that lentigo maligna melanomas and superficial spreading melanomas are generally thinner than nodular melano-

mas, and, further, that all these types of melanomas had equivalent survival rates at equal thicknesses. The only possible exception was acral lentiginous melanoma, which had a high rate of metastases, even with tumors <0.76 mm in thickness. Among the 35 patients with acral lentiginous melanoma, almost one third (11 out of 35) had regional metastases at first presentation, and the 5-year survival rate of the 24 pathologic stage I patients was only 60%.

MULTIFACTORIAL ANALYSIS

The relative influence on survival of different prognostic factors was tested in a multifactorial regression analysis described by Kalbfleisch and Prentice.[5] Tumor thickness was the most predictive prognostic factor (p < 0.001; Table 33-7). The sex of the patient and the anatomical site of the primary

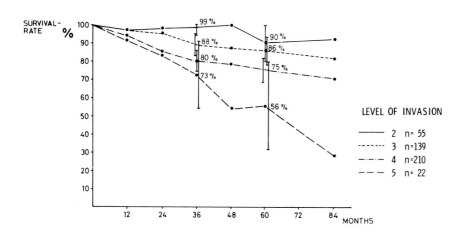

FIG. 33–6 Cumulative survival rates according to level of invasion of the primary tumor.

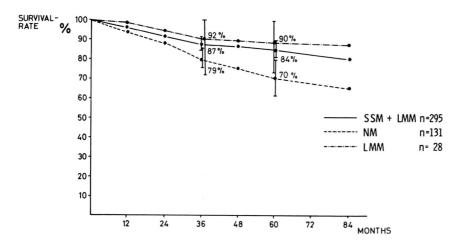

FIG. 33–7 Cumulative survival rates according to the growth pattern of the primary lesion; P < 0.05.

TABLE 33–7
RESULTS OF MULTIVARIATE ANALYSIS OF PROGNOSTIC FACTORS

Factor	X^2	P
Thickness	41.30	0.001
Sex	10.42	0.01
Anatomical site	3.89	0.05
Level of invasion	4.52	NS
Growth pattern	0.48	NS
Ulceration	0.57	NS

NS = not statistically significant

TABLE 33–8
PARAMETRIC MODEL AND RISK-INTERPRETATION

Factor	Relative Risk
Thickness	
0.76 mm–1.50 mm	1.1*
1.51 mm–3.00 mm	2.6*
>3.00 mm	6.3*
Sex	
Men vs women	1.7
Site	
Trunk vs extremities	1.6

*Relative risk versus tumor $\leq$ 0.75 mm in thickness

Note: Relative risk for different tumor thicknesses is given in relation to risk for tumors $\leq$ 0.76 mm thick. In melanomas between 0.76 mm and 1.50 mm in thickness, relative risk is not significantly greater than 1 and therefore not greater than the risk for the smallest melanomas.

lesion also both significantly influenced prognosis. Stepwise selection of these factors revealed their interdependence as well as the loss of predictive value if their order was reversed in the multivariate analysis. Factors highly correlated to tumor thickness, such as presence of ulceration, growth pattern, and level of invasion, failed to improve the prediction further.

Integration of the major predictive factors—tumor thickness, sex of patient, and anatomical site of primary lesion—were used in interpreting the prognosis. The relative risk of dying from a melanoma <0.76 mm in thickness was set at 1. Table 33-8 shows that melanomas between 0.76 mm and 1.5 mm in thickness have a similar relative risk. Men have a relative risk 1.7 times greater than women do, while melanomas of the trunk carry a risk 1.6 times greater than melanomas of the extremities. These calculations also show that the variables of sex and site have an equally strong influence on progno-

sis. These results contrast partially with earlier studies,[10] where the differences in prognosis for men and women appeared to be related to different distribution of melanomas between trunk and extremities and not to a sex-specific behavior of the tumor.

Similar results have been observed by Weidner[13] in an analysis of patients participating in the German Malignant Melanoma Working Group Study. In a study of 1191 patients with high-risk melanomas (>1.5 mm thick), he found no significant difference in the 5-year survival rates for men and women with the same tumor location, but highly significant differences in the 5-year survival for anatomical site (Table 33-9). This means that patient survival for melanomas of comparable mi-

TABLE 33-9
DIRECT COMPARISON OF 5-YEAR SURVIVAL RATES (%) OF PATIENTS WITH CLINICAL STAGE I MELANOMAS ACCORDING TO SEX AND SITE

Site	Women	Men	P value Women versus Men	P value Trunk versus Extremities
Trunk				
Erlangen, 1983	75% (n = 46)	68% (n = 84)	NS	NS
German Melanoma Working Group[13]*	51% (n = 102)	45% (n = 129)	NS	p < 0.01
Extremities				
Erlangen, 1983	87% (n = 224)	77% (n = 72)	NS	NS
German Melanoma Working Group[13]*	70% (n = 441)	65% (n = 93)	NS	p < 0.01

*Only melanomas >1.5 mm in thickness

NS = not statistically significant

croscopic invasion is mainly owing to differences in the anatomical site of the primary melanoma and not so much to sex-specific differences in biologic behavior of the tumor. In the group of patients who could be used for risk interpretation, the survival rates in extremity and trunk melanomas in the Erlangen series were directly compared for men and women (Table 33-9). No significant differences could be found in the survival rates between the sexes as to tumor site either on extremities or the trunk. Unfortunately, patient groups were too small to allow a valid statistical evaluation. The main reason for the sex difference in prognosis is probably that the location is closely correlated with sex, since 83% of the women had extremity lesions and 54% of the men had trunk lesions. Whether the sex of the patient is only of minor clinical importance for tumors of the same location needs confirmation by additional studies.

TREATMENT

PRIMARY MELANOMA

The primary melanoma was widely excised with a 5-cm margin of skin as measured on the tension-free specimen. A wide excision is especially recommended in melanomas measuring >1.5 mm in thickness. Different plastic surgical procedures are used to cover the defect. Very good results are obtained with split-thickness skin grafts on limbs. For tumors on the trunk, wound closure using a skin flap is the preferred treatment, or a primary skin closure can be used in certain anatomical locations. For tumors of fingers and toes, a partial amputation

is necessary. The level of amputation is dictated by the site of the primary tumor and the digit involved so that maximum function is preserved.

The original recommendations of Breslow and Macht[1] that thin melanomas (<0.76 mm thick) could be excised with a narrower margin of excision were substantiated in a retrospective study on 64 such patients treated at this institution. There was 100% survival at 5 years of those patients in whom the width of excision was <2 cm (Fig. 33-8). Similar results were obtained in 68 patients with tumors <1.5 mm in thickness in whom the width of excision was <2 cm. Five-year survival rates in these patients were nearly 100% (Fig. 33-8). None of these 141 patients had a local tumor recurrence. On the basis of these results, it is suggested that wide excision with a 5-cm margin is no longer necessary for melanomas <1.5 mm in thickness.

REGIONAL LYMPH NODES

The value of therapeutic dissection of clinically suspected lymph node metastases is undisputed. There is, however, controversy about the indications for elective lymph node dissection (ELND).[9] It must be emphasized that there is a direct relationship between the incidence of regional lymph node metastases and either tumor thickness or level of invasion. In superficial melanomas (those ≤1.5 mm thick), the probability of occult regional metastases is so small that ELND is not indicated. For thicker melanomas (those >1.5 mm thick), studies from this institution indicated that the incidence of occult lymph node metastases was 40% or greater.[9] In these patients, ELND is justifiable and necessary. Since this was a retrospective analysis, a definitive

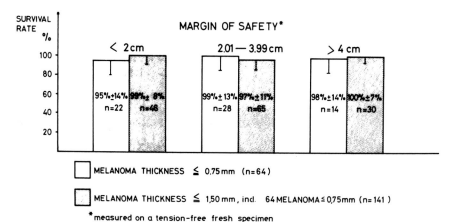

FIG. 33–8 Five-year survival rates in clinical stage I melanoma patients according to width of primary tumor excision.

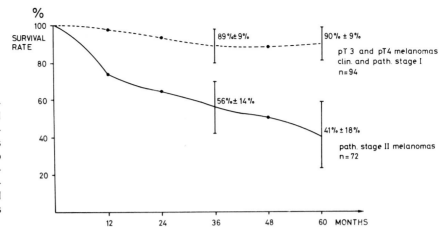

FIG. 33–9 Age-corrected cumulative survival rates in 94 clinical and pathologic stage I and 72 pathologic stage II melanoma patients with extremity primary tumors who received wide local excision, elective dissection, and adjuvant hyperthermic perfusion. All clinical stage I patients had primary tumors > 1.5-mm thick (pT3 and pT4).

conclusion cannot be made. For this reason, this institution is participating in the WHO Melanoma Group randomized, prospective protocol evaluating ELND for trunk melanomas >2 mm in thickness.

HYPERTHERMIC LIMB PERFUSION

In 1975, this institution was the first in Germany to use hyperthermic limb perfusion routinely in the treatment of melanoma.[11] The perfusion is performed according to the technique of Schraffordt Koops and associates[7] with some modifications.[11] When indicated (melanomas thicker than 1.5 mm or Clark's level IV and V), patients undergoing hyperthermic perfusion also had either therapeutic or elective lymph node dissection (ELND). Between 1975 and 1981, 195 perfusions were performed in patients considered to have potentially curable melanoma. A 5-year survival rate of 90% was achieved in 94 stage I patients with melanomas >1.5 mm in thickness or levels IV and V (Fig. 33-9). In 72 patients with regional lymph node metastases, the 5-year survival rate was 41%. This latter rate was clearly better than that previously obtained at this institution with surgery alone.[11]

Excellent results were obtained in 39 patients with satellitosis. Just under 50% of these patients (15 of 39) had complete disappearance of the metastases.

IMMUNOTHERAPY AND CHEMOTHERAPY

All patients with clinical stage I melanomas received, as adjuvant therapy, a prophylactic sensitization by local treatment of the operative scar with dinitrochlorbenzol (DNCB). In patients who de-

veloped skin metastases, threshold doses of DNCB were used. Weidner and Djawari[14] have reported on the early favorable results, but the long-term benefits of DNCB application are yet to be evaluated.

Immunotherapy with BCG (Bacillus Calmette-Guérin) has been abandoned after disappointing results. Systemic chemotherapy with dacarbazine (DTIC) or cis platinum has been used as a last resort in young patients with multiple distant metastases. The results of systemic chemotherapy have also been disappointing.

REFERENCES

1. Breslow A, Macht SD: Optimal size of resection margin for thin cutaneous melanoma. Surg Gynecol Obstet 145:720, 1977
2. Drepper H, Tilkorn H: The surgical treatment of the primary melanoma adjusted to the prognosis. XIIIth European Federation Congress ICS, West Berlin, Germany, 1983
3. Hermanek P, Hornstein OP, Tonak J, Weidner F: Malignes Melanom, Invasionstiefe und Melanomtyp. Beitr Path 157:269, 1976
4. Jung EO: Licht und Hautkrebse: Sitzungsbericht der Heidelberger Akademie der Wissenschaften. New York, Springer-Verlag, 1982
5. Kalbfleisch JD, Prentice RL: The statistical analysis of failure time data. New York, John Wiley & Sons, 1980
6. Magnus K: Incidence of malignant melanoma of the skin in Norway 1955–1970. Cancer 32:1275, 1973
7. Schraffordt Koops H, Oldhoff J, van der Ploeg E, Vermey A, Eibergen R, Beekhuis H: Some aspects of the treatment of primary malignant melanoma of the

extremities by isolated regional perfusion. Cancer 39:27, 1977

8. Swerdlow AJ: Incidence of malignant melanoma of the skin in England and Wales and its relationship to sunshine. Br Med J 2:1324, 1979

9. Tonak J, Gall FP, Hermanek P: Die prophylaktische Lymphknotendissektion beim malignen Melanom. Deutsch Med Wochenschr 51:1782, 1980

10. Tonak J, Hermanek P: Die unterschiedliche Prognose von Rumpf- und Extremitätenmelanomen. Lebensversicherungsmedizin 35:61, 1983

11. Tonak J, Weidner F, Hoferichter S, Altendorf A: Er- langer Therapieschema beim malignen Melanom. In Weidner F, Tonak J (eds): Das maligne Melanom der Haut, p 177. Erlangen, Perimed, 1981

12. Wagner G, Becker N: Die Krebssterblichkeit in Mitteleuropa. Deutsches Ärzteblatt 79:41, 1982

13. Weidner F: 8-year-survival in malignant melanoma related to sex and tumor location. Dermatologica 162:51, 1981

14. Weidner F, Djawari D: Adjuvante DNCB-Immuntherapie beim malignen Melanom. Hautkr. 54:436, 1979

KAM-HING LAM
JOHN WONG

Melanoma in Hong Kong: Experience at the Queen Mary Hospital

34

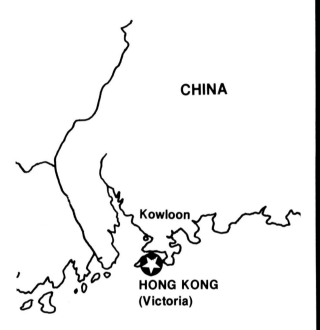

There is a paucity of published data about melanoma in Chinese. This is largely because the incidence is low and cancer registration is not compulsory. However, some melanoma data have recently been accumulated at the Queen Mary Hospital in Hong Kong.

Hong Kong is a British Protectorate. It is situated between the 22nd and 23rd parallels of north latitude and 114th and 115th parallels of east longitude and is entirely in the subtropical zone. The area of Hong Kong is 1064 square kilometers, and the population is 5.3 million. Persons of Chinese descent constitute 98% of the population.

Medical records were available for 26 patients with malignant melanoma who were admitted to the Department of Surgery, University of Hong Kong, Queen Mary Hospital, Hong Kong (Table 34-1). This represented a small proportion of all patients with melanoma seen in Hong Kong. It is likely that the majority of the early lesions were treated elsewhere and extensive and recurrent tumors were referred to this center. Follow-up of patients after treatment has been exceedingly difficult. This is probably because of the lack of concern of the patients themselves and their inability to take time off from work. Tracing patients has not been fruitful in spite of the small size of the country. Change of address is seldom given; thus, follow-up data have been incomplete.

EPIDEMIOLOGY

The incidence of melanoma is low among Asians as compared with white-skinned and black-skinned persons.[2] However, among the Asian populations,

TABLE 34–1
CLINICAL AND PATHOLOGIC DATA FOR MELANOMA PATIENTS TREATED IN HONG KONG

| Characteristics | Presenting Pathologic Stage | | | |
	Stage I	Stage II	Stage III	Total
Clinical				
Number of patients	4	15	2	21
Year of diagnosis				
≤ 1960	25%	7%	0%	10%
1961–1965	0%	13%	0%	10%
1966–1970	0%	13%	0%	10%
1971–1975	25%	40%	50%	38%
1976–1980	50%	27%	50%	33%
Median age	39 yr	57 yr	73 yr	56 yr
Sex				
Male	75%	60%	50%	62%
Female	25%	40%	50%	38%
Primary lesion site				
Female lower extremity	25%	33%	50%	33%
Male lower extremity	0%	27%	0%	19%
Female upper extremity	0%	7%	0%	5%
Male upper extremity	0%	20%	50%	19%
Female head and neck	0%	0%	0%	0%
Male head and neck	25%	0%	0%	5%
Female trunk	0%	0%	0%	0%
Male trunk	50%	13%	0%	19%
Pathologic				
Level of invasion				
II	25%	7%		12%
III	25%	7%		12%
IV	0%	7%		6%
V	50%	79%		70%
Ulceration				
Yes	25%	77%	0%	65%
No	75%	23%	0%	35%
Growth pattern				
Nodular	50%	73%	100%	71%
Superficial spreading	50%	27%	0%	29%
Lentigo maligna	0%	0%	0%	0%

the Chinese have the highest incidence. Collective data from cancer registries showed that the incidence of melanoma in Chinese men and women was 0.6 and 0.3×10^5, respectively.[2]

During the 3-year period from 1977 to 1979, the Cancer Registry of the Medical and Health Department in Hong Kong recorded 144 melanomas. Notification of cancer in Hong Kong is voluntary, so this probably constitutes an underestimation. In the same period, 660 cases of other types of skin cancer were registered. Thus, melanoma represents 18% of all skin cancers in this registry. Expressed as incidence $\times 10^5$ (Table 34-2), there was only a marginally higher incidence for men. During this 1977 to 1979 period, the Cancer Registry recorded between 40 and 60 new cases of melanoma each year, giving an incidence of between 0.8 and 1.4×10^5 (Table 34-2).

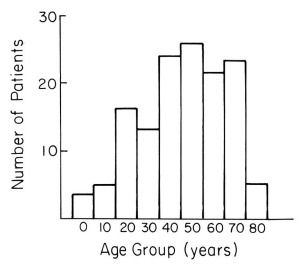

FIG. 34–1 Age distribution of 144 cases of melanoma of the skin (1977 to 1979).

PROGNOSTIC FACTORS

CLINICAL FACTORS

Of the 26 patients seen at the Queen Mary Hospital, 5 had melanoma arising from the mucous membranes (4 from the anorectum and 1 from the hard palate). Of the remaining 21 patients with cutaneous melanoma, 6 had previous treatment elsewhere, while the remaining 15 had their initial treatment at Queen Mary Hospital. The majority of patients presented with advanced primary melanomas, most of whom had metastatic disease (Table 34-1). In 11 patients (52%), the tumor was located on the lower limb, eight being on the plantar surface (38%) and one on the dorsum of the foot.

Data from the 144 patients in the Cancer Registry indicated that melanomas occurred in all age groups (Fig. 34-1). The median age for all patients was about 50 years, with the majority of patients ranging between 40 and 60 years of age.

PATHOLOGIC FACTORS

Pathologic details were available for 17 of the 21 cutaneous melanomas. Although the numbers are small, it is clear that most of the lesions were quite advanced. Most of the lesions (70%) invaded into the subcutaneous tissues (level V), were ulcerated (65%), and had a nodular growth pattern (71%). Not surprisingly, the majority of patients had nodal metastases (stage II), and only 4 patients (19%) had stage I disease, but even these were advanced (Table 34-1).

SURGICAL MANAGEMENT

The stage I patients were treated with a wide excision using a margin of at least 3 cm. No elective lymphadenectomies were performed. Two of the four patients so treated developed nodal metastases

TABLE 34–2
INCIDENCE OF MELANOMA OF SKIN IN HONG KONG

| Year | Men | | Women | |
	Number of Patients	Incidence Per 10^5 Inhabitants Per Year	Number of Patients	Incidence Per 10^5 Inhabitants Per Year
1977	33	1.4	25	1.0
1978	25	1.1	22	1.0
1979	20	0.8	19	0.8

(at 4 and 10 months), while the other two were lost to follow-up after 6 months.

The stage II patients were generally treated with wide excision of the primary lesion and a therapeutic lymphadenectomy. The primary lesions of the extremity were so advanced that they required coverage with cross leg flaps, and three required amputation. Despite optimal surgical management, only 1 of these 13 patients has lived beyond 5 years. The two patients who presented with advanced distant metastases (stage III) were untreated.

MANAGEMENT OF ANORECTAL MELANOMA

In the period under study, 4 of the 26 melanomas occurred in the anorectum. Their clinical management has been previously described.[1] Two ulcerative, fungating lesions were located at the anal verge, while the other two were polypoid lesions situated at 4 cm and 7 cm proximally in the rectum.

In three of these patients, lymph node or liver metastases were present at the time of diagnosis. These patients received palliative treatment. The one patient in our series with no clinical evidence of metastases underwent an abdominoperineal resection. However, this patient died from extensive metastatic disease 3 years later.

COMMENT

Melanoma in Chinese patients is substantially different from melanoma in Caucasian patients because of the higher proportion of plantar and anorectal melanomas. The sole of the foot was the most common site of melanoma in the Hong Kong series (38%). This contrasts markedly with the low proportion (1% to 5%) of plantar melanomas in white-skinned persons.[6] The concentration of plantar melanomas in Chinese is similar to that of other dark-skinned ethnic groups, including the Japanese,[7] the Hawaiians,[3] the American black,[6] and the African black.[5]

Trauma has been proposed as an etiologic factor predisposing to melanoma arising on the feet. This may apply to the people of Hong Kong, since the footwear of the majority of the lower social class is sandals and slippers, which expose the feet to risk of trauma.

Anorectal melanomas usually have a fatal outcome, since in both our series and those of other institutions[4,8] results were extremely poor. It is not possible to discern whether the higher proportion of anorectal melanomas in our series is caused by referral patterns, an actual increased incidence of mucosal melanomas in Chinese patients (compared with Caucasian patients), or the low frequency of cutaneous melanomas in sites other than hands and feet.

REFERENCES

1. Boey J, Choi TK, Wong J, Ong GB: The surgical management of anorectal malignant melanoma. Aust NZ J Surg 51:132, 1981
2. Crombie IK: Racial differences in melanoma incidence. Br J Cancer 40:185, 1979
3. Hinds MW: Anatomic distribution of malignant melanoma of the skin among non-Caucasians in Hawaii. Br J Cancer 40:497, 1979
4. Husa A, Hockerstedt K: Anorectal malignant melanoma. Acta Chir Scand 140:68, 1974
5. Lewis MG: Malignant melanoma in Uganda: The relationship between pigmentation and malignant melanoma on the soles of the feet. Br J Cancer 21:483, 1967
6. Reintgen DS, McCarty KM, Cox EB, Seigler HF: Malignant melanoma in black American and white American populations. JAMA 248:1856, 1982
7. Seiji M, Takematsu H, Hosokawa M, Obata M, Tomita Y, Kato T, Takahashi M, Mihm MC Jr: Acral melanoma in Japan. J Invest Dermatol (in press)
8. Wanebo HJ, Woodruff JM, Farr GH, Quan SH: Anorectal melanoma. Cancer 47:1891, 1981

HIDEAKI TAKEMATSU
YASUSHI TOMITA
TAIZO KATO
MASAAKI TAKAHASHI
RIKIYA ABE
MAKOTO SEIJI

Melanoma in Japan: Experience at Tohoku University Hospital, Sendai

35

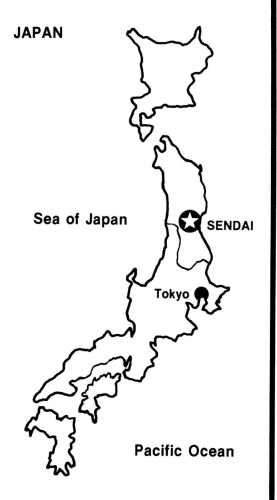

JAPAN

Sea of Japan

SENDAI

Tokyo

Pacific Ocean

Tohoku University is the main referral center of the Tohoku District of Japan, which is located between the 37th and the 42nd parallels of north latitude. Sendai is on a latitude of 38°N, has a local population of more than 600,000, and has four seasons. The clinical records and histologic materials for inclusive series of 81 patients with melanoma registered during the 12-year period (1969–1980) at the Department of Dermatology, Tohoku University School of Medicine, were reviewed. All but one were Japanese.

Sixty-four of the 81 patients had primary cutaneous melanoma (79%), 14 (17%) had mucosal melanoma, and 3 (4%) had occult primary melanoma with nodal metastases. One patient had Clark's level I melanoma and was excluded from the analysis.

Of the 64 cases of cutaneous melanoma, 32 patients (50%) were treated initially at this department. On an average, 5 to 6 patients have been treated each year over the past 10 years. There have not been significant changes in anatomical sites, sex ratio, or stage of disease. Each patient was followed at 2- to 3-month intervals for the first 2 years and annually thereafter. Follow-up data were also obtained by questionnaire.

This analysis was based on reexamination of representative sections of the lesions. Original histologic slides or paraffin blocks of the primary melanoma were obtained, and all this material was reviewed.

EPIDEMIOLOGY

The factor of race is highly related to the incidence and anatomical sites of melanoma.[1,3,5,6,7,11,12] Although melanoma occurs much less frequently in the Japanese than in white-skinned persons, the number of cases in Japan has increased steadily over recent years.[9] Although the incidence of melanoma in Japan is not available, the annual mortality rate from melanoma can be calculated from statistics collected by the Ministry of Health and Welfare of Japan. The data collected by the Miyagi Cancer Society provide the annual mortality rate from melanoma in Miyagi Prefecture, where Sendai is located and where the population is about 2 million. The mortality rate from melanoma in Japan increased almost linearly between 1960 and 1980 (Fig. 35-1). It rose more than threefold from 0.06×10^5 in 1960 to 0.21×10^5 in 1980. In Miyagi Prefecture, although there had been some fluctuations in the mor-

tality rate, an upward trend could be seen (Fig. 35-2).

Review of the literature showed that among the Japanese there was a tendency for involvement of the palm, sole, nail bed, and mucous membrane. These types of melanoma have been described as

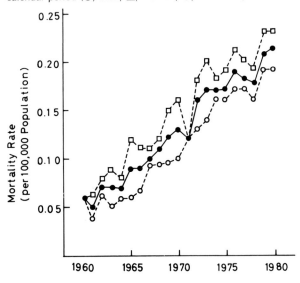

FIG. 35–1 Mortality rate from melanoma in Japan according to calendar period (○, men; □, women; ●, combined).

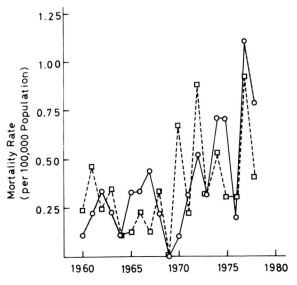

FIG. 35–2 Mortality rate from melanoma in Miyagi Prefecture according to calendar period (○, men; □, women).

palmar-plantar-mucosal melanoma.[4] Recently, the term *acral lentiginous melanoma* (ALM) has been used to define this category of melanoma.[8,13] Although ALM has been regarded as among the most aggressive forms of cutaneous melanoma, it has not been clear whether this growth pattern is inherently any worse prognostically than the other growth patterns. Studies from this department and the Melanoma Research Group in Japan revealed that there is a high incidence (54%) of ALM in Japan, but a low incidence (2%) of lentigo maligna melanoma (LMM) and superficial spreading melanoma (SSM).[13]

In the present study, the most common anatomical site of cutaneous melanoma was the lower extremity (Table 35-1). Melanoma occurred predominantly on the sole (39%), and 22% were subungual melanomas of the hands or feet. There were

TABLE 35–1
CLINICAL AND PATHOLOGIC DATA FOR MELANOMA PATIENTS TREATED AT TOHOKU UNIVERSITY SCHOOL OF MEDICINE, SENDAI, JAPAN

	Presenting Pathologic Stage			
Characteristics	*Stage I*	*Stage II*	*Stage III*	*Total*
Clinical				
Number of patients	36	19	9	64
Year of diagnosis				
≤1960	0%	0%	0%	0%
1961–1965	0%	0%	0%	0%
1966–1970	6%	0%	0%	3%
1971–1975	31%	47%	44%	38%
1976–1980	64%	53%	56%	59%
Median age	61 yr	58 yr	60 yr	60 yr
Sex				
Male	67%	42%	55%	58%
Female	33%	58%	45%	42%
Primary lesion site				
Female lower extremity	19%	42%	33%	28%
Male lower extremity	36%	32%	11%	31%
Female upper extremity	8%	16%	0%	9%
Male upper extremity	22%	5%	33%	19%
Female head and neck	6%	0%	0%	5%
Male head and neck	6%	0%	0%	3%
Female trunk	0%	0%	11%	2%
Male trunk	3%	0%	11%	3%
Other	0%	0%	0%	0%
Pathologic				
Breslow's tumor thickness				
<0.76 mm	19%	18%	0%	18%
0.76 mm–1.49 mm	31%	9%	0%	24%
1.50 mm–2.49 mm	13%	9%	50%	13%
2.50 mm–3.99 mm	16%	27%	0%	18%
≥4.00 mm	22%	36%	50%	27%
Median tumor thickness	3.0 mm	4.7 mm	2.9 mm	3.4 mm
Level of invasion				
II	13%	25%	0%	14%
III	24%	0%	0%	16%
IV	36%	25%	50%	35%
V	27%	50%	50%	35%
Ulceration				
Yes	56%	53%	63%	56%
No	44%	47%	37%	44%
Growth pattern				
Nodular	27%	32%	56%	32%
Superficial spreading	3%	0%	0%	2%
Lentigo maligna	3%	0%	0%	2%
Acral melanoma	67%	68%	44%	64%

41 melanomas in the acral regions, constituting 64% of all cases of cutaneous melanoma (Table 35-1). Melanoma in the acral regions was seen almost twice as often in men as in women. All these melanomas were ALM. In contrast to the melanoma in whites, melanomas on the trunk in men and those on the lower legs in women were uncommon in the Japanese.

There was an increase in the primary melanoma thickness in stages II and III disease compared with the thickness of primary melanoma in stage I disease. A very high incidence of regional or distant metastases (58%) was found among stage I melanoma patients after surgery.

There were 20 patients with nodular melanoma (NM), constituting 32% of the cases in this study. Of the patients with NM, 8 were men and 12 were women. Most of these NM occurred on the extremities (15 of 20). There was one patient with an SSM and one with an LMM, the one with SSM being white-skinned.

The clinical and pathologic features of ALM and NM are shown in Table 35-2. Patients with stages II and III NM constituted 55% of all NM lesions in this series. Of the patients with ALM, 41% were stage II and III cases.

PROGNOSTIC FACTORS

STAGE OF DISEASE

Status of the regional or distant lymph nodes was the most important prognostic factor. Patients with localized melanoma had a 5-year survival rate of 65%, whereas in patients with nodal metastases (stage II) this rate was 14%. Patients with distant metastases (stage III) had a 2-year survival rate of only 14% (Table 35-3).

PROGNOSIS IN PATIENTS WITH LOCALIZED MELANOMA (STAGE I)

Actuarial survival curves showed significant differences among all Clark's levels (Fig. 35-3) and among some thickness groups (Fig. 35-4). Patients with ulceration appeared to have a poorer prognosis (Fig. 35-5). Survival was better for the 24 patients with ALM compared with the 9 patients with NM (Fig. 35-6). The median thickness for stage I NM was greater than that for stage I ALM, but there was a higher proportion of ulcerated lesions among NM (Table 35-2). In addition to those 36 stage I patients listed in Table 35-1, there were 2 other patients with conjunctival melanoma who are alive more than 6 years after diagnosis.

PROGNOSIS IN PATIENTS WITH METASTATIC MELANOMA (STAGES II AND III)

The median thickness for stage II melanomas was 4.7 mm, compared with 3.0 mm for stage I disease (Table 35-1). The differences among Clark's levels of invasion and among melanoma thickness categories were reflected by differences in survival rates (Fig. 35-7). There were 3 patients with melanoma less than 0.76 mm in thickness who developed nodal

TABLE 35–2
A COMPARISON OF CLINICAL AND PATHOLOGIC FACTORS IN ACRAL LENTIGINOUS AND NODULAR MELANOMA

Factors	Stage I		Stage II		Stage III	
	Acral	Nodular	Acral	Nodular	Acral	Nodular
Number of patients	24	9	13	6	4	5
Sex (%)						
Men	71	56	46	17	75	40
Women	29	44	54	83	25	60
Mean age (years)	64	55	61	53		
Anatomical site %						
Hands and feet	100	44	100	33	100	20
Extremity	0	33	0	50	0	40
Trunk	0	0	0	0	0	40
Head and neck	0	22	0	17	0	0
Tumor thickness (mm)						
Mean	1.8	4.0	3.5	6.0		
Median	1.4	3.5	3.4	3.0		
	(0.2–12.0)	(1.4–12.0)	(0.3–7.0)	(1.2–17.0)		
Ulceration (%)						
Yes	58	67	45	67	50	75
No	42	33	55	33	50	25

or distant metastases. One man had plantar melanoma; one man, subungual melanoma; and one woman, melanoma on the ventral aspect of the great toe, in which there were areas of regression. All these patients are still alive (Fig. 35-7). In stage II disease, the presence of ulceration did not signify a poorer prognosis. Patients with ALM had essentially the same survival rate as NM patients. The mean thickness for stage II NM was greater than that for stage II ALM (see Table 35-3).

The median survival for the 9 stage III patients was 12 months, with an actuarial survival at 1 and 2 years of 50% and 14%, respectively (Table 35-3). Metastases occurred most commonly in the distant lymph nodes and the brain, most patients dying from the latter.

TREATMENT

The treatment policy in this department for stage I melanoma is wide local excision of the primary tu-

FIG. 35–5 Actuarial survival curves according to presence or absence of ulceration in stage I melanoma.

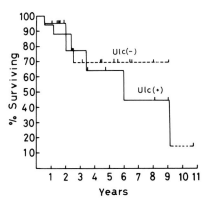

FIG. 35–6 Actuarial survival curves according to growth pattern in stage I melanoma (AL, acral lentiginous; NM, nodular melanoma).

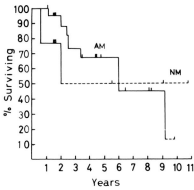

FIG. 35–3 Actuarial survival curves according to level of invasion in stage I melanoma.

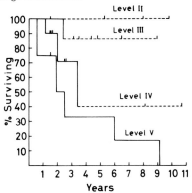

FIG. 35–4 Actuarial survival curves according to tumor thickness in stage I melanoma.

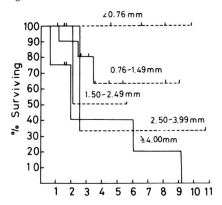

FIG. 35–7 Actuarial survival curves according to level of invasion and tumor thickness in stage II melanoma.

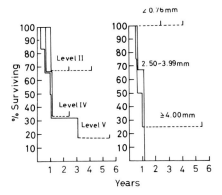

mor, elective regional node dissection, and chemotherapy before and after the operation. The primary melanoma is excised with a 3-cm to 5-cm margin, except where constrained by anatomical barriers. The deep incision includes the underlying fascia, and the defect is covered with a split-thickness skin graft. Subungual melanoma is treated by amputation at the metacarpophalangeal or metatarsophalangeal joint. The lymphadenectomy and the primary melanoma excision are performed under the same anesthesia. Lymphadenectomy in the cases of lower-limb melanoma consists of removal of inguinocrural and iliac nodes up to the aortic bifurcation; in cases of upper-limb melanoma, the opera-

TABLE 35–3
ACTUARIAL SURVIVAL DATA FOR MELANOMA PATIENTS TREATED AT TOHOKU UNIVERSITY SCHOOL OF MEDICINE, SENDAI, JAPAN

	Survival Rates	
Survival Data	*5-Year*	*10-Year*
Stage I		
Overall survival	65%	40%
Sex		
Male	62%	0%
Female	100%	100%
Primary lesion site		
Lower extremity	73%	33%
Upper extremity	50%	0%
Head and neck	50%	—
Trunk	—	—
Tumor thickness		
<0.76 mm	100%	—
0.76 mm–1.49 mm	50%	—
1.50 mm–2.49 mm	50%	0%
2.50 mm–3.99 mm	50%	100%
≥4.00 mm	67%	0%
Level of invasion		
II	100%	
III	67%	
IV	50%	50%
V	50%	0%
Ulceration		
Yes	63%	25%
No	67%	
	1-Year	*3-Year*	*5-Year*
Stage II			
Overall survival	64%	25%	14%
Tumor thickness			
<1.50 mm	100%	50%	
1.50 mm–3.99 mm	75%		
≥4.0 mm	25%	25%	25%
Number of positive nodes			
1			
2–4	100%	60%	25%
>4			
Ulceration			
Yes	78%	57%	17%
No	63%	29%	
	6-Month	*1-Year*	*2-Year*
Stage III			
Overall survival	63%	50%	14%

tion is an axillary dissection up to the subclavicular muscle. All these lymphadenectomies have been performed by one of the authors (R.A.). The standard chemotherapy regimen consisted of the following 5-day schedule: dacarbazine (DTIC), 200 mg on days 1 to 5; AC nitrosourea, 100 mg on day 1; and vincristine, 1 mg on day 1. If nodal metastases are found, this regimen is repeated at 2- to 3-month intervals for the first year and at 6-month intervals for the next 2 years. Stage III melanoma patients have received DTIC chemotherapy at 1- to 2-month intervals. A partial tumor response was seen in about one third of the patients. Neither surgery nor radiation therapy was used.

MUCOSAL MELANOMAS

The characteristics of the 11 patients with mucosal melanomas are shown in Table 35-4. In women with melanoma of the genitalia, the two with stage I disease received a radical vulvectomy combined with a node dissection, while the other three with stage III disease received only chemotherapy. Patients with melanoma of the nasal mucosa, gingiva, and lip were treated by appropriate excision of the tumor, while the patient with the primary esophageal melanoma was treated by esophagectomy. All these patients have died with the exception of one patient with vaginal melanoma, but the follow-up of this patient is short.

DISCUSSION

These analyses showed that in this department there was a high incidence of melanoma in the acral regions (51%) and mucous membranes (17%). Similarly, in a study of 490 cutaneous melanomas made by the Melanoma Research Group in Japan,[13] 46% were found to be located on the hands or feet (Table 35-5). There were four times as many melanomas on the feet as on the hands.

Interestingly, the male predominance in distribution of melanomas involving the hands and feet (51% men versus 40% women) in these Japanese patients is strikingly different from all reported series of extremity melanomas of white-skinned persons, where the vast majority of melanomas occur in women.

TABLE 35-4
MUCOSAL MELANOMAS

Site	Sex	Age (Years)	Stage	Status
Vagina	F	75	III	Dead, 6 months
Vagina	F	56	III	Dead, 7 months
Vagina	F	73	III	Dead, 16 months
Vagina	F	65	I	Dead, 15 months
Vagina	F	48	I	Alive, 15 months
Nose	F	68	I	Dead, 16 months
Nose	F	26	I	Dead, 54 months
Gingiva	F	37	III	Dead, 8 months
Gingiva	F	76	II	Dead, 12 months
Esophagus	M	66	II	Dead, 9 months
Lip	F	42	II	Dead, 63 months

TABLE 35-5
RATIOS OF MELANOMAS ON THE HANDS AND FEET IN JAPAN*

Regions	Male	Female	Total
Hands	16 (6.4%)	30 (12.5%)	46 (9.4%)
Feet	112 (44.8%)	65 (27.1%)	177 (36.1%)
Others	122 (48.8%)	145 (60.4%)	267 (54.5%)
Total	250 (100%)	240 (100%)	490 (100%)

*The Melanoma Research Group in Japan consists of the following: U. Miura (Hokkaido University); M. Seiji (Tohoku University); K. Ueno (Tukuba University); S. Ikeda (Saitama Medical School); S. Okamoto (Chiba University); A. Kukita (Tokyo University); H. Hatano (Keio University); K. Ishihara (Cancer Center); R. Nagai (Yokohama City University); R. Fukushiro (Kanazawa University); E. Sano (Osaka University); Y. Mishima (Kobe University); E. Fujita (Yamaguchi University); Y. Miki (Ehime University); H. Urabe (Kyushu University); R. Arao (Kumamoto University).

The incidence of ALM is considerably higher in Japanese and in African blacks than in whites. Figure 35-8 shows the striking difference in distribution of growth patterns between 126 patients in this department and 3691 patients from the Sydney Melanoma Unit. Mucosal melanomas are frequently referenced in the Japanese literature.[8] However, because of the scarcity of other epidemiologic data on mucosal melanomas, it is hard to make any comparison between the incidences among the Japanese and whites.[10]

The clinical stage of disease was the most significant determinant of survival. Within stage I, Clark's level of invasion, melanoma thickness, ulceration, and growth pattern influenced survival. In this series, patients with ALM had a more favorable prognosis than those with NM both in stage I and stage II disease. The Melanoma Research Group in Japan[8,13] found that the 5-year survival rate for pa-

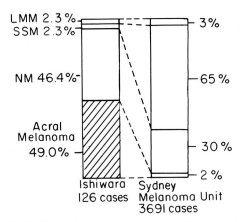

FIG. 35–8 Comparison of melanoma growth patterns in 126 Japanese patients from Tohoku University and 3691 Caucasion patients from SMU.

tients with plantar melanoma was almost equal to that for patients with other types of melanoma when matched by level of invasion. Because NM were thicker and had a higher incidence of ulceration than ALM within each stage in the present series, patients with NM had a poorer prognosis.

Kerl and associates[2] found that in whites with ALM, there was a 5-year survival rate of 100% at Clark's level II, 55% at level III, and 35% at levels IV and V, respectively. Thus, prognosis for whites and Japanese with ALM was similar.

The problem of whether or not to perform an elective lymph node dissection in patients with clinically uninvolved regional lymph nodes is a controversial issue. Since a prophylactic lymph node dissection was performed for all patients with clinical stage I disease, the efficacy of prophylactic lymph node dissection could not be assessed. Pathologic examination of the nodes revealed a very high incidence (58%) of metastases in patients with clinical stage I disease. Thus, immediate regional lymph node dissection may be indicated in patients with stage I ALM. The rationale for chemotherapy in these high-risk patients is a theoretical one. Since small metastases have a better blood supply and a faster growth rate than larger metastases, they may be more sensitive to chemotherapy. Therefore, it has been the policy of this department to administer adjuvant or prophylactic chemotherapy to stage I and stage II patients before and after initial surgery.

REFERENCES

1. Hosokawa M, Kato T, Seiji M, Abe R: Plantar malignant melanoma: Statistical and clinicopathological studies. J Dermatol 7:137, 1980
2. Kerl H, Hodl S, Stettner H: Acral lentiginous melanoma. In Ackerman AB (ed): Pathology of Malignant Melanoma, p 217. New York, Masson, 1981
3. Ohsumi T, Seiji M: Statistical study on malignant melanoma in Japan (1970–1976). Tohoku J Exp Med 121:355, 1977
4. Seiji M, Mihm MC Jr, Sober AJ, Takahashi M, Kato T, Fitzpatrick TB: Malignant melanoma of the palmar-plantar-subungual-mucosal type: Clinical and histopathological features. In Klaus SN (ed): Vol 5, p 95. Basel, Karger, 1979
5. Seiji M, Ohsumi T: Statistical study on malignant melanoma in Japan (1961–1970). Tohoku J Exp Med 107:115, 1972
6. Seiji M, Takahashi M: Malignant melanoma with adjacent intraepidermal proliferation. Tohoku J Exp Med 114:93, 1974
7. Seiji M, Takahashi M: Plantar malignant melanoma. J Dermatol 2:163, 1975
8. Seiji M, Takahashi M: Acral melanoma in Japan. Hum Pathol 13:607, 1982
9. Seiji M, Takematsu H, Hosokawa M, Obata M, Tomita Y, Kato T, Takahashi M, Mihm MC Jr: Acral melanoma in Japan. J Invest Dermatol 80:565, 1983
10. Takagi M, Ishikawa G, Mori W: Primary malignant melanoma of the oral cavity in Japan: With special reference to mucosal melanosis. Cancer 34:358, 1974
11. Takahashi M, Seiji M: Malignant melanoma in Japan. Jpn J Clin Oncol 6:33, 1974
12. Takahashi M, Seiji M: Acral melanoma in Japan. In MacKie RN (ed): Pigment Cell, vol 6, p 150. Basel, Karger, 1983.
13. Takahashi M, Seiji M, Tomita Y, Kato T: Acral melanoma in Japan. In Seiji M (ed): Pigment Cell 1981, p 555. Proceedings of the XIth International Pigment Cell Conference, Sendai, Japan, 1980. Tokyo, University of Tokyo Press, 1981

CHARLES M. BALCH
SENG-JAW SOONG
HELEN M. SHAW

A Comparison of Worldwide Melanoma Data

36

Epidemiology and Presenting Features of Melanoma

Prognostic Factors

   Stage I

   Stage II

   Stage III

Treatment Results

Summary

This chapter summarizes some of the clinical and pathologic features of melanoma, results of prognostic factors analysis, and recommendations for surgical treatment from 14 melanoma centers located in nine countries (see Chaps. 21 through 35). All centers contributed data in a standardized format to permit a more accurate comparison of results. Without such standardization of data presentation, spurious interpretations could easily occur. For example, overall survival rates would be higher in those centers with an increased incidence of lentigo maligna melanoma or those that had included level I melanomas, while it would be lower in those centers with an increased incidence of more advanced stages or thicknesses of melanoma. Several centers had previously reported their results, which included level I melanomas (melanoma *in situ*), but in this book they have recalculated their data to allow for a more accurate comparative analysis restricted to invasive melanomas. A brief description of each center reporting data is listed in Table 36-1.

This is the first attempt to compile a large data base from treatment centers worldwide. It consists of 15,798 stage I and 2,116 stage II melanoma patients. Considerable effort was spent arranging the data presentation in a uniform manner for purposes of comparison. It should be emphasized at the outset, however, that substantial heterogeneity of the data still exists. The nature of the referral practice varied from center to center based on the specialty nature of the hospital or the surgical practice within a general hospital (*e.g.*, general surgery, surgical oncology, plastic surgery). Patients were diagnosed in different years, with some data bases consisting of patients treated primarily in the 1960s, while others were predominantly treated in the 1970s. Varying proportions of the data were accumulated prospectively, while a few were strictly retrospective in na-

TABLE 36–1
DESCRIPTION OF MELANOMA CENTERS REPORTING DATA (CHAPTERS 21 TO 35)

Reporting Centers	Designation in Figures and Tables*	Geographic Location of Reporting Center	Number of Patients Contributed			Data Base	Referral Pattern	Chapter
			Stage I	Stage II	Stage III			
Sydney Melanoma Unit, New South Wales, Australia	Sydney	34°S/151°E	3025	366		Hospital	Sydney Metropolitan Area, also State of New South Wales	21
Queensland Melanoma Project, Queensland, Australia	Brisbane	27°S/153°E	1174	64	10	Population-based registry	Entire state of Queensland (1963–1969)	22
Survey of American College of Surgeons	American College of Surgeons (ACS)		4190	482	144	1980 Survey	A national survey of 614 hospitals from 48 states, District of Columbia, and Puerto Rico	23
University of Alabama in Birmingham, Alabama, USA	Alabama	33°N/87°W	783	119	17	Hospital	Predominantly from the state of Alabama, also four surrounding states	24
Duke Medical Center, Durham, North Carolina, USA	Duke	36°N/79°W	2470	418	61	Hospital	Predominantly from the state of North Carolina, also five surrounding states	25
University of California at Los Angeles, California, USA	University of California at Los Angeles (UCLA)	34°N/118°N		150		Hospital	Predominantly from Southern California	26
Mayo Clinic, Rochester, Minnesota, USA	Mayo	44°N/93°W	777	209		Hospital	90% from the state of Minnesota, also six surrounding states	27

TABLE 36–1 *(continued)*
DESCRIPTION OF MELANOMA CENTERS REPORTING DATA (CHAPTERS 21 TO 35)

Reporting Centers	Designation in Figures and Tables*	Geographic Location of Reporting Center	Number of Patients Contributed			Data Base	Referral Pattern	Chapter
			Stage I	Stage II	Stage III			
Melanoma Clinical Cooperative Group, USA	Harvard/ New York University (NYU)	Boston— 42°N/71°N; New York —41°N/ 74°W	598	33	3	Hospital	Predominantly from the states of Massachusetts and New York	28
National Cancer Institute of Milan, Milan, Italy	Milan	45°N/9°E	234	45	3	Hospital	70% from the Milan metropolitan area and the remainder from Northern Italy	29
Odense University Hospital, Odense, Denmark	Odense	55°N/10°E	632	11	5	Hospital	Southwestern districts of Denmark	30
University of Göteborg, Göteborg, Sweden	Göteborg	58°N/12°E	573			Hospital	City of Göteborg and surrounding region in Southwestern Sweden	31
West of Scotland	Glasgow	56°N/4°W	847			Population-based registry	West of Scotland	32
University of Erlangen– Nürnberg, Federal Republic of Germany	Erlangen	49°N/11°E	455	185	22	Hospital	Predominantly from Northern Bavaria (largely trunk melanoma)	33
University of Hong Kong, Queen Mary Hospital, Hong Kong	Hong Kong	22°N/114°E	4	15	2	Hospital	Entire territory of Hong Kong	34
Tohoku University Hospital, Sendai, Japan	Tohoku	38°N/141°E	36	19	9	Hospital	Predominantly from the Miyagi Prefecture	35

*For the purpose of abbreviation only, the university or institution of the principal investigator(s) is used.

ture. Most of the data were based on the experience at a single referring medical center, but the data from the West of Scotland and from Queensland, Australia, were population-based studies and the American College of Surgeons' data consisted of a survey involving almost one third of the melanomas diagnosed throughout the United States during the year 1980. Almost all of the centers calculated survival rates using actuarial methods, but the figures from the Scottish center (Chap. 32) used crude survival rates, and the Swedish calculations were based on absolute survival rates; thus, they are not directly comparable with survival figures from the other centers. Some centers presented data confined to only one stage of disease. Nevertheless, many of these limitations could be accounted for when comparing the overall data, and the important factors

were available for analysis in most cases (listed in the first and second tables in each of the chapters).

The results of this analysis demonstrate a significant diversity in melanoma. However, these differences can largely be accounted for by grouping patients according to known prognostic parameters, as described below. The comparisons of dominant prognostic variables showed consistent results from center to center despite the heterogeneity of the patient populations.

EPIDEMIOLOGY AND PRESENTING FEATURES OF MELANOMA

Much of the information regarding epidemiology has been incorporated into Chapter 17. It should be emphasized that many centers have different climatic conditions, latitude of residence, and mixture of ethnic groups. The incidence of melanoma ranged from 0.8×10^5 in Hong Kong to 30.6×10^5 in Queensland, Australia. Where incidence data were available over time, it was increasing in the geographic areas of all reporting melanoma centers except in Minnesota.

According to the American College of Surgeons' survey (Chap. 23), 81% of patients presenting with melanoma described a change in a mole. There is also a recurring theme in these chapters about changing trends of melanoma (see also Chap. 18). It is clear that patients around the world are presenting with an earlier stage of disease and with thinner, less ulcerative melanomas. Approximately 84% of patients at most centers had stage I (local-

ized) melanoma except at the Milan, Italy, center, where only 57% of patients had stage I melanoma.

There were some substantial differences among stage I patients from different countries in terms of their clinical and pathologic features (Table 36-2). Figures 36-1 to 36-7 show incidence data for age, sex, site, thickness, ulceration, and growth pattern from the centers reporting the lowest, highest, and average figures, respectively. In Japan, melanomas were typically acral lentiginous lesions occurring on the sole of the foot. There was a higher proportion of extremity melanomas in women from Scotland and Italy (Table 36-2). In Italy, melanomas were thicker and more ulcerated, and Swedish patients had the highest proportion of lentigo maligna melanomas (LMM). The incidence of thin melanomas in

TABLE 36–2
COMPARISON OF STAGE I MELANOMA FEATURES FROM SELECTED MELANOMA CENTERS WORLDWIDE*

	All 14 Centers[†]	Sydney	Duke	Brisbane	Glasgow	Alabama	Milan	Tohoku
Number of Patients	15,798	3025	2470	1174	847	783	234	36
Median Age (yr)	48	44	47	47	43	48	49	**61**
Percent Females	54%	53%	50%	58%	**67%**	52%	**61%**	**33%**
Percent Extremity	46%	48%	**39%**	51%	**60%**	42%	**57%**	**85%**
Percent Lentigo Maligna	7%	3%	4%	9%	**12%**	5%	5%	3%
Percent Superficial Spreading	65%	67%	68%	71%	73%	**50%**	**75%**	**3%**
Percent <0.76 mm	28%	27%	32%	32%	**20%**	31%	**7%**	**19%**
Percent Ulceration	29%	**21%**	35%	26%	NA[‡]	34%	**52%**	**56%**

*Boldface indicates substantial deviations from the median or average
[†] Average values for all 14 centers reporting stage I data
[‡] NA = not available

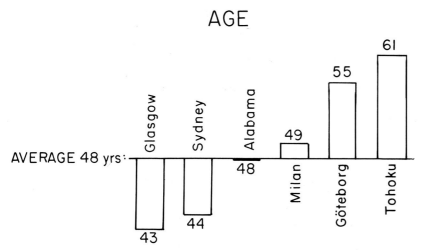

FIG. 36–1   Median age of stage I melanoma patients from selected centers. The average of 48 years was calculated based on all reporting centers.

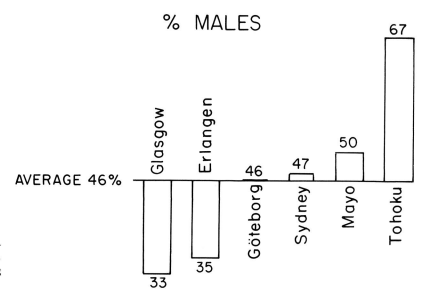

FIG. 36–2 Percentage of stage I melanomas for males. The average of 46% was calculated based on all reporting centers.

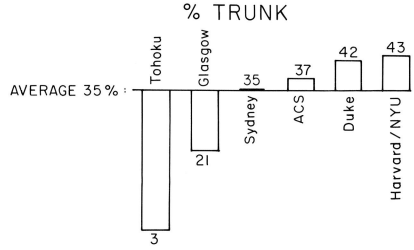

FIG. 36–3 Percentage of stage I trunk melanomas from selected centers. The average of 35% was calculated based on all reporting centers.

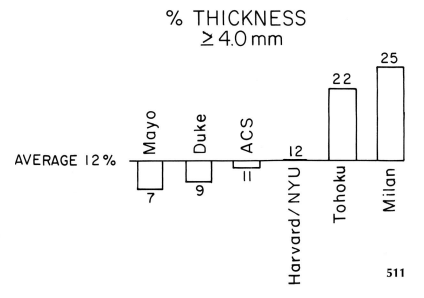

FIG. 36–4 Percentage of stage I melanoma patients with tumor thickness equal to or greater than 4.0 mm from selected centers. The average of 12% was calculated based on all reporting centers.

511

% ULCERATION

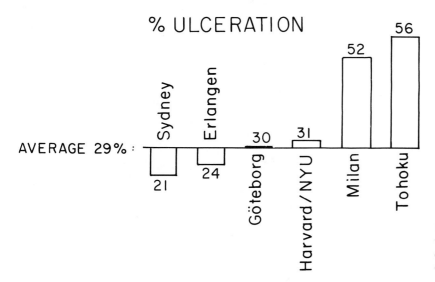

FIG. 36–5 Percentage of stage I patients with ulcerated lesions from selected centers. The average of 29% was calculated based on all reporting centers.

% SUPERFICIAL SPREADING

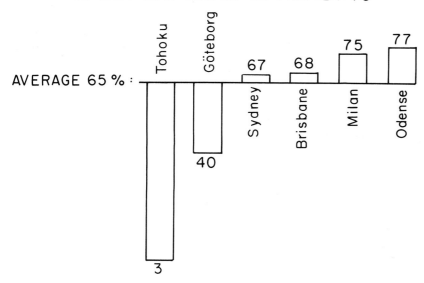

FIG. 36–6 Percentage of stage I superficial spreading melanomas from selected centers. The average of 65% was calculated based on all reporting centers.

% LMM

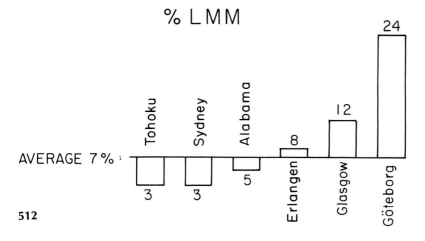

FIG. 36–7 Percentage of stage I lentigo maligna melanoma from selected centers. The average of 7% was calculated based on all reporting centers.

centers reporting recent patient entry indicates that 24% to 33% of patients have prognostically favorable melanomas measuring less than 0.76 mm. Melanoma patients in Queensland, Australia, tended to have thinner lesions and had the best 5-year survival rate (85%) (Fig. 36-8).

It is clear that melanoma occurs predominantly in the white-skinned population. Only 1% to 3% of melanoma patients from those centers reporting data from the United States and Australia were dark-skinned. Melanomas occurring in Orientals and black-skinned patients occur predominantly in low-pigmentation areas, particularly on the sole of the foot. In most of these centers reporting data, the incidence of melanoma arising on the sole ranged from 50% to 73% in dark-skinned patients (see Chaps. 23, 24, 25, and 35). This compares with only a 3% incidence in white-skinned persons. In most instances, these were thicker lesions and were associated more frequently with nodal metastases at the time of first presentation compared with melanomas arising in white-skinned patients. The analyses from Duke Medical Center (Chap. 25) suggested that there were some differences in the biologic behavior among black-skinned patients, whereas similar analysis from Alabama (Chap. 24) suggested that this was simply because melanoma in these patients occurred in unfavorable locations and prognosis in black- and white-skinned patients with comparable lesions is similar.

PROGNOSTIC FACTORS

STAGE I

The overall prognosis for stage I patients was good, with an average 5-year survival of 79% for pooled data from all centers (Table 36-3; Fig. 36-8).

The survival rates for individual centers varied according to such features as sex, tumor site, thickness, level of invasion, and ulceration by single-factor analysis (see Table 36-3). There are numerous interactions among these prognostic factors, however, so that results of multifactorial analyses were more reliable. Eight centers performed a prognostic factors analysis for stage I melanoma using a multivariate analysis technique. Overall, the most significant predictive variables (in descending order) were (1) tumor thickness, (2) tumor ulceration, (3) tumor site, (4) patient's sex, and (5) tumor growth pattern (Table 36-4).

The two most important clinical features of melanoma were the anatomical site of the tumor and the sex of the patient. There is considerable correlation between these two prognostic variables, but most centers identified the site of the primary melanoma as a relatively more important factor for predicting outcome compared with the patient's sex (e.g., Sydney, Alabama, Duke, Harvard/NYU). The Danish center analysis identified the patient's sex to be more important prognostically. It is clear that women have melanomas arising in more favorable sites and the tumors are thinner and less ulcerative, and women have a lower stage of disease at first presentation. Even in patients with stage II melanoma, there does not appear to be any female superiority when matched for prognostic factors, according to the analysis from Sydney.

Among pathologic factors, tumor thickness and ulceration were the two most dominant features in all the eight reporting centers performing this comparative analysis (Table 36-4). In each of the centers where thickness and level of invasion were directly compared, tumor thickness was a relatively more accurate and reproducible prognostic parameter compared with the level of invasion. Percentages of patients with ulcerative melanomas ranged between 21% and 56% among different centers. When

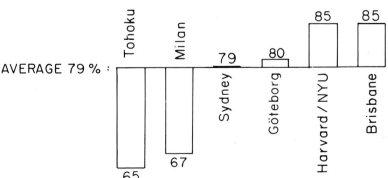

FIG. 36–8 The overall 5-year survival for all stage I melanoma patients from selected centers. The average of 79% was calculated based on all reporting centers.

TABLE 36–3
FIVE-YEAR SURVIVAL RATES (%) FOR STAGE I MELANOMA PATIENTS

	All Centers	Sydney	Duke	Brisbane	Alabama	Mayo	Odense	Harvard/NYU	Göteborg	Erlangen	Milan	Tohoku
Overall	79	79	81	85	77	83	82	85	80	81	67	65
Sex												
Male	72	69	76	79	75	80	76	81	75	75	62	62
Female	83	84	85	90	78	87	85	90	84	84	70	100
Site												
Lower extremity	85	84	86	90	73	86	85	92	82	83	78	73
Upper extremity	87	82	93	90	93	91	84	89	90	89	47	50
Head and neck	74	72	67	83	72	70	81	82	83	88	64	50
Trunk	75	71	80	79	70	84	78	80	75	69	53	NA*
Thickness												
<0.76 mm	96	95	93	97	98	98	98	99	96	96	100	100
0.76 mm–1.49 mm	87	84	85	92	87	93	91	95	90	100	86	50
1.50 mm–2.49 mm	75	73	74	83	76	78	78	84	80	79	78	50
2.50 mm–3.99 mm	66	64	68	77	73	61	73	70	73	NA	70	50
≥4.00 mm	47	37	54	48	55	45	58	44	35	NA	30	67
Level												
II	95	96	93	NA	93	98	97	99	96	89	96	100
III	82	78	87	NA	81	89	88	95	83	84	72	67
IV	71	74	68	NA	77	77	73	75	73	78	57	50
V	49	52	54	NA	50	NA	57	39	36	63	27	50
Ulceration												
Present	60	57	63	68	69	NA	65	68	57	70	59	63
Absent	86	88	85	91	85	NA	92	93	90	87	72	67

*NA = not available

TABLE 36-4
MAJOR PROGNOSTIC FACTORS DETERMINED BY MULTIFACTORIAL ANALYSIS FOR STAGE I MELANOMA
(LISTED IN RANK ORDER BY CENTER)

Center	Number of Patients	Thickness	Ulceration	Site	Sex	Growth Pattern	Level of Invasion	Other
Sydney	3025	3	1	2	NS*	NS	4	
Duke	2470	3	4	2	NS	1	NS	
Alabama	783	1	2	3	NS	NS	NS	
Odense	632	+[†]	1	NS	+	NA[‡]	+	Inflammation Biopsy
Harvard/NYU	598	1	+	2	NS	NS	NS	Microsatellite
Göteborg	573	2	1	NS	NS	+	+	Tumor diameter
Erlangen	455	1	NS	2.5	2.5	NS	NS	
Milan	234	1	NS	3	NS	2	NS	

* Not a significant predictive factor

[†] Major factor but rank order not given

[‡] Not analyzed as a separate factor

ulceration was present, it indicated a strikingly more aggressive type of melanoma, even after accounting for other prognostic features, including tumor thickness. Thus, six of eight centers that performed a multivariate analysis ranked ulceration among the first three most dominant prognostic factors. In fact, this was the single most important feature predicting outcome in several of the centers.

Nodular melanomas were associated with a much worse prognosis than other growth patterns in many of the data sets. This is probably because nodular melanomas are thicker lesions, since there were no significant differences in survival rates between nodular and superficial spreading melanomas of similar thickness (see Chap. 19). This does not mean that accounting for growth patterns is unimportant, since several centers identified it as a major prognostic parameter (Duke, Göteborg, and Milan). Some centers suggested that lentigo maligna melanomas were associated with a more favorable prognosis than the other growth patterns even after accounting for tumor thickness. This may be important to take into consideration, since the incidence of LMM lesions was higher in Sweden and Scotland compared with that of other centers (Fig. 36-7). It is recognized that the diagnosis of this growth pattern is subjective and that this may account for some of the differences in incidence. It is interesting to note that the incidence of LMM lesions has increased in Sweden but not in the neighboring country of Denmark. Acral lentiginous melanomas have only recently been recognized as a separate entity and were reported in only a few centers. However, the Japanese center reported the majority of their melanomas to be of this type (see Chap. 35).

STAGE II

Data for 2116 stage II melanoma patients could be compiled from a total of 13 reporting centers. Clinical and pathologic features of stage II patients are listed in Table 36-5. These melanomas are more common in men, are thicker, more ulcerated, and often have a nodular growth pattern (Table 36-5). In Japanese and Chinese patients, stage II melanomas occurred predominantly on the extremities and were thicker than average. The average overall 5-year survival was 36%, ranging from 27% in Brisbane to 42% at Duke Medical Center (Table 36-6). Patients with clinically occult nodal metastases detected by pathologic examination and those with a single metastatic node fared the best. Among these patients, survival rates were better when associated with a single metastatic node (51%), a melanoma less than 1.5 mm in thickness (49%), and without ulceration (47%) (Table 36-6). Five out of six centers that performed a prognostic factors analysis for stage II melanoma identified the most significant factor as the number of metastatic nodes. A significant factor in most of these analyses was also either ulceration or tumor thickness, or both (Table 36-7).

STAGE III

Data about patients with distant metastases (stage III) were analyzed only from Alabama and Milan. The number and site of metastases appeared to be the dominant prognostic features of stage III melanoma.

TABLE 36–5
CLINICAL AND PATHOLOGIC FEATURES OF METASTATIC MELANOMA IN REGIONAL NODES (STAGE II)

	All Centers	Duke	Sydney	ACS	Mayo	Erlangen	UCLA	Alabama	Brisbane	Milan	Harvard/ NYU	Tohoku	Hong Kong	Odense
Number of Patients	2116	418	366	482	209	185	150	119	64	45	33	19	15	11
Median Age (yr)	50	49	44	52	54	52	48	51	53	49	51	58	57	56
Percent Female	38	39	30	36	48	41	40	34	31	42	30	58	40	45
Site (%)														
Extremities	41	30	45	34		62		44	53	36	21	95	87	22
Head and neck	14	16	17	15		4		15	11	20	21	0		11
Trunk	35	30	35	41		30		40	36	44	58	0	13	67
Thickness (%)														
<0.76 mm	8	10	6	15	8	1	10	5	5	10	6	18		0
≥4.0 mm	34	30	48	26	21		14	46	48	59	58	36		56
Median (mm)	3.3	3.3	3.6		2.4		2.1	3.8	3.7	5.8	4.5	4.7		4.0
Ulceration Present (%)	54	55	50			38	53	65	69	66	76	53	77	91
Growth Pattern (%)														
Nodular	52	46	57	59	49	52	25	75	70	51	27	32	73	45
SSM	43	49	40	36	50	35	73	25	25	49	58	0	27	55

TABLE 36–6
FIVE-YEAR SURVIVAL RATES % FOR PATIENTS WITH NODAL METASTASES (STAGE II)

| Center | Number of Patients | Overall | Primary Melanoma | | | | Metastatic Nodes | |
| | | | Thickness | | Ulceration | | | |
			< 1.5 mm	≥ 4.0 mm	Absent	Present	1	≥ 4
Milan	530	33	50*	21*	35*	21*	50	18
Duke	418	42	55	47	52	35	55	16
Sydney	366	37	46	23	55	23		
Erlangen	185	33	51	22	49	38	50	16
UCLA	150	37	49	0	47	34	45	15
Alabama	119	38	40	33	62	24	57	15
Brisbane	64	27	29	16	34	24	33	25
All Centers	1832	36	49	26	47	28	51	17

* Based on a subset of patients

TABLE 36–7
DOMINANT PROGNOSTIC FACTORS FOR NODAL METASTASES (STAGE II)
DETERMINED BY MULTIFACTORIAL ANALYSIS

Center	Number of Patients	Factor
Milan*	530	Number of nodes, capsular invasion
Duke	418	Number of nodes, ulceration
Sydney[†]	366	Ulceration, tumor thickness
UCLA	150	Number of nodes, tumor thickness
Alabama	119	Number of nodes, ulceration
Harvard/NYU[‡]	46	Number of nodes, tumor thickness

* Data about primary melanoma are not available.

[†] Data for number of metastatic nodes are not available.

[‡] Clinical stage I, pathologic stage II patients only.

TREATMENT RESULTS

There is a growing consensus about the surgical management of melanoma, especially with regard to margins of excision around the primary melanoma. However, considerable differences of opinion still exist, and a scientifically acquired data base is needed. A summary of recommendations from each of the centers regarding excision margins around the primary melanoma is listed in Table 36-8. Most centers recommend narrower margins of excision for thin melanomas measuring less than 0.76 mm to 1 mm in thickness (Table 36-8).

The issue of elective lymph node dissection for clinically negative lymph nodes is controversial, as reflected by the varying recommendations among the treatment centers. This is discussed further in Chapter 8. At least three centers demonstrated that there is some benefit from elective lymph node dis-

section in a multifactorial analysis (Alabama, Duke, and Sydney). As a result, many of the reporting centers from the United States and Australia recommend this procedure on a selected basis, particularly for those with intermediate thickness melanomas.

Criteria for making treatment decisions are based primarily on the following properties of the primary lesion: measured tumor thickness, the growth pattern, the site, and the presence of ulceration. Most reporting centers from Europe do not recommend elective lymph node dissection. All the centers recommend lymphadenectomy for patients with clinically suspicious nodal metastases.

The currently available drugs and immunotherapeutic agents for patients with nodal metastases have not had a major impact on survival, and most centers do not recommend adjuvant therapy as standard treatment, while several of them are investigating newer forms of immunotherapy or hormone therapy.

TABLE 36–8
SUMMARY OF TREATMENT RECOMMENDATIONS FOR STAGE I MELANOMA

Center	Primary Melanoma		Regional Nodes
	Usual Excision Margins (cm)	Margins in cms for Thin melanomas (e.g., <1.0 mm)	Immediate (Elective) Dissection
Sydney	3	1–2	Selectively
Brisbane	>3	2	Selectively
Alabama	3	2	Selectively
Duke	NS*	NS	Selectively
Mayo	5	1.5–2	No[†]
Harvard/NYU	3	1.5	Selectively
Milan	3–5	NS	No
Odense	5	NS	No
Göteborg	5	NS	No
Glasgow	3	NS	No
Erlangen	5	2	Selectively
Hong Kong	3	NS	No
Tohoku	3–5	NS	Always

* Not specifically stated in the text

[†] Selectively for head and neck melanomas

SUMMARY

A collaborative data analysis was performed on 15,798 stage I and 2,116 stage II melanoma patients treated at 14 major melanoma treatment centers from nine countries. The average 5-year survival rate for stage I melanoma was 79% (range 65%–85%), excluding all level I melanomas. There were significant differences in stage I melanoma patients both clinically and pathologically. In Japan, melanomas were typically acral lentiginous lesions occurring on the sole of the foot. In Italy, melanomas were thicker and more ulcerative. Swedish patients had the highest proportion of lentigo maligna melanomas (24%). Melanomas in Queensland, Australia tended to be thinner and patients there had the best 5-year survival rate (85%). Among the 8 centers that performed a prognostic factors analysis for stage I melanomas, the most significant predictive variables (in descending order) were: (1) tumor thickness, (2) ulceration, (3) site, (4) sex, and (5) growth pattern.

The average 5-year survival rate for stage II melanoma patients was 34% (range 27%–42%). The most significant prognostic factor in all studies was the number of metastatic nodes, while ulceration or tumor thickness, or both, were also significant factors in most analyses.

The incidence of melanoma ranged from 0.8×10^5 in Hong Kong to 28×10^5 in Queensland, Australia. Incidence is increasing in the areas of all reporting melanoma centers except in Minnesota. Most of the increase appears to be due to thinner melanomas with a superficial spreading growth pattern.

From this comparative analysis, it is clear that several paradoxical differences exist in melanoma between European countries of relatively close proximity and similar latitude. These differences are valid, since they involved nonsubjective parameters such as age and sex of patients and the thickness of their primary tumors. There was a marked preponderance of female melanoma patients in Scotland, Germany, Italy, and Denmark, but virtually no preponderance in neighboring Sweden. As a result of the female preponderance in these four countries, a high proportion of extremity melanomas were treated there. Tumors treated in Scotland and Italy were twice as thick as those treated in the other three European countries. Patients from the European mainland were considerably older than those from Scotland. There were no major disparities in the type of melanoma treated in various parts of the American and Australian continents.

The results indicate a significant heterogeneity of melanoma that is increasing in frequency among different ethnic groups and latitude of residence. However, these differences can be largely accounted for by grouping patients among known prognostic parameters.

Index

Index

An *f* following a page number indicates a figure; a *t* indicates tabular material.